Third Edition

Medical Transcription
Fundamentals & Practice

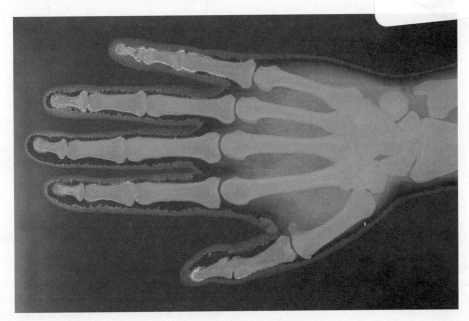

Health Professions Institute

Sally Crenshaw Pitman, M.A.

John H. Dirckx, M.D.

Ellen B. Drake, CMT, FAAMT

Linda C. Campbell, CMT, FAAMT

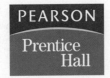

PEARSON
Prentice
Hall

Upper Saddle River,
New Jersey 07458

Publisher: Julie Levin Alexander
Publisher's Assistant: Regina Bruno
Executive Editor: Joan Gill
Development Editor: Andrea Edwards, Triple SSS Press Media Development, Inc.
Assistant Editor: Bronwen Glowacki
Director of Marketing: Karen Allman
Senior Marketing Manager: Harper Coles
Marketing Coordinator: Michael Sirinides
Marketing Assistant: Wayne Celia, Jr.
Managing Production Editor: Patrick Walsh
Production Liaison: Julie Li
Media Product Manager: John Jordan
Manager of Media Production: Amy Peltier
New Media Project Manager: Tina Rudowski

Manufacturing Manager: Ilene Sanford
Manufacturing Buyer: Pat Brown
Senior Design Coordinator: Christopher Weigand
Interior Designer: K and M Design
Cover Designer: Rob Aleman
Cover Image: Getty Images Inc./Stone Allstock
Director, Image Resource Center: Melinda Reo
Manager, Rights and Permissions: Zina Arabia
Manager, Visual Research: Beth Brenzel
Manager, Cover Visual Research and Permissions: Karen Sanatar
Image Permission Coordinator: Annette Linder
Composition: Sally C. Pitman, Health Professions Institute
Printing and Binding: Courier Corporation
Cover Printer: Phoenix Color Corporation

Pearson Education, Inc., Upper Saddle River, N.J.
Pearson Education Ltd
Pearson Education Singapore, Pte. Ltd
Pearson Education, Canada, Ltd

Pearson Education—Japan
Pearson Education Australia PTY, Ltd
Pearson Education North Asia Ltd
Pearson Educacion de Mexico, S.A. de C.V.
Pearson Education Malaysia, Pte. Ltd

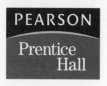

10   9   8
ISBN 0-13-188143-4

Contents

PART ONE
Fundamentals of Medical Transcription   1

Chapter 1   Medical Fundamentals   3

Chapter 2   Perspectives on Medical Transcription   47

Chapter 3   Style Guide   77

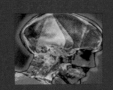
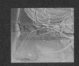

PART TWO
The Practice of Medical Transcription 115

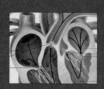
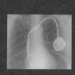

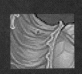
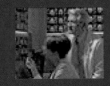

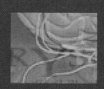
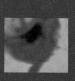

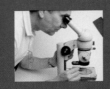

Preface

Welcome to the third edition of *Medical Transcription Fundamentals & Practice,* the most comprehensive transcription learning system available in a single package. We've designed this course for learners with no prior experience as well as those looking for refresher training. This course is ideal as a module within programs of medical assisting, medical or legal transcription, and business technology.

Medical Transcription Fundamentals & Practice was written to provide a reasonably priced, comprehensive, authentic training course at a basic or introductory level. It is short and compact, yet it provides a broad overview of medical transcription as a career. In a compressed format, it reviews key knowledge in anatomy, medical vocabulary, clinical medicine, common diseases, diagnostic and surgical procedures, laboratory procedures, and pharmacology. No other book or course that we know of provides such a succinct, yet thorough, introduction to medical transcription.

In this book, students will read real-world contributions from medical transcription practitioners and physicians. In fact, the text is a compilation of writings by CMTs, MT practitioners, and physicians who have played important roles in the medical transcription profession. On the accompanying CD, students will be able to transcribe reports from authentic physician dictation.

The combination of coordinated medical readings with transcription practice in the related specialty or body system is a sound teaching methodology unequaled by other products at this level. This approach was pioneered by Health Professions Institute and has been refined over time to provide medical transcription training that enables students who successfully complete this program to transcribe for physicians and clinics. In addition, it provides a strong foundation for students who want to continue with advanced training in order to qualify to work in acute care and sit for credentialing exams offered by the professional association for medical transcription.

A unique feature of this text is the inclusion of abundant essays and commentary, many of them humorous or light-hearted, from physicians and MTs in the field. These features may be included as medical content, boxed sidebars, and the Spotlight on transcription in each chapter. Students will be exposed to a variety of voices—voices of icons from the past and present community of medical transcriptionists. Though varied, these voices present a unified picture of medical transcription as a fulfilling and rewarding career choice.

This third edition of *Medical Transcription Fundamentals & Practice* reflects the feedback and recommendations of many current users. We have endeavored to incorporate most of the suggestions we received from both reviewers and users. Those familiar with the course will be happily surprised at the new and updated content and the new look of the book with its expanded use of four-color illustrations and real-world vignettes for added interest. Those using the course for the first time will be impressed with its usefulness and comprehensiveness.

The textbook is divided into two parts. Part One consists of three chapters that introduce students to the fundamentals of medical transcription. Chapter 1 gives an overview of the profession, work environments, the healthcare record, and technology and starts students on their journey to understand the importance and structure of the medical documents they transcribe. Chapter 2 expands on ethics and professionalism and the transcriptionist's role in documentation. Chapter 3 is a style guide that students will be able to use throughout the course to ensure that their transcripts conform to the standards recommended in the *AAMT Book of Style.*

Part Two consists of 14 chapters, each addressing a specialty or body system. The specialty/body system approach for transcription training is a proven effective strategy that incorporates coordinated reading and learning activities combined with hands-on transcription practice of progressive difficulty. These chapters have been organized in a "top-down" fashion, beginning with skin, then ENT and ophthalmology, progressing to the organ systems, then the musculoskeletal and nervous systems, and ending with pathology and radiology.

Each chapter in Part Two has a standard content. At the beginning of each chapter are a brief review of anatomy and medical vocabulary and a section that compares lay terms to their medical counterparts. Next come medical readings, including an overview of the content of the history and physical examination pertaining to the body system or specialty, common diseases, diagnostic and surgical procedures, laboratory procedures, and pharmacology. The final section of each chapter includes transcription tips that specifically relate to typical problems encountered in transcribing the specialty, abundant exercises, sample reports, and transcription practice instructions. A special feature of each chapter is the Spotlight on medical transcription that provides a student with real-world insights from medical transcription practitioners.

Physician Dictations

Perhaps the most important component of this course is the unique combination of authentic physician dictation by medical specialty, coordinated readings and exercises by medical specialty, and supplementary information vital to every medical transcription student. This instructional technique provides a distinct learning advantage over programs using professional readers as dictators. It is only by transcribing actual medical dictation that a student develops the selective hearing skills and experience necessary to gain competency as a medical transcriptionist.

The dictation is sequenced from simple to complex, encompassing a full spectrum of terminology for each medical specialty. Within the general framework for this course, students are exposed to many dictating variables in style and punctuation as well as genuine distractions such as hospital noises and voices in the background. Men and women physicians and regional and foreign accents have been included.

The 150 dictated reports include chart notes, letters, initial office evaluations, consultations, history and physical examinations, discharge summaries, operative reports, emergency department reports, procedure notes, and diagnostic studies from each of the medical specialties. The dictations and accompanying transcripts have been carefully reviewed by certified medical transcriptionists (CMTs), educators, and physicians to ensure that the reports reflect an accurate and representative sample of each medical specialty.

Features of the Textbook

Spotlights provide a glimpse into the practice of transcribing in each specialty, and Transcription Tips offer handy suggestions to improve accuracy and avoid the error traps students and new MTs often encounter.

Proofreading Skills provide students with the opportunity to practice correction of style, spelling, and grammar errors—important skills for the medical transcriptionist.

Skills Challenge offers various end-of-chapter exercises to reinforce content. Bloopers provide a light touch and point out humorous yet common errors made in transcription.

Sample Reports offer model transcribed reports prepared according to the recommendations of *The AAMT Book of Style for Medical Transcription*, 2nd ed. (Modesto, CA: American Association for Medical Transcription, 2002), and Transcription Practice prompts students to apply concepts by transcribing the accompanying dictation.

A Complete Learning Package

This edition breaks new ground with a carefully coordinated package including the textbook, an interactive CD-ROM, an innovative companion World Wide Web site, and transcript answer keys.

Interactive CD-ROM. By combining all dictations along with on-screen audio controls, a word-processor with timing systems, and a wealth of workbook-style exercises as well as links to the book, the CD-ROM allows students to listen and transcribe without need of a special transcribing machine. At the instructor's discretion, students may be given access to the transcript keys and compare their work to the keys in a split-screen format, giving them immediate feedback on their errors. The CD-ROM also contains numerous resources for the student accessible by means of drop-down menus.

Foot Pedal. A custom-built foot pedal works with the audio medical dictations on CD-ROM to function much like a traditional transcribing machine. To purchase either a USB foot pedal or a game port foot pedal, visit **http://www.USBFootPedals.com** or call 866-447-4786. Alternative contact information: Health Professions Institute, 209-551-2112 or **http://www.hpisum.com**.

Medical Transcription Central (http://www.prenhall. com/medtrans). Prentice Hall's free Web site featuring software downloads, dictation bloopers, up-to-date word lists, and more.

Instructor's Guide and Transcript Keys. Available for instructors. The *Instructor's Guide* contains answers to exercises in the textbook, suggestions for using the text, supplementary readings for teachers, and post-transcription exercises to help the students engage the content. The latter grew out of Ellen Drake's experience in teaching the *MTF&P* course at Seminole Community College, Sanford, Florida.

What's New

A reorganized format allows for greater teaching flexibility. Important readings on relevant professional and human interest issues appear in Part One, and medical specialties are grouped in distinct chapters in Part Two. The order of the specialties/body systems has been changed and follows a linear progression, basically from the head to the feet. However, each chapter is self-contained and instructors may choose to follow a different order of specialties in their teaching.

Color has been added, both to the text and to the illustrations. Four-color illustrations abound throughout. The number of illustrations used in this edition is nearly quadrupled over the previous edition.

Original writings from physicians, renowned authors, and medical transcriptionists have been added as sidebars in tinted boxes. The reader will find numerous new inclusions from the writings of John H. Dirckx, M.D., a highly respected physician consultant to the industry. There are new contributions from Richard Lederer, humorist, NPR columnist, and English language guru. Readers will enjoy the "Medical Short-Tongue" excerpts in Chapter 3, by Perri Klass, M.D., written first as a fourth-year medical student; she is now a noted author of many books from the physician's point of view.

Those who enjoy all the new forensic shows on television will find Sidney Moormeister's "Careers in Death Investigation—Is One Right for You?" in Chapter 16 right up their alley. New articles by Renee Priest, an MT humorist, will entertain and inform. An article by Lea Sims, AAMT's Director of Communications, on her first-hand experience visiting a hospital with a full EHR environment will provide a unique insight into the future of medical documentation.

An extensive Glossary has been added, and a comprehensive Quick-Reference Word List at the back of the textbook contains words and phrases from medical transcripts, including specialty terms and medical jargon not readily found in dictionaries and other references. Also new to this edition is a table of Normal Lab Values for reference. An extensive Index will help students find topics and illustrations quickly.

In Chapters 1 and 2, the information on the career, the industry, the healthcare record, and technology has been updated and expanded. HIPAA, the electronic health record, and speech recognition are addressed. Advances in technology, sometimes looked at as negatively impacting the future of medical transcription, are addressed frankly and, we believe, realistically.

Chapter 3, Style Guide, has been greatly expanded and reorganized. As the dictations were reviewed, every attempt was made to ensure that the Style Guide covers every style, punctuation, or editing issue that arises. Each chapter in Part Two contains Style Guide activities to be completed prior to transcription so that students are adequately prepared as they encounter issues in the dictations.

In Part Two, Chapters 4 through 17, the sections on Common Diseases, Diagnostic and Surgical Procedures, Laboratory Procedures, and Pharmacology have all been reviewed, revised, and updated. New content has been added throughout the text.

A significant new feature of this edition is the end-of-chapter pretranscription activities. Students are given assignments in the Style Guide, problem-solving "hypothetical" scenarios, and pretranscription research assignments that will better prepare them for transcription of the dictations. Rather than an after-the-fact, wish-I'd-known-that-before feeling after transcribing, students will be armed with foundational knowledge that will allow them to maximize learning when transcribing the dictations.

Finally, new dictations have been provided. The transcript keys have been prepared in accordance with the current edition of the *AAMT Book of Style* and carefully edited and footnoted to highlight teaching moments.

The goal of *Medical Transcription Fundamentals & Practice*, third edition, is to familiarize students with the transcription of dictation in the basic medical and surgical specialties. Students seeking employment as medical transcriptionists will find that this course prepares them for entry-level positions in physician offices or medical group practices, clinics, and specialty departments.

Students wishing to become Registered Medical Transcriptionists (RMT) and Certified Medical Transcriptionists (CMT) and expand their employment options to hospitals and transcription services will want to continue their education through advanced training.

As comprehensive as this course is, the authors assume that students will have had at least a medical terminology and perhaps anatomy course prior to embarking on this course of study. The medical terminology and anatomy content of this program is intended for review and not in-depth study. Students should be required to have a medical and an English dictionary. A pharmacology reference is optional but would be helpful.

This edition of *Medical Transcription Fundamentals & Practice* represents a major revision of the entire course—text, supplemental materials, and dictation—and we believe instructors and students will find it an engaging and effective course of study.

Acknowledgments

Medical Transcription Fundamentals & Practice, third edition, has been greatly expanded to meet the needs of medical transcription students of the twenty-first century. The new arrangement of material is designed to enhance learning in each medical specialty, and extensive material has been added on common diseases. The new material makes this short course in medical transcription timely and up-to-date.

What makes this transcription course unique is not only the inclusion of authentic physician dictation but also the pertinent medical readings by physicians, the interesting articles by medical transcriptionists about the profession, and the challenging exercises and learning tools.

New exercises on the dictations as well as post-transcription exercises were developed for this edition by Ellen Drake, CMT, who also extensively edited the textbook and the transcript keys. New dictations were carefully selected and professionally edited by Linda Campbell, CMT, who also edited the transcripts and proofread the textbook. Special thanks go to John H. Dirckx, M.D., for his scholarly and astute editing of the medical transcripts.

Impressive and relevant materials have been assembled from other publications by Health Professions Institute. The textbook includes numerous excerpts from the writings of John H. Dirckx, M.D., author of *Human Diseases, H&P: A Nonphysician's Guide to the Medical History and Physical Examination, and Laboratory Tests and Diagnostic Procedures in Medicine,* as well as many timeless articles published in *Perspectives on the Medical Transcription Profession.* In addition, sections on pharmacology were drawn from Susan M. Turley's *Understanding Pharmacology for Health Professionals,* third edition (Prentice Hall Health, 2003).

Humorous and interesting essays on medical transcription have been reprinted from Judith Marshall's collection of essays, *Medicate Me,* illustrated by Cindy Stevens, and *Medicate Me Again.* Interesting, informative, and humorous essays by many outstanding authors in the medical transcription profession are drawn from *Perspectives on the Medical Transcription* and *The SUM Program for Medical Transcription Training.* The fine contributions of many of the leaders in the medical transcription profession are noted in the list of Resources in the appendix.

We are most grateful to Joan Gill, executive editor of Health Professions at Prentice Hall Health, who enthusiastically supports medical transcription as an important health profession. She has spearheaded the revision of *Medical Transcription Fundamentals & Practice* in the past year and pushed for full-color illustrations in the text, and her encouragement of our efforts to provide quality education for medical transcription students has contributed greatly to the success of this book.

Many thanks to the staff and associates of Prentice Hall Health for the dynamic graphic design and layout and for the glorious four-color art and medical illustrations that add so much to the textbook.

Art Acknowledgments

Bonnie Fremgen and Suzanne S. Frucht, *Medical Terminology: A Living Language,* 3rd ed. (Upper Saddle River, NJ: Pearson Prentice Hall, 2003).

Jane Rice, *Medical Terminology with Human Anatomy,* 5th ed. (Upper Saddle River, NJ: Pearson Prentice Hall, 2005).

Other illustrative art for chapter and part openers was taken from Medical Perspectives and Medicine & Health Care collections from EyeWire Photography.

Special photos of medical transcriptionists at work were provided by Linda Campbell, Autumn and Brett Marler, and Philips Dictation Systems.

Humorous illustrations by Cindy Stevens were taken from Judith Marshall, *Medicate Me* (Modesto, CA: Health Professions Institute, 1987).

Sally Crenshaw Pitman, M.A.
Editor & Publisher
Health Professions Institute
Modesto, California

A Note to Students

To make the most of this course of study, it is important that you understand the features of this course and how best to maximize your training. Please read the Preface to familiarize yourself with the content and features of the course. Take the time to page through the book, looking at the different features and especially become familiar with the appendiceal material following Chapter 17 (Resources, Glossary, Quick-Reference Word List, a table of Normal Lab Values, and an Index).

It is also important for you to familiarize yourself with the features on the CD-ROM, with its interactive programming by Georgia and Dave Green of Horus Development. Click on each drop-down menu and then click on each feature in the menu. Make friends with the Help menu. Some students have completed the entire course in the past without knowing some of the features on the CD-ROM that would have made their study and transcription time much more productive.

Prior to transcribing the specialty dictations, you should read the entire chapter, complete the exercises, and study the Transcription Tips and the Sample Reports.

A new feature in this edition of *Medical Transcription Fundamentals & Practice* is the inclusion of exercises and activities that relate specifically to the dictations you will be transcribing. These include Using the Style Guide, Problem Solving, and Preparatory Research. These activities are to be completed prior to transcribing the dictations. In addition, your instructor may assign additional exercises called Engaging the Content to be completed after transcription of the dictations has been completed.

Using the Style Guide. This alerts you to style issues you may encounter with each dictation assignment. There is some repetition in that similar issues may occur within several specialties, but this will help to reinforce your learning. Over time, you will learn to be efficient at using the Style Guide, and you'll avoid style mistakes you might otherwise make.

Problem Solving. The problem-solving questions are primarily intended to forewarn you about the stumbling blocks, hurdles, and pitfalls that occur with authentic physician dictation. For the most part, these questions have no definitive answers, which initially will be disconcerting if you're like most students. Students sometimes want black and white answers, and it's unfortunate when an education system teaches students that memorization and regurgitation of facts is learning, but it is not.

The ability to solve problems and use critical thinking is of primary importance in medical transcription. These exercises are intended to help you develop those skills. Your answers and the way you address the problem when it occurs in dictation will demonstrate whether you have an informed and logical approach to editing, physician misspeaks, and risk management issues. One hopes your answers will become more mature and sophisticated as you progress through the course.

Preparatory Research. Any information requested in these questions not readily available in the textbook or required references can easily be found using Internet search engines such as Google or on-line medical dictionaries. These questions anticipate auditory discrimination problems and refresh and reinforce vocabulary so you will avoid the usual errors that beginning medical transcription students make. They also prepare you for analysis of and interacting with the content of the medical report.

When first introduced to dictation and medical transcription, you have myriad things to remember. You're learning intellectual and physical coordination skills you've never had to use before. You're struggling with format and style and punctuating occasionally nonstandard syntax "on the fly." And, of course, you're developing auditory discrimination and trying to recognize what you hear as vocabulary you've actually studied in medical terminology. With all these things to do, it's easy to develop a kind of "remote control" habit of just typing sounds and failing to connect with the meaning of the words coming into your ears and brain.

It's important that you take time to understand the medical content of the reports you're transcribing. By doing so, you begin to make connections between symptoms and diseases, diseases and diagnostic procedures, diseases and treatments, drugs and interactions, diagnoses and outcomes. These are the connections that enable the experienced transcriptionist to decipher difficult or garbled dictation and to spot and report inconsistencies, omissions, and risk management issues.

Engaging the Content. To help you focus on the content of the dictations you're transcribing, your instructor may assign exercises from the *Instructor's Guide* called Engaging the Content. Some of the questions do nothing more than encourage you to interpret the medical content into lay language. Others focus on auditory discrimination skills. Some require you to see relationships and corollaries. Almost all require you to justify your answers using information contained in the medical content of the report. All the questions will help to develop your problem-solving and critical thinking skills and make you better transcriptionists.

I hope you find these new activities of benefit. These are techniques I have been developing throughout my years of teaching. I've found that my students have become better and better thinkers as I find more ways for them to engage the content.

Ellen Drake, CMT, FAAMT
Adjunct Professor
Seminole Community College
Sanford, FL

About the Authors

Medical Transcription Fundamentals & Practice, third edition, was written and developed by the editorial staff and associates of Health Professions Institute (HPI), Modesto, California.

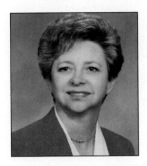

Sally C. Pitman, M.A., is editor and publisher of Health Professions Institute. Since 1985 she has published 10 editions of *Vera Pyle's Current Medical Terminology)* and numerous periodicals, primarily the quarterly *Perspectives on the Medical Transcription Profession* since 1990. She edited and published *The SUM Program for Medical Transcription Training* and numerous other educational materials for medical transcriptionists, teachers, supervisors, and business owners. She owned a medical transcription service for 10 years (until 1982), having previously taught English in a community college for five years. She was a founding director of AAMT (1978-1984), editor and publisher of all AAMT publications for eight years (until September 1986), author of *The eMpTy Laugh Book* (AAMT, 1981), and co-author of the *Style Guide for Medical Transcription* (AAMT, 1985). She was also the founder and executive director of the Medical Transcription Industry Alliance (MTIA) in the early 1990s. In 2006 she received the Lifetime Achievement Award from MTIA, recognizing her service in the medical transcription profession over the past 30 years. She and her husband Leon have two children and six grandchildren.

Ellen Drake, CMT, FAAMT, Director of Education and Certification of the American Association for Medical Transcription (AAMT), has worked closely with Health Professions Institute to develop many books and training materials over the past 15 years. She has written numerous articles on medical transcription, and she

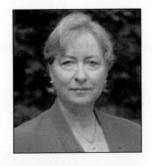

is a frequent speaker at seminars and conferences for medical transcription educators and practitioners. She is a former medical transcription program director and is now an adjunct professor at Seminole Community College in Sanford, Florida. She has a B.A. in English education and taught high school English for five years. She co-authors (with Randy Drake) *Saunders Pharmaceutical Word Book*, published annually since 1992 by W. B. Saunders Elsevier (St. Louis).

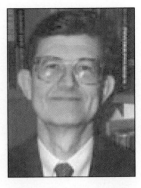

John H. Dirckx, M.D., retired in 2003 after 35 years as director of the student health center at the University of Dayton, Ohio. His long-standing interest in classical and modern languages has led to the writing of several books and numerous articles on the language, literature, and history of medicine. He is the author of *The Language of Medicine: Its Evolution, Structure, and Dynamics*, 2nd ed. (New York: Praeger Publishers, 1983); *H&P: A Nonphysician's Guide to the Medical History and Physical Examination*, 3rd ed. (HPI, 2001), *Human Diseases*, 2nd ed. (HPI, 2003); and *Laboratory Tests & Diagnostic Procedures in Medicine* (HPI, 2004). He is a frequent contributor of educational articles on medicine and medical language to medical transcription periodicals, including *Perspectives on the Medical Transcription Profession* (published by HPI) and *Journal of AAMT* (American Association for Medical Transcription), and is medical consultant for *The SUM Program for Medical Transcription Training* developed by Health Professions Institute. He has served as consulting or contributing editor to several medical journals and to Lippincott Williams & Wilkins, publisher of Stedman's references, and the G. & C. Merriam Company, publisher of the Merriam-Webster dictionaries. His short fiction appears regularly in national magazines. His hobbies include book-collecting and music. He and his wife Joyce have five daughters and ten grandchildren.

Linda C. Campbell, CMT, FAAMT, served as HPI Director of New Product Development for almost 20 years. In this capacity she contributed to the development of *The SUM Program for Medical Transcription Training, Student Syllabus, Teacher's Manual,* and *The Medical Transcription Workbook*. In addition, she contributed to three

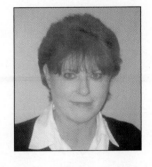

editions of *Medical Transcription Fundamenals & Practice* published by Prentice Hall Health. She has been in the medical transcription field for over 30 years, having worked as a medical transcriptionist for hospitals, transcription companies, and in self-employment. She has written and edited many articles and books and presented seminars and workshops for medical transcription teachers and practitioners. She works with medical facilities and educational institutions to implement medical transcription training programs and advises individuals in self-directed study.

List of Figures

Part One

Fundamentals of Medical Transcription

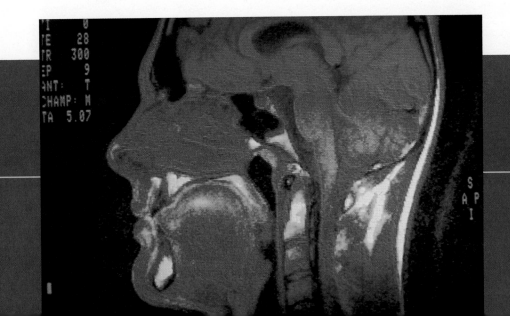

Medical Fundamentals

Chapter Outline

Learning Objectives

- Describe the professional healthcare team and what attributes distinguish the professional medical transcriptionist.
- Identify and describe the various types of dictated medical reports.
- List several purposes of the healthcare record. Describe its various components.
- Identify the chief tools of the medical transcriptionist.
- Describe digital dictation systems.
- Describe various types of reference books used by medical transcriptionists.

- List several different work environments, and give pros and cons for each.
- Identify and describe the two main parts of the history and physical examination.
- Tell why laboratory tests are important and why medical transcriptionists should know reference values.
- Identify various drug forms. Describe common routes of administration of drugs.
- Define *therapeutic effect* and *side effect*.

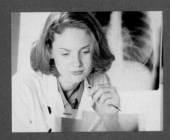
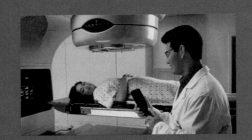
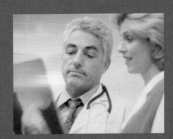

Transcribing Medical Dictation

The Medical Transcription Profession

The medical transcriptionist (MT) is a vital member of the professional healthcare team. While not as visible to the general public as those members of the team providing hands-on care, such as physicians, nurses, therapists, technicians, dietitians, and other healthcare support staff, the medical transcriptionist plays an important role in documenting the quality of patient care and the continuity and accuracy of the healthcare record.

Medical transcriptionists (MTs) provide an important service to both physician and patient by transcribing dictated medical reports that document a patient's medical care and condition. These may include office chart notes, history and physical examinations, consultations, letters, memos, admission notes, emergency department notes, operative reports, discharge summaries, and many specialized laboratory, imaging, and other diagnostic studies. Medical transcriptionists transcribe reports from a variety of medical specialties, and each day's work presents a unique challenge and opportunity for learning.

Medical transcriptionists contribute to quality patient care through their commitment to excellence. Because each dictated report represents a part of a patient's healthcare record, the medical transcriptionist transcribes it with care, demonstrating an extensive knowledge of medical terminology, anatomy, pharmacology, human diseases, surgical procedures, diagnostic studies, and laboratory tests in order to produce an accurate and complete permanent medical record.

A mastery of English grammar, structure, and style, a knowledge of transcription practices, skill in typing, spelling, and proofreading, and the highest professional standards contribute to the medical transcriptionist's ability to interpret, translate, and edit medical dictation for content and clarity.

With the advent of the electronic health record, it is anticipated that the medical transcriptionist's role will evolve into a more technological-based position which will require advanced clinical knowledge, greater problem-solving skills, and mastery of a variety of computer software programs such as database management and spreadsheet programs.

For all these reasons, medical transcriptionists must be critical thinkers, that is, they must be able to use their interpretive medical language skills and the context clues in the report to detect and correct errors, to make decisions about leaving blanks and flagging, and to spot potential risk management issues.

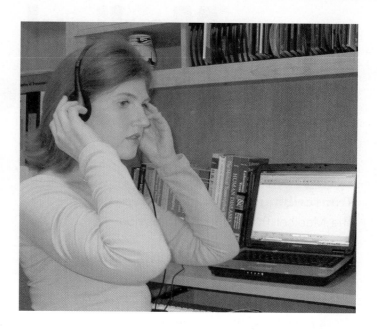

Medical transcriptionists work in a variety of settings, including medical centers, general and specialty hospitals, clinics and group practices, radiology and pathology offices, medical transcription services, government facilities, insurance companies, home offices, and other environments. A large percentage of MTs working for the above organizations work from home.

Some medical transcriptionists combine their transcription skills with clinical skills to work as medical assistants. Others become supervisors, managers, college teachers, quality assurance specialists, proofreaders, and speech recognition editors. In the future, MTs may have even more responsibility for making sure that the electronic health record is complete and medically accurate.

Medical transcriptionists' earnings vary according to geographic area, skill level, place of employment, and method of compensation. Transcriptionists working for companies in large metropolitan areas generally earn more than those in smaller cities. Experienced transcriptionists who are paid on production often earn more than those who are compensated on an hourly basis.

Some facilities have incentive pay plans where transcriptionists are paid a bonus over and above the minimum production level and base pay for that facility. Generally speaking, entry-level transcriptionists can expect to earn at least twice the hourly minimum wage in larger cities, perhaps less in other areas. Experienced transcriptionists and those paid on production usually earn significantly more.

Job opportunities exist all over the United States and Canada and in American hospitals in foreign countries. In addition to choice of work setting, transcriptionists can often find part-time or full-time employment with flexible scheduling. Furthermore, through the miracle of technology and high-speed Internet access, transcriptionists may live in the Deep South and work for a transcription service in the Pacific Northwest. A transcriptionist may move from the East Coast to the West Coast and never change employers.

Advances in technology have also made it possible for people with a variety of disabilities to become medical transcriptionists. There are blind and visually impaired MTs as well as MTs confined to wheelchairs.

The Healthcare Record

The healthcare record is a legal record detailing the healthcare services rendered to a patient. The healthcare record contains reports of dictated diagnostic studies, progress notes (which may be handwritten or electronic) made by all the clinical staff who attend the patient, machine-generated diagnostic reports, and documentation necessary for reimbursement. The record may be paper, stored digitally in electronic format in a computer, or a combination of the two.

The healthcare record is the property of the hospital or the medical facility or office in which it originated, and it cannot be removed from the premises without a subpoena or court order. In a hospital, and usually in a large multi-specialty health maintenance organization (HMO), it is maintained in a health information department usually headed by a registered health information administrator (RHIA). Other duties in the health information department are performed by a registered health information technician (RHIT). RHIAs and RHITs are certified by the American Health Information Management Association (AHIMA).

Purpose of the healthcare record. The healthcare record is a measurement of care rendered in a medical facility. It is utilized to plan, communicate, and evaluate the quality of care given to each patient. It is "proof of work done," containing documentation to meet federal, state, and the Joint Commission on Accreditation of Healthcare Organizations (JCAHO) standards and regulations, as well as those for reimbursement and third-party payer requirements.

The healthcare record is maintained for medicolegal protection for the patient, facility, staff, and physician. It is used for research, compiling statistics, and evaluation of healthcare delivery.

Origin of the healthcare record. In hospitals, the healthcare record begins in the admissions department, outpatient registration, or the emergency department (ED). Patients having surgery as outpatients check in at outpatient registration, which registers elective sur-

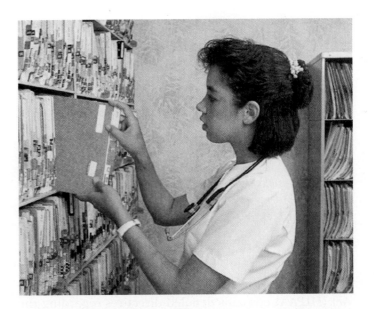

gery outpatients and clinic patients. These patients, after observation, may also be admitted. Patients may also enter the hospital after evaluation in the emergency department, which collects patient identification and demographic information. The correct spelling of the patient's legal name and birth date are critical elements to determine positive patient identification. This information is used to assign a healthcare record number that is maintained for the lifetime of the patient and should be recorded on all transcribed reports.

Additional identification entries on patients are address, next of kin, birthplace, Social Security number, occupation, sex, marital status, ethnic origin, religious preference, and admitting diagnosis. Financial entries include the patient's employer, job title, address of company, insurance company, person responsible for emergency notification and payments, type of coverage, insurance identification number, and type of payment plan. All this information is recorded on an admission sheet or patient demographic face sheet.

Consents and privacy notice. These departments also have responsibility for obtaining forms which include the patient's consent for treatment and outline of patient's responsibilities, including billing, and the assurance that confidentiality will be protected. Throughout a patient's care, additional informed consents for surgery, procedures, invasive diagnostic tests, transfer, etc., will be obtained as appropriate.

Admissions clerks will also often ask a patient about to be admitted if he or she has a "living will," a healthcare declaration that simply documents a person's wishes concerning treatment when those wishes can no longer be personally communicated. Some hospitals and physician offices provide a form for patients to complete if they do not already have a living will.

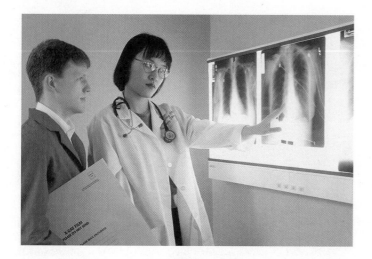

The **Health Insurance Portability and Accountability Act (HIPAA)** contains detailed directives regarding the confidentiality of all data contained in healthcare records. Under the terms of this legislation, a provider of healthcare must inform each patient of the extent of privacy protection, including exceptions (for example, sharing of historical or diagnostic information among physicians in a group practice), and must obtain the patient's signed authorization for any transfer of information to a third party, except as so set forth.

Medical transcriptionists have always been taught to keep the contents of medical records confidential, but until HIPAA, there was no definitive federal regulation governing the confidentiality of medical records. HIPAA makes it illegal to disclose protected health information (PHI).

The Privacy Rule of HIPAA defines PHI as individually identifiable health information (including that of non-U.S. citizens), held or maintained by a covered entity (for example, a hospital or physician) or its business associates (for example, a medical transcription service) acting for the covered entity (CE), that is transmitted or maintained in any form or medium. This includes identifiable demographic and other information relating to the past, present, or future physical or mental health or condition of an individual, or the provision or payment of healthcare to an individual that is created or received by a healthcare provider, health plan, employer, or healthcare clearinghouse. For purposes of the Privacy Rule, genetic information is considered to be health information.

The Privacy Rule does not protect individually identifiable health information that is held or maintained by entities other than covered entities or business associates (BAs) that create, use, or receive such information on behalf of the covered entity.

Examples of information protected by the Privacy Rule include the following: patient's name and address, Social Security number, birthday, ethnic origin, medical number, and the following when this information can be linked back to an identifiable individual: health background, lab test results, healthcare and x-rays, provider's name, notes taken by a doctor or nurse, diagnosis, and medical records.

It is now recommended that patients keep copies of their own medical reports in order to have a complete personal health record (PHR) available to emergency departments, hospitals, and their doctors. A PHR can help improve the quality of care a person receives by reducing or eliminating duplicate tests and allowing patients to receive faster, safer treatment and care in an emergency. In short, a PHR helps people play a more active role in their own healthcare. There are many Web sites that provide a way for individuals to safely store their PHR on the Internet. One such site that is free is MyPHR (**www.myphr.com**), hosted by AHIMA.

Physician orders. A patient is admitted and treated only on the order of an attending physician. The admission includes orders for diagnostic tests, medications, and treatments. Pharmacy orders may be entered electronically for safety reasons. Paper-based forms are usually multipart with a copy for the department.

Diagnostic tests. From the physician's orders, the nurses generate a requisition for diagnostic tests. These are sent to the appropriate department, whose personnel perform the tests and document the results. Typical diagnostic results include the following.

Laboratory: Lab slips include the results of urinalyses, complete blood counts, electrolytes, chemistries, specimens, and blood transfusions. Pathology and autopsy results are also the responsibility of this department.

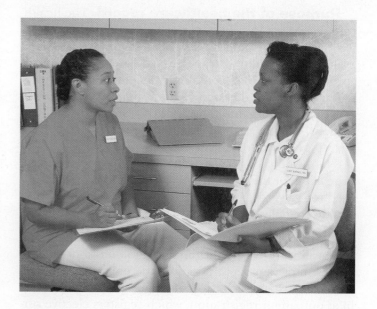

Radiology: Dictated reports include the clinical history, findings, and conclusion for any x-rays performed.

Cardiology: Electrocardiograms, Holter monitor, and exercise stress test results are dictated, or reports are machine generated.

Neurophysiology: Electroencephalograms, electromyograms, and sleep disorder results are dictated or machine generated.

Nursing entries. Nurses assess patients on admission by completing an admission history and physical, establish a patient care plan, and set up forms for documentation of graphic information such as vital signs (temperature, pulse, respiration, blood pressure, and weight). Intake and output of fluids, diet and hygiene records, medication records, as well as specialized forms for monitoring diabetes, operating room checklists, operating room record, recovery room record, and nurses' notes and observations become a part of every patient's healthcare record.

Physician entries. The physician dictates the patient's History and Physical, which includes the Chief Complaint, History of Present Illness, Past Medical History, Family History, Social History, Review of Systems, Physical Examination, Assessment, and Plan.

The physician may call in consultants as appropriate to assist in the patient's care. The consultant writes or dictates a consultation which includes a comprehensive review of the healthcare record and complete physical examination and recommendations. The physician writes or dictates progress notes which include all pertinent plans and observations during the patient's care. If the patient has a diagnostic procedure or a surgical procedure performed, the surgeon dictates preoperative and postoperative diagnoses, the name of the procedure, assistant, findings, technique, and outcome. The anesthesiologist completes a preanesthesia and postanesthesia evaluation.

At the conclusion of the patient's hospitalization, the physician writes or dictates a comprehensive discharge summary which includes a brief history, course of the hospitalization, conclusions, followup instructions and discharge medications, diagnoses, complications, and any surgical procedures.

Therapist entries. Physical, respiratory, occupational, speech, vocational, and recreational therapists, and social workers who might be requested to assist in the patient's care, write or dictate an initial evaluation and plans, ongoing progress notes, and a final summary with followup instructions.

Ancillary personnel entries. Dietary personnel, discharge planners, utilization review managers, and others participating in the patient's care make a record of progress notes on each of their visits. Thus, the health information department and medical transcription are vitally linked in the delivery of healthcare.

The Medical Reports

A variety of medical reports are generated every day in physician offices, clinics, and hospitals. Medical transcriptionists should be familiar with those dictated in each work setting.

Physicians in private practice frequently dictate office chart notes, letters, initial office evaluations, and history and physical examinations. Medical reports dictated in hospitals and medical centers are numerous in category; however, they invariably include dictations from the "basic four" reports: History and Physical Examination, Consultation Report, Operative Report, and Discharge Summary. Emergency department reports, hospital progress notes, and diagnostic studies are often dictated as well. (See Sample Reports, pp. 35-43.) Every treatment, every diagnostic study, and every procedure must be documented in one way or another and placed in the patient's chart or permanent medical record.

Chart note. The chart note (also called progress note or followup note) is dictated by a physician after talking with, meeting with, or examining a patient, usually in an outpatient setting, although progress notes may also be dictated on hospital inpatients. The chart note contains a concise description of the patient's presenting problem, physical findings, and the physician's plan of treatment, and may also include the results of laboratory tests. (See Sample Reports, p. 36.)

Chart notes or progress notes become a permanent part of the patient's medical record. Chart notes can vary in length from one sentence to one or more pages, with the average note being two to four paragraphs long. Chart notes are sometimes dictated in an informal, staccato style using clipped sentences, abbreviations, and brief forms. There are numerous formats for dictated chart notes. SOAP notes are those dictated in the SOAP format (an acronym for Subjective, Objective, Assessment, and Plan, which are headings within the note) (see p. 36).

Although formats vary from office to office, chart notes and progress notes should include the date of visit, patient's name, the patient's ID number, a signature line for the physician, and the transcriptionist's initials.

Letter. Physicians frequently dictate letters to communicate patient information to other physicians, insurance companies, patients' employers, and government offices. Medical transcriptionists need to be familiar with the various standard business letter formats. A dictator may express a preference for a specific letter format, although the full-block format (with the parts of the letter lined up on the left margin) is the one most commonly used. The patient's name and identification number are included in the Re (regarding) line. (See Sample Reports, p. 35.)

Referral letters and consultation letters are not mere business letters; they are medical documents in letter form and as such should be transcribed with the same high degree of skill and accuracy as other medical reports. A copy of each letter must be kept and incorporated into the patient's medical record.

Initial office evaluation. Performed in the physician's office or clinic setting, the initial office evaluation is dictated after the physician sees a patient for the first time. It contains essentially the same information as the history and physical examination, although the physical examination in an initial office evaluation may be limited to specific areas of disease.

Demographic data. All hospital reports contain a certain amount of information about the patient called demographic data. Although formats vary, the demographic data usually include the patient's name, ID number, the date of admission (and date of discharge if a discharge summary), and the name of the admitting physician. At the end of the report, there should be a blank space for the signature of the dictator (and attending or supervising physician if different), the date of dictation and transcription, and the initials of the dictator and transcriptionist. The following reports are contained within a patient's hospital chart or record.

History and Physical Examination (H&P). Shortly before or after a patient is admitted to the hospital, the physician obtains the patient's subjective history and conducts an objective physical examination. These findings are then dictated by category and usually include the following (see Sample Reports, pp. 37-38).

Chief Complaint. This is the patient's main presenting problem and the reason for which the patient is seeking medical help. It can be a short sentence or a paragraph in length. Usually, the chief complaint is a rephrase of the patient's statement to the physician, but sometimes the dictator will quote the patient's exact words ("I fainted."). This is particularly true for psychiatric reports. When the patient's exact words are used, the statement is set off with quotation marks. The dictator may say "quote unquote" at the beginning of the sentence, and the MT must decide which dictation to put in quotation marks.

History of Present Illness. The history of present illness is a description of the events leading to the patient's presentation to the physician (or admission to

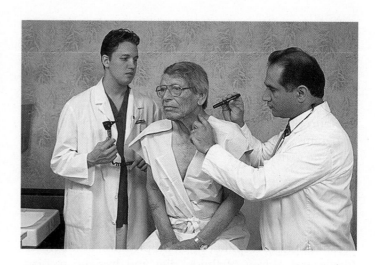

the hospital). It can be a few lines to one or two paragraphs in length. Some of the material dictated under this heading may appear to be past history because it could have happened in the distant past, but if it relates to the admitting complaint or complaints, then it will likely be included in the history of the present illness.

Past Medical History. This category includes all medical and surgical problems from childhood to the present, including medications and allergies.

Family History is the medical condition of parents, other family members, and blood relatives. A complete family history (often not elicited) includes the age and state of health of all the immediate family members.

Social History contains a description of the patient's personal information—occupation, lifestyle, and habits. Asbestos and hazardous chemical exposure, for example, contain medical implications. The patient's use of caffeine, nicotine, alcohol, and prescription or illicit drugs are described here.

Review of Systems. The review of systems is *subjective*, that is, it reflects the patient's perception of symptoms as the physician asks questions about the major organ systems. Because this section reports on the patient's symptoms, physicians sometimes misspeak and say "review of symptoms" instead of "review of systems." The systems reviewed usually include Head, Eyes, Ears, Nose, Throat (HEENT); Cardiovascular (CV); Respiratory; Gastrointestinal (GI); Genitourinary (GU); Neuromuscular; Psychiatric; and occasionally Integumentary (Skin).

Physical Examination. The physical examination details the physician's *objective* findings on examination of the patient. The following subheadings are usually dictated: General Appearance, Vital Signs, Skin, HEENT (Head, Eyes, Ears, Nose, and Throat), Neck, Chest (Breasts, Heart, and Lungs), Abdomen, Back, Extremities, Genitalia or Pelvic, Rectal, Neurologic, and occasionally Mental Status Exam.

In addition, the History and Physical Examination often includes an Admitting Diagnosis or Impression, and often a proposed Treatment Plan. The History and Physical report is also known as the Admission History and Physical. More detailed information about the History and Physical Examination is covered later in this chapter.

Emergency department report. An emergency department report is much like an initial office evaluation, except that the patient is seen and treated in an emergency department of a hospital or acute care clinic. The Presenting Complaint, Present Illness, Physical Examination, and Course of Treatment are usually dictated. Sometimes the patient's condition is serious enough to warrant admission to the hospital, but more often the patient is seen, evaluated, treated, and then released to home with a recommended treatment plan.

Consultation. A consultation occurs when one physician requests the evaluation, opinion, and recommendations of another physician (almost always a board-certified specialist) in the care and treatment of a patient. The consultant bears no responsibility for patient care and, in fact, no doctor-patient relationship is established by the consultant until or unless the patient's care is either turned over to or shared with the consultant by the requesting physician. A consultation report must be generated by the consultant for each consultation service provided (see Sample Reports, pp. 39-40). The report becomes part of the consultant's records, part of the requesting physician's medical records, and, if the consultation was performed in a facility, part of the facility's medical records.

The report usually contains the subheadings Brief History of the Present Illness, Findings, Pertinent Laboratory Work, Working Diagnosis or Impression, and a

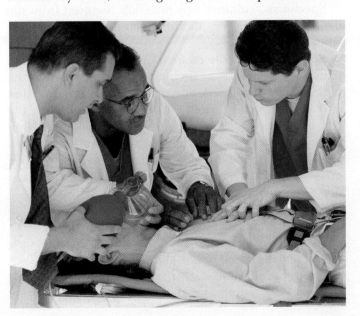

Recommended Course of Treatment. The Consultation Report may be dictated in letter format and is to be transcribed on the stationery of the physician's office or the medical facility or on preprinted consultation forms, which usually require the date of consultation, the name of the requesting physician, the name of the consulting physician, and the reason for consultation.

Operative report. After a surgical procedure is performed, a detailed description of the operation is dictated. Surgical procedures are carried out in hospitals, outpatient surgery centers, and occasionally in a physician's office (see Figure 1-1).

The format used in dictating an operative report will depend to some extent on the surgeon's specialty and training, on the nature of the procedure, and on local conventions and institutional guidelines. The following discussion is based on an idealized format, some parts of which would be appropriate only for certain types of surgery. In addition, some pieces of information presented here under separate headings are regularly included by some dictators as part of the account of the operative procedure. (See Sample Reports, pp. 41-42.)

Often a printed form or template is used for operative reports, containing a heading with spaces for entering the following information.

Identifying data. The operative report must contain, as an absolute minimum, the name of the patient and any case or admission number assigned by the hospital for record-keeping purposes; the name of the surgeon; and the date on which the procedure was performed.

Name of procedure. Generally, standard procedural terminology must be used, and in addition to the name of the operation, a code number, for insurance and statistical purposes, may be required to be entered by the surgeon or by a clerk.

Preoperative diagnosis. The surgeon's provisional assessment of the patient's condition before beginning the operation, including the disease or condition that is the principal reason for the surgery. Again, standard terminology is required, followed by appropriate coding.

Postoperative diagnosis. A more definitive and precise diagnosis established at or after operation, but often the same as the preoperative diagnosis.

Names of surgeon(s) and anesthesiologist(s). The surgeon, any surgical assistants, and the anesthesiologist(s) are ordinarily identified somewhere in the operative record. The name of the person dictating the operative report (who may not be the principal surgeon) will also appear at the end of the dictation. In some institutions, nurses or technicians assisting in the operating room are also identified.

Indications, history. Here the dictator elaborates on the preoperative diagnosis and explains the reasons

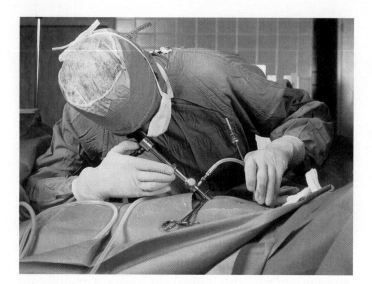

Figure 1-1
Laparoscopic Cholecystectomy

that led to surgery on this patient and the choice of procedure and techniques used. This part of the operative report is not to be confused with the full clinical history of the patient contained elsewhere in the hospital record and perhaps dictated by someone other than the surgeon.

Clinical status, physical examination. This information is a continuation of the preceding and may appear under the same heading. The surgeon describes the patient's physical condition (including results of pertinent laboratory tests or x-rays), particularly as it has a bearing on the need for surgery and the choice of procedure. Again, this is not to be confused with the complete physical examination report contained elsewhere in the patient's record.

Operative report. The dictator's description of the actual surgical procedure may be given as a continuous narrative or may be presented under two or more of the following headings.

Anesthesia. A simple statement of the type of anesthetic used. The dictator may say simply "general" or "spinal," knowing that detailed information about the anesthetic will be recorded by the anesthesiologist.

Position. The position of the patient on the operating table is often passed over in silence unless some special positioning is required by the nature of the procedure.

Skin preparation. Scrubbing of the skin is usually a routine procedure carried out by an assistant or technician. The surgeon may record the name of the soap or disinfectant used and any special procedures used for sterile draping.

Incision. Under this heading the surgeon records the anatomic location and orientation of the incision by which access was gained to the operative site; for example, "right upper quadrant oblique" or "median sternotomy."

Procedure, technique. A detailed, step-by-step narrative of the operation from beginning to end. Although parts of the operative report may be quite routine, each operation varies in some details from others, and a thorough and accurate report will reflect this uniqueness. The surgeon ordinarily includes in this narrative a record of the findings and some comment on their bearing on the choice of procedure and their implications for the future health of the patient.

Grafts, implants. Any foreign objects or materials left in the patient, including grafts, artificial cardiac valves, stents, artificial joints, orthopedic fixation devices, pacemakers, shunts, mesh, screws, wire, and cement, must be fully identified. The brand names, chemical nature, origin, sizes, shapes, adjustments or settings, and exact anatomic location of such materials are all an essential part of the record.

Closure. The repair of the incision and of any dissection or structural alterations performed during the surgery is described. Each layer of the body wall is closed separately, often with a different type of stitch and a different suture material for each layer. The skin may be closed with metal clips or adhesive strips.

Operative findings. When not incorporated in the operative report, this information appears under its own heading at some point in the dictation.

Drains, packs, dressings. These are devices or materials temporarily placed in or on the patient during or at the conclusion of the procedure. Since they must later be removed, recording their presence is of critical importance. Splints, casts, and other externally applied devices such as suction apparatus for evacuation of bleeding from the operative site may also be reported here.

Tourniquet time. The number of minutes during which blood flow to an extremity was shut off by a tourniquet.

Specimens, cultures. Any materials removed from the patient during surgery and intended to be submitted for laboratory study.

Sponge and needle counts. In order that no foreign material or object may be inadvertently left inside the patient, it is standard practice for sponges, needles, and certain other articles to be counted before the commencement of surgery and again just before the surgeon begins to close the wound. Usually two persons perform the counts together for greater security. The surgeon does not begin closure of the wound until the sponge and needle counts are reported correct.

Estimated blood loss. Various measures are used during an operation to monitor blood loss, including close observation of blood absorbed by sponges and measurement of blood in the trap of the suction machine.

Fluids administered. Intravenous fluids, including whole blood, administered during the procedure are sometimes recorded in the operative report. This information is also part of the anesthesia record.

Condition of patient at conclusion of operation. The surgeon reports that the patient left the operating room in satisfactory condition, or if this is not so, records any significant health problems occasioned by the surgery or anesthesia.

Complications. Under this heading the surgeon lists any unexpected and untoward consequences of the surgical procedure, such as accidental injury to healthy tissues or organs, extensive hemorrhage, or adverse reactions to anesthesia.

Postoperative plan. The surgeon's intentions regarding postoperative care, including inhalation therapy, physical therapy, graded resumption of activities, followup examinations, and so on.

Discharge summary. This report is sometimes referred to as a clinical resumé. By the time a patient is ready for discharge from the hospital, a variety of treatment modalities have been carried out. The Discharge Summary is the medical document that summarizes the patient's course in the hospital and may be short if the patient's stay in the hospital was brief and uncomplicated. (See Sample Reports, p. 43.)

Most reports include a summary of the admission and discharge diagnoses, procedures or operations performed (if any), brief review of the patient's history, the physician's findings on physical examination, a report of laboratory work performed and pertinent findings, the patient's hospital course, discharge medications, and the discharge plan or disposition. This actual summary of the patient's hospital course becomes a part of the hospital's medical record for that patient, but is also sent to and becomes a

permanent part of the admitting physician's medical record for that patient. Discharge summaries can be extremely important in terms of followup care after the patient is discharged.

A transfer summary is a modified form of discharge summary that is prepared by the treating physician when a patient is discharged to a nursing home, a skilled nursing facility, or another hospital to ensure continuity of care.

Technology

As important as technology is to the field of medical transcription, it is pointless without the most important but often overlooked asset—the brain. This anecdote from Vera Pyle sums it all up:

> Some 30 years ago, our hospital got the prototype of one of the first word processing machines. Our medical record director brought in a group of interns and residents to see this marvel. Pointing to the machine proudly, she said, "And this is the machine that transcribes your reports." Not so! I thought then, and now. The machines we use are simply tools. Without the knowledge contained in the mind of the transcriptionist, the machines are impotent. The transcriptionist is the mind behind the machine.

The field of medical transcription has seen many changes in the area of dictation and transcription technologies that have dramatically altered *how* transcriptionists do what they do. No one has a crystal ball and can predict with certainty what future technological changes will bring. However, experts in the field anticipate that future technological developments, not the least of which is the electronic health record, will dramatically change *what* transcriptionists do. For this reason, it is important to emphasize again that it is medical transcriptionists' interpretive medical language skills, their reasoning and problem-solving abilities, and their attention to quality and detail that will ensure their place in the future, regardless of what it brings.

Dictation and transcription systems. We still see some Mylar tape cassette dictation systems in place today, but most have been replaced with digital dictation systems. A digital dictation system works much the same as a compact disc (CD). The end result is a dictation that is without any hiss or other extraneous sounds found on regular Mylar tape. In the digital dictation system, voice files are stored in "digital" (computer) format rather than "analog" (tape) format, and the dictation is usually free from mechanical noise. The computer on which the digital voice files are stored may be in the same room as the

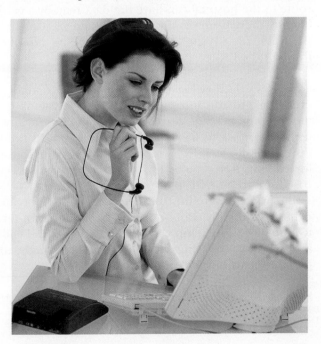

dictator or in a room on the other side of the country through the Internet.

To dictate medical reports, doctors may use a hardwired dictation unit, an ordinary phone, a handheld pocket-sized digital recorder, or a headset with microphone attachment. With digital dictation, the physician is usually required to key in a personal ID number, a patient identification number, and a report type number, or the physician may swipe a bar code encoded with all the patient's demographic data. On some systems, this electronic information can be imported directly into a report without intervention by the transcriptionist. However, the MT still needs to verify that the information is correct.

The transcriptionist may access digital dictation by working on a proprietary dictation system that is local or on a personal computer in the next room or across the country. If remote, the dictation probably will be transferred via the Internet, either in encrypted form or via a secure FTP (file transfer protocol) site.

Foot pedals may be connected to a computer via serial port or, more likely, a USB connection. These pedals operate the **.wav player** on the transcriptionist's computer or a proprietary player. A stereo headset is plugged into the speaker output. With these accessories, the computer completely replaces the transcriber that is necessary for playing Mylar cassette tapes.

The Competitive *Edge*

In May 2005 I took a trip in a time machine. I was transported to a reality that awaits all of healthcare in the not-too-distant future. As a participant and presenter at the *Exploring the Digital Hospital* event in Indianapolis, I was taken on a tour of the Indiana Heart Hospital, a facility that was designed and built from the ground up in partnership with General Electric to function on an entirely digital platform. Although the facility has a handful of procedures that still require paper (they are quick to tell you that they are "paper light" rather than "paperless"), the majority of all information functions are handled via integrated digital systems. When you consider the magnitude of transitioning all hospital systems to this reality, it is amazing that they have coordinated this in such a short time. They have been operational for less than two years.

Physicians and nurses use stationary or mobile tablets to enter data from an up-to-date computerized physician order entry (CPOE) system for physician-directed order entry to templated progress notes and nurses' notes. Medications are scanned via bar codes from the point of order to delivery at the patient bedside. The facility does not house a full-service laboratory because almost all primary labs can be done via handheld analyzers *at the patient's bedside.* Patients have an integrated education system via the television in their rooms—they can watch educational videos with interactive questions and order their own meals from an on-screen menu. They do not have scheduled tray delivery at this facility. Patients order their meals at will, and their orders are coordinated via the computer, where dietary restrictions are verified before food delivery.

Physicians can log in to the hospital from their tablets anywhere, whether in their practice setting or at home, and can quickly view any patient's current data.

This includes viewing their ongoing telemetry, vital signs, etc., as though they were sitting in the room. Orders and updates can be entered, and those modifications are immediately transmitted to the patient's record and to all of the integrated systems that rely on those orders. The facility houses voice-recognition (VR) technology and a digital dictation system, where some physicians are working strictly to train VR and others to use a back-end scenario with MT editors.

Given the ability to have enroute data (including a 12-lead ECG) transmitted digitally from ambulance to the emergency department, the Indiana Heart Hospital boasts a "door to balloon" time of 30 minutes (often less). This means that a patient with suspected myocardial infarction (MI) whose telemetry confirms this en route to the hospital can have the data read by a cardiologist (there is one in the ER 24/7) and go straight to the cath lab within 30 minutes of being admitted through the ER.

From the architectural layout of the facility, which addresses workflow issues better than any hospital I've ever seen, to the integrated technology systems that monitor and manage virtually everything, this facility is truly *amazing*. This was *enabling* technology at its finest. Providers who have every tool at their fingertips to care for patients were enabled to streamline processes, cut costs, and trim inefficiencies.

But most important, the investment in this reality (which admittedly could not have happened without a technology partnership with GE) has given this facility a *competitive edge.* It has become, not surprisingly, the premier heart hospital in that region.

Source: Lea Sims, "The Competitive Edge," *JAAMT* (Vol. 24, No. 4), August 2005, p. 203.

Keyboards. The input of data, whether via traditional or ergonomic keyboard, Dvorak keyboard, steno machine keyboard, or speech recognition system, proves once again that it's *the mind behind the machine*, not the machine, that produces quality transcription.

Speech recognition. Speech recognition (SR) is sometimes referred to as voice recognition (which actually refers to voice identification, such as that used as a security pass code). For close to two decades, it has been predicted that speech recognition would replace medical transcriptionists. Today, industry experts, including the more candid vendors of SR products, recognize that the technology is still far from perfect. Why? Because it has no brain. Widely used in medical transcription, speech recognition has been found to be another technological advancement that improves productivity and helps transcriptionists avoid repetitive stress-related injury, but it doesn't replace them. Many MTs are working today as speech recognition editors, correcting not only grammar and punctuation errors but medical content errors that are due to mistranslation.

Templates and "normals." MTs have used templates (basically, report outlines containing the headings and some routine phraseology) to improve their productivity for many years. Combined with speech recognition, doctors use templates in a similar way. Normals are typically diagnostic studies, procedure notes, and operative reports that are always the same except for a few specific details. Sometimes, doctors create the normals and will dictate something like, "Use my normal bypass for internal mammary to right coronary artery, and make the following changes." Transcriptionists may develop their own normals because they've recognized repetitive dictation. These may be entire reports or "boiler plate" paragraphs which they pull into a report and then edit to reflect any changes in dictation.

Point and click. "Point and click" refers to templated, computerized forms with check boxes that a physician simply clicks on to indicate positive and negative findings. There is usually an option to include some unstructured content which may be entered by the physician or dictated for transcription that is later incorporated into the form.

Electronic health record. The electronic health record (EHR) may be called by a variety of similar names, including electronic medical record (EMR). President George W. Bush mandated that the EHR be made a reality by 2010. Basically, it consists of a database system that incorporates the patient's medical record along with some other management features. It may also incorporate clinical and diagnostic data to support decision-making and diagnosis.

Data are brought into the electronic record by means of all the technologies previously discussed. Clinicians, nurses, technologists, and other patient caregivers may enter data into a patient's record. The data is stored in "chunks," and for a traditional printed report to be generated, someone must tell the system which chunks to export and in what order to create the report. Also, because of the way the data are stored, there need to be checks and balances to make sure that the record is complete. Because of the medical transcriptionist's medical knowledge, superior language skills, attention to detail, and critical thinking abilities, industry experts see a key role for MTs in the management of the EHR.

References

Medical transcriptionists are known for their love of words and their use of medical references. Today, unlike 15-20 years ago, there are many excellent references (both printed and electronic) available for the medical transcriptionist—medical dictionaries, medical specialty word and phrase references, medical abbreviation references, and medical style manuals.

Each type of reference fills a particular need. A *medical dictionary* confirms correct spellings and provides definitions to help the medical transcriptionist differentiate between similar-sounding words; however, it does not contain many specialty words, abbreviations, and surgical instruments. *Medical specialty word and phrase references* contain terms from one medical specialty or a group of related specialties and include slang, surgical instruments, drugs, new and unusual terms, abbreviations, and laboratory tests for that specialty. These types of references are also called spellers because they do not contain definitions. Their usefulness for students and inexperienced transcriptionists is limited. If you use them to find the spelling of an unfamiliar word, be sure to look up the word in a dictionary and make sure that meaning fits the context before using the term. *Medical abbreviation references* contain common and unusual abbreviations and their expansions from all medical specialties. *Medical style manuals* give suggestions on how to handle questions of format, punctuation, grammar, spelling, and style in medical reports.

Evaluating reference books. Learn to evaluate reference books for quality and appropriateness by examining the contents. For example, are words extracted from a preexisting large database (unauthored books) or researched and compiled by experienced transcriptionists? The former types of books may not include as many phrases and cross-referencing as the latter. Some unauthored books are, however, reviewed by a team of

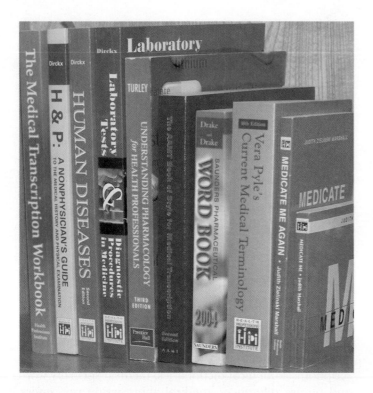

A word of caution here: Many word and phrase books include both the nonpreferred and the preferred spelling of a term. Often the nonpreferred spelling comes first alphabetically. Never choose a word from a speller unless you are sure of the meaning and that you have the preferred spelling.

Similar to the above, identify and translate abbreviations correctly. You must consider context. If you cannot be sure of the translation of an abbreviation, draw a blank line and put the abbreviation in parentheses.

When word searching, do not guess at a word just to fill in a blank. A blank does not reflect poorly on the medical transcriptionist who has thoroughly researched the question. Leaving a blank is the correct thing to do when all reference books and other sources have been exhausted. Remember, the integrity and accuracy of the medical record is far more important than never leaving a blank. The latter is not a realistic goal, even for experienced medical transcriptionists.

In class or at work, learn to use even the references you're not fond of. You may be stuck sometime and that may be all you have.

practicing MTs, and these would be preferable to those with no MT input.

Check the copyright date. This is important in references where the terminology changes rapidly, especially drug and surgery references. Who are the authors, editors, contributors, and what are their credentials? Is the publisher known for publishing quality references, and does it have a special division for medical transcription? What are the organizational features of the book? Is it user-friendly?

Become completely familiar with the front matter of every reference you use or acquire. Some MTs have used the *Saunders Pharmaceutical Word Book* for 10 years and still don't know that the authors' e-mail address and the URL for monthly updates are in the preface.

Pay special attention to any instructions on how to use the book. Do you know the meanings of standard reference terms such as *see* and *see also*, *q.v.* (which see) and *cf.* (compare)? Check the table of contents, appendices, indexes, and other features of each reference book. These features, too, can help you evaluate whether the reference book you are using is a good one or not.

When you look up a term, don't just check the spelling and type or paste it into your document. There are way too many soundalikes in medical language. Read the definition to make sure you have chosen the correct term. Never put a word whose meaning you do not know into a report. Learn to identify and take the time to read the etymology (origin) of a word. Often, this will help you create a mnemonic for remembering it.

Honing your research skills. No medical transcription practitioner or student should be without up-to-date references. A basic library should include a full-sized medical dictionary, an English dictionary, a current drug reference that includes indications and dosages, laboratory and diagnostic studies reference books, and an abbreviation book. Specialty and surgical word and phrase books can be added as necessary.

Electronic spell-checking programs, if sufficiently extensive and specialized, can help avoid misspellings of both technical and nontechnical words but cannot distinguish between homophones (*discreet/discrete, their/there*). As a rule, we recommend that students not use spell-checking programs while they are training. It's important to look up words in references as they transcribe, and then to proofread carefully after completing each report.

Not all unfamiliar dictated words are medical. It is important to remember that many physicians have extensive vocabularies and may dictate English words that are new to the transcriptionist. Thus, an English dictionary is an essential reference. If a reference book cannot provide the answer to a drug question, the medical transcriptionist may even seek help from a pharmacist. No medical transcription practitioner or student should be without up-to-date reference sources.

Take time to examine the medical reference books available to you as you begin this course. Word-searching, or locating the medical word that is correct in both spelling and meaning, is a skill that takes time and practice to develop.

The following suggestions will help you develop research skills that will serve you well as a student and on the job. These suggestions focus on spelling and locating terms as well as on selecting and evaluating reference books.

You need to understand phonics and know which sounds are represented by which letters or combinations of letters. Most medical and English dictionaries have guidelines for pronunciation but that's not enough. You need to know that every vowel can sound like almost every other vowel. Consonant sounds fall into groups of letters that are formed in different ways, depending on the way the letters are formed in the mouth. For example, *b, d, p,* and *t* can be difficult to distinguish from one another as can *b* and *v* or *s* and *f. X* is pronounced like a *z* at the beginning of a word (*xiphoid*). How many letters or combinations of letters can you think of that make a *k* sound? Which ones can make an *s* sound?

Take *ghoti* as an example of how different sounds can be rendered in English. *Ghoti* is pronounced "fish." How can this be? The *gh* is pronounced *f* as in the word *enough*. The *o* is pronounced like the short *i* in women. The *ti* is pronounced as *sh*, as in emo*tion*. Ghoti = fish!

Once you find a difficult-to-spell word, analyze it. If you find that it was because it contains a letter or letter combination that sounds like a different letter, make a note of it.

Remember that a fair number of words contain silent letters (the final *e* on many words is silent) and may even begin with a silent letter. Examples of words with silent letters include *pneumonia, psychiatric, psyllium, ptosis* (all silent *p*); *mnemonic* (silent *m*); *phthisis* ("tysis"); *gnathodynia* (silent *g*); *rhinorrhagia* and *rhonchi* (silent *h*); *euphoria* (silent *e*), and *scybala* (silent *c* ["SI-ba-la"]).

When you find words with silent letters, especially at the beginning, you might write these words in the margins of the dictionary or appropriate word and phrase book at the place it would be if it were spelled like you thought it was spelled. Be sure to write it correctly spelled, however!

A final spelling stumbling block is doubled letters. Examples are *desiccate, parallel, diarrhea* (doubled *r* and a silent *h*).

For all difficult-to-spell words, try to think of memory aids (mnemonic devices) to help you remember the spelling. In *parallel*, for example, the two *l*s remind you of parallel bars used in gymnastics. If you can't think of a mnemonic (speaking of silent letters—the *m* is silent), typing the word correctly 10, 20, or 50 times will help you learn the correct spelling.

Medical dictionaries rarely list every form of a word. You need to understand spelling rules well enough to be able to correctly add plural, noun, adjective, and adverb, and sometimes verb, endings when only one form of a word can be found.

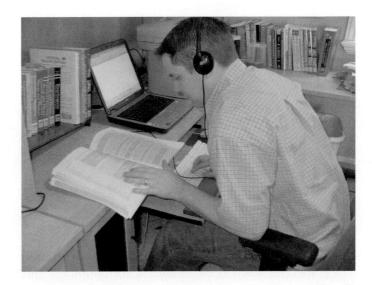

Learn to recognize and keep a list of coined (made-up) words (nouns turned into verbs and adjectives or vice versa), slang terms, and brief forms. Some coined words are acceptable if they follow the rules for forming words and there is no simple, ready substitute. For example, *coumadinize* has become a fairly standard term. Other coined words are not so acceptable. The footnotes in the transcript keys will help you identify which is which.

Slang usually consists of unacceptable brief forms such as *lytes* (electrolytes), *dig* (digoxin or digitalis), and *tic* (diverticulum). These words are not acceptable because they are either obscure, can have multiple meanings, or the brief form has been pulled from the middle or end of a longer term.

Learn to break sounds into appropriate syllables and words. Breaking the sound into syllables, writing the syllables phonetically, and analyzing by comparing to known word parts (prefixes, suffixes, and root words) can help. In your medical terminology course, pay particular attention to how these word parts are combined and what combining vowels are used, if any, to connect one part to another. There are no exact rules for putting two combining terms together, but often, in anatomy at least, combining forms are put together proximal to distal (*glenohumeral*), anterior to posterior (*anteroposterior*), or cephalad (top) to caudal (bottom) (*esophagogastroduodenoscopy*).

Medical dictionaries and most spellers do not supply the part of speech of a term. Learn to recognize parts of speech by word endings and clues in the definition. For example, a definition that begins with an article (*a, an,* or *the*) will be a noun. If the definition begins with *to,* it will be a verb. If it begins with *pertaining to* or *relating to,* it will be an adjective.

Identify the preferred spelling when more than one spelling is given. When a term has an alternative spelling, it is customary to use the spelling accompanied by the definition. If both spellings are accompanied by definitions, either may be used. Some dictionaries, especially English dictionaries, may put two spellings separated by a comma as the main entry. In that case, the first spelling is preferred. So, if you look up a word and the definition says "See [another spelling]," the *see* spelling is the one you'd use. If there is a complete definition with both spellings, then usually either spelling is acceptable.

Learn to recognize what type of word you're looking for so that you will know which reference book to use first. Context will help you determine whether the word is a drug, a surgical instrument, a laboratory test, or x-ray procedure, etc. While all specialties can be touched upon in a single history and physical examination, contextual clues (including format headings) should help you determine which specialty word book to choose for symptoms and diseases.

Learn to distinguish among trade (brand), generic, and chemical names of drugs, and also to distinguish between drug names and drug classes. This will save time if your main drug reference is the *Physicians' Desk Reference (PDR)*. Memorize the spellings of the 200 most-prescribed drugs and their indications. A list can be found in the appendices of the *Saunders Pharmaceutical Word Book* and on the Internet. This will save you hours of research time.

Find lists of the most commonly misspelled English and medical words and memorize the spellings and definitions. Study lists of English and medical homophones (soundalikes) and know which to use when.

Distinguish between Latin and English anatomical terms. English adjectives precede the noun, but in Latin the noun comes first. This is important because when you look up a phrase, you want to look up the noun. For example, to find *bullous emphysema*, look under *emphysema* (the noun), not *bullous*. To find *Parkinson disease*, look under *disease*. The adjectives will be subentries below the noun.

In Latin phrases, the noun is followed by the adjective: *tensor fasciae latae, ligamentum flavum*. Look under the first

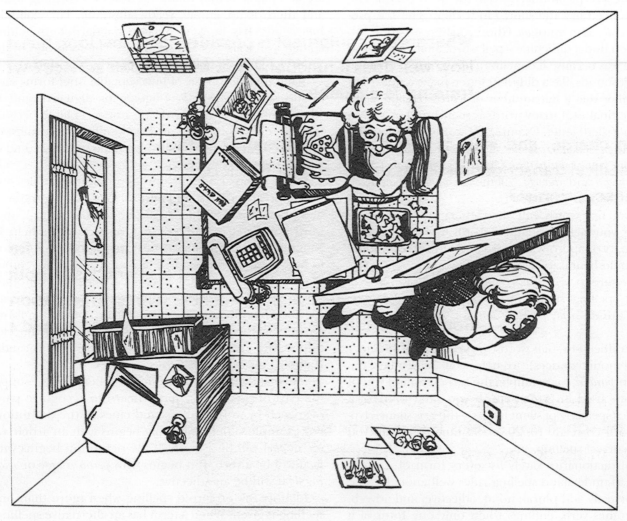

"I don't care what it pays; are there windows?"
Source: Judith Marshall, *Medicate Me*, illustrated by Cindy Stevens

word. Another exception is bacterial names: the genus is given first, followed by the species: *Clostridium difficile, Neisseria gonorrhoeae.*

If you are looking for the name of a muscle, look under both *musculus* and *muscle.* Other Latin/English entries include *ligamentum* and *ligament, fissura* and *fissure, arteria* and *artery.*

Learn the synonyms for main entries. For example, a doctor might dictate a disease, but you cannot find the term under *disease* in the dictionary; try *syndrome.* *Test* and *sign* are often interchangeable as are *sign* and *reflex.* *Procedure* and *operation* may be interchanged. *Tendons* and *ligaments* may be named for the bones or muscles to which they are attached.

Learn Latin/English equivalents too: bone and os, muscle and musculus, nerve and nervus. Sometimes English and Latin are mixed as in the *rectus adominis muscle.* *Abdominis* doesn't sound like an English word, so you can assume it's Latin and look under *musculus* to find the correct spelling.

Learn the uses and limitations of the Internet. If you cannot find a term or phrase after consulting the appropriate reference books, a Google (or other search engine) search may be the next best choice. Know that there is no such thing as *style* on the Internet. Words are capitalized, hyphenated, closed, or open without regard to correctness. Misspellings are rampant. The Internet is lawless. It can be a remarkable research tool and resource, but it's not infallible. Books aren't either, but at least they've been edited and proofread in an attempt to make them as accurate as possible. It's a good idea, once you find a term you've been searching for on the Internet, to see if you can now find it in an appropriate reference.

Work Environments

Medical transcriptionists (MTs) work for hospitals, multispecialty clinics, physician practices, transcription companies, home offices, radiology clinics, pathology laboratories, tumor boards, law offices, and even veterinary hospitals. Some work as employees; others prefer the independence of being "freelance" MTs or independent contractors (ICs). Qualified MTs may eventually become supervisors, managers, quality assurance specialists, proofreaders, speech recognition editors, and teachers, while others may establish their own transcription companies. In the not-too-distant future, some transcriptionists may become healthcare data integration analysts—ensuring the accuracy, completeness, and continuity of the patient's healthcare record.

Hospitals and medical centers. In the recent past, medical transcriptionists employed by hospitals worked under the direct supervision of a health infor-

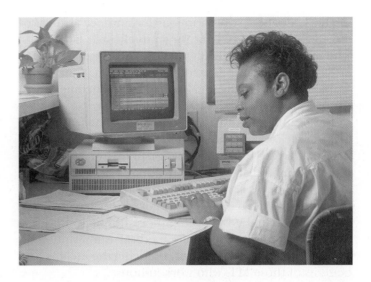

mation managers. Today, it is common for a hospital's transcription staff to be centralized in its own department, in some instances physically remote from the health information management department. Many hospitals have sent their transcriptionists home to work remotely or outsourced their transcription to a medical transcription service.

Most modern hospital transcription departments are headed by transcription supervisors who may or may not be medical transcriptionists. This supervisor may work under the auspices of the health information administrator or may report directly to a hospital administrator. However, MTs who perform specialty transcription, such as radiology or pathology, may work within or adjacent to those departments.

In large teaching hospitals, some medical transcriptionists function as secretaries/transcriptionists in the offices of physicians who act as department heads for the various medical specialties within the institution.

Hospitals may offer competitive salary and benefit packages, particularly larger hospitals in metropolitan areas. In addition, many offer some type of incentive pay plan that has the potential to increase income for productive MTs.

Hospitals offer opportunities for advancement into supervisory positions for motivated employees. Hospital transcription provides a wide range of dictation types, covering all medical specialties and challenging areas of interest to transcriptionists. Facilities and equipment are often state of the art.

Traditionally, hospital employment has offered job security and stable work schedules. In addition, some hospitals include in their benefit packages the payment of professional membership dues and/or registration fees for continuing education events such as conventions and seminars.

Even when working remotely, many hospital transcriptionists have access to the hospital's server, allowing them to check a patient's prescriptions for an unclear drug or dosage or laboratory data for unintelligible lab results. Similar reports by a difficult physician may be consulted in order to fill in blanks caused by unclear dictation. Demographic data is usually imported into the document with the press of a single key or key combination.

Disadvantages of working in the hospital setting may include lack of autonomy, inflexible scheduling, lower wages, a lackluster environment, supervisory personnel who are unfamiliar with or unsympathetic to the needs of transcriptionists, and the frustration of dealing with hospital bureaucracies. With the advent of managed care and its associated cost-cutting, more hospitals are looking toward outsourcing their medical transcription to transcription services or simply reducing the income and benefits of those MTs who work in-house.

A medical transcription student, almost without exception, is not prepared to move directly from coursework to the hospital setting as a transcriptionist. It is virtually impossible to prepare most students to transcribe with the accuracy and efficiency required by the inpatient transcription departments. Students may want to find positions transcribing for a solo physician, for a group practice, or for a transcription service. Once you have achieved enough experience to be productive and efficient, then the hospital setting is a realistic goal.

Physician offices and clinics. The small office environment can be decidedly more personal, often providing a family-like atmosphere. Employees in such environments may enjoy medical and retirement benefits and a predictable income, although with the decline in physician income due to managed care, some offices no longer offer benefits to their employees.

Physician office or clinic hours may more readily accommodate the needs of MTs with school-age children, seldom requiring weekend work. In addition, transcriptionists may enjoy the direct contact with physicians, who may be more appreciative of their work, more accessible for questions, and more willing to take the time to teach and offer feedback—a real advantage to the new MT.

While the transcriptionist in a physician's office or clinic may become more proficient with practice, there are less likely to be opportunities for advancement in this environment, and the dictation will offer less of a challenge to the MT hoping to increase knowledge and skills.

Transcription services. Employees of transcription companies often enjoy competitive rates of pay. Because they transcribe a variety of dictation from different accounts (physician offices, clinics, hospitals), their skills are continually challenged. Transcriptionists working in a service's office usually enjoy a comfortable

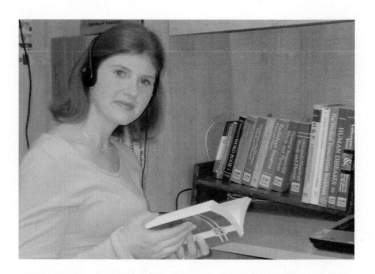

environment, and there may be greater flexibility of work schedules.

Disadvantages of working for a transcription service can include absence of immediate feedback concerning questions about dictation. The same resources an off-site employee of a hospital has access to are usually unavailable to the employee of a service working on the same account. Client specifications and physician lists are often out-of-date or incomplete. Each client often has its own formats and specifications, and being switched from one client to another may adversely affect production.

Compensation may be based entirely on production, so that a day of poor-quality dictation, lack of dictation available for transcription, or personal illness can wreak havoc with the transcriptionist's income. Benefit packages may not be as comprehensive as those offered by a hospital, and health insurance is often unavailable. However, a number of transcription services are responding to the shortage of qualified transcriptionists by offering attractive benefit packages.

At-home employees. Many hospitals and transcription services employ home-based workers who transcribe exclusively for those employers, using the employer's equipment and working under the employer's direction. Such employment may offer medical and retirement benefits as well as a predictable income.

Disadvantages of at-home employment, however, may be the same as those experienced by freelance medical transcriptionists working from home.

Freelance transcriptionists. These transcriptionists function as independent contractors, most often working from home, although some prefer to maintain offices outside their homes. Because they are solo workers, few of them can individually handle the volume of a hospital account, but some transcribe hospital overflow (the excess of dictation that cannot be handled by a hospital's in-house transcriptionists).

Advantages of freelancing include a sense of accomplishment and independence, high self-esteem, pride in entrepreneurship, and the opportunity to work flexible hours. For those who choose to work at home, the advantages also include decreased costs for transportation and office wardrobe.

For the freelance MT, disadvantages can also include the burden of having to handle all areas of a business, including bookkeeping, arranging for pickup of dictation and delivery of finished work to each client's office, and the need for finding other MTs to cover during times of overload, vacation, or sickness. Also a disadvantage is the unpredictable level of income, difficulty with financial planning, lack of affordable medical benefits, and the necessity for complying with the IRS and other regulatory agencies. Unless children are old enough to fend for themselves, childcare is still a necessity.

The transcriptionist working from home must be prepared to practice self-discipline and deal with distractions created by family members, neighbors, solicitors, and the telephone. Some at-home MTs complain that they are never able to "get away" from their work, household chores, or family concerns that demand their attention. Finally, there is often a sense of isolation, and the inability to ask questions or network with other transcriptionists and physicians can prove frustrating.

Other employment settings. Medical transcriptionists are often employed by insurance companies or government facilities. Others combine their transcription skills with clinical skills to function as medical assistants. Still others work in medical research facilities or tumor registries. In law offices that specialize in personal injury or medical malpractice cases, medical transcriptionists may be employed to analyze discrepancies in health records and translate medical language in a chart into lay language for attorneys.

Within all of these settings, MTs may also perform transcription, or they may act as supervisors, managers, or quality assurance experts. In addition, many are called upon to teach medical transcription within hospitals, in community colleges, at vocational/technical schools, or in court-reporting schools. A few MTs have found alternative job pathways in dictating reports for physicians, as well as serving as researchers, editors, consultants, and authors in the areas of the publishing industry that service medical transcription.

Externship, apprenticeship, and trainee positions. Many companies offer externship, apprenticeship, or trainee positions for graduates of good medical transcription programs. Such programs provide the opportunity to become familiar with client specifications, technology, and office procedures without the pressure of production quotas.

Medical Readings

History and Physical Examination

Physical Diagnosis

by John H. Dirckx, M.D.

The term *diagnosis* (from Greek *diagignosko*, to judge, discriminate) has several closely related meanings in medicine, which few of us take the trouble to distinguish in practice.

Diagnosis means, first, the intellectual process of analyzing, identifying, or explaining a disease. In this sense, diagnosis forms the subject matter of the branch of medicine called Physical Diagnosis.

Secondly, in a more concrete sense, diagnosis means the explanation proposed for a given patient's problems. Thus we speak of "arriving at a diagnosis" or of "making a tentative diagnosis of pancreatitis."

Thirdly, diagnosis is often used synonymously with disease or the name of a particular disease: "Her diagnosis is multiple sclerosis." "Patients with this diagnosis often progress to renal failure."

The techniques used by the physician to gather data for a diagnosis are embodied in the two procedures known as history and physical examination. The history is an account of the subjective experiences—the *symptoms*—that constitute this episode of illness, as perceived by the patient and elicited by the diagnostician's careful, methodical questioning. Physical examination is the process whereby the physician seeks and observes objective changes and abnormalities—the *signs* of illness. It is not generally appreciated by lay persons that

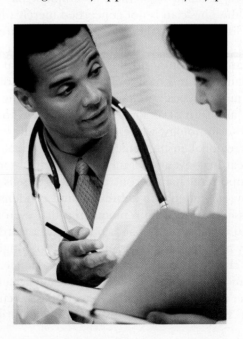

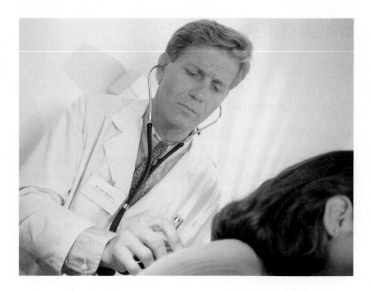

a skillfully obtained history usually supplies both a larger number of diagnostic clues and more useful and specific ones than the physical examination.

Much may depend on formally established, quasi-legal requirements—forms to be filled out for a prospective employer or insurer, or hospital staff bylaws to be complied with.

Usually there is some overlapping of content between the history and the physical examination. The physician does not wait until the history is completed to start observing the patient, nor do the questions stop once the examination starts.

The report of a thorough history and physical contains more negative than positive statements: "He has had a mild chronic cough for many years but denies hemoptysis, purulent sputum, chest pain, dyspnea on exertion, orthopnea, asthma, bronchitis, or emphysema." This is because the physician is not concerned merely with compiling a list of abnormalities. A complete picture of the patient's condition must also indicate which common or relevant symptoms and signs are not present.

The language in which a physician writes or dictates a history and physical contains many recurring terms, phrases, and formulas. Some of these pertain to formal medical terminology, while others are highly informal, perhaps regional, institutional, or even individual, and do not appear in conventional medical reference works.

An important characteristic of this language is its rigid economy, its tendency to abbreviate and condense wherever possible. It must be remembered that even a physician who dictates many pages of medical records a day probably produces at least as many pages of longhand in hospital charts and office or clinic records. Hence, written abbreviations crop up constantly in dictated material, as when the physician dictates, "a mass in the subcu" for "a mass in the subcutaneous tissue," or "nocturia times

three" (which would appear as "nocturia x3" in a longhand note), meaning that the patient gets up three times a night to urinate.

Compression of ideas and omission of connectives and even of whole phrases yield a terse and seemingly incoherent style of prose. "The heart is regular at 82 without murmurs, clicks, or rubs." "The face is symmetrical and the tongue protrudes in the midline." The physician who passes abruptly from a description of a painful, red, light-sensitive eye to the remark that the patient gives no history of pain or swelling in joints has not slipped a mental cog. The dictator has merely omitted a connecting phrase rendered unnecessary by the fact that any other physician reading these remarks will know that arthritis occurs in several syndromes along with iritis (the tentative diagnosis in this patient).

Adding to the difficulty of the workaday language of physicians is its heavy use of long, arcane, abstract words. This is not the place to explore the reasons why physicians feel compelled to say "experienced epistaxis" instead of "had a nosebleed," but the fact must be recognized that, in clinical records, technical words and phrases often replace simpler and plainer forms of expression.

As in nonmedical settings, the grammar of dictated material tends to be exceedingly loose, with many incomplete sentences and syntactic breaks. The extent to which a transcriptionist amends and refurbishes what is dictated will depend on local conventions and institutional guidelines.

History. As a rule, the physician compiles the medical history by questioning the patient. At times, however, much or all of the information must be obtained from someone else; considerable historical material may be drawn from written records. With experience, a physician learns to word questions so that they can be understood by a person of average intelligence, do not give offense or provoke hostility, elicit a maximum amount of relevant information with a minimum expenditure of time and effort, and do not suggest or invite specific answers. (A question like "You haven't had any sexual problems, have you?" virtually demands a negative reply.) Often the patient's response to one question determines what will be asked next, or how it will be asked. Little by little, a tolerably complete understanding of the medical picture, as perceived by the patient, emerges.

It must be emphasized that, although a standard format is almost always followed in recording the patient's history, the information may have been obtained in much different order, perhaps even on more than one occasion or from a variety of sources. The answer to a dozen questions may be compressed into a single telling phrase.

The physician often translates the patient's statements into medical jargon. Thus, "I threw up at least five times" becomes, "He experienced emesis times five." On the other hand, the physician may make a point of quoting the patient's words exactly ("It feels like my intestines are all tangled around my heart.") or may fall into a colloquial style of dictation, unconsciously echoing the language actually used in interviewing the patient ("Since then he has had no more bellyache and is eating fine.").

In building up a complete picture of any given symptom, the physician asks a number of fairly standard questions. For example, with respect to pain—probably the commonest and most general presenting symptom—the physician inquires as to its quality, intensity, onset, duration, intermittency, location, and radiation, as well as any aggravating or alleviating factors, prior episodes of similar pain, and associated symptoms.

From the start, the physician has a mental agenda or outline of information to be obtained, but the sequence and wording of the questions depends partly on the way the patient answers. Had the patient been a professor of law or a teenaged girl, the phrasing and even the purport of some of the questions would have been different, even though the same basic range of information was being sought.

Physical examination. As with the history, the scope and character of the physical examination performed on a given patient in a given instance depend on circumstances. A Boy Scout camp physical may be rushed through in less than one minute; thorough assessment of the nervous system alone in a patient suspected of having early multiple sclerosis can take more than an hour.

The term *physical examination,* by convention, includes only those procedures performed directly by the physician relying on the five senses, with the aid of a few simple handheld instruments. Although x-ray and laboratory studies, electrocardiography and electromyography, various kinds of scans, or other elaborate techniques may be absolutely essential to a precise and accurate diagnosis, they are not considered part of the physical examination.

The scope and nature of the history and physical depend on several variables. The patient's complaints give direction and focus to both history-taking and examination. The physician's field of specialization often determines the type and extent of diagnostic maneuvers employed. The setting of the examination—doctor's office or clinic, hospital emergency department, intensive care unit, or the patient's home—will have a bearing on what is done and not done. The patient's condition—whether alert, confused, belligerent, or unconscious—will influence the type of history that can be obtained and the degree of cooperation that can be enlisted during examination.

Virtually all diagnostic maneuvers employed in the physical examination are variations on the four basic classical techniques: *inspection* (looking), *palpation* (feeling), *auscultation* (listening), and *percussion* (tapping).

Laboratory Tests

In the past decade there has been a dramatic increase in both the number of new diagnostic laboratory tests as well as in the complexity of the tests offered. This explosive growth in the field of laboratory medicine has been due to the demand by physicians for new and improved diagnostic procedures, combined with the ever-expanding capacity of modern technology to meet the demand with increasingly sophisticated laboratory methods and equipment.

On a daily basis medical transcriptionists come in contact with dictation which details the results of laboratory tests performed on patients. In order to accurately transcribe this material, it is important to be familiar with the names and abbreviations of many laboratory tests, the reasons they are offered, and the meaning of the results.

Laboratory tests can be performed in many different settings: clinics, physicians' offices, health fairs, and sometimes even at home by patients themselves, though the greatest number of laboratory tests are performed within the hospital setting. Hospital laboratories are equipped with the most technologically advanced and automated equipment to handle hundreds of tests each day. The largest hospitals perform all standard laboratory tests as well as many uncommon ones which may be requested by smaller hospitals or clinics whose facilities are not equipped to handle unusual tests.

The laboratory of a hospital is divided into many smaller departments which perform specialized laboratory tests. This division of labor is also reflected to a great extent on the average laboratory slip which is used to report the results of laboratory tests. Various sections on the lab slip include hematology, blood bank, chemistry, coagulation, urinalysis, stool examination, microbiology, and cytology.

Hematology is concerned with the study of the formed components or cells of the blood. These cells include mature red blood cells, white blood cells, and platelets, as well as their immature forms. The function of the red blood cell is to carry oxygen from the lungs to the body tissues. The function of the white blood cell is to fight any foreign substances that enter the body, such as bacteria. Platelets function along with the coagulation factors in the blood to form a blood clot at the site of tissue injury. White blood cells are further differentiated into groups which have diagnostic value. These include lymphocytes, monocytes, neutrophils, eosinophils, basophils, and bands or immature neutrophils.

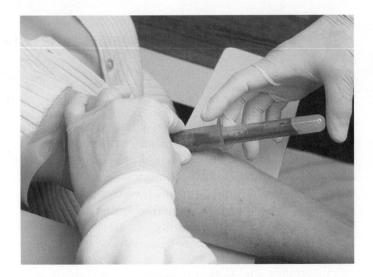

There are many brief forms, slang, and special terms associated with the blood. Brief forms are acceptable in medical reports, but transcriptionists should always spell out in full any slang words that are dictated. For example, *monos* is an acceptable brief form for *monocytes*, but *lytes* is a slang term that must be translated *electrolytes* in medical reports. (See *Brief Forms and Medical Slang* section in Chapter 3.)

A complete blood count (CBC) includes tests that measure red blood cell and white blood cell levels. A CBC with differential also measures the levels of all of the different types of white blood cells. Other common tests are the hemoglobin and hematocrit (which is often dictated as *H&H* but must be written out in full), which are indicative of the oxygen-carrying capacity of the blood as well as the percentage of red blood cells per blood sample. Normally the hematocrit is about three times greater than the hemoglobin level for the same patient, so that if the patient's hemoglobin level was reported as 15, you could expect that the hematocrit would be approximately 45.

The chemistry section of the laboratory performs tests on many different electrolytes, fats, and other substances found in the serum, or clear fluid which separates from a clotted blood sample. Blood chemistries include tests for electrolytes: sodium, potassium, calcium, and chloride. Lipids (fatty substances) include cholesterol and triglycerides. Other substances tested include bilirubin, ALT (formerly SGPT), AST (formerly SGOT), and LDH which are used to evaluate liver function. BUN and creatinine are useful indicators of kidney function. Uric acid levels are tested to diagnose the medical condition of gout. An elevated serum acid phosphatase is useful in detecting prostatic cancer.

Often the physician orders a combination of tests under one name. For example, by checking a box next to the entry "serum lipid profile" on the laboratory slip, the physician can order the tests for cholesterol, triglycerides, total lipids, and lipoproteins.

The microbiology department of the laboratory identifies infectious organisms through the use of microscopes and culture and sensitivity testing. Specimens for testing are obtained from urine, stool, blood, sputum, wound drainage, or other body fluids. A sample of the specimen is smeared onto a culture medium and incubated at 37°C for sufficient time to allow bacterial growth to occur. Antibiotic disks placed on the media of the culture plates permit evaluation of the sensitivity of the bacteria cultured to specific antibiotics. Antibiotic disks to which the bacteria are sensitive are surrounded by a ring or zone of inhibition of bacterial growth. Bacteria that are resistant to an antibiotic show no inhibition of growth around the disk.

A rapid method to tentatively identify a pathogenic bacterium is to smear a sample on a slide and then stain the slide with the Gram stain. This stain differentiates between organisms that are gram-positive and those that are gram-negative. The shape of the bacterium can provide further clues to the identity of the organism. The acid-fast stain is used to identify mycobacteria specifically.

Physicians order laboratory tests to be performed on patients for a variety of reasons:

1. To diagnose disease in a patient who is ill.

2. To screen for hidden diseases. Well-known examples include use of the Pap smear to identify cervical cancer, and the self-administered test for occult or hidden blood in the stool as an indicator of colon cancer.

3. To assess the extent of damage from disease processes.

4. To monitor the effectiveness of treatment prescribed by the physician.

5. To monitor blood levels of certain medications. Periodic blood samples can ensure that drug levels in the blood remain within the therapeutic range.

6. To monitor the course of a disease.

7. To confirm freedom from disease, or to detect recurrence, after a cure has apparently been achieved.

Laboratory test results are measured and reported most often in **SI** (Système International) **units**, including submultiples of the meter (centimeters, millimeters, cubic centimeters), the liter (milliliters), the gram (milligrams, micrograms), and the equivalent (milliequivalents).

If the reported value falls within the range observed in normal individuals, it is considered normal. If it falls outside of this range, it is considered abnormal. The age and sex of a patient cause variation in the normal range of laboratory values.

The accepted normal range for a particular laboratory test also varies from one laboratory to another, due to differences in equipment and methodology used in testing. Therefore, lab slips usually give the accepted normal range for that particular facility. The normal value is printed next to the blank space for the reported value for the individual patient. When transcribing, it is not unusual for the medical transcriptionist to hear the physician say, "Normal for our laboratory is . . . ," after dictating a patient's test result.

The transcription of laboratory test terminology presents certain challenges for the medical transcriptionist. Correctly transcribing the name of a laboratory test or its abbreviation is just the first step. Numerical results must be transcribed with absolute accuracy. Care must be taken to place decimal points accurately and to transcribe units of measure correctly.

It is also necessary to understand why a test was ordered and what the results indicate. Some dictations contain considerable detail concerning the test process, the use of special stains or dyes, as well as the significance of the results.

As a student, you will want to study this critical area of medical transcription diligently. As a practicing medical transcriptionist, you will always be increasing your knowledge of laboratory tests and procedures, as the technology of medicine increases daily.

Pharmacology

"Pharmacology is a fascinating and multifaceted discipline that impacts not only our professional careers but our personal lives as well. From our role as members of the healthcare team to that of consumers, pharmacology plays a part in our lives." So begins the preface to *Understanding Pharmacology for Health Professionals*, by Susan M. Turley, and it well describes the subject of pharmacology.

Simply stated, pharmacology is the study of drugs and their interactions with living organisms. The term *pharmacology* comes from a Greek word meaning *medicine*. The term *drug* is derived from a Dutch word which means *dry* and refers to the use of dried herbs and plants as the first medicines. The Latin word for *drug* is *medicina*, from which we derive our term *medicine*. Pharmacology is concerned with the nature of drugs and medications, their actions in the body, drug dosages, side effects of drugs, and so on. Drugs are used to prevent, treat, and cure diseases, and in some instances to diagnose diseases.

Drug forms. Different forms of a drug are appropriate for different routes of administration. Some common manufactured drug forms are tablets, capsules, transdermal patches, suppositories, creams, ointments, lotions, powders, oral suspensions, sprays, and

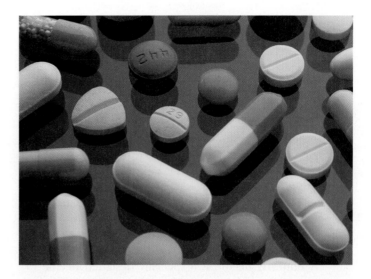

foams. Some drugs are ineffective when administered in a certain form or by a certain route; other drugs may seriously injure the patient if administered in certain forms or by a certain route.

1. **Tablet**. This drug form contains dried, powdered, active drug as well as binders and fillers to provide bulk and ensure proper tablet size. A **scored** tablet has an indented line running across the middle. It can be easily broken into two pieces with a knife to produce two doses. **Enteric** tablets are covered with a special coating that resists stomach acid but dissolves in the alkaline environment of the small intestine to avoid irritating the stomach (e.g., Ecotrin). **Slow-release** tablets are manufactured to provide a continuous, sustained release of certain drugs. Often this is abbreviated as **XR (extended release)**, **SR (slow release)** or **LA (long acting)** and included in the trade name of the drug (e.g., Dilacor XR, Dilatrate-SR, Cardizem LA, all used in the prophylaxis of angina pectoris). **Caplets** are coated tablets in the form of capsules. Tablets can also be designed to be dissolved in water before being taken orally (e.g., Alka-Seltzer effervescent tablets). Some over-the-counter drugs come in the form of **lozenges**. These tablets are formed of a hardened base of sugar and water containing the drug and other flavorings. They are never swallowed, but are allowed to dissolve slowly in the mouth to release the drug topically to the tissues of the mouth and throat (e.g. Cepacol lozenges for sore throat). In prescriptions, *tablet* is sometimes abbreviated as *tab* or *tabs*.

2. **Capsule**. This drug form comes in two varieties. The first is a soft gelatin shell manufactured in one piece in which the drug is in a liquid form inside the shell (e.g., docusate [Colace, Surfak], a stool softener; fat-soluble vitamins such as A and E). The second type of capsule is a hard shell manufactured in two pieces which fit together and hold the drug, which is in a powdered or granular

Needle *Classification*

Needles are classified according to gauge and length. The gauge is the inside diameter of the needle. The lower the gauge number, the larger the inside diameter will be. For example, a 15-gauge needle is used for blood donation to allow the blood to flow freely through the needle and to decrease turbulence and damage to the red blood cells. An 18- to 22-gauge needle is used for intramuscular injections in adults. A 27-gauge needle is used for an intravenous line in a premature infant. The inside diameter of a needle is also known as the **bore**. The term *bore* is synonymous with *gauge*, but the bore is designated only as either small or large.

A **butterfly needle** is a specially designed needle of short length and high gauge with color-coded tabs of plastic on each side of the needle. These tabs facilitate control of the needle during insertion. This needle gets its name because the tabs on either side of the needle make it appear like the wings of a butterfly. Butterfly needles are most often used to start intravenous lines on premature infants or on elderly patients with poor veins.

Susan M. Turley
Understanding Pharmacology for Health Professionals

form. Many nonprescription cold remedies and pain medications were manufactured in this form until some Tylenol capsules were reported to be contaminated with cyanide in the early 1980s. Now, most pharmaceutical companies manufacture their nonprescription pain medications in a tablet or caplet form. Many prescription drugs, however, are still manufactured as hard-shell capsules. In written prescriptions, *capsule* is sometimes abbreviated as *cap* or *caps*.

3. **Cream**. A cream is a semisolid emulsion of oil (such as lanolin or petroleum) and water, the main ingredient being water. Emulsifying agents are added to keep the oil and water well mixed. Many topical drugs are manufactured in a cream base (e.g., hydrocortisone cream for skin inflammation).

4. **Ointment**. An ointment is a semisolid emulsion of drug, oil (such as lanolin or petroleum, and water, the main ingredient being oil. Many topical drugs are manufactured in an ointment base (e.g., Kenalog ointment for skin inflammation). Specially formulated ophthalmic ointments are made to be applied topically to the eye without causing irritation.

5. **Lotion**. A lotion is a semisolid suspension of drug dissolved in a thickened water base (e.g., calamine lotion for itching).

6. **Gel**. A gel is a semisolid suspension in which the drug particles are suspended in a thickened water base (e.g., MetroGel for acne rosacea).

7. **Powder**. A powder is a finely ground form of an active drug. Powdered drugs can be in capsules but also can be manufactured in glass vials where they must be reconstituted with sterile water before being injected (e.g., intravenous ampicillin, an antibiotic). Powders can also come in packets; the packet is opened and the powder is reconstituted for oral use (e.g., Metamucil, a laxative). Powders can also be sprinkled on topically or sprayed on (e.g., Tinactin, an antifungal drug for the skin). Powders can also be inhaled into the lungs with the help of a special inhalation device (e.g., Serevent Diskus, a bronchodilator).

8. **Liquid.** Liquids come in the form of either solutions or suspensions. **Solutions** contain the drug dissolved in a water base. Solutions never need to be mixed as the drug-to-water concentration is always the same in every part of the solution, even after prolonged standing. Solutions come in many forms: elixirs, syrups, tinctures, liquid sprays, and foams.

Elixirs are solutions that contain an alcohol and water base with added sugar and flavoring (e.g., Tylenol elixir for fever and pain). Elixirs are commonly used for pediatric or elderly patients who cannot swallow the tablet or capsule form of a drug.

Syrups are solutions that contain no alcohol and are a concentrated solution of sugar, water, and flavorings. Syrups are sweeter and more viscous (thicker) than elixirs. Most over-the-counter cough medications have a syrup base which not only carries the drug but acts to soothe inflamed mucous membranes in the throat (e.g., guaifenesin [Robitussin] for coughs).

Liquid sprays contain a solution of drug combined with water or alcohol; they are sprayed by a pump or aerosol propellant. Spray liquid drugs are commonly used for topical application (e.g., Afrin nasal spray, a decongestant).

Foams contain a solution of drug that is expanded by tiny aerosol bubbles (e.g., Cortifoam, a hydrocortisone product used in the treatment of proctitis).

Suspensions contain fine, undissolved particles of drug suspended in a water base. With prolonged standing, these fine particles gradually settle to the bottom of the container. It is always important to shake suspensions well before using them, a fact that is noted on the label of these drugs (e.g., Maalox antacid). An **emulsion** is a suspension in which the drug is mixed with fat particles and water (e.g., Intralipid intravenous fat solution).

Two general terms used to describe a liquid are *aqueous* (from the Latin word *aqua*, water), meaning of watery consistency, and *viscous*, which designates a nonwatery or thick liquid.

9. **Suppository**. A suppository is composed of a solid base of glycerin or cocoa butter that contains the drug. It is manufactured in appropriate sizes for rectal or vaginal insertion and in adult and pediatric sizes. Vaginal suppositories are most often used to treat vaginal infections. Rectal suppositories can deliver topical medicine to the rectal mucosa or can be used to administer drugs to patients who are vomiting and cannot take oral medication.

10. **Transdermal**. The transdermal form of a drug is a multilayered disk consisting of a drug reservoir, a porous membrane, and an adhesive layer to hold it to the skin. The porous membrane regulates the amount of drug released into the skin. These drugs are often known as *transdermal patches*.

11. **Pellet/Bead**. A drug can be implanted in the body in the form of a pellet or bead that slowly releases the drug to the surrounding tissues (e.g., gentamicin beads [Septopal] on a surgical wire are inserted into the bone to treat chronic osteomyelitis).

Routes of drug administration. There are various routes of drug administration. These include oral, sublingual, nasogastric, gastrostomy or jejunostomy, rectal, vaginal, topical, transdermal, inhalation, parenteral, subcutaneous, intramuscular, intravenous, endotracheal, intra-arterial, intra-articular, intracardiac, intradermal, intrathecal, umbilical artery or vein.

1. **Oral**. The oral route is the most convenient route of administration and the most commonly used. Tablets, capsules, and liquids are all given orally. Even patients who have difficulty swallowing a tablet or capsule can usually take the liquid form of a drug without problems. Infants are given drugs in a liquid form mixed with a small amount of formula and administered through a nipple. Even unconscious patients can be given liquid medication through a nasogastric (NG) tube. The oral route is routinely abbreviated as *PO* or *p.o.* (Latin for *per os*, meaning *through the mouth*).

Disadvantages of the oral route include the following: Some drugs (e.g., interferons, hormones such as insulin, and antibiotics such as gentamicin) are inactivated by stomach acid and cannot be given orally. After oral administration, some drugs (e.g., lidocaine [Xylocaine] for cardiac arrhythmias) are metabolized so quickly by the liver that a therapeutic blood level cannot be achieved. Some drugs (e.g., tetracycline) cannot be taken with certain foods and drinks because they combine chemically to form an insoluble complex. Other drugs (e.g., MAO inhibitors for depression) cannot be taken with certain foods or drinks because they produce adverse side effects.

What Is *Half-life?*

Half-life is the time required for drug levels in the serum to decrease from 100% to 50%. The half-life of a drug can be significantly prolonged when liver or kidney disease decreases metabolism and excretion of a drug. The shorter a drug's half-life, the more frequently it must be administered to sustain therapeutic levels.

Drugs with a short half-life may be manufactured in a slow-release form to provide sustained drug levels with less frequent doses. Digoxin (Lanoxin) has a half-life of approximately 30 hours. Elderly patients with decreased liver and kidney function often develop toxicity from this drug.

Susan M. Turley
Understanding Pharmacology for Health Professionals

2. **Sublingual**. Sublingual administration involves placing the drug (usually in a tablet form) under the tongue and allowing it to slowly dissolve. The tablet is not swallowed (because this would become oral administration). The drug is absorbed quickly through oral mucous membranes and into the large blood vessels under the tongue. The sublingual route provides a faster therapeutic effect than the oral route (e.g., nitroglycerin tablets for treating angina).

3. **Nasogastric** (abbreviated *NG*). This route is used to administer drugs to patients who cannot take oral medications. Nasogastric administration is accomplished with a nasogastric tube that passes from the nose through the esophagus and into the stomach. Only liquid drugs can be given by this route.

4. **Gastrostomy or jejunostomy**. These routes are used to administer drugs to patients who cannot take oral medications. These routes use a surgically implanted feeding tube to deliver liquid drugs directly into the stomach (gastrostomy) or jejunum (jejunostomy).

5. **Rectal**. This route is reserved for certain clinical situations, such as when the patient is vomiting and/or the medication cannot be given by injection (e.g., Tylenol suppositories). Absorption of a drug via the rectal route of administration is slow and often unpredictable, so this route is not used often. However, the rectal route is the preferred route when drugs are administered locally to relieve constipation (e.g., Fleet enema) or treat hemorrhoids (e.g., Anusol) or ulcerative colitis (Proctofoam-HC).

6. **Vaginal**. The vaginal route is used to treat vaginal infections and vaginitis by means of creams and suppositories (e.g., Monistat 7 suppositories, Premarin vaginal cream). Contraceptive foams are inserted vaginally as well.

7. **Topical**. When a drug is applied directly to the skin or to the mucous membranes of the eyes, ears, nose, or mouth, it is administered via the topical route. The effects of the drug are generally local (e.g., bacitracin antibiotic ointment for skin abrasions, Sudafed nasal decongestant spray, Timoptic eye drops for glaucoma).

Some sites of topical administration are abbreviated as follows:

AD	*auris dextra*	right ear
AS	*auris sinistra*	left ear
AU	*auris uterque*	each ear
OD	*oculus dexter*	right eye
OS	*oculus sinister*	left eye
OU	*oculus uterque*	each eye

Note. Although physicians continue to dictate the above traditional abbreviations, JCAHO directs that they be expanded in medical reports to avoid confusion with similar abbreviations. Thus, medical transcriptionists need to know their proper translation.

8. **Transdermal**. This route of administration differs from the topical route in that the drug is applied to the skin via physical delivery through a porous membrane, and the therapeutic effects are felt systemically, not just at the site of administration. Drugs delivered by the transdermal route are usually manufactured in the form of a patch. A transdermal patch is worn on the skin and releases the drug slowly over a 24-hour period, providing sustained therapeutic blood levels (e.g., Transderm-Nitro for prevention of angina pectoris).

9. **Inhalation**. This route of administration involves the inhaling of a drug that is in a gas, liquid, or powder form. The drug is absorbed through the alveoli of the lungs (e.g., nitrous oxide, a general anesthetic; albuterol [Proventil], a bronchodilator).

10. **Parenteral**. Parenteral is a general term, taken from two Greek words, *para* and *enteron*, which literally mean *apart from the intestine.* Technically, *parenteral* administration means all routes of administration other than oral, but in clinical usage, parenteral commonly includes the following routes of administration: subcutaneous, intramuscular, and intravenous, and other less frequently used routes: endotracheal, intra-arterial, intra-articular, intracardiac, intradermal, intrathecal, and injection into the umbilical artery or vein (see Figure 1-2).

Subcutaneous administration involves the injection of liquid into the subcutaneous tissue (the fatty layer of tissue just under the dermis of the skin but above the muscle

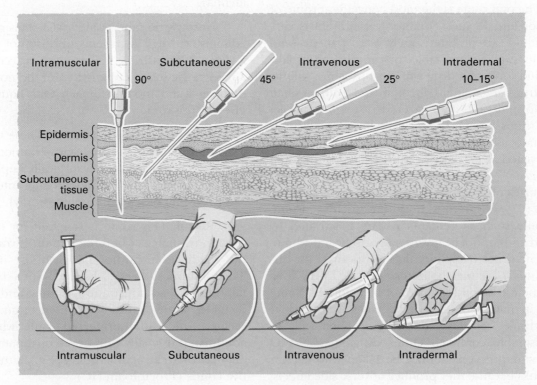

Figure 1-2
Angle of Needle Insertion for Four Types of Injection

layer) (e.g., insulin for diabetes mellitus, allergy shots). There are few blood vessels in this layer, so drugs are absorbed more slowly by this route than when given by intramuscular injection. Diabetics who inject insulin use approximately 10 to 12 different areas on the upper arms, thighs, and abdomen and rotate the site of each subcutaneous insulin injection. The term *subcutaneous* is abbreviated *subcu*.

Intramuscular (abbreviated *IM*) administration involves the injection of a liquid into the belly (area of greatest mass) of a large muscle. The large muscles of the body are well supplied with blood vessels, and drugs are absorbed more quickly by this route than when given by subcutaneous injection. There are five intramuscular injection sites that can be used; injection at other sites invites damage to adjacent nerves and blood vessels.

deltoid, located on the upper arm, lateral aspect.

vastus lateralis, located on the midthigh, lateral aspect.

rectus femoris, located on the midthigh, anterior aspect.

ventrogluteal, located on the side of the hip .

dorsogluteal, located in the upper outer quadrant of each buttock.

Some drugs cannot be given by intramuscular injection because they are not water soluble and would form precipitate particles in the tissue (e.g., Valium and Librium, antianxiety drugs). Examples of drugs given intramuscularly: Demerol for pain, vitamin B_{12} for pernicious anemia, Garamycin for bacterial infections.

Intravenous (abbreviated *IV*) administration of a drug involves the injection of a liquid directly into a vein. The therapeutic effect of drugs given intravenously can often be seen immediately. This is because the drug does not need to be absorbed from tissue or muscle before it can exert an effect. IV administration can be done in one of three ways. The injection of a single dose of a drug (**bolus**) may be given through a **port** (rubber stopper) into an existing intravenous line. This is often referred to as **IV push** because the drug is manually pushed into the IV line in a short period of time. A drug may also be mixed with the fluid in an IV bag or bottle and administered continuously over several hours. This is known as **IV drip**. A drug may also be mixed in a very small IV bag or bottle and administered over an hour or less by IV drip. This small secondary IV bag or bottle is connected through tubing to a port in the existing primary IV line. This method is known as **IV piggyback** administration.

Examples of drugs given intravenously include thiopental (Pentothal) for induction of general anesthesia, diazepam (Valium) to control continuous epileptic seizures, and most chemotherapy drugs.

Orphan *Drugs*

An orphan drug is a drug or biological product for the diagnosis, treatment, or prevention of a rare disease or condition. A rare disease is one that affects less than 200,000 persons or for which there is no reasonable expectation that the cost of development and testing will be recovered through U.S. sales of the product.

Federal subsidies are provided to the manufacturer or sponsor for the development of orphan drugs. Applications for orphan status are made through the FDA, and may be made during drug development or after marketing approval.

Ellen Drake and Randy Drake
Saunders Pharmaceutical Word Book

Other parenteral routes that have specialized uses include the following:

endotracheal This route is used during emergency resuscitation measures (e.g., Adrenalin) and to deliver pulmonary drugs to intubated patients via the endotracheal tube.

intra-arterial This route is used occasionally for direct injection of a chemotherapeutic agent to a tumor area. Generally, arterial lines are used for continuous monitoring of arterial blood pressure and are not used to administer drugs.

intra-articular This route is used only to inject specific drugs, such as corticosteroids, into the joint to decrease severe inflammation and pain caused by a chronic disease such as arthritis. The Greek word *arthron* means *joint*.

intracardiac This route is used only during emergency resuscitative measures (e.g., epinephrine is given directly through the chest wall into the heart to stimulate the heart muscle during cardiac arrest).

intradermal This route involves the injection of a liquid into the dermis, the layer of skin just below the epidermis. The epidermis itself is only about 1 mm (less than 1/20 of an inch) thick; therefore, when an intradermal injection is correctly positioned, the tip of the needle is still plainly visible through the skin (e.g., Mantoux test for tuberculosis).

intrathecal Intrathecal administration involves the injection of a liquid within the sheath or meninges of the spinal cord into the cerebrospinal fluid (e.g., spinal anesthesia). *Theka* is Greek for *sheath*.

umbilical artery or vein This route is accessible only in newborn infants before the umbilical cord has dried. It is used to administer fluids and draw blood. It is generally not used to give drugs. Instead, an IV line is

Drug *References*

A *pharmacopeia* is a collection or compendium of information about all of the drugs in use in a particular country. The *United States Pharmacopeia (USP)* was compiled by 11 physicians in 1820 and was the first comprehensive drug reference in the United States.

The *National Formulary (NF)* was first published in 1888 by the American Pharmaceutical Association. Since 1979, these two references have been combined into one volume, called the *USP/NF.*

The *USP/NF* contains standards for manufacturing drugs (strength, purity, uniformity, labeling, storage, etc.), as well as information about drugs, dietary supplements, and various types of medical products.

Susan M. Turley
Understanding Pharmacology for Health Professionals

inserted peripherally in the hand, foot, or scalp for drug administration.

Some drugs may be approved for use via more than one route and are manufactured in different forms appropriate for those different routes. Each route of administration has distinct advantages and disadvantages. A drug given by one route may be therapeutic, while given by another route it may be ineffective, harmful, or even fatal. Therefore, every drug prescription or drug order always includes the form of the drug as well as the route of administration.

Drugs exert their effects in a number of ways and at a number of sites within the body. Basically, drugs act in two ways: locally or systemically. A local effect is limited to the site of administration and those tissues immediately surrounding it. Drugs applied topically are an example of those that exert a local effect. A systemic drug effect is not limited to the site of application but can be felt throughout the body, particularly evident in certain organs and tissues. Drugs taken intravenously and intramuscularly always exert a systemic effect. Drugs taken orally and subcutaneously usually exert a systemic effect.

All drugs have an intended therapeutic effect and a side effect. The therapeutic effect is the drug's main action for which it was prescribed by the physician. The therapeutic effect will cure a disease, decrease disease symptoms, or prevent a disease. The perfect drug would have a complete therapeutic effect perfectly suited for its use with no side effects. Unfortunately, this perfect drug does not

exist. Side effects vary widely with the type of drug administered. They may be mild or quite severe. Many drugs, for example, exert gastrointestinal side effects which include anorexia, nausea, vomiting, or diarrhea. Common side effects expressed in the central nervous system include drowsiness, excitement, or depression.

Drugs may react with other drugs in the system to cause side effects. Many patients are treated with more than one drug at a time. In particular, elderly patients with chronic medical problems may consume a number of medications several times a day. Some drugs react to each other in a particular way to either accentuate or diminish the action of each.

Drug references. Drug reference books are an important resource for medical transcriptionists. Experienced transcriptionists often purchase their own drug reference books every year or two to keep up-to-date on new drugs.

Drugs are used to treat many medical and surgical conditions. Some people, particularly those who are elderly, take as many as 10 or more medications each day. Therefore, it is critical that medical transcriptionists be familiar with drugs, their indications and dosages, and how to research new or unusual drug names in drug reference books.

Pharmaceutical companies use three different names to describe a drug: the **chemical name** (which is a complicated formula describing the drug's molecular structure), the **generic name** (a shorter name assigned to the drug chemical), and the **trade** or **brand name** (the copyrighted name selected by the pharmaceutical company). The brand name is easy to pronounce, may indicate what the drug is used for or how often it is taken, and is selected for its appeal to prescribing physicians. A generic drug may have several trade names copyrighted by different manufacturers.

Generic drug names are always written in lowercase letters, while trade name drugs have an initial capital letter. Some trade name drugs also have internal capitalization (such as pHisoHex), although in most instances it is acceptable to type such words with initial capitalization only (Phisohex).

Medical transcriptionists use several types of drug references frequently. Some contain short lists of drugs in alphabetical order, while others are much more comprehensive. The experienced medical transcriptionist has at least two types of drug references available: a quick-reference A to Z drug book, and a comprehensive book that gives indications and contraindications to drug therapies.

Spotlight on

How Doctors Dictate

by Judith Marshall

How sweet doctors were in their youth. They sounded like this:

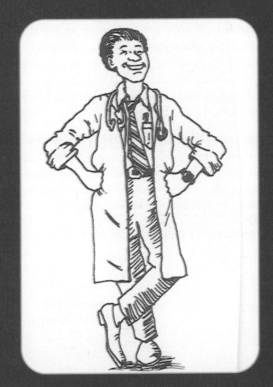

This is Dr. Cackleberry. Good evening. I am about to do my first physical, testing, testing, hope you can hear me. I want to do this right. I will spell all the medical words for you. This is a 36-year-old white female with BP 120/70 make a capital B and a capital P and the number 120 and a diagonal line, that is, uh, slash, I think, over the 70. That is 7-0.

Doctor learned and grew and became a successful physician in private practice, dictating to the same old transcriptionist—me.

This is the big C here with a letter to, what date is this, the 7th of October, no, the 8th, 6th, whatever, you check that. Letter to looks like S. Voinovich, somewhere in Newton, look it up, re that Blount woman, I forget her name. Dear so and so, thank you for referring this pleasant 74-year-old female to me who was complaining of cardiac symptoms with no other problems. Then fill in the usual blah blah and so forth, normal exam, add the meds from the front of the chart, that's a good girl, signature, so and so and a copy to Frankel in Chicopee, he is some sort of osteopath.

And I told you I'm in to my broker and not in to my wife, not the other way around. Now a letter to—

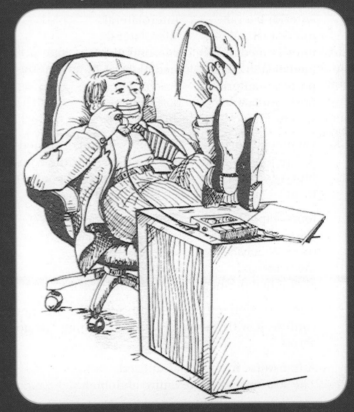

Source: Judith Marshall, *Medicate Me*, illustrated by Cindy Stevens

TRANSCRIPTION**TIPS**

1. Directions can be expressed as adverbs by adding the suffix *-ly*.

anterior	anteriorly
posterior	posteriorly
inferior	inferiorly
superior	superiorly
distal	distally
proximal	proximally
lateral	laterally
medial	medially

2. Two directions used together to designate a direction can be either hyphenated or combined into a single word. Notice the spelling changes in the combined form. *Note:* This is the physician's option, not the transcriptionist's. The transcriptionist should transcribe what is dictated.

anterior-posterior	anteroposterior
anterior-lateral	anterolateral
inferior-lateral	inferolateral
inferior-medial	inferomedial
medial-lateral	mediolateral
posterior-anterior	posteroanterior
posterior-lateral	posterolateral
superior-lateral	superolateral

3. **Combined forms** are frequently dictated in medical reports. It is acceptable to use either the combined form or the standard (often hyphenated) form when it is uncertain which is dictated.

femoral-popliteal	femoropopliteal
tracheal-bronchial	tracheobronchial
ureteral-pelvic	ureteropelvic
medical-legal	medicolegal
abdominal-perineal	abdominoperineal

4. The direction *transverse* is an adjective. Do not confuse it with the verb *traverse* meaning "to go across."

   A transverse incision was utilized.
   The scar traversed the entire abdomen.

5. **Homonyms** are words that are pronounced in the same way but are spelled differently and have different meanings. Well-known English homonyms include:

sight	site
bare	bear
stationary	stationery
principal	principle
their	there

6. Common medical homonyms include:

coarse	course
humeral	humoral
ileum	ilium
viscus	viscous
perineal	peroneal

7. Soundalike words are similar to homonyms but may have a slightly different pronunciation. Soundalike words are, however, quite difficult to distinguish when dictated by a physician. Therefore, distinguishing soundalike words and selecting the one with the correct meaning is a critical skill for medical transcriptionists listening to a dictated report.

8. Common soundalikes include prefixes such as *intra-* and *inter-*, *hypo-* and *hyper-*, as well as suffixes such as *-tomy*, *-ostomy*, *-ectomy*, and *-scope*, *-scopy*. Making the wrong choice of prefix or suffix can drastically change the medical meaning of a word.

9. Common soundalike words include:

advice	advise
affect	effect
elicit	illicit
than	then
in	on
prostate	prostrate
oral	aural
abduction	adduction
bile	bowel
ascitic	acidic
facial	fascial
perineal	peritoneal
ureteral	urethral

10. *Prefixes* and *suffixes* must be selected correctly based on the medical meaning of the report, even when what is dictated is unclear. Many prefixes and suffixes can sound the same when dictated: *intra-* and *inter-*, *-tomy* and *-stomy*, *-scopy* and *-scope*. Failing to differentiate between *hypokalemia* (low blood potassium) and *hyperkalemia* (elevated blood potassium) in transcribing is a serious medical error. Likewise, failing to differentiate between *gastroscopy*, *gastrotomy*, and *gastrostomy* will convey an entirely wrong medical meaning.

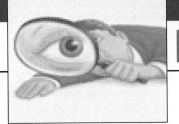

Proofreading Skills

How to Proofread

Professional medical transcriptionists function with minimum supervision while producing maximum results in both quantity and quality. While the majority of working transcriptionists have an immediate supervisor responsible for quality control, the attitude of transcriptionists should be one of independence and responsibility for their work. Professionals take pride in the accuracy and completeness of their own work and gain satisfaction from a job well done, both in quality and quantity.

Proofreading is a critical skill for medical transcriptionists. Proofreading involves looking for mistakes of all types in the transcribed document and correcting them. The usual types of errors that occur include omitting important dictated words, selecting the wrong English or medical word, misspelling words, and making typographical, grammatical, or punctuation errors.

As with all other skills, proofreading skills can be improved with practice. As your instructor points out errors in your transcripts, you may begin to see trends in the errors you make. If you find that you miss few medical words but misspell many English words, you will know to pay particular attention to English words as you proofread your next transcript.

Most students proofread too superficially when they begin transcribing. Here is a four-step method to help you achieve the best results from your proofreading.

1. The conscientious use of reference books is the first step toward good proofreading. Look words up as you encounter them. Do not save all your word searching until the end of the report when you will have forgotten how some of the words sounded at the beginning of the dictation.

2. Lightly proofread what you are transcribing as it appears on the screen of your monitor. Your eyes will begin to do this automatically as you perfect your proofreading skills. This method helps you catch missed words and typographical errors as they occur. Print out your transcript. It is much easier to proofread the transcript in hard copy than it is on the screen.

3. If you cannot find a word, leave a blank of appropriate length depending on how long or short the word sounds. If permitted to do so by your instructor, in parentheses after the blank, transcribe a phonetic rendering for the word(s) you heard. In this electronic age, it is difficult to attach a **flag** (formerly a sheet of paper clipped to the transcript or a sticky note placed on the transcript) which identifies all blanks,

which lines of the transcript they are located on, and what the dictated word sounded like to you. On the job, you will be told how to handle blanks. In the classroom, ask your instructor how to handle them.

4. As a final step in proofreading, use a medical or English spell-checker if your word processor has one and your instructor allows you to do so. Be aware, however, that the spell-checker will not catch errors such as transcribing *no* instead of *not* or transcribing *ilium* instead of *ileum*.

Proofreading is a skill that requires continual practice to perfect. There are several components to proofreading, all of which must be mastered by the medical transcriptionist. Careful proofreading is the key to eliminating the following errors.

Omitting important dictated words. Beginning medical transcriptionists often try to improve their transcription speed too soon—before they are able to listen and remember blocks of dictation. As they try to keep up with the dictating voice, they inadvertently omit some of the dictated words. By adjusting the speed control on the transcriber unit, the transcriptionist can begin slowly, assure that no dictated words are overlooked, and then slowly increase the speed of the dictation which will, in turn, increase transcription speed.

Selecting the wrong medical or English word. Because the quality of an electronic recording does not perfectly reproduce the human voice, it is easy for words and phrases to be garbled or to sound like something quite different from what they are. Therefore, transcriptionists never just transcribe what they *think* they hear; they transcribe only what makes sense in the context of the report. By careful word searching and verifying word definitions, medical transcriptionists avoid selecting the wrong English or medical word.

A wrong medical word can convey a wrong diagnosis for a patient, and that error is carried in the patient's permanent medical record. The professional medical transcriptionist NEVER transcribes anything that does not make sense and/or cannot be verified in a reference book.

Misspelling words. The misspelling of a medical word can be as serious an error as selecting the wrong medical word. Misspellings of both medical and English words can be avoided by careful proofreading and by using the spell-checker function on the word processor. Experienced medical transcriptionists know that electronic spell-checkers cannot be relied upon to locate all of the errors in a document.

Typographical errors. Typographical errors are often the result of carelessness or attempting to type fast rather than focusing on accuracy. You will catch most of these errors through careful proofreading, especially if some time elapses between the time of the transcription and the time of proofreading. Word processing spell-checkers will also help to catch transposed letters and other kinds of typos.

Grammatical errors. Subject-verb agreement errors and other grammatical errors are commonly made by dictating physicians, and it is the job of the transcriptionist to correct them. Sometimes grammatical errors are hard to catch when transcribing, and thus must be identified through careful proofreading.

Punctuation errors. Punctuation is an important part of a correctly transcribed sentence. Incorrectly placed commas can, at times, actually change the medical meaning of a sentence. Chapter 3, Style Guide, provides transcription guidelines to review the grammar, punctuation, style, and format rules that contribute to the correct transcription of a medical report. (See the section on *Editing and Proofreading* in Chapter 3.)

Proofreading cannot be done quickly or haphazardly. It is often more productive to proofread your transcript several hours or even a day after you generate it so that errors will become more obvious. This is a trick that beginning medical transcriptionists can use to strengthen their ability to find errors; however, on the job, transcriptionists are expected to proofread their work as they are transcribing it and do a final proofreading check as soon as they finish the entire document.

Instructions: In proofreading exercises throughout the text, the student is instructed to circle or identify misspelled and missing medical and English words and write the correct words in the numbered spaces opposite the text. For illustration purposes in this example, the errors appear in boldface type on the left, and the corrections are listed in the right column.

1.	HISTORY	1	
2.	The patient was admitted with a **cheif** complaint	2	chief — misspelling
3.	of shortness of breath and chest pain. She is an	3	
4.	84-year-old **femail** with a history of hypertension and	4	female — misspelling
5.	coronary artery disease, recently **dischraged** post	5	discharged — misspelling
6.	admission for congestive heart failure. Her	6	
7.	admission then was **remakable** for pulmonary	7	remarkable — misspelling
8.	edema, and she responded well to diuresis.	8	
9.		9	
10.	The patient has been **doingwell** since discharge and	10	doing well — typo; space omitted
11.	was taking her discharge medications until this a.m.,	11	
12.	when she woke up with shortness of breath and	12	
13.	deep sternal chest pain that radiated **tward** her left	13	toward — misspelling
14.	arm. Associated symptoms at this time included	14	
15.	diaphoresis, **nausea mild** headache, and shortness	15	nausea, mild — punctuation; omitted comma
16.	of breath. She denied palpitations, tachycardia, or	16	
17.	emesis.	17	
18.		18	
19.	The pain persisted and she **present** to the	19	presented — wrong verb tense
20.	emergency department, where she was noted to have	20	
21.	a blood pressure of 164/112. Previous to coming	21	
22.	into the ED, she had taken sublingual nitroglycerin	22	
23.	without response. On EKG monitor she was noted to	23	
24.	have a rate of 85 and rare PVCs. She was given oxy-	24	
25.	gen, 40 mg of IV Lasix, and 10 mg of **sublingal**	25	sublingual — misspelling
26.	nifedipine, with resolution of her chest pain and	26	
27.	improvement in breathing. She still has mild left	27	
28.	shoulder discomfort but is otherwise **comtorble**.	28	comfortable — misspelling

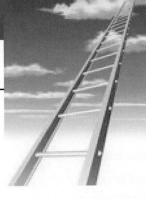

SkillsChallenge

Completion Exercise

Instructions: Complete the following questions and write brief definitions as needed. Consult the readings in Chapter 1.

1. List three skills that contribute to the medical transcriptionist's ability to interpret, translate, and edit medical dictation.

_____

_____

_____

_____

2. List the "basic four" medical reports.

_____

_____

_____

_____

3. List three purposes of the patient health record.

_____

_____

_____

4. List three important tools of the medical transcriptionists' trade.

_____

_____

_____

5. List four environments in which medical transcriptionists work.

_____

_____

_____

_____

6. Write a brief definition for each of the following:

Chief Complaint_____

_____

_____

History of Present Illness_____

_____

Past Medical History_____

_____

Family History_____

_____

Social History_____

_____

Review of Systems_____

_____

_____

Physical Examination_____

_____

_____

7. Give four reasons why laboratory tests are done.

_____

_____

_____

_____

8. List four types of drug forms.

_____

_____

_____

_____

9. List four routes of drug administration.

_____

_____

_____

_____

Soundalikes Exercise

Instructions: In the following sentences circle the correct soundalike from the words in parentheses.

1. The patient was (counseled, councilled) to get psychiatric help.

2. The patient expressed strong (decent, descent, dissent) to the recommended bypass operation.

3. Venous (access, assess, excess, axis) was needed for IV administration of antibiotics, so a heparin lock was placed.

4. (Accept, except) for a slight weakness in the left arm, the patient had no residual symptoms of stroke.

5. Because penicillin was not (affective, effective), the patient was put on another antibiotic.

6. The patient's wife made an (allusion, elusion, illusion) to possible alcoholism by stating that the patient drank a six-pack a day, but the patient denied a drinking problem.

7. My (advice, advise) to the patient was to drink plenty of liquids, get lots of sleep, and take aspirin for pain.

8. The patient complained of (a symptomatic, asymptomatic) cough for the last month, but it was nonproductive.

9. I would (assess, access, excess, axis) his chances of surviving the operation at 50:50.

10. The surgical (cite, sight, site) was dressed with a sterile bandage.

11. The patient was not (conscious, conscience) after the head injury.

12. Moderate exercise would certainly (complement, compliment) the patient's post-CABG therapy.

Directions of the Body

Instructions: Match the direction of the body in Column A with its definition in Column B.

Column A

1. ____ toward the front of the body
2. ____ toward the back of the body
3. ____ toward the midline
4. ____ toward the side
5. ____ away from the center; toward the periphery
6. ____ within the body
7. ____ toward the body surface

Column B

A. anterior
B. distal
C. internal (or deep)
D. lateral
E. medial
F. posterior
G. superficial

Prefixes and Suffixes

Instructions: Match the definitions in Column A with the prefix or suffix in Column B.

Column A

1. ____ the study of
2. ____ a tumor
3. ____ toward
4. ____ development or form
5. ____ inflammation of
6. ____ pain
7. ____ without
8. ____ discharge, flow
9. ____ enlargement of
10. ____ across
11. ____ self
12. ____ a disease condition
13. ____ within
14. ____ new opening created surgically
15. ____ beside or near
16. ____ cutting out
17. ____ increased in amount
18. ____ an abnormal condition
19. ____ an instrument used to record
20. ____ painful or difficult
21. ____ a surgical repair
22. ____ process of examining visually
23. ____ located above
24. ____ making an incision into
25. ____ coming after
26. ____ false

Column B

A. -itis
B. auto-
C. post-
D. -logy
E. -tomy
F. -pathy
G. intra-
H. -algia
I. -scopy
J. supra-
K. -graph
L. a-
M. -megaly
N. -plasty
O. trans-
P. -oma
Q. ad-
R. -osis
S. dys-
T. -stomy
U. pseudo-
V. -plasia
W. hyper-
X. -ectomy
Y. para-
Z. -rrhea

Sample Reports

Sample medical reports appear on the following pages, illustrating a variety of reports. Fictional names are provided for illustration of proper format, and no resemblance to actual persons is intended. Sample transcripts were prepared according to the *AAMT Book of Style*, where possible.

Letter, Block Format

October 1, XXXX

Stanley Lessing, MD
1829 Apache Way
Cheyenne, CA 95555

Re: Laverne DeFazio

Dear Dr. Lessing:

I have seen the above-named patient for several visits since her colonoscopy, and I wanted to update you about what has transpired. After the colonoscopy, I increased the Azulfidine to 500 mg q.i.d. I also sent stool for *C. difficile*, which was negative, and ordered an upper GI with a small bowel series. This showed a small sliding-type hiatal hernia with rapid transit time through the small bowel. The remainder of the exam was normal.

I saw this patient again 3 months later, at which time she had a fever and sweats with temperature of 103 degrees. I referred her to your office to further assess whether the Azulfidine or Crohn's is the source of her fever. Also, when she took Lomotil for loose stools, she became obstipated. Metamucil may help avoid rebound constipation.

Thank you for allowing me to participate in this very lovely patient's care and management.

Very truly yours,

James Wood, MD

JW:hpi
D: 10/2/XXXX
T: 10/3/XXXX

cc: Leland Hill, MD

Chart Note

PALMA, MARIA
June 28, XXXX

The patient was seen today for skin testing, and all of her skin tests are negative. It is my impression, therefore, that she has intrinsic asthma.

She is to discontinue the Theo-24, as she has been experiencing episodes of tachycardia and anxiety. Switch to Proventil 2 mg tablets 4 times daily for wheezing. Return to see me again in 2 months.

SONIA VAN HALA, MD

SVH:hpi
d: 6/28/XXXX
t: 6/29/XXXX

SOAP Note

SUMMERS, JENNIFER
#802741
October 1, XXXX

SUBJECTIVE
Patient is here for routine gynecologic examination. She is on Ortho-Novum and is having no difficulty with the pill. She forgets to take the pill occasionally.

OBJECTIVE
Breasts reveal no masses or tenderness. Abdomen negative. Pelvic exam was entirely negative. Pap smear taken.

ASSESSMENT
Normal gynecologic examination.

PLAN
Advised to use alternative forms of contraception when she misses a pill. Given a refill of Ortho-Novum 1/35. To return in 9 months.

HIYAS FONTE, MD

HF:hpi

JEFFREY, THOMAS
April 8, XXXX

HISTORY
This 38-year-old male was admitted through the emergency department with a history of less than 1 day of acute ureteral colic on the left side. Patient had an intravenous pyelogram in the emergency department earlier today, which shows partial to complete obstruction of the left ureter at the ureterovesical junction with a large stone, approximately 8 x 5 mm, lodged at the ureterovesical junction. Patient has no other calcifications visible. Patient denies any previous history of urinary tract stones or other genitourinary problems except for prostatitis a couple of years ago. Patient has no other significant medical problems.

PAST MEDICAL HISTORY
Otherwise negative.

ALLERGIES
None.

REVIEW OF SYSTEMS:
HEENT on the system review is essentially unremarkable. He denies headache. He has a moderate hearing deficit.
Respiratory: No upper respiratory symptoms; no cough, congestion, or hemoptysis.
Cardiac: All symptoms are denied.
Gastrointestinal: There has been no history of hematemesis or melena. She denies significant fatty food intolerance.
Genitourinary: Ureteral colic as noted in the history.
Neuromuscular: Without complaint.
Musculoskeletal: Moderate arthritis.
Endocrine: No dysuria, polyuria, or polydipsia.
Hematologic: There is no history of anemia.
Integumentary: No significant skin problem.

MEDICATIONS
None. Follows usual diet.

FAMILY HISTORY
No familial history of kidney stones or other significant hereditary disease.

PHYSICAL EXAMINATION
GENERAL: Physical exam reveals a well-nourished, well-developed male in no acute distress.
HEENT: Eyes: Pupils equal, round, react to light. Ears, nose, and throat clear.
NECK: Neck supple. No jugular venous distention or bruit.
LUNGS: Lungs clear to percussion and auscultation.
HEART: Regular rhythm, no murmur.
ABDOMEN: Abdomen soft. Slight left costovertebral angle tenderness, slight left lower quadrant tenderness. No rebound.
GENITALIA: Genitalia within normal limits. Penis: Normal male.
EXTREMITIES: No cyanosis, clubbing, or edema.
NEUROLOGIC: Neurologically oriented x3 with no gross deficits.

(continued)

JEFFREY, THOMAS
April 8, XXXX
Page 2

IMPRESSION
Left lower ureteral stone with obstruction.

RECOMMENDATION
Hydration, analgesia, observation, and if stone does not pass within 72 hours or less, will probably recommend patient for ureteroscopy and stone basketing and, if needed, ultrasonic lithotripsy. If the stone cannot be mobilized downward, push-back and extracorporeal shock wave lithotripsy might be considered.

SONYA PITT, MD

SP:hpi
D: 4/8/XXXX
T: 4/8/XXXX

Consultation Report

FLINT, SHIRLEY
#989898
December 15, XXXX
Attending: Barry Topham, MD

HISTORY

The patient was admitted with a chief complaint of shortness of breath and chest pain. She is an 84-year-old female with a history of hypertension and coronary artery disease, recently discharged post admission for congestive heart failure. Her admission then was remarkable for pulmonary edema, and she responded well to diuresis.

The patient has been doing well since discharge and was taking her discharge medications until this a.m., when she woke up with shortness of breath and deep sternal chest pain that radiated toward her left arm. Associated symptoms at this time included diaphoresis, nausea, mild headache, and shortness of breath. She denied palpitations, tachycardia, or emesis.

The pain persisted and she presented to the emergency department, where she was noted to have a blood pressure of 164/112. Previous to coming into the ED, she had taken sublingual nitroglycerin without response. On EKG monitor she was noted to have a rate of 85 and rare PVCs. She was given oxygen, 40 mg of IV Lasix, and 10 mg of sublingual nifedipine, with resolution of her chest pain and improvement in breathing. She still has mild left shoulder discomfort but is otherwise comfortable.

PAST MEDICAL HISTORY

The past medical history is well documented in past admissions and is notable for:
1. Type 2 diabetes mellitus, treated with oral agents.
2. Coronary artery disease, status post subendocardial myocardial infarction 2 years ago.
3. Episodes of atrial fibrillation on multiple occasions in the past.
4. Hypertension.
5. Anemia, unknown type.

MEDICATIONS ON ADMISSION

Glipizide 5 mg b.i.d., Lasix 40 mg b.i.d., Nitrodisc 16 mg q.d., Capoten 12.5 mg b.i.d., Procardia 10 mg t.i.d., KCl 20 mEq b.i.d., Naprosyn 375 mg b.i.d.

PHYSICAL EXAMINATION

General: A pleasant, obese female who is comfortable.
Vital signs: Current blood pressure is 118/60, respiratory rate 22, temperature 97.5, and heart rate 88.
HEENT: Extraocular muscles intact. Pupils irregular with postsurgical changes right eye. Ears, nose, and throat clear.
Neck: Supple.
Chest: Bibasilar rales with nonlabored respirations.
Cardiovascular: Carotids with mild delay and sustained upstroke. Bilateral bruits or radiated murmurs also noted. Jugular venous pressure 7 cm. The point of maximal impulse (PMI) was not palpable. Regular rate with rare ectopic beats. S1, S2 normal. Positive S4. No S3. Grade 2/6 systolic murmur heard at the lower left sternal border. Distal pulses intact and fair.
Abdomen: Soft. Positive bowel sounds. She had a pulsatile midline mass consistent with a possible abdominal aortic aneurysm that did have an overlying bruit. She had no hepatosplenomegaly or other mass.
Extremities: Extremities revealed 1+ edema to midshin, but extremities were without clubbing, cyanosis, or edema.
Rectal: Deferred.
Pelvic: Deferred.
Neurologic: Neurological examination was nonfocal.

(continued)

FLINT, SHIRLEY
#989898
December 15, XXXX
Attending: Barry Topham, MD
Page 2

LABORATORY
Laboratory was remarkable for a potassium of 4.0, a BUN of 94, a creatinine of 3.2, glucose of 112, hemoglobin 10, hematocrit 32, and a white count of 8.4. Platelets were normal. EKG revealed sinus rhythm at 80 with an axis of +15 and normal intervals. Left ventricular hypertrophy was identified. She had ST-segment elevation in I, II, aVL, and V4 through V6, which is unchanged, and she has a Q in lead III.

IMPRESSION
1. Chest pain with shortness of breath. Rule out congestive heart failure.
2. Possible abdominal aortic aneurysm.
3. Anemia.
4. Renal insufficiency.

PLAN
Usual rule out myocardial infarction protocol with serial EKGs and CPKs. Continue supplemental oxygen at 2 L, and obtain arterial blood gases to document PO_2. Continue Lasix. Recommend abdominal ultrasound to document the size of the aneurysm. Suggest the usual iron studies and stool guaiac to follow anemia. The worsening of the renal function could be due to congestive heart failure, and this will be followed.

MARIANNE SMITH, MD

MS:hpi
d: 12/15/XXXX
t: 12/16/XXXX

MENLOVE, LYNN
575662
Date of surgery: 9/15/XXXX

PREOPERATIVE DIAGNOSIS
Cholelithiasis; recurrent biliary colic; chronic cholecystitis.

POSTOPERATIVE DIAGNOSIS
Cholelithiasis; recurrent biliary colic; chronic cholecystitis.

PROCEDURE PERFORMED
Laparoscopic cholecystectomy.

ANESTHESIA
General endotracheal anesthesia.

INDICATIONS
Presented for evaluation of recurrent, intermittent biliary colic. She needed a laparoscopic cholecystectomy in treatment
for her symptoms.

PROCEDURE
After satisfactory general anesthesia was accomplished, a nasogastric tube and Foley catheter were placed for
decompression of the stomach and urinary bladder. The anterior abdominal wall was sterilely prepped and draped.
A curvilinear infraumbilical incision was made and the fascia grasped with two Kocher clamps. Two #1 PDS sutures
were placed to assist with retraction of the fascia, and the Hasson trocar was placed in an incision in the fascia. The
placement of the Hasson was preceded by digital examination of the peritoneal cavity to ensure that there were no
periumbilical adhesions to the anterior abdominal wall. Pneumoperitoneum was established, and the camera was
placed through the Hasson retractor for placement of the other trocars under direct visualization. A 10-mm epigastric
port was placed, and two lateral 5-mm ports were placed in the subcostal plane. Graspers were placed through the
lateral ports and used to retract the fundus of the gallbladder over the edge of the liver and to retract the body to
facilitate dissection of the hilar structures. Before this could be accomplished, some thin, filmy adhesions between the
omentum and the gallbladder were taken down bluntly with the dissector. Then attention was directed to dissection of
the hilar structures.

The cystic artery and cystic duct were isolated, doubly clipped proximally and doubly clipped distally, and then divided
with the parrot scissors. Dissection was commenced with cautery, and the gallbladder was removed from the hilar
structures to the fundus. The camera was moved to the epigastric port, and the gallbladder was removed through
the Hasson umbilical port. The gallbladder was inspected and indeed found to have all the clips in the appropriate
place. There was an approximately 2-cm stone in the gallbladder. The Hasson retractor was replaced in the umbilical
port and the camera was replaced through this. Inspection of the right upper quadrant revealed the hilar clips to

(continued)

MENLOVE, LYNN
#575662
Date of surgery: 9/15/XXXX
Page 2

be in good position. The right upper quadrant was copiously irrigated with saline and aspirated. Of note, there was no spillage of stones during the case; however, one of the graspers had disrupted the gallbladder wall early in the case, and there was some minimal spillage of clear yellow bile. All of this was irrigated and aspirated at the conclusion of the case.

The lateral ports were removed and revealed no bleeding. The epigastric port was removed and also revealed no bleeding. The Hasson retractor was withdrawn and pneumoperitoneum evacuated. The PDS sutures at the umbilical fascia were approximated to close the fascial defect, and an additional #1 PDS suture was placed to completely close this fascial defect. All skin incisions were closed with a running subcuticular 4-0 Vicryl suture. Steri-Strips were applied. The patient tolerated the procedure well and was returned to the recovery room in stable condition.

TONI DALY, MD

TD:hpi
d: 9/15/XXXX
t: 9/16/XXXX

Discharge Summary

HUGHES, SCOTT
#898989
Admitted: 12/1/XXXX
Discharged: 12/3/XXXX

ADMITTING DIAGNOSIS
Fracture of right tibia, closed.

DISCHARGE DIAGNOSIS
Fracture of right tibia, closed.

OPERATION PERFORMED
Open reduction and internal fixation with Lottes nail, right tibia.

HISTORY
The patient was playing baseball on the day of admission. He was hit at second base and sustained an injury to his right leg with immediate pain and swelling. He was brought to the emergency department and diagnosed as having fractured his right tibia.

PHYSICAL EXAMINATION
The fracture site was tender to palpation. He had good sensation and circulation in the leg, but marked swelling was present.

X-RAYS
Multiple views of the tibia revealed there was a stairstep-type fracture at the distal portion of the middle one third of the tibia.

HOSPITAL COURSE
On the day of admission, the patient was taken to surgery and a Lottes nail inserted to fix the fracture. The patient's postoperative course was essentially benign. He was placed in a long leg cast and gradually ambulated on crutches.

DISCHARGE PLAN
The patient will remain on crutches for the next 6 weeks. At that time another set of x-rays will be carried out to assess the progress of healing. The patient is to call our office immediately if he notices increased pain, swelling, or duskiness of the toes.

DISABILITY
The patient is disabled for his usual activities as a plumber.

DISCHARGE MEDICATIONS
Tylenol No. 3, one p.o. q.4h. p.r.n. pain.

JOYCE GARDEN, MD

JG:hpi
d: 12/3/XXXX
t: 12/4/XXXX

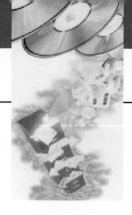

Transcription Practice

How to Transcribe Medical Dictation

As you transcribe, remember that you are beginning a new physical skill that requires the coordination of your eyes, ears, fingers (if you use hand controls), and foot (if you use a foot pedal). You may already be an accomplished typist, and that will give you an advantage. We recommend that students have a copy-typing speed of at least 45 words per minute before attempting to transcribe. However, the skills needed to copy type and transcribe are somewhat different, and you should expect your transcription to be slow and halting in the beginning.

Try this exercise: Cross your arms across your chest in a way that is comfortable. Now try to cross your arms so that the other arm is uppermost. This can be quite awkward for some people. You may find yourself repeatedly trying to "arrange" your arms to get them right.

Just as it feels unfamiliar to cross your arms in a different way than you are accustomed to, it may also feel awkward to transcribe what you *hear* rather than *copy-type* what you see. Although the keyboard is the same, the way in which you interact with it is significantly different, requiring coordination of timing of the eyes, ears, fingers, and use of a foot pedal or hand control connected to the desktop.

As you begin to transcribe, do not try to type fast at first, but strive first for accuracy of medical words, grammar, punctuation, and format. All of these constitute another group of new variables that you must constantly consider, evaluate, and take time to master. Understanding the scope and details of all of these variables in the transcription process can seem overwhelming at first, but your diligence will be rewarded later as you add speed to your new skill of accuracy.

Transcribe each dictation carefully, stopping as often as necessary to look up new and unfamiliar words for spelling and meaning. Word searching is time well spent and is NEVER wasted, as it strengthens and builds one of the most important skills you bring to transcription.

Start slowly and proceed carefully and thoughtfully, taking advantage of every opportunity to learn, memorize, and understand new medical material. Most importantly, be encouraged by your progress. Speed will come naturally as you gain knowledge and experience, and soon you will see the fruits of your efforts as you transcribe new reports confidently, accurately, and quickly.

Error Analysis

The most common errors committed by students include omitting important dictated words, selecting the wrong words (both medical and English), misspellings, typographical errors, and grammatical and punctuation mistakes. The solutions listed below will help you assess the kinds of errors you are making and show you how to minimize them.

Omitted dictated word. Listen carefully to the dictation and slow your pace. Do not attempt to increase your transcription speed until these errors are minimized.

Wrong word. Take care in checking word definitions. The definition must match the context of the report.

Misspelled word. Mentally spell the corrected word several times. Highlight it in your dictionary or write the word in your personal notebook so that you will be aware of it each time you look it up.

Typographical error. Your proofreading is at fault. Allow time to elapse between the time you transcribe the report and the time you proofread it.

Grammatical error. If a physician makes a grammatical error, you are expected to correct it. If your transcription contains a significant number of these types of errors, a review of basic English is in order—for you, not the physician, unfortunately.

Punctuation error. The most serious punctuation errors are those that alter medical meaning. If you make a significant number of these kinds of errors, a review of basic punctuation would be useful. There may be several acceptable but different ways to punctuate some sentences without changing the medical meaning.

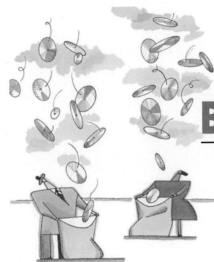

BLOOPERS

Incorrect	Correct
At the close of the procedure there was no breathing noted.	At the close of the procedure there was no bleeding noted.
The patient underwent a two-ball ligation.	The patient underwent a tubal ligation.
The wound was treated with icepicks.	The wound was treated with ice packs.
There was a palpable mask in the abdomen.	There was a palpable mass in the abdomen.
The patient had congenial syphilis.	The patient had congenital syphilis.
The liver itch was palpable.	The liver edge was palpable.
The patient was sexually impudent.	The patient was sexually impotent.
The ankle was edentulous.	The ankle was edematous.
The patient was in the sublime position.	The patient was in the supine position.

Perspectives on Medical Transcription

Learning Objectives

- Describe three ways in which silent letters in the spelling of English words complicate the process of medical transcription.
- Describe the ways in which the medical transcriptionist must edit mispronunciations, slips of the tongue, malapropisms, and other dictating errors.
- Discuss two important points in accepting and dispensing criticism.
- List two reasons why medical transcriptionists will not be replaced by technology.

- Discuss the most common errors of grammar made by ESL physicians and how the medical transcriptionist corrects them for accuracy and completeness.
- Discuss how the dictating practices of some physicians impact the transcription process.
- Cite two reasons why laughter is important in medical transcription.

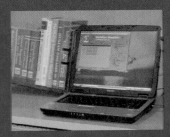
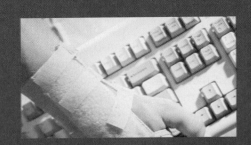
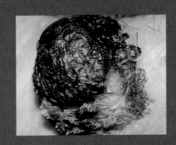

Ethics and Professionalism

A Doctor's View

Dictation and Transcription: Adventures in Thought Transference

by John H. Dirckx, M.D.

> The pronunciation is the actual living form or forms of a word, that is, the word itself, of which the current spelling is only a current symbolization. . . . (General Explanations, *The Oxford English Dictionary*)

Every time I read this passage, I am struck anew by the realization that the sequences of letters we put down on paper are not words, but only visible representations of those evanescent sequences of vocal sound that are the only true words. When we speak of "the written word," we are indulging in metaphor: words are heard but not seen. Indeed, most of the world's 3,000 languages are exclusively spoken languages having no writing systems.

I offer these reflections to introduce an inquiry into the nature of the **dictation-transcription process**, a form of communication unique among human activities. The dictator expresses thoughts in speech (which is electronically recorded) and the transcriptionist puts those thoughts on paper by converting sounds heard to conventional symbols.

The product of the transcriptionist's effort is not, however, a mere phonetic record of what is heard on the tape but rather a rendering of the dictator's thoughts in finished English prose. That is, instead of making a perfectly faithful record of speech sounds heard, the transcriptionist performs various analytic and interpretive functions and modifies the record by a complex series of deletions, additions, alterations, and emendations. Moreover, this editorial activity is performed simultaneously at several levels: *phonetic* (recognition and interpretation of speech sounds and their correct representation in writing), *conceptual* (monitoring of word choice, grammar, and style), and *formal* (punctuation, consistency of form, appropriate units of measure).

Even at what I have called the phonetic level, the transcriptionist constantly discriminates and amends on the basis of context, so that even here there is nothing mechanical or automatic about the transcription process.

Silent letters may not be the most difficult feature of English spelling, but they are surely the most paradoxic. For a phonetic writing system to include symbols that are essential to the spelling of certain words, and that nevertheless represent no sounds heard in those words, is a palpable absurdity. Yet there is hardly a letter in our alphabet that does not figure in the spelling of some word without being represented in its pronunciation.

Suffice it to say that the relation between speech sounds and the symbols that convention requires us to use to represent them is erratic, almost haphazard. That is why the transcriptionist cannot simply match a symbol to a sound heard, as in making a stenographic (shorthand) record, where, for example, *f*, *ph*, and *gh* (in *enough*) are all represented by the same symbol, while the *b*'s of *doubt* and *subtle* are not represented at all.

The same, only different. A frequent source of difficulty in transcription is the existence of homonyms or, more precisely, of homophones. **Homonyms** are two or more words that are spelled and pronounced the same but differ in meaning—for example, mole "small mammal"; mole "pigmented nevus"; mole "uterine neoplasm"; mole "breakwater"; mole "unit of measure based on molecular weight."

Strictly speaking, a set like this should cause no trouble, because even if the transcriptionist should mistake the meaning, the spelling would be the same.

Similarly, **homographs** (words spelled the same but pronounced differently) should create no ambiguity in dictation. A special kind of homograph results from variation in placement of syllable stress: *tínnitus-tinnítus, ángina-angína, fácet-facét*. The American transcriptionist may sometimes be startled by a British dictator's placement of stress in such words as *cervícal, éphedrine, labóratory,* and *skelétal*.

But it is **homophones** that demand alertness and judgment—words that sound the same but are spelled differently. Sometimes the difference is plain from the context ("I guessed he was a guest when he discussed his disgust") and sometimes it is not ("Dr. Templeton is losing his patience/patients"). Many homophone pairs are created by our custom of reducing unaccented vowels to a neutral "uh" sound. We hear this sound, for example, in the second syllables of both *callus* and *callous, mucus* and *mucous, villus* and *villous*. Only the context tells the transcriptionist whether to type the noun form in *-us* or the adjective form in *-ous*. In the same way, *instillation* may be indistinguishable from *installation, perineal* from *peroneal, have* from *of*.

Styles of pronunciation that are characteristic of certain regional or ethnic dialects may create homophones in the dictation of some speakers. One person may fail to distinguish between *finally* and *finely*, another between *then* and *than*, a third between *his* and *he's*, a fourth between *long* and *lung*. The practice of dropping final *l* or *r* or both can erase the differences between such pairs as *sulfa/sulfur* and *femoral-popliteal/femoropopliteal*, and place the transcriptionist in peril of creating such monstrosities as *musculo-dystrophy* and *normal tensive*.

In my part of the country, a sizable segment of the populace practices *itacism*. This term, originally denoting an analogous dialectal variation in Greek, refers to a raising of the short *e* sound in a tonic (stressed) syllable so that it sounds like short *i*. Thus, for example, *attend, get, men*, and *shelter* are pronounced as if they were spelled *attind, git, min*, and *shilter*.

Although this causes little or no inconvenience in the examples I have used, the wholesale disappearance of tonic short *e* does create some ambiguities that must be averted by further modifications of the language. For instance, persons who pronounce *pen* exactly like *pin* customarily distinguish the former word by saying *inkpen* (pronounced "inkpin"). (Less than a week after making notes for the above paragraph, I saw in a local antique shop a box of old fountain pens labeled "Inkpins $1.00.")

Homophony is not confined to pairs of words. A phrase may sound almost exactly like another phrase of entirely different, even opposite meaning. Two notorious examples—*had no carcinoma* for *adenocarcinoma* and *prepped and raped* for *prepped and draped*—have passed into legend. Whole books of such blunders, many of them no doubt spurious, have been published. A frequent source of difficulty is the unaccented *a* at the beginning of words: *atonic bladder* vs. *a tonic bladder, a symmetric swelling* vs. *asymmetric swelling*.

Besides discriminating between homophones, the transcriptionist performs a variety of what might be called normalizing operations, that is, recognizing variant pronunciations and reducing them to their conventional forms before putting them on paper. The range of such deviations is enormous. Some result from congenital or acquired speech impediments such as tongue-tie or obstruction of the nasal passages by hypertrophic adenoids or chronic allergic rhinitis. Some are due to dialectal variations (a few of which I have already mentioned) or to speech habits learned in childhood, such as substituting a glottal catch (momentary closure of the vocal cords) for *t* at the end of a syllable.

A large number of deviant pronunciations arise from the structure of the human vocal apparatus and the difficulty or awkwardness of producing certain sound sequences. The omission of the first *d* sound in *Wednesday* and the rearrangement of sounds in *comfortable* (="comftorble") are examples of such changes. In rapid speech, *cysts* and *tests* often come out "cyss" and "tess." We also tend to insert extraneous sounds into our speech to smooth certain transitions. Some of these inserted sounds are virtually standard (*compfort, intsulin*), some are dialectal (*hematoma-r of the rectus sheath, mower* [=more]), and some are decidedly substandard (*athaletic, drownding*).

Frank mispronunciations include both the mishandling of English phonetics by non-native speakers and isolated errors (most of them acquired by imitation) such as *phalynx, larnyx, ishium*, and *meninjocele*. Here may also be mentioned certain recurring deviations from correct pronunciation that have been adopted as an affectation by certain speakers. Among these are the bizarre plurals *abscesses, processes*, and other words pronounced to rhyme with *neuroses*, and the compulsive gallicization of words having no connection with French (*centimeter, centrifuge, difficile*, and *mitrale*).

To recapitulate, in turning a phonetic (speech) record into a written one, the transcriptionist inserts "silent" letters, suppresses extraneous sounds (including "uh"), selects the correct one of several alternative spellings, and recognizes deviant pronunciations—all in the light of a sustained monitoring of the context and a thorough understanding of medicine, medical terminology, dictating conventions, and human frailty.

In other words. Although nearly everyone takes it for granted that the kinds of editing I have been discussing thus far are part of the transcription process, many question the propriety of the transcriptionist's judging and altering the factual content of a dictation, correcting the dictator's grammar and syntax, and touching up the style to improve clarity and coherence. Yet such adjustments are manifestly necessary, not only in dictation by non-native speakers of English but in the vast majority of all dictations.

By choosing to dictate a document rather than write it out, the dictator not only sidesteps many of the mechanical tasks associated with composition but implicitly delegates these tasks to the transcriptionist. No dictators have such perfect powers of concentration that they never accidentally repeat themselves, never inadvertently substitute one word for another, never leave a sentence unfinished. Sooner or later the most alert and cautious dictator makes each of these mistakes, and others besides. Clearly these normal human lapses ought not to be reproduced in the transcript, and just as clearly the duty of identifying and correcting them devolves on the transcriptionist.

Just as mispronounced words and names must be spelled correctly by the transcriptionist, erroneous spellings supplied by the dictator must be ignored.

When the intrusive word sounds something like the right one, it is called a *malapropism* (after Mrs. Malaprop, a character in an eighteenth-century comedy by Sheridan). Some malapropisms evidently result from momentary lapses: *pericardial infusion* (for *effusion*). Others are permanent features of the dictator's vocabulary, as was the case with Mrs. Malaprop: *melanotic* (for *melenic*) *stools; with regards* (for *regard*) *to*.

One of the medical transcriptionist's greatest challenges is dealing correctly with **slang terms** used by dictators. These terms vary in propriety; some may be left in the record while others must be replaced with more formal terminology. The transcriptionist must therefore not only distinguish the acceptable from the inappropriate but also understand the latter and be able to supply suitable alternatives.

Among the few vestiges of grammatical inflection in modern English are changes in the form of nouns and verbs to signify whether they are **singular or plural**: *one stitch, two stitches; he stitches, they stitch.* Not surprisingly, most of the purely grammatical errors committed by dictators are faults of subject-verb agreement. Such errors are common in everyday speech and even writing. As the mind constructs a sentence phrase by phrase, grammatical forms are apt to be selected on the basis of ideas rather than of words. Often a singular noun is used when the speaker is actually "thinking plural" and goes on to use a plural verb: "The right and left lung (lungs) are congested." "No definite site of his occult GI bleeding were (was) identified."

A permanent medical document dictated by one professional and transcribed by another is expected to conform to certain norms of precision, clarity, coherence, and taste. Where the dictator's competence or diligence falls short, the transcriptionist must supply the deficiency. Again the task requires a broad base of knowledge about the subject of the dictation and considerable skill in composition and editing. Most transcriptionists perform this operation so deftly and unobtrusively that the majority of dictators never even suspect that their dictation has undergone revision (or that it needed it).

A matter of form. The third level at which the transcriptionist exercises a discriminating and editorial function is that of **format or layout**, including punctuation and consistency in the use of abbreviations, numerals, and units of measure. In general the transcriptionist's decisions on these points are unrelated to anything heard in the dictation. It is true that dictators often supply directions for formatting and punctuation, but many of these (such as calling each new line a "paragraph" or separating complete sentences with a "comma") must simply be ignored by the transcriptionist. Other directions, while not actually incorrect, may violate the canons of English composition or introduce inconsistencies.

Armed with basic keyboarding skills and a knowledge of the rules of punctuation, the transcriptionist creates the format of a report and supplies commas and periods as needed in the very act of transcribing the dictation. Numerals and units of measure are typed according to established conventions and in consistent fashion regardless of how they occur in the dictation. Thus "six tenths" becomes *0.6* and "four and a half milliliters" becomes *4.5 mL.*

No one can master the lore of a craft so perfectly as never to be at a loss for a word, a meaning, a rule, a spelling. A crucial requirement for the practice of most professions is knowing where to look up what one doesn't remember or can't understand. The medical transcriptionist depends heavily on dictionaries, drug references, word books, and personal files or notebooks to supply authoritative answers to questions raised by the dictation.

While it is all too easy for transcriptionists and dictators alike to take it for granted that transcription is "writing down what somebody said," it should be evident from my remarks that it is only by penetrating and sharing the dictator's thoughts that the transcriptionist can produce an accurate and otherwise fully satisfactory transcript.

Fuller awareness of the breadth, intricacy, and difficulty of medical transcription should heighten the respect of dictators and others outside the profession for those who practice it. Transcriptionists themselves can be proud of their hard-won and socially valuable competence in a field demanding both technical and intellectual virtuosity.

A Transcriptionist's View

What is it like to *be* a medical transcriptionist? How do medical transcriptionists look at their immediate world and the medical community at large? The readings in this section portray "life as a medical transcriptionist" with all the real-life drama, humor, romance, and sense of self and professionalism that distinguish the myriad individuals who choose medical transcription as a career.

The Mind Behind the Machine

by Vera Pyle

Let me introduce you to medical transcription and medical transcriptionists. You will notice that I use the term "transcriptionist," not "transcriber." A transcriber is the machine that plays a dictated report through our headsets so that we may transcribe it. It is NOT the person who transcribes. A medical transcriptionist is "the mind behind the machine."

If there is one thing that transcriptionists are known for, it is our love for words. This is the common thread in our profession. It is what makes us professionals.

If I were cast away on a desert island, the book I would probably want to take with me is an unabridged English dictionary, and I could be happy for years. Transcriptionists can get lost in a dictionary. We look up a word and we see something else that looks interesting, and then we look up another word, and so on. Words are truly exciting. I would much rather have a dozen new medical words all researched and defined than a five-pound box of candy. I hope that you too will come to share this feeling.

Some years ago I was transcribing the manuscript of a textbook by a physician for whom I had worked in the past. He is a well-educated, extremely literate person. He is a published poet, a musician, a composer, a teacher—a real Renaissance man. So it was with some trepidation that I presumed to suggest changes. I transcribed the page the way he dictated it, and then I gave him my version as well. He read it and beamed. "This is a tremendous improvement," he said. "You know, Vera, together we could rule the world."

It was a charming proposition. However, it is not my ambition to rule the world. All I want is recognition for what I know and how accurately and intelligently I can convey that information—my contribution to the delivery of the best possible healthcare for a patient.

Some 30 years ago, our hospital got the prototype of one of the first word processing machines. Our medical record director brought in a group of interns and residents to see this marvel. Pointing to the machine proudly, she said, "And this is the machine that transcribes your reports." Not so, I thought then, and now.

The machines we use are simply tools. Without the knowledge contained in the mind of the transcriptionist, the machines are impotent. The transcriptionist is *the mind behind the machine*.

Professionalism and the Medical Transcriptionist

by Kathy Donneson

What is professionalism? What qualities distinguish a professional from a nonprofessional? Professionals may be judged by their attitudes and conduct as they relate to matters of work, interpersonal relationships, and ethics.

Medical transcriptionists work independently and produce a product (the transcribed medical document) which reflects their care, integrity, and skill.

Professional medical transcriptionists function with minimal supervision while producing maximum results in both quantity and quality. While the majority of working transcriptionists do have an immediate supervisor responsible for quality control, the attitude of each transcriptionist should be one of independence and responsibility for his or her own work. Professionals take pride in the accuracy and completeness of their own work and gain satisfaction from a job well done, both in quality and quantity.

Professional medical transcriptionists demonstrate responsibility in their day-to-day working judgments by combining past experience, the powers of deductive thinking, and a vast store of medical knowledge to

Tape *Dancing*

Whenever medical transcriptionists get together and talk about our work, we often chat about "that rhythm," those perfect blends of great physicians, mellifluous tones, equipment without snaps and crackles in the headset and without sticky keys and broken pedals—that rhythm. When every word you hear, you know, when every spelling is there in your head or at your fingertips in the proper reference source—whizzing along, getting that upbeat feeling, *that* rhythm. Each of us has felt it. Fortissimo, pianissimo, largo or molto vivace, on it goes. . . .

So where is the music? It's all in our perspective. It's how *we* view it first. A mining expedition? A treasure hunt each day in an ocean of words? A challenge? Do your days pass in a blur of disco-like beat or hum along in ballad form? It doesn't matter. What matters are the voices, whether they are staccato or monumentally dull-pitched. The voices form the very fabric of what we do.

We have to be alert and oriented times three even when the dictating physician isn't. And typing speed, while nice to possess, isn't the answer. All the technology in the world isn't going to make that medicolegal document correct—only you can do that with your expertise.

Judith Marshall
Medicate Me

produce an accurate medical record. Taking the time to consult up-to-date references or other healthcare professionals is the distinguishing feature between the professional and others who cannot be bothered to be medically accurate as they carelessly and thoughtlessly transcribe.

Professional medical transcriptionists demonstrate ethical values when dealing with confidential or personal information contained in the medical record. The professional resists gossiping about personal information contained in medical records and protects the right to privacy and confidentiality for each patient.

Professional medical transcriptionists demonstrate a disciplined work attitude with dedication to the needs of the patient before personal needs.

Professional medical transcriptionists display a commitment to continuing education by setting a high standard of performance and knowledge. The professional welcomes new knowledge and readily participates in educational efforts, not only for personal enrichment, but also for the collective benefit of the entire healthcare team.

Professional medical transcriptionists view co-workers as valuable members of the healthcare team, treating them with dignity and courtesy.

Through their conduct and attitude, professional medical transcriptionists can demonstrate to the public and other medical professionals that they are indeed disciplined, knowledgeable, and dedicated members of the healthcare team.

What Is a Medical Transcriptionist?

by Judith Marshall

Medical transcriptionists are very special people. We are workers who sign our initials on each finished product; we are craftspersons in a modern age. We are the experts in the complicated machinery of today—word processing units, computers, and digital dictation.

But more importantly, we are the practitioners of communication. We are the magicians of medical terminology, the masters of grammar and punctuation, and our expertise flows through related areas of pharmacology and the sophisticated new instruments from the operating room. We are the trained ears who create sense out of many diverse accents, and sometimes, just plain nonsense.

And one of the hallmarks of a medical transcriptionist is the willingness to share. Like the great cooks of the world who share their recipes, we try to help the newcomer, the student fledgling, and each other with the tricks of the trade—how to check under *ph* when the word sounds like it begins with *f*, how to find something under *disease* or *syndrome* when all we hear is a proper name.

I think we all evidence, to a great degree, a commonality of compassion. Marching across our view each day are life and death, struggle with disease, social problems, and sometimes (thank goodness) the human comedy.

We have our ethics and we have our morals. Medical transcriptionists know more about a patient than anyone else except the physician. We practice discretion. We wade through gallons of urinalyses and rivers of blood samples, and we know the chemical state of the patient as well as the most intimate details of the social history.

Although we may be half-crazed after a morning of 30 T&A's (tonsillectomies and adenoidectomies) or cataract extractions, or 30 chest x-rays (all of which were normal), we just appear to have a glazed, bored look.

But when we transcribe a birth record, often the medical transcriptionist breathes a silent "welcome on board, kid" to the new arrival. When a discharge summary becomes a death summary, often we are saddened, no matter how old the patient.

When transcribing surgery, major or minor, when we hear "The patienttoleratedtheproceduriwellandleftthe-operatingroomingoodcondition," we often think, "Good," not just because the report is over but because it was a successful surgery.

And in the medical offices, how fortunate the patient is to have a friendly personal relationship with the guardian of the medical record, the medical transcriptionist. Like the personnel in the drug company, the insurance company, and the laboratory, the dedicated professional in transcription serves the healthcare consumer—the patient.

So, if you know that *café au lait* is not a Spanish cheer, that *peau d'orange* is not orange sauce for a duck, that *bilirubin* is not the name of a little boy, that a *CABG* ("cabbage") *patch* has nothing to do with Br'er Rabbit, that *Takahashi* is not a new Japanese car, and if you know the great tunnels of Boston and New York, the Callahan Tunnel, the Sumner Tunnel, and the carpal tunnel—you speak the language of medical transcription professionals.

Criticism

by Marcy Diehl

Criticism first became a subject for conversation in my life about 30 years ago when I went to work for a prominent thoracic and cardiovascular surgeon. During the course of the interview, he asked me if I was able to take criticism gracefully. Well, I was stumped. No one had ever asked before; they had just handed it out, and I really didn't known how gracefully I had accepted what I had had so far. It depended on who was dishing it out, I guess.

I thought about my response, worrying that my prospective job somehow hinged on what I had to say one way or the other. I felt he would have liked for me to say something like "Oh, I love criticism" or even "I never need it!" Evidently I gave the right answer, however (he did hire me), when I replied, "Well, I guess we'll have to find out, won't we?" This answer implied to him that he would hire me and that we would both see how his criticism and my acceptance of it went along.

But I was now on the alert. I was forewarned that criticism was, in fact, a big possibility, and I worked very hard against the day when "we" would find out how gracefully I could accept it. I really didn't know where it would come from. There were a lot of possibilities; the day seemed fraught with them.

That was just the first day.

By the second day, I found out. That was the day my first transcripts were returned. Large permanent blue-black ink circles covered the many carefully prepared documents. It was hard to be graceful when I looked at the ruination of a half-day's labors (actually, half a night, too, as I had spent long hours at home researching unfamiliar words).

We had weeks of that, and I was getting discouraged; still graceful, I presume, but discouraged. The errors were becoming fewer and fewer, but that didn't seem to help much, since I wanted them to disappear. It was harder and harder to face up to them somehow, now that I was feeling more secure in the job. Grace was wearing thin. He never said anything. I never said anything. I just retyped. A lot.

Then two things happened. The surgeon's wife came into the office on Saturday morning when he proofread and busily marked up my work. She watched, appalled. Monday morning shortly after I arrived for work, she called "to see how you're taking it." "Fine," I said. She was relieved, and reported that she had talked to him about it, feeling that he had been too harsh. "Well," he said, "she won't learn if I don't teach her, and she's worth teaching."

I learned about grace that day. He took his precious time to teach and to help me. He had a B.S. in journalism and knew his Greek and Latin roots to a fine degree as well. I was pretty much humbled by his constant criticism, his love of perfection, and his belief in my potential for growth.

All of our lives we are both subjected to and the dispensers of criticism. If we can remember to accept it with the spirit in which it is given, realizing it took some time to critique our performance and that it was done because of our ultimate potential, we then must accept it not only with grace but with thanks.

Secondly, we must try to remember to give our criticism only with graciousness, knowing that we can help someone in whom we see the potential for personal or professional betterment, and not criticize to showcase our own skills. If we cannot criticize fairly, with love and in private, then we need to withhold it.

This is a lifelong relationship—us and criticism. We never should feel we have outgrown the need. If we protect ourselves by not doing anything new anymore, sticking to only what we do perfectly, then we will no longer grow in grace and wisdom.

How I Became a Medical Transcriptionist

by Bron Taylor

When I started my shift today, I turned on the computer, adjusted the ergonomic chair and keyboard tray from my desk partner's settings to mine, and changed the monitor to a fresh set of colors. Then I checked my electronic mailbox. I found a format for a new type of clinic note, which I downloaded, quickly read, and filed in my procedure manual. Next I looked at the statistics and saw that we were very caught up, so I relaxed a bit. I felt a little like an airline pilot, booting up and adjusting all this powerful equipment.

When I turned on my digital transcriber, my first piece of work was a stat discharge summary. During the dictation, the doctor mentioned the Kleihauer-Betke test. As it

had been many months since I'd last heard this, I thought I'd better check it. Was it really Kleihauer or Kleihaure? I could have left my terminal and found it in a reference book, or asked a co-worker, but as I was working on a stat, I used our on-line Homemade Dictionary instead, confirming that I had all the vowels in the right places (yes; Kleihauer), and within seconds I was back in the report.

When I was through, I phoned from the off-site office where I work to the transcription unit at the medical center, to let them know a stat was being printed; it was already coming off the printer and was quickly tubed to the floor. Only then did it strike me—the contrast between the equipment I used in the early 1970s, and the high-tech equipment of 1996 [the time of this article]. . . .

I was 28 years old when I discovered there was such a thing as transcription. I was extremely fortunate in how I discovered it, and yet I don't think my story is that different from that of others who have been doing this work for more than 20 years. There were no formal training courses when we started. One way or another, we stumbled onto the existence of the job; usually someone in a position to give us a chance to learn, someone who always needed more MTs, became aware of us and made the connection for us. Some didn't have this kind of mentoring and had to gamble that they could learn on the job, promising skills they didn't have but quickly developed.

I'd gone to college straight out of high school and married straight out of college, so I was 28 and unskilled when I was finally looking for my first job in the early 1970s, after an amicable divorce. After a long search, I finally found an entry-level job in the file room at a university teaching hospital. As I'd always loved everything about medicine, and would have gone to medical school had my math skills been strong, I was pleased to be working in a medical center, right in the midst of the real thing.

During the day there would be slow times when nobody wanted a record from my rows of files. I'd pull a thick chart and read it without looking at the name on it. One day a woman I knew only as "that nice lady who works in the back somewhere" caught me at it, but was smiling. Soon we were talking whenever she came looking for a chart, and she elicited from me that I'd been pre-med, loved to read, loved medicine, and, curiously, couldn't type. Why would she want to know that, I wondered. I had met Vera Pyle.

Soon I started working weekends, and part of my job was to change a broad band of tape when a bell rang. I didn't have the vaguest idea what I was doing, but carefully followed instructions. Vera Pyle was often in on weekends, and one day she asked if I'd like to be shown around the transcription department. "Yes," I said. So she showed me the cubicles, the Correcting Selectric typewriters, the reference material (at great length, as I was awed), and the Homemade Dictionary. She told me

The Medical *Editor*

Many of us were not even aware transcription existed as a profession until we fell into it. Some individuals were put in front of a typewriter and learned on the job with little to no references. Some were medical assistants or doctor's office secretaries who were pushed into it as part of their duties. Some went to school and earned degrees or certificates to obtain employment in this field. Whatever the circumstances, we all found ourselves here in a profession we are very passionate about.

Not all of us share the same roles. We are transcriptionists, editors, trainers, educators, consultants, supervisors, managers, and service owners; however, we are ALL medical documentation specialists.

Just as the profession of transcription continues to evolve, so must the skills and knowledge base of the transcriptionists. The once very green and inexperienced MT continues to learn, grow, and evolve into an experienced MT and then possibly moves on to become lead MT, trainer, QA editor, or even a supervisor or manager. When does this miraculous transformation occur? Does an MT simply wake up one morning and *presto!* is an editor? It takes years of experience to fine-tune the skills necessary, and continuing education is a necessity to remain relevant in the work force.

For the experienced MT, think back to when you were a new MT. Remember listening over and over to the same phrase in a dictation and not having a clue what Dr. Speedracer was trying to say? If you were in an office or hospital setting, you remember the trainer or the MT you asked to come "have a listen." You remember that person very confidently looking at you and telling you exactly what the doctor just dictated, and you wondered how on earth he/she understood that. You proceed to listen AGAIN, but this time knowing what it is, you hear it clear as day, all the while looking at that experienced MT with astonishment. Fast forward 6 months or so, and a new MT asks you to listen to that same doctor. You listen to it once and then look at them without hesitation and tell them exactly what was just dictated. Remember that same look of astonishment from them when they "get it"?

Many MTs have the privilege of working from home; however, one of the greatest challenges for a new person working from home is that you do not have the advantage of having that "second ear." A good transcription company will have a system set up for every new person to be assigned to a trainer or editor—that second ear. This allows work done by a student to be sent to an experienced person to proof the work prior to delivery to the facility and also for a relatively new but learning MT to have a trouble spot in a dictation filled in. This allows for continuing education for the new MT. It is critical that feedback be provided and is timely to assist in their training. This evolution in technology and in the profession has created a need for qualified MTs to serve as editors and trainers, all healthcare documentation specialists.

The skills needed to be a great transcriptionist are the very foundation of a healthcare documentation specialist: excellent proofreading skills, at least two years of acute-care experience, a good ear, proficient research abilities, and strong communication skills.

One of the great benefits of being a transcriptionist or an editor is that we all learn something new every day, but even more so as an editor. As you listen to dictation and review transcribed documents done by a student or new person, proofreading skills are enhanced, and you have the ability to learn from others' mistakes. There are skill-building exercises available to help hone these skills.

Editing medical reports is where superb communication skills come into play. Corrected reports and constructive feedback are critical to the success of students and new MTs. The first reports are strewn with blanks and incorrect terms. As time progresses and the communication cycle continues, you will see fewer and fewer blanks and incorrect terms. You will see perfect reports eventually come through, and the gratitude of the new MT or student is immeasurable. You share in their accomplishments.

An often-overlooked role of the MT of the future is that of editor. The increased use of offshore transcription has created a demand for experienced MTs to serve as editors who understand the idiosyncrasies of the English language, ones who understand the difference between a veteran who was "deployed to Iraq" versus one who was "decoyed to a rack."

As speech recognition technology continues to improve, so will the demand for experienced MTs to serve as medical editors. There will always be the clinician who is unable to use speech recognition for a myriad of reasons, so there will always be the need for the essential MT skill set; however, the MT of the future needs to transform into much more—a hybrid MT. That MT must develop editing skills.

Source: April Martin, "Evolution of the Healthcare Documentation Specialist," *Plexus*, Vol. 1, Issue 6, November 2005, pp. 8-9.

how the dictionary had been developed in the transcription unit and how it was kept up-to-date. Any MT could make entries, but they had to be verified and not just "doctors' spelling." I wondered what that meant. She explained about the tape equipment and why I was changing belts. She asked me again if I could type, and I had to say no. It felt as if a door was closing.

The campus newspaper printed an article about transcriptionists, including Vera Pyle, and I read it again and again, not even realizing that I wanted to do this so badly I couldn't even admit it to myself. Vera could see that, though. In our talks she'd told me the ingredients for a good transcriptionist. One had to love medicine, love researching words, have a good feel for English grammar, and a good ear for accents. One had to respect the patient behind the paper of the medical record and never ever *guess* what a physician was saying. I can do that, I thought to myself, but couldn't type, so I didn't even consider it. Sometimes I'd listen to the sound of fast typing from the transcription department in action, and it seemed hopeless. I didn't realize then that typing was the least of it.

The university normally required an MT to have two years of acute care hospital experience before hiring, but Vera Pyle received permission to train me and a co-worker from the hospital laundry. She asked us if we'd commit to work on transcription for an hour each day if she agreed to teach us. We were speechless. We promised to read reports, read journals, and work as hard as we could to learn.

Over the years I learned transcription and then went on to learn transcription theory, editing, and editing theory, opening the door not only to a career I've enjoyed but to work as a writer and editor.

I was very tentative at first, in a room with such experts. The first documents I produced were thanks to a resident physician who was afraid of the phone, who handwrote all her consultations which then had to be copy-typed. None of the MTs wanted to do her work, which mystified me then, but now I understand. Happily for me, she was a pediatric endocrinologist with good handwriting, so my first documents were thick with complex lab work and gave me a sense of format. As Vera realized, of course, doing all of this copy-typing was good practice for my beginning typing skills. I typed as much as I could in the clerical part of the day.

During my "transcription hour," I'd work until I'd asked everyone in the room at least one question, like "Is there such a thing as Betadine?" After that I dared not bother anyone twice, so I'd retype the work. Of course, I quickly did learn how to type, and I'm now as irritable as anyone when someone walks into a room full of MTs, listens to rapid typing, and says, "Oooh, how fast do you type?"

Every piece of work I did, Vera proofread. I think I had some of the most intensive proofreading anyone has ever had. I wanted to capture every nuance, every subtlety. I liked the medical center's style, demanding full sentences in every part of the report with consistent tenses, with lab work written in narrative style and divided into the correct categories. BUN and creatinine were put in a separate sentence from electrolytes, never mind what the dictator said. We were expected to know that a differential was not part of a routine CBC and punctuate accordingly. Work coming out of our unit didn't look or read like something sent by Western Union. (It has taken me many years to lighten up and accept that in some cases a telegraphic or clipped style communicates just as well, and using it is not a moral failing.)

Now it's many years later. I've helped to write, edit, and proofread many books, and had many articles published by three publishers. I'm just as pleased with transcription and just as proud to be an MT and just as curious as to what the next dictation will reveal as I was at the beginning. Vera gave me a strong foundation, and when I later went to work as a proofreader for a large service, in pathology, in radiology, and at home for researchers. I was rarely challenged as I had been working for her at the university medical center.

Why do we have a rule "never guess"? Because a wrong guess, a soundalike but incorrect medication, will go into someone's permanent record, and be picked up and repeated, and could cause harm. The same rule that applies to everyone in the medical profession—Hippocrates' "First, do no harm"—applies to us too. Transcription decisions are made based on what in the end will best serve the patient.

Many of us were given a chance to learn transcription by a manager who needed more MTs and saw potential in someone with no experience. Very few of us knew that this niche in the medical field existed until one day we stumbled on it by accident. I don't think too many of us as children said, "I want to be a medical transcriptionist when I grow up." I'm glad that such good teaching materials exist now, and that transcription teachers are everywhere, with that field becoming a profession in itself. This raises the level of transcription and everyone benefits.

Patient Confidentiality

by Linda C. Campbell

Medical transcriptionists are pledged to protect the privacy and confidentiality of the individual health record. They must never acknowledge or disclose that they are privy to personal, medical, or social patient information. Even if a patient is a relative, friend, or celebrity, the details of every report must remain absolutely confidential. This is true in every work setting.

A privately owned medical transcription company once ran an ad in several allied health publications picturing a home-based medical transcriptionist in her bathrobe, gossiping on the telephone to her friend, with a crying baby nearby in a playpen. The caption read, "Madge, you won't believe what I just found out about your neighbor!" The implication was, of course, that a medical transcriptionist working at home is more likely to breach confidentiality than one who is working in an office or within the confines of a hospital. Is this a valid conclusion?

In the past, medical transcriptionists who "came up through the ranks"—that is, those who were trained and then practiced medical transcription solely in the hospital or clinic environment—were often directly involved in some way with patients' medical records. This may have included accessing patient charts to find specific information or even "charting" transcribed reports (physically placing transcribed reports in patient charts). The need for confidentiality of the patient health record was well understood within this environment.

Today there are many practicing medical transcriptionists who have never set foot in a hospital health information or transcription department. Having learned their craft in a college setting or private company, they have gone on to work in transcription services or at home and have never worked directly with patient charts. These transcriptionists may have signed confidentiality agreements in which they commit to hold all patient information in the strictest confidence. But merely signing a confidentiality agreement does not necessarily mean that they truly understand all that the term "breach" encompasses. Because breach of confidentiality is one of the few areas in health information management where the transcriptionist can be held liable, its importance cannot be overstated.

The following are true case histories that describe encounters with health information. Which are breaches of confidentiality? Case reviews follow each case history.

1. A transcriptionist sees the name of a friend on a hospital inpatient roster. He phones the patient's room and says, "I heard you're in the hospital. Would you like a visitor this evening?"

Case review. Unless the patient gave the hospital permission to release his name and room number, the transcriptionist is breaching confidential patient information by contacting his friend in the hospital. It doesn't matter that the transcriptionist avoided telling his friend where he got the information—the patient has the right to privacy. This incident indicates either inadequate education regarding the extent of confidentiality, or lack of professionalism on the part of the transcriptionist.

2. A transcriptionist overhears two lab technicians discussing a patient by name. Because she transcribed the patient's operative report earlier, the transcriptionist is familiar with the patient's history. As she listens to their conversation, she realizes they have inaccurate information. "You've got it wrong," she interjects. "The woman in 413 had a therapeutic abortion, not just a D&C."

Case review. It's certainly possible that the transcriptionist felt it was all right to set the record straight with fellow workers; however, it was not her prerogative to do so under these circumstances. The information did not promote patient care and could even be construed as gossip. Knowledge obtained from transcribing a report should not be discussed with co-workers and must never be related to anyone other than those with a valid need to know.

3. A physician admits an Elvis impersonator for facial plastic surgery. The medical transcriptionists on the evening shift eagerly locate the chart after the patient is discharged to look at the "before" and "after" pictures.

Case review. Curiosity does not justify the violation of confidential patient information.

4. Your mother has had quintuple bypass surgery. You are a medical transcriptionist working at home, and you want to help your mother better understand her medical condition. You call your friends in the health information department of the hospital where she is a patient and ask them to make photocopies for you of any report they transcribe on your mother.

Case review. The home worker is not utilizing proper channels to obtain report transcripts on her mother. The health information sought might be legally obtainable, but it must be procured in accordance with regulations. Even if the patient is a relative or friend, the details of every report must remain absolutely confidential; thus, the appropriate action on the part of hospital staff would be to deny the request.

5. A transcriptionist employed by a private company transcribes what she believes to be a sexual abuse case. The physician fails to report the case to the proper authorities. The transcriptionist contacts state authorities and relates the incident.

Case review. This is a very serious breach of confidentiality. Even where state laws mandate the reporting of suspected child abuse, that reporting is the responsibility of the hospital or the examining physician, not the transcriptionist. (What actually transpired in this incident is that the transcriptionist was in error about the validity of the child abuse, and she was successfully sued for violation of confidentiality.)

6. You transcribe at home for a private practice physician. He uses your call-in line and frequently dictates from

The Gourmet *Medical Transcriptionist*

All right, I confess. I'm the one who sends dinner menus to my friends; lunch menus too. I also have to admit that it is unnerving to hear the disembodied voice of my boss on my message service, enunciating very clearly and sternly, "Nae, you cannot fool me. I know darn well you are there. It is the first of the month and your cooking magazines just came. STOP reading and START transcribing right now!" Well, honestly, I did plan to get back to work just as soon as I finished that fascinating article on gutting and cleaning squid.

No matter what kind of dictation we transcribe—acute care or chart notes—the words we listen to daily, in all their graphic detail, have a profound and direct impact on the food we plan to eat. Let's face it, transcribing bowel resections and the odd proctoscopy or two does not make that hunk of liver, thoughtlessly tossed in the sink to thaw, look appetizing at all. In fact, the sight of it will undoubtedly quell any desire to come near the kitchen for a very long time.

It is important to realize that there is an art to this, a subtle matching of words and ingredients. While I cannot be considered an expert, I have had considerable experience in making those critical dinner menu decisions. Sometimes the determining factor is a dictator's accent, some tiny little thing in the patient history, and sometimes just a background noise. I do have to admit that acute-care dictation, with its wide variety of accents, dictators, and different reports, is a virtual cornucopia of fertile food for thought.

For instance, the proctoscopy . . . every now and then I get a French physician who makes a proctoscopy sound positively romantic. The sound of those sibilant syllables can lead me directly to mental visions of mussels gently steamed in white wine, crusty French bread, real butter, and little green cornichon pickles for tartness.

A certain Asian dictator had me considering stir fry one day until I remembered there were no shrimp in the freezer. I continued transcribing until I heard the sound of a radiologist from Pakistan and remembered I had some cans of white beans on hand, pita bread, and eggplant in the garden. A Southern physician is sure to trigger a frenzy of black-eyed peas, cornbread, ham slices, or maybe buttermilk biscuits, collards, fried chicken, and sliced tomatoes from the garden with a tiny sprinkling of olive oil.

One of my favorites (I keep these ingredients on hand because I have this dictator frequently) is a surgeon from Jamaica. Just the way those vowels roll around, the cadence of his spoken words, you can bet we are having jerk chicken done on the grill.

Patient names can do it as well. A woman from Hungary created quite a dilemma for me as I had no paprika in the spice rack. A desperate phone call to a friend finally solved that problem. You simply cannot make a proper goulash without paprika!

No matter how you look at it, this matching up stuff is not easy. The consequences of a mismatch are immediately obvious. A little forethought and planning are essential ingredients in the process. Just because you hear island music in the background of a dictation does not mean the family is going to be particularly enthusiastic about recreating an official version of a Hawaiian cooking pit in the front yard. The desire to create authenticity is most certainly going to suffer a setback if someone has to put on rubber boots and slog through the swamp searching for the right palm tree to cut down in order to produce a genuine hearts of palm salad.

Asian dictators bring out my creative side. I have discovered that it is possible to use up practically anything lurking in the refrigerator just by plopping it in a wok. So it was indeed disheartening when the family simply sat in silence when I presented them with a truly inspired dish of baby corn, shiitaki mushrooms, and fried softshell crab.

I still cannot figure out why those blue corn tortillas, lovingly created one night because one of my dictators happened to examine a native American Indian, remained untouched. It is true that they were slightly more gray than blue, with a texture reminiscent of fried washing machine lint, but that is no excuse.

While I cannot exactly blame that 90-year-old Polish patient (he kept singing Polish ditties during his neurological exam), it is certainly true that Southern smoked sausage does not blend with sauerkraut and caraway seeds as well as kielbasa would have. I did discover that chicken gizzards make a suitable substitution for sweetbreads in a dish from Provence. But someone forgot to mention that when making a cassoulet, it is essential to use a really DEEP dish because, if you don't, those beans and juices just ooze to the bottom of the oven, making a stink you would not believe.

I am constantly amazed when I read threads on Internet message boards on how boring medical transcription can be, typing the same thing day after day, same procedures, same words. I never seem to have that problem. After all, there is always that evening meal to plan ahead for, and who knows what might spark the creative juices!

Renee Priest
Perspectives on the Medical Transcription Profession

his cellular phone, where he isn't bothered by office noise or children at home.

Case review. The physician and the transcription company owner may be unaware of the fact that cellular phones are not secure. These transmissions can be intercepted by anyone with inexpensive eavesdropping equipment. The dictation should be done only on traditional phone lines and not from cars, portable phones, or airplanes.

7. A medical transcription service owner in a large metropolitan area is interviewing job applicants. One applicant proudly shows the service owner samples of work she has transcribed at a different facility in the same town. The service owner observes that patient names appear on the reports.

Case review. The applicant not only violated patient confidentiality by taking documents from a facility, but she left the patient names on the documents. The service owner who spoke with this applicant advised her that showing work samples was inappropriate since the sample documents could have been someone else's work. Furthermore, the service owner stated that he would not hire the applicant under any circumstances because she had blatantly violated patient confidentiality by not removing or obscuring the names in the documents.

Protecting confidentiality. During World War II there was a popular slogan that was printed and posted prominently: "Loose lips sink ships." In other words, the slightest breach of confidentiality may cause irreparable damage. There are several steps that you as the transcriptionist can take to promote the confidentiality of the patient healthcare record.

1. Use document shredders to dispose of discarded health information sheets, photocopied documents, or other printed matter containing confidential health information that is no longer needed.
2. Clarify standards for the use of demographic information which is computer-downloaded to other settings.
3. Adhere to the length of time that documents can be retained in computer hard drives by employees or outside contractors and the means by which confidential information is deleted.
4. Verify guidelines for archiving, and adhere to security measures that must be taken when modeming, faxing, or using other unsecured communication lines.
5. Use passwords and encryption methods where appropriate.
6. If you are working in an environment that is not secure from prying eyes, whether at home or in an office, use privacy screens. These prohibit anyone from reading the monitor who is not sitting directly in front of it.

7. Never leave your desk with confidential information on the monitor screen.
8. Make sure that your environment is secure from intruders. A hospital in California went to great expense to implement state-of-the-art computers networked to their satellite facilities, running sophisticated software programs, then neglected to provide adequate locks and alarm systems. A resulting break-in resulted in the theft of millions of dollars' worth of computer equipment—and an untold amount of confidential patient information—when the thieves just walked out with computers in hand.

Finally, understand that the penalties for violation of confidential patient information will probably include immediate dismissal or termination of contract and legal liability for violations. In other words, you can be fired and sued.

Because confidentiality is a critical issue, your employer will inform you of the facility's policy about patient confidentiality. The employer may also require you to sign a **confidentiality statement** and will inform you of the penalties for violating patient confidentiality. In most facilities a breach of patient confidentiality is grounds for immediate dismissal from the job. See the article on HIPAA (p. 6) for further discussion of issues of confidentiality and protected health information.

Transcribing Foreign Accents

by Susan Dooley and Ellen Drake

As more foreign-born physicians and other allied health professionals for whom English is a second language become a part of the American healthcare scene, medical transcriptionists are faced with an increasing number of ESL (English as a second language) dictators. This is a scary experience for newcomers to the MT profession, and even seasoned MTs often find transcribing for ESL dictators to be a major challenge.

Successfully translating the dictation of those who are foreign-born requires one to become familiar with the speech patterns of various nationalities, bearing in mind that English is a very difficult language that has few hard-and-fast rules. One must give credit to those ESL dictators who do their best to communicate clearly in what is essentially two languages rolled into one—English/medical.

The syntax in many foreign languages is entirely different from what is found in English, and ESL dictators often have difficulty wrapping their tongues around sounds that are not common in their own languages. For example, there is no *p* sound in Arabic, and for many healthcare professionals whose native language is Arabic, a *p* sound may be converted to a *b* sound. A transcriptionist who worked for a time in Saudi Arabia reported that she was confused by the request from a resident physician for what sounded like a *boberglib*, and it was only after much discussion that she was able to determine that the young man was seeking a paper clip.

Foreign-accented dictation seems very daunting at first. Approach it as a challenge. Believe it or not, the accent that seems totally unintelligible at first will eventually become second nature. Remember—the more versatile and capable you are as a transcriptionist, the more valuable you will be in the employment market.

Sometimes it helps to make a game of it. Perhaps a dictator will sound like Roseanna Danna, Ricky Ricardo, or Crocodile Dundee to you. Relating an accent to a familiar character from TV or the movies can, silly as it seems, help get your ears "into the rhythm" of the accent of a foreign dictator. It may help you to listen ahead; the dictator may repeat the word in question more clearly, or context clues may help you to choose the correct word.

It is a good idea to keep your own list of foreign pronunciations of English words. In your notebook, write the word phonetically the way it sounded to you, write the word correctly spelled, and note the nationality of the dictator if you know it. This practice will increase your awareness of pronunciation variants and improve your ability to understand foreign dictators.

General anomalies. Often, in an attempt to be clear in dictation, the speaker may pronounce final consonants so that it sounds like there is an added syllable at the end of a word, like *chestah* for *chest*. Sometimes, *ed* endings are made into separate syllables; the word *explained*, for example, is pronounced *ex-plain-ed*.

It's also very common for speakers to place emphasis on the wrong syllable of a word, like *ba-SI-tra-cin* instead of *ba-ci-TRA-sin* (bacitracin), or *ter-EE-ter-EE* for *TER-i-tor-ee* (territory). Additional examples are *deb-BRISS* for *debris* (correctly pronounced *de-BREE*), *per-i-TON-eum* for *per-i-to-NE-um* (also, *peri-TON-eal*), *rezi-DOO-al* for *re-SIJ-oo-al* (residual), *cap-PI-lar-ees* for *CAP-i-lar-ees* (capillaries), *ce-fo-TOX-i-ME* for *cefotoxime*, *ce-FIX-i-ME* for *cefixime*, *obi-SI-ty* for *obesity*, *vera-PAM-il* for *verapamil*.

Sometimes several words may sound like one word because the dictator does not pause between them. Conversely, one word may sound like several words, or pauses may occur so that syllables from one word appear to be part of the following word, as in *intap* [pause]*ering* dose for *in tapering dose*. When all else fails, try to write out the sounds you hear, syllable by syllable. Once the sounds are on paper, you may more readily see that several words are involved.

Watch for interchange of personal pronouns—sometimes the dictator refers to the patient as *he* for *she* or may use the possessive *his* and *her* for the opposite sex in the same report.

In some languages, there are no articles; thus, when translating to English, the speaker may drop *a*, *an*, or *the* preceding a noun. In languages where an article precedes every noun, the speaker may add articles when translating into English. These articles may occasionally sound like part of the trailing word rather than a separate word. If the word you are hearing has an initial vowel sound, you may want to drop off the initial sound and determine if what is left is a complete word.

Word endings such as *-s*, *-ed*, *-al*, and *-ive* may not be pronounced. The transcriptionist should use the proper noun, adjective, or verbal form of a word called for in the sentence, even if the dictator did not. Also, the final sounds of some words ending in *m* may be dropped—for example, *spaz* for *spasm*, *neoplaz* for *neoplasm*. Internal syllables may be omitted as well; thus, *transluminal* may become *transminal*.

A *schwa* (∂ like a soft short *e*) sound may be added in the middle of a word, creating an extra syllable. Examples: *ad-∂-van-tage*, *ad-∂-ven-ture*, *ad-∂-vance*. Some dictators may use word endings not used in English—*abdomens* for *abdomen*, *feets* for *feet*, or *childs* for *children*.

Foreign physicians may choose an incorrect word that is similar in meaning to the one intended but does not exactly fit. For example, they may say *look* for *see*, *prolonged* for *extended*. One gastroenterologist consistently dictated on a colonoscopy report that the scope was "slided up" the colon. This could be edited to *slid*, but a better edit might be *advanced*.

Unfamiliar words and expressions may be used that the transcriptionist thinks must be a mistake but are not. One Indian physician dictated, "Please *vide* (VI-DEE) the anesthesia record," the word *vide* a Latin term meaning "see."

Many Spanish dialects add an *eh* sound before words that begin with the letter *s*, so that skin becomes *eskin*, spine becomes *espine*, stone becomes *estone*, etc. *Eh* is often used by foreign dictators the way Americans use *uh*, as a filler when thinking.

Pronunciations that cannot be categorized. An East Indian physician pronounced *trivial* as *tri-gal* or *tri-ger*, both syllables receiving equally heavy accent. *Basically* was pronounced *vesi-CA-ee*. One physician pronounced a patient's name like *Fuller*, spelled what sounded like *F-O-W-E-R*; the patient's name was *Fowler*. A phrase sounding like *double-up pain* (a somewhat logical and reasonable-sounding expression for a foreign dictator) was actually *developed pain*.

Punctuation. The punctuation mark comma (,) may be pronounced *KO-ma*, which sounds just like the medical word *coma*. Sometimes foreign speakers use the term *point* to indicate a *period* (.), *two points* to indicate a *colon* (:), *dot* to mean a *period* (.), *stop* or *full stop* to mean a *period* (.). For European speakers, *stop* can also mean a *comma* (,). East Indians often say *perrid* with the rolled *r* for *period* (.).

Note: When the word *period* is dictated, it does not always signify a punctuation mark; it may be that you are to type the word. For example, "The patient denied any new complaints during this period." You might also hear *new line* for *new sentence* or *new paragraph*.

Both native and foreign speakers of English frequently dictate the wrong punctuation. You should edit for correctness. Foreign dictators tend to place adverbs and adjectives according to their native syntax, not ours. For example, a Spanish speaker might say, "A polyp, large, was in the colon," instead of "A large polyp was in the colon," or "tolerated well the procedure," instead of "tolerated the procedure well." Edit them to the correct English syntax.

Prepositions can also be a problem for foreign dictators. "Patient agreed *for* the discharge," should be edited to "The patient agreed *to* the discharge." *In* and *on* are also frequently confused.

Remember that when one learns a new language, one tends to use the rules of syntax from one's native language, whether they are correct or not. For this reason, always be prepared for grammatical errors and know how to correct them.

Feeling the Need for Speed

by Georgia Green

Which is more important to success in the medical transcription field: quality or production? The answer should be obvious. It doesn't matter how many reports you can produce in an hour, a day, or an entire pay period if those reports contain medical inaccuracies or if misspellings, typos, and errors in grammar and punctuation compromise their readability. That doesn't mean productivity is not an issue. Speed does count when it comes to the size of a paycheck based on production wages and even more so when mandated minimum production requirements determine whether or not you will continue to be employed. So how can a medical transcription student increase production without jeopardizing quality?

Proceed with caution. This article gives specific suggestions for improving your productivity, but these suggestions must be prefaced with this cautionary note: Speed should be the furthest thing from your mind until the last stages of training. Traditional speed-building techniques work by eliminating redundancies, but it is these same redundancies that are an essential element of fundamental transcription training. Taking shortcuts of

any kind undermines the learning process, with the end result being decreased overall production and quality. Looking up the same term for a second, third, or fourth time is not a wasted effort but an investment in building your fund of medical knowledge.

Until you have committed to memory the widest possible range of medical concepts and its associated vocabulary, avoid spell-checkers, macros, expanders, or templates. Electronic references that link terms with their definitions are fine for student use. If you keep a quick reference word list, manual or electronic, jot down a brief definition with each entry to reinforce these connections in your mind every time you consult the list.

After completing the entire *Medical Transcription Fundamentals & Practice* course, transcribing each report twice and achieving an acceptable accuracy score on the final attempt, you can focus your attention on speed-building techniques in random practice sessions before moving to more advanced training.

Defining terms. It is important to understand the difference between *production* and *productivity*. Your total output, whether lines, characters, or number of reports, during your regularly scheduled workday is your production. Productivity, on the other hand, is a measure of your rate of production over a standard unit of time, e.g., lines per hour. If you work more hours per day, you increase your production but not your productivity. However, as your proficiency as an MT improves, you can increase both your productivity AND your production.

Let's look at a student whose productivity is 100 lines per hour. If that student's total production for a particular 8-hour workday is only 400 lines, there is a discrepancy of 4 hours. Perhaps it was necessary to slow down in order to accommodate a difficult dictator or two or three. But there is still a large chunk of time spent with an idle keyboard. Some of this downtime is a necessary part of the job—researching new terms, reviewing instructions for format and style, overcoming the occasional problem with hardware or software, and time spent mastering a new work procedure or productivity technique.

When it is appropriate to turn your attention to increasing your speed, keep a notepad next to your keyboard and keep track of time away from the keyboard so you can analyze it later. Use a chart with columns to designate various types of "down time"—word research, technical problems, consulting another person, and so on—and then just make check marks in each column to indicate each 5-minute block spent in an activity away from the keyboard.

Investment in your fund of medical knowledge. Even the clearest dictation can stump you if you encounter a term that is unfamiliar. And if you don't understand the concept behind a term, you can't be sure that what you are hearing is correct. A deficit in your internal medical knowledge database correlates directly with both the amount of time you spend researching unfamiliar terms and the number of mistakes you will make in selecting the right term. The best defense is a well-rounded program of study that includes academic coursework in the structure and function of the human body, human diseases, physical diagnosis and treatment, pharmacology, laboratory medicine, and more.

Practice makes perfect. There are so many different ways to express the same idea, and for each of these variations in expression there are hundreds of ways for an individual dictator to render a passage containing that idea in a nearly incomprehensible manner. The only way you can gain a reasonable level of competency is to engage in as much practice as possible, transcribing each report as many times as necessary to achieve mastery not only of the content but also the nuances of a particular dictator's voice and style, many of which are missed on a single pass at a report.

Once you enter the workplace, you lose this wonderful opportunity for true mastery unless you are lucky enough to encounter a supervisor or mentor who understands this concept and makes work assignments that include enough repetition to allow you the opportunity for continued mastery. While you are still a student, it is crucial that you understand the role of retranscription in "training your ear." Never take shortcuts here.

Comma chameleon. Does your understanding of grammar and punctuation allow you to supply necessary commas or correct verb tense as you transcribe, without consulting a style guide each time? Sometimes a dictator does mangle a sentence so badly that it will stop an English teacher in his tracks, but most of the time you should be able to make minor fixes without interrupting your rhythm. If this isn't a problem for you, this is one productivity leak you don't have to worry about. If it is a problem, don't worry—you can overcome it with some remedial work in grammar.

Grammar guides are invaluable and you should study them (a quick on-line guide is available at **http://www.grammarbook.com/**), but your study should include not just a review of rules but plenty of exercises, including bare-bones sentence diagramming. When you really get a solid understanding of sentence structure and why words and phrases are arranged the way they are, punctuation will fall into place much more easily. Here is a great Web site that can guide you through the basics of sentence diagramming: **http://www.geocities.com/ gene_moutoux/diagrams.htm**. Capital Community College hosts a comprehensive grammar site at **http://webster.commnet.edu/grammar/index.htm**. They provide a

section on diagramming sentences, but be sure to click the links for quizzes and for PowerPoint presentations and see everything they have to offer.

If you are enrolled in a formal program of study, don't forget to ask your instructor for advice. Your school may offer a nuts and bolts grammar course, and your instructor can help you find the course that is right for you.

Plug all the leaks. Close your eyes for a moment and imagine this scenario: You are transcribing along without a hitch, then all of a sudden you come to a grinding halt. Either you didn't hear something at all or what you heard didn't make sense. What do you do? Back it up and play again. And again. And again. Slower. Faster. Reread the sentence, the paragraph. Scan the whole report. Play the dictation forward and finish the paragraph or even the report. Should you grab a book? Which book? Should someone else listen?

We Take *Ourselves with Us*

My friend Judy tells the story of her six-year-old daughter who talked all the time in class instead of doing her work. She asked the teacher if her daughter could move to another seat where she would not be as likely to talk so much. The teacher observed, "Wherever Ann Marie goes, *she takes herself with her.*"

Perhaps that is why some of us have the same difficulties wherever we go—we take ourselves with us. Most of us blame everything and everybody but ourselves for our failures. "I lost that job because . . . " "I lost that account because . . . " "That relationship failed because . . . " We aren't happy in our jobs so we change jobs, thinking the job is the problem. Then we have the same or similar problems in the next job, and think another job is the answer. Or we can't get along with a client, so we dump that one, and sign up another. Or one consulting job after another is unsatisfactory, and we always blame the client. We think if we just change jobs, or change cities, or change clients, or change friends or family, things will work out.

If our personal insight enabled us to recognize that "wherever we go, we take ourselves with us," then perhaps we could better see who or what needs to be changed. Without self-awareness of our strengths and weaknesses, and using that knowledge to our advantage, we can't successfully control our speed, or strategies for moving forward, on the racetrack of life or business.

Sally C. Pitman
Perspectives on the Medical Transcription Profession

The answer may be "all of the above" or "none of the above," depending upon the circumstances, but developing an efficient process can contribute greatly to your productivity at the latter part of your training and as you transition to the work environment. An "efficient process" might also be referred to as "time management" as it refers to how you handle the inevitable constant interruptions in work flow that occur when you must pause on an unclear word or phrase, replay it, research it, ask for help, etc. If you waste 10 minutes at a time on only a dozen words during your transcription session, that totals two hours in lost production. Could that time have been cut down to one hour or even to just half an hour if your process was more efficient? When you are producing high-quality lines but far less than anticipated, this is usually the area that needs attention.

Most experienced productive MTs have an efficient process in place even if they aren't consciously aware of it and cannot explain it to you, and each MT will have his or her own twists that make that process unique. There is no single "one size fits all" process, but you can start with a guideline and gradually develop the process that you find most efficient for you. Here is one you can use as a starting point and customize it to meet your own style and available resources:

1. When you have stopped on a word, relisten to it one or two times.

2. Stop and ask yourself why you can't hear it—is it mumbled, too fast or too slow, obscured in some way, or is it a term you think you can hear clearly enough but just don't know? If you can hear it, but don't know it, skip down to #5.

3. If appropriate, speed up and slow down the dictation to see if this makes a difference. If the word was said too rapidly, say it aloud yourself syllable by syllable, fast and slow. Write down a phonetic equivalent and look at it. Does anything come to mind?

4. Reread the sentence the term occurs in or even the paragraph to develop a context. Ask yourself what kind of word should go here if you had to guess—is it a drug name, a body part, an English word?

5. Choose the right reference book for the job. If it is a drug name, go to a drug book, if it is an English word, try *Webster's*, if it is a body part go to your full-size medical dictionary. If you think it is a new term or if you have already checked your medical dictionary, check *Vera Pyle's Current Medical Terminology* (new, difficult, and hard-to-find terminology with definitions). Go to the appropriate specialty word book or general phrase index to narrow down your choices after consulting the medical dictionary—and then come back to the medical dictionary to confirm the meaning. Context is everything.

6. If you didn't hear enough of the word to look it up and you have an electronic reference, try a wild card search (refer to your software for instructions).

7. If the term seems to be part of a phrase, be sure to look up the parts you do hear as the term may appear as a cross-reference. If it is the name of a ligament, look also under *muscle* and *tendon* as you may find clues there.

8. STOP—don't spend more than five minutes researching in your books. Leave a blank (ideally with a phonetic "sounds like") and finish transcribing the report. Then come back to it. Many terms are repeated later in the report.

9. Come back to any missing terms at the end of the report and see if you can hear it now, given that you now know the whole context of the report and are more familiar with the dictator's voice.

10. If you come up empty, now is the time where judgment is required. Does it seem reasonable to leave a blank? This depends on both the expectations for your performance (is this practice dictation, a test, on the job under full QA review, or are you on your own?) and the circumstances of the dictation itself. Ask yourself if a more skilled MT would have been able to fill in this blank. If the dictation truly is garbled, very heavily accented, or obscured in some way, any MT may have had trouble. Leave the blank. Did you leave too many blanks in this report and how many blanks constitute too many? Again, consider your expectations. If you feel you are not ready to abandon the search for the term, give yourself 10 more minutes and include any Internet research within this time limit.

11. Make a note about how the term sounded and its context so you can research it later if no feedback is forthcoming from your teacher or supervisor.

Developing good judgment. The ability to make independent judgments grows out of a combination of confidence in your skills and awareness of your limitations—and definitely impacts your "process," as noted above. This can't be taught from a book per se but can be enhanced through the use of critical thinking exercises. Consider the old adage about giving a man a fish versus teaching him how to fish. If you learn not just how to solve a problem in a particular situation but instead develop a mental framework for addressing problems in varying circumstances, you are able to think independently and will be able to exercise reasonable MT judgment without a teacher standing by. A good source of critical thinking exercises can be found in *H&P: A Nonphysician's Guide to the Medical History and Physical Examination* available at **www.hpisum.com**.

Smoking those keys. One of the first things you learn when you begin transcribing is that your keyboarding speed on a copy-typing exercise has little to do with the speed at which you will transcribe. In fact, the faster your raw typing speed, the greater the percentage of speed loss. A 100-wpm typist will feel much more discouragement than a 45-wpm typist. Nevertheless, good keyboarding skills are prerequisite for any MT. Generally, keyboarding speed picks up naturally over time, but if it doesn't, this area may need attention. One has to be able to move quickly through dictation that flows smoothly to make up for time lost on the more challenging parts. Keyboarding speed in and of itself should be assessed periodically apart from actual transcribing speed, and any deficits that are discovered should be addressed. Luckily, an inexpensive software program can add 20 wpm onto your baseline keyboarding speed in just a couple of weeks.

Adding to your MT toolbox. As you near the end of training and AFTER you have addressed all the impediments to production discussed in this article, it is time to look at the myriad of tools used by experienced medical transcriptionists to enhance their productivity. Abbreviation expansion tools built into your word processing program or obtained through third party software can dramatically increase your production—after you have mastered all the basics presented here.

Employment Issues

Job Searching

by Ellen Drake

If you're like most students, you've been thinking about the job you want since your first days as a student, how much you're going to make, and how you're going to spend all that money. You probably have also been planning ahead and preparing your resumé, practicing for interviews, and learning all that you can so that you can make the best impression possible on a potential employer and live up to that impression.

Maybe you're not that well prepared, but it is foolish to wait until you have a certificate or diploma in hand to think about applying for a job. If you want to work as a medical transcriptionist in a local clinic, physician office, or hospital, you should be participating in the local professional association activities and getting to know MTs and supervisors.

If your school does not plan field trips to various hospitals and clinics, you may try to call transcription supervisors and ask if they have time to show you around their department. If working for a doctor's office appeals to you, talk to a few physician office transcriptionists and ask them for advice. Follow up with a handwritten, personal thank you note (not a preprinted card).

You may hear conflicting stories and sometimes negative comments about job openings, but don't be discouraged. The need for medical transcriptionists is well documented throughout the country. Even the want ads in the newspapers don't tell the whole story because many job openings are only periodically advertised or not advertised at all. The employers who need qualified transcriptionists often choose not to advertise because of the large number of unqualified applicants who respond or the fact that they pay a lot for the ads with no results.

A number of Internet sites list transcription openings. Use a search engine to find them. A suggested search might be "medical transcription classifieds." Be skeptical about what you read in some medical transcription forums and chat rooms, however. Some "job openings" are little more than scams to entice you into a poor training program. Although some transcription services may require you to purchase your own computer and ancillary equipment, any equipment specific to that company's operation should be provided by the company. If anyone asks you for money before you can begin to work, run away!

Be aware that opportunities for transcription jobs are numerous and varied. Besides hospitals and doctors' offices, those needing qualified MTs include clinics, HMOs, freestanding surgical and radiology centers, laboratories, medical transcription services, nursing homes and visiting nurse associations, physical therapy centers, psychologists, podiatrists, chiropractors, and insurance companies. Even some dentists and veterinarians are now hiring transcriptionists.

One of the statements students often encounter is "I hire only experienced transcriptionists." This can be very discouraging. If every employer hires only experienced workers, how does one get experience? If your school offers work experience through internships, externships, or practicums as part of the medical transcription program, these usually improve your employability (and should be listed on your resumé under the heading "Experience").

If a school-sponsored work experience is not provided, you may want to create your own trainee position by agreeing to work in an office for two to four weeks at no charge, giving a potential employer a no-risk opportunity to see that your skills are sufficient for the job. Yes, you need to pay bills and eat, but sometimes it's necessary to look at the long-term benefits of just a short time more of sacrifice.

There are many sources of information to help you in preparing a resumé, writing an application letter, and putting your best foot forward in an interview. Your school may have classes to help you. The counseling office or learning/tutoring center at your school may be able to help. The library has numerous references, and even some student dictionaries give advice in the appendix on preparing resumés.

Application letters. Application letters are written to accompany resumés, indicate the job you want, highlight your strengths, and state your availability for an interview. They should be only a page long, no more. If you are sending your resumé to the Human Resources Department of a large clinic or hospital, you may want to send a copy to the transcription supervisor as well, or at the very least, telephone to say that you have sent your resumé to the Human Resources Department. Be sure to proofread your letter and resumé carefully. In the area of transcription, quality is all-important, and many supervisors would look no further than the first error before discarding your application.

Resumés. The purpose of your resumé is to persuade an employer to interview you. It must look professional and present your qualifications in the best possible manner. It should be specific for the position for which you are applying. A resumé should be limited to one page if possible and should contain the following categories of information:

1. **Personal data**: Name, address, telephone number. Age and marital status are not included.

2. **Educational background**: Include name of schools, degrees, areas of special training, academic awards. You might also mention the medical specialties covered in your training program and that the dictation you transcribed was actual physician dictation (not reports read by actors or other readers).

3. **Work experience**: If work experience is unrelated to the position applied for, explain how the experience you've gained in the jobs you've held can be applied to the position you are seeking. Include any internship or practicum experience, and give dates.

4. **References**: Just list names and addresses; don't include actual letters at this point. Take the letters of recommendation to your interview. Be sure that you have contacted each of your references to be sure it is okay for you to list them. You do not want to list anyone who may give you a noncommittal or even negative recommendation.

5. **Professional affiliations**: Be sure to include professional association membership on the national, state/regional, and local level, any offices held, awards, and published works.

Portfolio. Some students create a portfolio to carry to an interview. A portfolio might include letters of reference and samples of your work. Be sure your work samples are of the highest quality and there is no patient/facility/physician identifiable information on any reports. It may also include copies of your certificate or diploma and awards, certificates of attendance at professional meetings, a more extensive description of the transcription you've

Sample *Application Letter*

September 13, XXXX

Sandra Comp, CMT, CMA-A
Transcription Supervisor
Sunshine Medical Clinic
32 South First Street
Orlando, FL 32801

Dear Ms. Comp:

I saw your advertisement in the *Florida Sentinel* for a Medical Transcriptionist I, and I hope that you will consider me for the position.

You may recall that I met you when our class toured the medical clinic last April. I was very impressed with your facilities, equipment, and the efficiency with which your employees worked. I decided then that Sunshine Medical Clinic would be a great place to work.

You no doubt are already aware of the quality of the transcription program at Florida Community College. You will see from my resumé that I was one of the top students in the program. My typing speed is 95 words per minute copy-typing, 80 words per minute on dictation. My grade point average is 3.90.

I am available for an interview at your convenience and look forward to speaking with you.
-
Sincerely yours,

Susan Bright
210 State Street
Orlando, FL 32820
(407) 555-9999

done, and copies of any evaluations your instructor or work experience supervisors may have given.

Professional credentials. Your ultimate professional goal is to become a Registered Medical Transcriptionist (RMT) and then a Certified Medical Transcriptionist (CMT). These are the professional designations awarded to individuals who have met credentialing requirements as specified by the American Association for Medical Transcription (AAMT).

The RMT exam is based on the level 1 AAMT Medical Transcriptionist Job Description and the competencies outlined in the AAMT Core Competencies and the AAMT Model Curriculum, and the CMT credential is level 2.

The AAMT RMT exam consists of both medical transcription-related knowledge items and transcription performance items. The medical transcription-related knowledge portion

of the exam consists of multiple-choice questions in certain specified content areas and percentages.

The transcription performance portion of the RMT exam consists of short items employing medical dictation and/or transcription that must be transcribed, proofread, and/or edited. It consists of dictation that is realistic and representative of that encountered under actual working conditions. Dictation is selected for its appropriate medical content. The practical portion of the exam is designed to test a candidate's knowledge, skills, and abilities to practice medical transcription effectively in today's healthcare environment. Emphasis in the practical portion of the exam is more on critical thinking skills rather than keyboarding, research, or other technical skills.

AAMT's mastery-level CMT examination was established to recognize individuals with specialized, advanced transcription competencies. Individuals interested in certification

Sample *Resumé*

Susan Bright
210 State Street
Orlando, FL 32820
(407) 555-9999

Education   Florida Community College, graduated 2006. Certificate in Medical Transcription. Other electives include Coding 1 and 2, Medical Law, and computer courses in word processing, dBase, spreadsheets, and desktop publishing.

Experience   **Medical Transcription Intern**, E. W. Jones, M.D., Orlando. August 2006. Transcribed dictated reports and correspondence, scheduled surgery, coded and filed insurance reports for prominent orthopedist.

Medical Transcription Intern, Health Information Management, Community Hospital, Sanford, Florida. July 2006. Transcribed dictated histories and physicals, clinical summaries, and operative reports from all specialties and staff physicians. Used Microsoft Word and became familiar with digital dictation and management system.

Student Assistant to Dean of Vocational Education, Florida Community College, August 1997 to August 1998. Answered phone, typed correspondence, did general filing.

References   Jane Emeritus, CMT, Medical Transcription Program Director, Florida Community College, Sanford, FL 32771. Phone (407) 555-2456.

E. W. Jones, M.D., 2013 Main St., Orlando, FL 32820. Phone (407) 555-2456.

Joan Flagg, RHIA, HIM Director, Community Hospital, Sanford, FL 32771. Phone (407) 555-2456.

Student Member: American Association for Medical Transcription, Florida Association for Medical Transcription, Central Florida AAMT Chapter, and Business/Vocational Students of America.

Awards: Medical Transcription Scholarship from Central Florida AAMT Chapter, Florida Vocational Honor Student Society award, and Outstanding Vocational Student award from Florida Community College.

Publications: "Origins of Cancer—Genetic or Virus," *The Communicator*, February 2005.

should gain substantial transcription experience before taking this examination. It is not recommended for recent graduates who have completed a transcription certificate program and have no other transcription experience.

It is not acceptable to use the designation MT (medical transcriptionist) or MLS (medical language specialist) after one's name because doing so gives the impression that the appellation carries the weight of a professional certification designation. *RMT* and *CMT* are the recognized professional credentialing designations for medical transcriptionists, and they may be used only if authorized through the American Association for Medical Transcription. See **www.aamt.org** for credentialing information.

Employment Enigmas

by Judy Hinickle

The possibilities of employment in the transcription field today have increased in scope and variety. Many people are faced with decisions or options not open to them even 10 years ago.

Transcriptionists are paid in various employment settings by the hour, by production, by a combination of the two, or with the profits of self-employment. All sorts of personal needs are taken into consideration with each. Do you need the security of hourly wages or a salary? Or would you rather take risks that you will make more money when paid by production or through self-employment? Does a spotlight on production statistics cause you too much stress, or do you thrive on the challenge?

What about the other areas of compensation? Benefits are a major method of compensation, but perhaps we should consider whether an employer is the best choice for obtaining maximum benefits. Would you take a job because of the medical insurance, or the profit sharing, or the pension plan? Or would you rather make a better wage with a job having no benefits and make your own provisions for insurance, investment, and retirement?

We should analyze benefit opportunities in the light of today's society. Employment is in a fickle state these days. Employees job-hop and employers "reorganize" constantly. The days of working for one employer 25 years have passed for most employees. Our society is restless and mobile. Jobs may last less than five years. Careers may last only 10 or 20 years, then new paths are embarked upon. Are employees asking for long-term benefits from short-term employers? Do employees cling to making employers responsible for too much of their future financial security—possibly *expecting* that empowerment, yet *resenting* it at the same time?

When looking at these wage and benefit issues, we need to consider trade-offs. If your choice of employment gives you none of the benefits which traditionally equate

to 25-33% of your wages, are you then getting that in cash and applying it to those benefits? As an independent contractor with no benefits, are you making that additional 25-33% after expenses so that you can pay your taxes and also purchase the insurance and a pension plan independently? If self-employed, do your wages and profit after expenses equal or exceed an equivalent wage and benefit package in a traditional setting?

There are, of course, lifestyle and personal benefits to be considered in alternate employment settings, but we must be careful not to shortchange our financial future with short-sightedness now.

Once we get past wage and investment issues, personal ability and satisfaction become important. What kind of work hours does your lifestyle require? How much responsibility do you want to accept? Do you like to supervise? Teach? Do you like to "plug in and tune out"? Would you rather not deal with people? Do you like taking risks? Do you think self-employment means there is no one to answer to? Do you want to work a certain number of hours per week and no more? All these questions are appropriate for various transcription opportunities.

Other issues surround our employment options:

Self-employment and independent contracting tend to result in uneven cash flow and unreasonable hours, and can perpetuate poor future financial planning.

Working at home takes great self-discipline and sometimes leads to a feeling of never getting away from work to relax.

Employing others includes tremendous responsibility for their financial well-being, the quality of their work, the standards of their work environment, and making available enough steady work and benefits to keep them with you. Healthy cash flow is all-important to meet these responsibilities, and the paperwork can be overwhelming. Skills in marketing, accounting, and managing personnel are required. Clients may not have the bureaucratic drawbacks of an institutional employer, but their quality and timeliness expectations and their erratic quantity demands can be even more distressing.

Working in a hospital or clinic setting can be anonymous, rigid, and sterile, with bureaucracy and remote supervision leaving you feeling unappreciated or without a sense of accomplishment.

Working in a transcription service can mean insecurity and a greater risk of layoffs.

Working in a small office can be limiting and dictatorial.

Does this mean there are no good employment opportunities for medical transcriptionists? Of course not! There are excellent employment opportunities, but, as in most aspects of our lives, we have to take some bad with the good.

Self-employment may offer a sense of achievement, freedom, flexibility, and more money if properly planned and executed. Long hours and uneven cash flow are accepted or compensated for in other ways.

Working at home can be done profitably with application of self-discipline to hours worked and hours played.

Employing others can create a sense of accomplishment, fulfilling a dream of doing something others cannot do, or cannot do as well. With proper planning and financial strategies, and many hours of hard work, cash flow and profit can come together. Marketing strategies can be utilized to equalize the work flow as much as possible. Clients can have clearly stated expectations met consistently.

Working in a hospital or clinic can offer security of hours and benefits, and opportunities for career advancement. Sometimes it offers other perks such as convention and workshop attendance. With good supervision the employee is not anonymous, can find flexibility, and may find fertile ground for creativity in a financially sound environment.

Working for a good transcription service can offer flexibility and excellent wages, generous benefits and profit sharing. Slow employment times may be compensated for during peak times. It may be especially profitable and fulfilling for part-time, high-energy professionals.

Working in a small office can provide personal contact with appreciative dictators on a daily basis—leaving you feeling appreciated and secure.

There are many things to consider in our employment decisions—certainly more than are described here. Within each opportunity we need to balance the wage and benefit issues with the personal fulfillment and family issues, and the spirit of independence with the risks of less security. Being aware of our own personal needs and giving them priority levels, while keeping a watchful eye on the future, will help ensure fruitful decisions.

Avoiding Work-Related Injuries

by Elaine Aamodt Abba

In recent years **repetitive stress injury** (RSI), also known as cumulative trauma disorder (CTD), has become one of the fastest growing occupational hazards in the United States. In the mid-1980s the Department of Labor statistics showed RSI accounting for 20% of all occupational injuries, but since then that figure has increased to over half.

Such injuries have long been common among butchers, carpenters, and assembly line workers; however, with the advent of widespread computer use, RSI has now become the scourge of the white-collar world as well. A job such as medical transcription is now done on computer,

Transcription *for Life*

Are you a lifer? Or do you know someone who is? A transcriptionist for life, that is. Medical transcription has been in my life for over 30 years, and yet I know few medical transcriptionists who think in terms of "transcription for life." Rather they think medical transcription is what they "do" or what they have done at various times in their life.

Many transcriptionists have said they never consciously made a commitment to "transcription for life" and are as surprised as I am that they have been medical transcriptionists so long. The transcriptionists who love what they do, and do it consistently well year after year, are those who exemplify that connection.

Some of the best transcriptionists I've known have had a love-hate relationship with medical transcription. For them medical transcription was almost like an addiction or obsession, something they *had* to do, although they were highly qualified to do many other things for a living. Others love it without reservation.

One of my friends, who worked at home so that she could smoke at her desk, approached each batch of dictation with a childlike glee and wonder. She was always tickled to receive the occasional box of dictation from a hospital outside the area. It was like a delightful holiday package to open and savor. At her desk she would reach into the box with trembling fingers and barely suppressed excitement, take out the first tape and pop it into her transcriber, hit the foot pedal and advance forward, holding her breath until she heard the first voice on the tape. Foreign accents, difficult reports, inconsiderate dictators—no matter. She could do anything, and did it with joy and equanimity. And she felt that way for over 40 years!

That's truly a medical transcriptionist for life whose fire is lit from within.

Sally C. Pitman
Perspectives on the Medical Transcription Profession

and unlike the typewriter of old, the computer allows its user to sit at the keyboard for entire shifts, striking keys four or five times per second without even the occasional break to change paper and ribbon or to hit the carriage return. Such a work environment can easily lead to repetitive stress injuries, and those involved in the transcription field must become aware of the possible risks as well as ways to avoid those risks.

Repetitive stress injuries arise precisely as their name indicates, from repetitive stress, and any job in which continuous repetitive motion is required is a potential offender. Among keyboard users, one of the most common cumulative trauma disorders is **carpal tunnel syndrome** (CTS) (see Chapter 14, Figure 14-8). In fact, it was estimated in 1990 that 15% of all workers in high-risk industries (such as medical transcription) would develop carpal tunnel syndrome.

Carpal tunnel syndrome develops when the median nerve leading to the hand becomes pinched by swollen tendons or tissue in the carpal tunnel—the narrow tunnel in the wrist formed by the carpal bones. The results are numbness, tingling, pain, or burning sensations in the fingers and hand.

CTS injuries vary both in severity and longevity. In some cases, symptoms subside with such self-help treatments as rubbing or shaking the hand, running warm or cold water over the hand, ice packing, elevation, or rest. Symptoms may return when the stressful motions of the job are resumed. In other cases, symptoms are more severe, often becoming especially painful at night, and can make even the simplest daily task, such as buttoning a shirt, strenuous if not impossible. If further damage is not prevented, pain can also travel to the shoulders, neck, and upper back.

Symptoms of carpal tunnel syndrome usually appear gradually and, in the early stages, are often hard to distinguish from arthritis. However, it is extremely important that anyone suspecting CTS development take preventive steps and see a doctor as soon as possible because symptoms that go ignored for several months can lead to permanent disability.

Not only is this a frightening prospect from a health perspective, it is also a potential financial disaster.

Spotlight on

Ergonomics: It's All in the Tushie

by Renee M. Priest

It starts out as an isolated creak or squeak now and then, mildly irritating, but nothing to get all excited about. Insidiously, day by day, that squeaking gradually gets louder, more obtrusive, and one day, just as you delicately poise yourself above the seat and lower the derriere down to its comfortable, well-worn place . . . the darn chair BREAKS! I have watched in awe as seemingly sensible, calm, mild-mannered MTs have thrown incredibly spectacular temper tantrums when this astonishing phenomenon occurs.

Of course this does not receive much publicity, but it is a sad, sad truth that right now, all over the United States, MTs are shamelessly abusing chairs—plopping those heinies down way past the time limit per day that the manufacturer recommends for sitting; exceeding the optimum weight limitation while transcribing with a *Dorland's*, three word books, and a couple of drug books piled in the lap; endlessly fiddling with all the screws, wing nuts, and levers that manipulate height, armrest position, and back support. This tragic and truly pitiful condition has been appropriately dubbed the WT (wear and tear) syndrome. Do not make the mistake of believing that press release the chair manufacturers recently sent out. This absolutely does not have anything to do with size, shape, or poundage of the posterior in question.

Consider the length of time it takes to properly squash, mash, wriggle, and baptize that chairseat with assorted liquids and foodstuffs into just the proper configuration for maximum comfort. Is it any wonder that when this dreaded breakdown occurs the MT is amazed to learn that the favored chair was long ago officially classified as a chair "dinosaur," no longer manufactured, irreplaceable! A designation that is guaranteed to provoke a frenzied rooting through junk drawers by those hapless MTs searching for Krazy Glue, duct tape, even looting the garage to locate the husband's welder. (Okay, okay, I will admit that some MTs are thrifty, which just might have a little something to do with this frantic behavior.) Nevertheless, there comes a time when, despite all resuscitation efforts, the MT is forced to admit that the pile of fabric, wood, and ball bearings sitting on the floor in front of the computer is simply not repairable anymore.

The search for just the right chair can rapidly evolve into a quest that takes on mythic proportions, sort of like the search by Indiana Jones and his father for the Holy Grail—with one tiny difference. Instead of outsmarting sneaky archaeology thieves, snakes, bats, and the odd camel or two, the MT quickly finds that he/she is engaged in a battle of wits with that most heinous of hucksters—the chair salesman on commission. The search for just the right headset, transcriber, or keyboard with the perfect touch simply pales by comparison with the convoluted

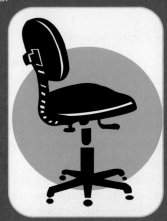

According to OSHA, one in every three workers' compensation dollars pays for RSIs. In all, insurers awarded an estimated 2.73 million workers' compensation claims for RSIs in 1993, costing employers more than $20 billion. Indirect costs to employers are estimated to be five times that amount—$100 billion. One major insurance company estimated the individual cost per claim to be $8,000, or double the average claim for other injuries or illnesses. In 2003, the Bureau of Labor statistics reported repetitive stress injury rates were 6.5 cases per 10,000 workers for a total of 57,420 injuries annually and a median 22 days of work lost.

These are the simple, easy-to-measure costs. More difficult to quantify is the suffering of the victims. I recently spoke with a transcriptionist in Texas who was plagued with CTS for over a year before doctors were able to diagnose her condition. During that year, because her pain was not diagnosed as resulting from a work-related injury, she was ineligible for worker compensation. (She had been told that pain without an actual diagnosis of injury was not an acceptable reason for missing work.) Unable to continue in her job, she was forced to go on unemployment until a diagnosis was finally made several months later. Since that time she has undergone surgery on both wrists, and while her condition has improved greatly, the damage done is permanent. Not only will she never be able to work at a keyboard again, she can no longer do simple household chores such as washing dishes or hanging clothes in the closet without experiencing excruciating pain. No price tag can be put on that kind of suffering.

chair-testing process. When one's tushie is going to grace the seat in question for hours and hours and hours, no effort should be too elaborate when it comes to choosing the "creme de la creme" of chairs.

I find it handy to assemble a simple assortment of testing devices before entering any office store to peruse the tempting array of chairs on display. This will help to minimize that impulse buy—"Oh look, the color of the seat cushion matches the rug in my office," resulting in the salesman whisking you out the door with the chair conveniently crammed into an 2" x 2" box, needing only "minimal assembly" once home.

One of my oversized baskets for harvesting vegetables works quite well to hold the implements I consider essential for a true test of a chair's suitability. Just ignore that nasty look the salesman is giving you as you whip out the tape measure to "size up" the width of the backside and compare it to the chair seat. Remember, it is no longer possible to allow that half-inch or so of overhang space when measuring. Chair manufacturers strategically place those armrest supports closer and closer to the seat cushion in a subliminal effort to undermine one's tushie self-esteem, thus provoking the desire to pay more money for the deluxe-size chair. Be aware that a salesman might attempt to tackle you as you are getting ready to douse that chair with a generous sampling of Coke or coffee. Wave that chair label claiming to be water- and stain-resistant at him and pour away.

Bringing children along is always a good idea. If necessary, borrow a few for the afternoon. Ages four through eight have proven the most successful for me. This will enable you to judge just how quickly you can restore all those ergonomic knobs and levers back to the optimum settings for ultimate comfort once the child is done spinning around in circles as fast as possible. This is also a good test of how quickly one can sponge that seat clean of the resultant eruption of stomach contents without any of it sinking into the foam padding. Do be sure to bend over and listen closely for the telltale squealing of ball bearings as those kids see how far and fast they can push those chairs from the desk, utilizing the "feet off the top drawer" maneuver as leverage. This will give one a very reasonable estimate of the rolling life of the ball bearings.

Animals also come in handy, and they fit in that basket quite nicely. Cats, guinea pigs, perhaps birds, especially ones who like to make deposits in strategic places. Trust me, if that fabric can hold up to the canines of a teething puppy, it's a keeper.

I really should warn you that the final test in my arsenal is not for the squeamish or the faint of heart. Those salesmen really become uncontrollable when one is bringing out the heated backpad to line the chair with; the vibrating massage mat for back and "glutes"; the icy cold orthopedic pads for sciatica; and the test of all tests . . . the donut. It is most important to make sure that the chairseat can accommodate that donut easily because sitting in a chair for eight hours, afflicted with external hemorrhoids, is a lesson in endurance that will quickly separate the truly dedicated (or extremely demented) MT from those who have common sense.

Source: *Perspectives on the Medical Transcription Profession*

Because carpal tunnel syndrome can be so debilitating and costly, in both human and financial terms, it is something that cannot be ignored in any high-risk field. And while treatments do exist, their results are not always guaranteed. As with most injuries, an ounce of prevention is worth a pound of cure.

Most preventive measures are fairly simple, but they must begin with education (both of management and employees) to be effective. There has to be an atmosphere in the workplace of understanding and an acknowledgment of CTS as a legitimate health concern. Too often employers do not take complaints about pain seriously, and employees are afraid to discuss or even admit discomfort for fear of losing their jobs. This kind of production-first, workers-last environment is not only dehumanizing, it greatly increases the risk for work-related injuries.

Fostering a positive environment, on the other hand, can lead to improved morale and higher productivity in the long run. The crucial element of education will help transcriptionists to recognize the signs and dangers of wrist pain while still in the early, reversible stages. Secondly, understanding and compassion will keep lines of communication open and allow supervisors and transcriptionists to work together to find ways of resolving a problem before it becomes a disaster.

Preventing injury. A good first step is evaluation of the work environment. The service owner or supervisor may want to have a physical therapist come into the workplace to counsel employees on the safest and most comfortable ways to perform their tasks.

A transcription service owner recently hired a physical therapist to counsel her employees in the office. With a biofeedback machine, the therapist was able to demonstrate for the transcriptionists how tension is built or released depending on chair position, hand position, screen position, and so on. In this way the transcriptionists became aware of the possible flaws in their usual working positions and consequently learned how to minimize stressful positions and movements.

Often medical transcriptionists who have been working for years feel that they have no need to make any adjustments. To an extent that may be true; a transcriptionist who has been working for 10 years or more and hasn't gotten CTS probably never will, according to the medical experts. However, all transcriptionists should be trained to minimize stress and to find the position with the lowest tension, reducing their risk for injury.

Sitting. The workplace must, of course, be completely adjustable. Chairs, for example, must be comfortable and fit their occupants. The jury is still out on what comprises the perfect chair; however, many ergonomists now say that a chair should be adaptable to the diversity of every human body type and seating preference that comes its way. The ergonomically correct chair, they say, should come with an operator's manual and have about 150 parts. Proper seating will not only help stave off CTS, it will also assist in prevention of lower back pain and other injuries.

Once seated, transcriptionists should have the computer screen at eye level so that they will not have to crane their necks this way or that. Wrists should be in a level position, and feet should be comfortably planted on an appropriate footrest. However, even this supposed cure-all position which was once touted as the only correct way to sit has its shortcomings.

According to Marvin Dainoff, Director of the Center for Ergonomic Research at Miami University in Ohio, "Static posture is the enemy." Dainoff explains that remaining perfectly still in any position for too long is not good for anyone. Small movements, called "micro-movements" (wiggling and fidgeting), are important in that they help relieve stress on the back, shoulders, hands, and wrists. This will not only help avert CTS, but also will help reduce other injuries related to long periods of sitting.

In *Sitting on the Job* (Houghton Mifflin, 1989), author Scott Donkin also recognizes the problem: "People who sit a great deal tend to develop weak abdominal, buttock, and front and inner thigh muscles. Their neck, shoulder, and back muscles tend to be tense, and their spinal movements are usually restricted." Exercise and the freedom to move about and to take stretching breaks are crucial in combating repetitive stress injury.

Breaks. Not only are breaks a vital part of CTS avoidance, but the manner in which breaks are taken actually makes a difference as well. Statistically, it appears that people working in a mentally or emotionally stressful environment are more prone to developing CTS due to the general effects of stress on the body. Psychologically, and consequently physically, it is therefore crucial that employers not only allow, but actually encourage or mandate frequent breaks for employees. The feeling that breaks are encouraged helps employees feel that their well-being is a top priority, which improves morale and can actually contribute to the healing effect in and of itself.

The *Los Angeles Times* office, where nearly 40% of its editorial staff was suffering from CTS to varying degrees, has seen positive results from having messages programmed into the computer terminals that automatically remind employees to take a break every 50 minutes. The newspaper office also provides a break room where employees have access to exercise equipment and a refrigerator with ice packs to help them ease the pressure in their wrists.

Self-help. If symptoms of CTS do appear, there are some self-help efforts that can be very effective. However, if implemented incorrectly these same efforts can actually do more harm than good. For example, wearing a forearm splint works well for some, but if used improperly, this same splint can increase pressure on the wrist and increase damage. Similarly, some researchers have asserted that a vitamin B_6 deficiency is a leading cause of CTS. However, trying to treat your CTS by taking B_6 supplements on your own can be extremely dangerous since high B_6 intake can lead to permanent nerve damage. Exercise is also important in combating CTS, but the wrong kinds of exercise will also lead to further damage. It is wise to consult a physician or physical therapist and to do plenty of research on your own while planning your attack on carpal tunnel syndrome.

If your office cannot afford state-of-the-art ergonomic chairs, fully adjustable work stations, and all the other available gadgetry, there are still many simple steps that can be implemented quickly and easily to reduce the chance of injury in your workplace.

A medical transcription service owner suffering from CTS found that a good wrist pad running along the lower edge of the keyboard was enough to get her back on the job. Such a pad helps prevent the wrists from flexing or bending in unhealthy ways and generally costs only about $30.

It is also important to give your hands frequent breaks from the keyboard in order to stretch. If possible, consult a physical therapist or physician to find out about specific exercises you can do both at home and at the keyboard to keep carpal tunnel syndrome at bay. You may also find such exercises in the popular literature. Scott Donkin's book, *Sitting on the Job*, contains detailed diagrams of exercises for back, neck, shoulder, and hands, as well as diagrams and descriptions of healthful sleeping positions, sitting positions, and even breathing exercises for relaxation.

While there are many new and innovative ergonomic products on the market, we must realize that, while these products can be very helpful, a major component in fighting carpal tunnel syndrome is attitude. Everyone involved must become educated about carpal tunnel syndrome and accept the fact that some fundamental changes will have to be made in the way we go about our work before this problem can be eliminated.

Humor in Medicine

Jest for the Health of It

by Richard Lederer, Ph.D.

An Austin, Texas, emergency medical technician answered a call at the home of an elderly woman whose sister had collapsed. As they were placing her into the ambulance, the lady wailed, "Oh, lawdy, lawdy. I know what's the matter with her. She done got the same thing what killed her brother. It's a heretical disease."

The technician asked what that would be, and the lady said, "The Smiling Mighty Jesus!"

When the EMT got the sister to the county hospital, she looked up the brother's medical records to find he had died of spinal meningitis.

A woman rushed into the lobby of a hospital and exclaimed, "Where's the fraternity ward?" The receptionist calmly replied, "You must mean the maternity ward."

The woman went on, "But I have to see the upturn." Patiently, the receptionist answered, "You must mean the intern."

Exasperated, the woman continued, "Fraternity, maternity, upturn, intern—I don't care wherever or whoever. Even though I use an IOU, and my husband has had a bisectomy, I haven't demonstrated for two months and I think I may be fragrant!"

That same woman later became three centimeters diluted and, narrowly avoiding a mess carriage, she ultimately went into contraptions. Her baby was born with its biblical cord wrapped around its arm, and she asked if she could have the child circumscribed before leaving the hospital.

It is ironic that the humor in hospitals, emergency departments, and doctors' offices—usually some of the scariest places—can be exceedingly hilarious. The giddy ghost of Mrs. Malaprop haunts medical halls and application forms, where we discover all manner of strange conditions, such as swollen asteroids, an erection nervosa, shudders (shingles!), and migrating headaches. All the malappropriate terms in this article were miscreated by anxious patients or hassled doctors and nurses.

A man went to his eye doctor, who told him he had a case of myopera and would have to wear contract lenses. That was a lot better than his friend who had had a cadillac removed from his eye. Still, when he worked at his computer, he would have to watch out for harbor tunnel syndrome. He worried that his authoritis of the joints might be a signal of Old Timer's disease and fretted that a genital heart defect was causing a myocardial infraction and trouble with his duodemon.

Another man was in the hospital passing gull stones from his bladder while the doctor was treating a cracked dish from his spine. After the operation, his glands were completely prostrated. A hyannis hernia, hanging hammeroids, inflammation of the strocum, and a blockage of his large intesticle could have rendered him impudent.

We're not talking about just a deviant septum here. These symptoms were enough to give a body heart populations, high pretension, a peppery ulcer, and postmortem depression—even a cerebral hemorrhoid. But at least that's better than a case of headlights (head lice), sea roses of the liver, cereal palsy, or sick as hell anemia. Any of these could cause one to slip into a comma.

A woman experienced itching of the virginia during administration, which led to pulps all up her virginal area and they had to void her reproductions. This was followed by a tubular litigation and, ultimately, mental pause. Mental pause can cause one to become a maniac depressive and act like a cyclopath.

She didn't worry about her very close veins, but she thought that a mammy-o-gram and Pabst smear might show if she had swollen nymph glands and fireballs of the eucharist. That's "fibroids of the uterus," and it's something you can't cure with simple acnepuncture, Heineken maneuver, or a bare minimum enema. Apparently, evasive surgery would be required. Afterward, she would recuperate in expensive care.

Seasoned Medical Transcriptionist Syndrome

by Renee Priest

When interviewing, examining, and performing diagnostic tests, patients with SMTS (seasoned medical transcriptionist syndrome) may or may not exhibit some or all of the following symptoms:

Patient is able to easily decipher dictation that sounds suspiciously like it is coming from underwater, where the dictator is thoroughly enjoying gazing at the colorful fish swimming around the Great Barrier Reef while dictating through a snorkel.

Patient's powers of concentration have been honed to such a fine degree that turning the stereo to level 10, with the house reverberating, and children pelting each other with ice because "someone" ate the last ice cream bar, cannot distract the patient's attention and not one keystroke is missed.

Patient instinctively corrects the word "bowl" to bowel, regardless of whether the document in question is referring to breakfast cereal or a colon resection.

Patient is well known to local emergency department personnel due to multiple visits for whiplash as patient repeatedly forgets to unplug the headset from the transcriber when jumping from the chair to reach for an obscure medical reference book.

Patient has developed a permanent list to the left or right, with chronic cervical and paraspinal tics and spasms due to the strain of trying to get as close to the sounds of dictation as possible.

Patient exhibits progressive loss of function in activities of daily living, accompanied by muscle atrophy and wasting, possibly due to maintaining a sitting position for 8 to 10 hours a day. Simple activities of daily living such as sweeping, folding laundry, or washing dishes are no longer within this patient's functional capabilities.

Patient is visibly distressed when reporting the ability to clearly hear the children whispering in the bedroom at 10:30 p.m., with the headset on and dictation playing, but states that upon removal of the headset, the children's voices are muffled, tinny sounding, and seem to be accompanied by various clicks, buzzes, and static-type noises.

Patient reports development of visual acuity defects, complaining of the inability to bring words and letters into proper focus unless they are written on white or blue background. As well, patient reports the need to use a magnifying glass to decipher medical record numbers on hospital record sheets, despite ophthalmology consultant report that vision is perfectly normal.

Patient is cooperative; however, displays some slight disorientation to time, place, and person. Patient routinely refers to the examiner as "the dictator." When asked if patient knows where he/she is, patient states, "halfway through that last 20-minute vascular surgery report."

Patient exhibits signs and symptoms of increased stress levels, emphasizing repeatedly that the examiner needs to "speed this up, my lines are due back in exactly one hour, and I have already had two hours of down time sitting in the waiting room until you got back from lunch. Do you have any idea what this is doing to my line count today?"

Patient is seemingly unaware of compulsive finger movements when speaking or listening to the examiner speak. Hands may be held at waist level as if poised over a keyboard. Patient seems unable to stop repeatedly interrupting the examiner to request that he/she spell a word or to dispute the proper use of medical terminology.

Patient exhibits signs and symptoms of obsessive "proofreading palsy," with inability to refrain from sneaking peeks at the medical chart held by the examiner.

Indeed, patient may appear more concerned with the chart than with discussing his/her medical condition.

Patient demonstrates a tendency for self-diagnosis, self-medication, and self-delusion. Making repeated assertions that "I know exactly what is wrong with me. Believe me, I could transcribe these symptoms in my sleep!"

Bloopers

by Sally C. Pitman

Most medical transcriptionists have a lively sense of humor, and we hear much to laugh about in a typical day's dictation. A sense of humor is essential for longevity in the field of medical transcription. While we are not insensitive to the gravity of the medical reports that we are transcribing, nevertheless we enjoy the comic relief afforded by the humor in medicine. Laughter helps us maintain a sense of balance and perspective.

Practically every transcription office has a central Funny File where the medical transcriptionists routinely record some of the misstatements, malapropisms, slips of the tongue, dangling modifiers, and other bits of humor in medical dictation. When an experienced medical transcriptionist occasionally has a lapse in consciousness—or takes a shortcut between the ears and the keyboard without the dictation going through the mind—an embarrassing gaffe can occur. Instead of typing "senile cataract," the transcriptionist may type "penile cataract"—a blooper.

Doctors and medical transcriptionists alike can be guilty of Freudian slips, and the results provide a good laugh when shared with one's colleagues. In fact, sharing a laugh with someone who understands the joke intensifies the fun of the error in dictation or transcription. When I am transcribing alone and have no one around to share the laughter with, my enjoyment is diminished. When a doctor dictated, "This is the second hospital admission for this 66-year-old white male who was found under the bed in his hotel room and was admitted to the hospital for evaluation of this problem," that struck me as hilarious. It would not have been nearly so funny if I had not been able to share it with someone.

Many years ago I was transcribing x-ray reports for hours on end, and doing it very mechanically by the end of the day. Suddenly, a sentence I had just transcribed registered in my brain. The radiologist had said, "The glenoid fossa is well seated in the acetabulum," and I had typed exactly what he said. I burst into laughter at the image this evoked and called the radiologist to tell him what he had dictated. Undaunted, he roared, "Yeah, you should've SEEN that guy!" The incident shows what can happen when even an experienced medical transcriptionist unthinkingly or mechanically types what doctors **say** rather than what they **mean**.

Surely every doctor has at one time or another said something like, "The patient smokes two beers a day and drinks two packs." Most physicians know they are not infallible and appreciate the transcriptionist's medical knowledge and editing ability. Though they may dictate half asleep in the middle of the night or after 10 hours of surgery, they are counting on us to be alert and, when necessary, to correct their mistakes.

Lest you think we are putting anyone down, let me say that we are not deriding doctors who make mistakes in dictation, or students or trainees who guess wrong in transcription, or experienced medical transcriptionists who occasionally err. But one reason these dictation and transcription bloopers are funny is that they are "inside jokes." We have to know the correct medical terms and have a vivid imagination for the quotes to be funny. The medical transcriptionist has to know that the glenoid fossa is in the shoulder joint and cannot be well seated in the *hip*—without grotesque results!

Doctors don't always just accidentally say funny things in the dictation, however. Frequently they crack jokes in an aside to the medical transcriptionists. We fondly remember the bicentennial tape dictated by our favorite radiologist in 1976. Also, the physician who dictated a clinic note on the Great Pumpkin one Halloween Day was clearly out to entertain us. And the transcriptionist can *hear* the laughter in the voice of the physician who dictated, "The only complaint of this 74-year-old woman is that the wind keeps blowing her off her motorcycle and she suffers aches and pains because of this."

Why are **bloopers** funny? I think lapses from correct medical terminology are funny when they evoke **concrete sensory images** that in context are humorous. The image of bunny fur (bony spur) on the spinal column is so incongruous that, when pictured on the x-ray, it evokes laughter.

Does humor have a place in medicine? Laughter can be the best medicine for whatever ails us. We can be tired, frustrated, overworked, depressed, and even ill, and something funny in the dictation—whether intentional or not—can make us laugh and bring us out of the doldrums. Laughter can renew our spirits and help us to work with renewed energy. It's the best medicine.

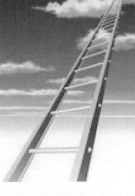

SkillsChallenge

Completion Exercise

Instructions: Complete the following listing questions.

1. Editorial activity is performed simultaneously at three levels. List them.

   _____

   _____

   _____

   _____

   _____

2. List four dictation errors or problems which the medical transcriptionist may need to edit or bring to the attention of the dictator or a supervisor.

   _____

   _____

   _____

   _____

   _____

   _____

   _____

3. List four of the most common errors of grammar made by ESL physicians and how the medical transcriptionist corrects them for accuracy and completeness.

   _____

   _____

   _____

   _____

   _____

   _____

   _____

4. Discuss two important points in accepting and dispensing criticism.

   _____

   _____

   _____

   _____

   _____

5. Cite two reasons why laughter is important in medical transcription.

   _____

   _____

   _____

   _____

6. List four important qualities demonstrated by professional medical transcriptionists.

   _____

   _____

   _____

   _____

   _____

   _____

   _____

   _____

   _____

   _____

Multiple Choice Exercise

Instructions: Choose the correct answer in each of the following multiple-choice questions. Write the letter for your answer in the space provided next to the number of the question.

___ 1. If the transcriptionist discovers through a dictated medical report that a close friend has been hospitalized, the MT should:
   A. Do nothing.
   B. Call upon the friend's pastor to make a hospital visit.
   C. Contact the health information manager to get permission to see the chart.
   D. Get permission from the family before visiting the patient.

___ 2. Discarded old copies of health records should be:
   A. Archived.
   B. Shredded.
   C. Sealed in a plastic bag.
   D. Put onto microfiche.

___ 3. Under normal circumstances, who has the right to breach a patient's confidentiality?
   A. The clergy.
   B. The health information manager.
   C. The patient himself/herself.
   D. The psychiatrist.

True/False Exercise

Instructions: Label the following true or false statements by placing a *T* for true or *F* for false in the blank next to the statement.

___ 1. Transcriptionists working at remote sites are not covered by the same rules relating to the maintenance of patient confidentiality as those who work on site.

___ 2. If your home office is in your living area, your computer screen should not face outward where it can be seen by others entering the room.

___ 3. No one should access a patient health record who does not have a legitimate need for the information contained therein.

___ 4. It is unfair for an employer to fire you because your son logged onto your computer and disseminated to a friend some confidential patient information that he found there.

___ 5. Learning to "think phonetically" will help the MT to understand foreign dictators.

___ 6. The MT should transcribe ESL dictation as dictated, rather than editing for proper grammar and syntax.

___ 7. Those who speak English as a second language often confuse the parts of speech.

___ 8. ESL dictators often refer to patients in the wrong gender.

___ 9. Carpal tunnel syndrome symptoms that are ignored can lead to permanent nerve damage.

___10. It is important to keep the wrists flexed while keyboarding to avoid compression of nerves.

___11. An ergonomic chair will not help stave off lower back pain and other injuries.

___12. Wiggling and fidgeting are important in that they help relieve stress on the back, shoulders, hands, and wrists.

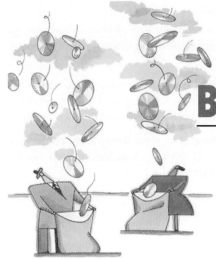

BLOOPERS

Incorrect	Correct
At the end of the operation the leg was elevated and sent to the recovery room.	At the end of the operation, the leg was elevated and the patient was sent to the recovery room.
The patient has been given pain for medication.	The patient has been given medication for pain.
The patient has no history of suicides.	The patient has no history of suicide attempts.
The patient refused an autopsy.	The patient's family refused an autopsy.
The patient has chest pain if she lies on her left side for over a year.	The patient has had chest pain for over a year when she lies on her left side.
She has some headache if she eats cheese or chocolate in the back of her head.	She has some headache in the back of her head if she eats cheese or chocolate.
She slipped on the ice and apparently her legs went in separate directions in early December.	She slipped on the ice in early December and apparently her legs went in separate directions.
Review of systems: Positive for shortness of breasts.	Review of systems: Positive for shortness of breath.
The lab test indicated abnormal lover function.	The lab test indicated abnormal liver function.
The patient was in a 30-day program which was a month in duration.	The patient was in a 30-day program.

Chapter 3

Style Guide

Chapter Outline

Learning Objectives

- Demonstrate knowledge of guidelines for grammar,
  punctuation, editing, and transcription practices
  by reviewing the examples from dictation and
  completing the exercises at the end of this chapter.

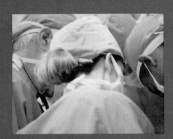
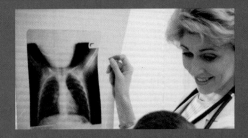
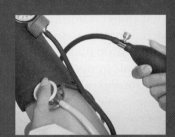

General Information

The transcript keys for *Medical Transcription Fundamentals & Practice (MTF&P)* were prepared with as little editing as possible. Many medical transcriptionists (MTs) would have edited much more extensively. Verbatim transcription was done as much as possible, even omitting articles (*a, an, the*), pronouns (*he, she, it*), prepositions (*in, with, for*), conjunctions (*and, but, or*), and helping verbs that were not dictated but could have been added for a smoother reading report.

Verbatim transcription is difficult to do because our ears, eyes, brains, and fingers often supply these tiny words even when they are not dictated. Furthermore, it is sometimes impossible to tell if a dictator is saying *a, an, the, then,* or merely saying *uh* or some other sound indicating a pause in thought. If students add in these small words, they should not be considered errors unless they change the medical meaning of the report.

Edits suggested or explained in the footnotes may or may not be made in the reports themselves. Like style, attitudes toward editing (when to edit, how much to edit) vary from facility to facility. The transcriptionist on the job would follow the employer's guidelines or dictator's preference, if known, or those guidelines specified by the transcription department where the dictation originated.

Grammar, punctuation, and style are frequently discussed as a single unit. There are, however, distinctions.

Grammar consists of the rules by which words are combined to construct and arrange sentences. It includes determining agreement between subject and verb, pronoun and antecedent, and adjective and noun; using the parts of speech appropriately; and spelling correctly and using words properly according to their meaning. Grammar rules are the least flexible and have few exceptions. Dictators often compose their thoughts "on the fly," so to speak, and may make frequent errors in grammar. It is the job of the medical transcriptionist (MT) to correct those errors.

Punctuation consists of symbols used as pointers in sentences and to enhance meaning. There is some flexibility in punctuation rules and more exceptions than in grammar rules. One of the skills MT students must learn is to apply punctuation to the spoken word as they transcribe. This can be difficult. MTs also often have to correct a dictated punctuation mark when it is wrong. At times, dictated sentences do not conform to standard sentence structure, making editing necessary and punctuation difficult to determine.

Style, on the other hand, is very flexible. A clear style contributes to clarity of meaning. Style varies according to context. Spoken language, formal written language, literature, journalism, medical journals, and medical reports all use different styles. Even two medical journals may differ in their style preferences. Preference is a good word to associate with style because that's what style is—a preferred way of writing or speaking. It is useful for institutions and organizations to have their preferences standardized in writing for uniformity and consistency in appearance.

Each institution, facility, or transcription service has its own guidelines for MTs. Some adopt a published style reference and add their own guidelines. Others may have their own in-house style guide. Still others may have nothing in writing, and MTs find out by trial and error what the quality assurance department requires. The guidelines in this chapter are for your use in transcribing *MTF&P* dictation. The styles and practices you encounter on the job may differ.

The following guidelines are not intended to be comprehensive but are general guidelines for the accurate transcription of the dictations accompanying this textbook. A medical transcription student or practicing MT should always have a comprehensive style guide, such as *The AAMT Book of Style for Medical Transcription*, latest edition (Modesto, CA: American Association for Medical Transcription), which we have used as our primary style reference.

You should read through this section before beginning to transcribe the dictations and again after you have transcribed a specialty. These guidelines will make more sense after you have transcribed a few reports. Pay special attention to the **Editing** and **Format** sections, as there is additional information in those sections specific to this unit. Guidelines are presented in alphabetical order by topic.

Abbreviations

See also **Brief Forms**.

1. Abbreviations practices vary from institution to institution. In the past, the Joint Commission on Accreditation of Health Organizations (JCAHO) had spelled-out rules for the use of abbreviations. Today, its only policy concerning abbreviations is in regard to those that have been designated as "dangerous" or "error-prone." Some departments and companies have lists of acceptable abbreviations and their translations. Others use such nebulous guidelines as "Do not use any abbreviations that are not widely known or immediately recognized by the reader."

2. It is a good idea for students to spell out most abbreviations (except for laboratory, diagnostic, and radiology tests and metric units of measure) so that they learn the proper expansions. On the job, abbreviation expanders will no doubt handle the required expansions,

but you still need to know the proper translation in order to create your expansion initially and in order to know that you have correctly interpreted the letters in the abbreviation. *H&P* sounds very much like *HNP*, but they do not mean the same thing and are not interchangeable.

3. In doctors' office notes, abbreviations are used much more liberally than in hospital and clinic records. As students, however, you should make an effort to know the correct translation of every abbreviation you transcribe and follow these general rules.

Abbreviations in dosages

When abbreviations are used with numbers for medication dosage times, use periods.

q.4 h. (every 4 hours)
 Note the space after the number.

Abbreviations that need not be expanded

1. Some abbreviations are rarely or never expanded. In rare instances, the translation of abbreviations may cause confusion rather than achieve clarity. This is particularly true for many laboratory, radiographic, and other diagnostic procedures as well as department or unit name abbreviations. These abbreviations and others like them do not need to be translated; if dictated in full, however, they should be transcribed as dictated.

ALT (alanine aminotransferase)
AST (aspartate aminotransferase)
CAT (computerized, or computed, axial tomography)
CBC (complete blood count)
CT scan (computed tomography scan)
ECG, EKG (electrocardiogram)
ER or ED (emergency room or department)
ICU (intensive care unit)
IM (intramuscular)
IV (intravenous)
IVP (intravenous pyelogram)
L5-S1 (5th lumbar vertebra and 1st sacral vertebra)
MRI (magnetic resonance imaging)
PT (prothrombin time)
PTT (partial thromboplastin time)
VDRL (Venereal Disease Research Laboratory)
WBC, WBCs (white blood count *or* white blood cells)

Note. Do not use abbreviations that can be translated more than one way (for example, CVA or PND) unless the abbreviation has been translated in the report already.

2. Some terms that appear to be abbreviations may not be readily translatable or may be brand names. The following abbreviations fall in this category:

DDD pacemaker
ST depression
T.E.D. hose

Body of the report

Expand most abbreviations on first use in the body of the report and place the abbreviation itself within parentheses. Subsequent uses of the abbreviation in the same report may be transcribed as dictated.

D: The patient was admitted with DOE and chest pain.
T: The patient was admitted with dyspnea on exertion (DOE) and chest pain.

D: Eyes: PERRLA. EOMI.
T: Eyes: Pupils equal, round, reactive to light and accommodation (PERRLA). Extraocular movements intact (EOMI).

Diagnoses

Expand almost all abbreviations used in all impressions and diagnoses; place the abbreviation itself within parentheses. If the abbreviation is repeated in the body of the report, transcribe as dictated.

D: ADMITTING IMPRESSION
 COPD.
T: ADMITTING IMPRESSION
 Chronic obstructive pulmonary disease (COPD).
D: FINAL DIAGNOSIS
 Status post CABG.
T: FINAL DIAGNOSIS
 Status post coronary artery bypass graft (CABG).

Error-prone abbreviations

1. The Institute for Safe Medication Practices (ISMP) publishes a list of error-prone abbreviations related to the prescribing and administering of drugs that are considered dangerous because they could be misread. From this list, the JCAHO has identified a "minimum list" of abbreviations that are *not* to be used. In addition, each organization must identify and apply at least three other "do not use" abbreviations, acronyms, and brief forms. Eventually, avoidance of the entire list will be implemented. **Listed below are the abbreviations you should avoid using in transcription** of the *Medical Transcription Fundamentals & Practice* reports.

If Dictated	Transcribe
AD	right ear
AS	left ear
AU	each ear
AZT	zidovudine
cc (cubic centimeters)	use *mL* with drug dosages (use *cc* with laboratory values)

If Dictated	Transcribe
D/C or DC	discharge or discontinue
HCTZ	hydrochlorothiazide
HS	half-strength
IU	international unit *or* unit
µg (microgram)	mcg
OD	right eye
OS	left eye
OU	each eye, both eyes
per os	p.o., by mouth, *or* orally
q.d.	daily *or* every day
q.h.s.	nightly *or* at bedtime
q.o.d.	every other day
/ (slash mark)	use *per* to separate doses
subq, sq, or SC	subcu *or* subcutaneous(ly)
U (for unit)	unit
zero after decimal	Do not insert a zero after the decimal unless dictated as part of a lab value.
zero before decimal	Always insert a zero before the decimal when the value is less than 1.

2. A complete list of error-prone abbreviations can be found at

> **http://www.ismp.org/**
> **http://www.jcaho.org/accredited+organizations/**
> **patient+ safety/04+npsg/04_faqs.htm**

Measurements

1. Abbreviate all metric and SI (International System of Measuring Units) units of measure when used with numerals. Expand English units of measure, except when used in tables. Expand metric and SI units of measure when not preceded by a numeral.

8 mEq	10.8 mV
5 cm	height 5 feet 6 inches
a few milliliters	several millimeters
6 mL	weight 120 pounds

2. When a measurement is dictated but the unit of measure omitted, it should be added if it can be done with certainty.

D: Height five six
T: Height 5 feet 6 inches

D: Decadron 0.75
T: Decadron 0.75 mg

Note: When *foot* is dictated for *feet*, transcribe *feet*.

Plural abbreviations

To make an abbreviation plural, simply add the letter *s* with no apostrophe if the abbreviation is in all capital letters.

> IVs were ordered to run to keep open (TKO).
> The patient stated she had had 6 BMs in less than 3 hours.
> The urinalysis revealed too-numerous-to-count WBCs.

Report headings

Expand abbreviations used in report headings and subheadings.

D: CC
T: CHIEF COMPLAINT

D: HPI
T: HISTORY OF PRESENT ILLNESS

D: Neuro
T: NEUROLOGIC

Note: It is acceptable to transcribe the abbreviation HEENT as a subheading.

Style for abbreviations

Medical abbreviations are written several ways. The three most common include all capital letters, a combination of capital and lowercase letters, and all lowercase letters with periods (primarily Latin terms used with drug dosages). Today, periods are rarely used in all-capital abbreviations unless it is a stated preference of an association or organization. Use periods in lowercase drug-related Latin abbreviations (b.i.d.) but not in non-Latin lowercase abbreviations (rbc/hpf). Generally speaking, although the style is acceptable, it is best to avoid lowercase abbreviations other than Latin abbreviations (p.r.n.) and units of measure (cm). The reason for this is that the lowercase abbreviations get lost in the text.

> ACLS (advanced cardiac life support)
> b.i.d. (twice a day)
> CBC (complete blood count)
> mmHg (millimeters of mercury)
> mV (millivolt)
> pCO_2, PCO_2, pO_2 (no subscripts in transcripts)
> pH
> p.o. or PO (by mouth; orally)
> p.r.n. (as needed)
> q.i.d. (four times a day)
> RBC (red blood cells)
> rbc/hpf (red blood cells per high power field)
> TED (thromboembolic disease)
> T.E.D. stockings (a brand name)
> t.i.d. (three times a day)
> WBC (white blood cells)

Medical *Short-Tongue*

"Mrs. Tolstoy is your basic LOL in NAD, admitted for a soft rule-out MI," the intern announces. I scribble that on my patient list. In other words Mrs. Tolstoy is a Little Old Lady in No Apparent Distress who is in the hospital to make sure she hasn't had a heart attack (rule out a myocardial infarction). And we think it's unlikely that she has had a heart attack (a *soft* rule-out).

If I learned nothing else during my first three months of working in the hospital as a medical student, I learned endless jargon and abbreviations. I started out in a state of primeval innocence, in which I didn't even know that "w/o CP, SOB, N/V" meant "without chest pain, shortness of breath, or nausea and vomiting." By the end I took the abbreviations so for granted that I would complain to my mother the English Professor, "And can you believe I had to put down *three* NG tubes last night?"

"You'll have to tell me what an NG tube is if you want me to sympathize properly," my mother said. NG, nasogastric—isn't it obvious?

I picked up not only the specific expressions but also the patterns of speech and the grammatical conventions; for example, you never say that a patient's blood pressure fell or that his cardiac enzymes rose. Instead, the patient is always the subject of the verb: "He dropped his pressure." "He bumped his enzymes." This sort of construction probably reflects the profound irritation of the intern when the nurses come in the middle of the night to say that Mr. Dickinson has disturbingly low blood pressure. "Oh, he's gonna hurt me bad tonight," the intern may say, inevitably angry at Mr. Dickinson for dropping his pressure and creating a problem. When chemotherapy fails to cure Mrs. Bacon's cancer, what we say is, "Mrs. Bacon failed chemotherapy."

"Well, we've already had one hit today, and we're up next, but at least we've got mostly stable players on our team." This means that our team (group of doctors and medical students) has already gotten one new admission today, and it is our turn again, so we'll get whoever is next admitted in emergency, but at least most of the patients we already have are fairly stable, that is, unlikely to drop their pressures or in any other way get suddenly sicker and hurt us bad.

Baseball metaphor is pervasive: A no-hitter is a night without any new admissions. A player is always a patient—a nitrate player is a patient on nitrates, a unit player is a patient in the intensive care unit and so on, until you reach the terminal player.

It is interesting to consider what it means to be winning, or doing well, in this perennial baseball game. When the intern hangs up the phone and announces, "I got a hit," that is not cause for congratulations. The team is not scoring points; rather, it is getting hit, being bombarded with new patients. The object of the game from the point of view of the doctors, considering the players for whom they are already responsible, is to get as few new hits as possible.

These special languages contribute to a sense of closeness and professional spirit among people who are under a great deal of stress. As a medical student, it was exciting for me to discover that I'd finally cracked the code, that I could understand what doctors said and wrote and could use the same formulations myself. Some people seem to become enamored of the jargon for its own sake, perhaps because they are so deeply thrilled with the idea of medicine, with the idea of themselves as doctors.

I knew a medical student who was referred to by the interns on the team as Mr. Eponym because he was so infatuated with eponymous terminology, the more obscure the better. He never said "capillary pulsations" if he could say "Quincke's pulses." He would lovingly mull over the multinamed syndromes—Wolff-Parkinson-White, Lown-Ganong-Levine, Henoch-Schoenlein—until the temptation to suggest Schleswig-Holstein or Stevenson-Kefauver or Baskin-Robbins became irresistible to his less reverent colleagues.

And there is the jargon that you don't ever want to hear yourself using. You know that your training is changing you, but there are certain changes you think would be going a little too far.

The resident was describing a man with devastating terminal pancreatic cancer. "Basically he's CTD," the resident concluded. I reminded myself that I had resolved not to be shy about asking when I didn't understand things. "CTD?" I asked timidly.

The resident smirked at me. "Circling. The Drain."

The images are vivid and terrible. "What happened to Mrs. Melville?"

"Oh, she boxed last night." To box is to die, of course.

Then there are the more pompous locutions that can make the beginning medical student nervous about the effects of medical training. A friend of mine was told by his resident, "A pregnant woman with sickle cell represents a failure of genetic counseling."

The more extreme forms aside, one most important function of medical jargon is to help doctors maintain some distance from their patients. By reformulating a patient's pain and problems into a language that the patient doesn't even speak, I suppose we are in some sense taking those pains and problems under our

Medical *Short-Tongue* (continued)

jurisdiction and also reducing their emotional impact. This linguistic separation between doctors and patients allows conversations to go on at the bedside that are unintelligible to the patient. "Naturally, we're worried about adeno-CA," the intern can say to the medical student, and lung cancer need never be mentioned.

There may be specific expressions I manage to avoid, but even as I remark them, promising myself I will never use them, I find that this language is becoming my professional speech. It no longer sounds strange in my ears—or coming from my mouth. And I am afraid

that as with any new language, to use it properly you must absorb not only the vocabulary but also the structure, the logic, the attitudes. At first you may notice these new and alien assumptions every time you put together a sentence, but with time and increased fluency, you stop being aware of them at all. And as you lose that awareness, for better or for worse, you move closer and closer to being a doctor instead of just talking like one.

Perri Klass, M.D.
Journal of AAMT (Summer 1985)
New York Times (October 4, 1984)

Note. Special styles used in publishing, such as small caps and subscripts or superscripts, are rarely used in transcription because special characters do not transmit well electronically.

Uncertain abbreviations

Never expand an abbreviation in a report if you are uncertain of the translation in the context of the report. If you cannot translate an abbreviation with confidence in its correct meaning, use the abbreviation and flag the report to the dictator's attention.

Examples of abbreviations with multiple translations:

CVA (cerebrovascular accident)
CVA (costovertebral angle)
CVA (cardiovascular accident) (rarely)

PND (paroxysmal nocturnal dyspnea)
PND (postnasal drip)

D: CHIEF COMPLAINT
    PND.
T: CHIEF COMPLAINT
    _____ (PND).

Note. There are many such abbreviations that can be confused. Always proceed with caution when translating abbreviations.

Words or phrases dictated in full

Do not abbreviate a word or phrase dictated in full; transcribe as dictated. An exception is metric units of measure, which are routinely abbreviated when used with numerals.

Acronyms

1. An acronym is a word formed from the first letters of other words and pronounced as a word.

AIDS (acquired immunodeficiency syndrome)
CABG (coronary artery bypass graft) (pronounced "cabbage")
CUSA (Cavitron ultrasonic aspirator)

2. Acronyms are initially formed with capital letters, but after they gain acceptance as words, they are sometimes converted to lowercase letters and their origin as initialisms is forgotten.

laser (light amplification by stimulated emission of radiation)
scuba (self-contained underwater breathing apparatus)

Agreement of Subject and Verb

1. Use a plural verb with a plural subject and a singular verb with a singular subject. If a compound subject is joined by *or*, the verb must agree with the subject *nearest* it. Delayed subjects, as in sentences that begin with *there*, can be particularly tricky.

2. Subject-verb agreement errors occur frequently in medical dictation, and it is the medical transcriptionist's responsibility to correct such errors. In the following examples, the subjects have a single underline, the verbs are in bold type.

At rest there **are** some occasional theta activity <u>ripples</u> in both temporal regions.
There **are** three small <u>ulcers</u> on the anterior wall of the stomach.
On chest x-ray no new suspicious <u>masses</u> or <u>change</u> in old density of suspicious nature **has occurred**.
No clustered <u>microcalcifications</u>, skin <u>thickening</u>, or nipple <u>retraction</u> **is** present.
There **were** copious <u>amounts</u> of urine draining from the vaginal vault.

No <u>evidence</u> of any thrombosis of the distal vessels, including popliteal, posterior tibial, peroneal, anterior tibial, and saphenous veins, **was seen.**

Wound care <u>instructions</u> as well as a prescription for Tylox q.4 h. p.r.n., #15, **were given** to the patient.

Note. Phrases beginning with *including* or *as well as* are not considered part of the subject and do not influence the number of the verb.

3. When the subject is a word that indicates a portion—percent, fraction, part, majority, some, all, none, remainder, portion, etc.—you must look at the object of the preposition to determine whether to use a singular or plural verb. If the object of the preposition is singular, use a singular verb. If the object of the preposition is plural, use a plural verb.

Some of the stones were little more than gravel.
Some of the specimen was so friable, it could not be saved for frozen section.

Collective nouns

Not all style guides agree about whether to use a singular or plural verb with a collective noun. Generally, if the sense of the noun is plural, the verb will be plural.

The patient's family understand that the patient's outlook is grim; they all agreed with the "Do Not Resuscitate" order.
A majority of the healthcare team agree that further inpatient care is needed for this patient.

Tip. The use of *they* in the first example is a clue to the choice of the plural verb with the collective noun *family*. In the second example, the article *a* in front of the collective noun *team* makes it plural, while *the* would have made it singular.

Compound subject joined by *and*

A plural verb must be used even if the word closest to the verb is singular.

Lab results and chest x-ray were both normal.
Febrile agglutinins and white blood count were elevated.

Compound subject joined by *or*

Make the verb agree in number with the closest noun.

No definite adenopathy or masses were felt.
No definite masses or adenopathy was felt.

Prepositions

The second most frequent occurrence of subject-verb agreement errors is the confusion of the object of a preposition with the subject of the sentence.

D: A new interstitial infiltrate in both midlung zones with some shagging of the cardiac borders are evident on chest x-ray.
T: A new interstitial infiltrate in both midlung zones with some shagging of the cardiac borders is evident on chest x-ray.

Pronoun and its antecedent

A pronoun must agree with its antecedent (the noun or pronoun to which it refers) in person (first, second, third), number, and gender. It has become politically correct to use plural pronouns, such as *they* or *their*, with singular nouns to avoid gender bias. Instead, minor recasting of the sentence can avoid pronoun-antecedent agreement errors and gender bias.

D: A *person* with diabetes must be especially wary of nonhealing ulcers on *their* toes. (The plural *their* does not agree with the singular noun *patient*).
T: *Patients* with diabetes must be especially wary of nonhealing ulcers on *their* toes.

Sentences beginning with *there*

Perhaps the most frequent occurrence of subject-verb agreement errors happens in sentences or clauses beginning with *there*. Because the verb precedes the subject in this construction, care must be taken to identify the correct subject(s). With compound subjects joined by *or*, the subject closest to the verb determines the number of the verb.

There is no thrush or oral lesions.
There are no oral lesions or thrush.
There are no stridors or meningismus.
There is no meningismus or stridors.

D: There is scattered hyperkeratotic lesions that the patient states are similar to the lesion resected on his right forearm.
T: There are scattered hyperkeratotic lesions that the patient states are similar to the lesion resected on his right forearm.

D: There are no definite palpable cervical, supraclavicular, axillary, epitrochlear, or inguinal adenopathy.
T: There is no definite palpable cervical, supraclavicular, axillary, epitrochlear, or inguinal adenopathy.

Subject farther from verb

The farther the subject is from the verb, the more difficult it is to identify.

D: There **is**, on examination of the skin over the abdomen, well-approximated incision <u>margins</u> without erythema, crepitus, fluctuancy, or induration and mild inconsistent left mid and lower quadrant <u>tenderness</u> without definite rebound.

T: There **are**, on examination of the skin over the abdomen, well-approximated incision <u>margins</u> without erythema, crepitus, fluctuancy, or induration and mild inconsistent left mid and lower quadrant <u>tenderness</u> without definite rebound.

D: No definite findings of egophony or rhonchi, wheezes, or rub was noted.

T: No definite findings of egophony or rhonchi, wheezes, or rub were noted.

Verbal phrases as subjects

It may be difficult to identify the subjects of sentences if the subjects themselves are verb forms. The verbals (*-ing* forms) functioning as subjects are underlined, and the verb is in bold type.

D: Driving or operating heavy machinery are to be avoided while on this medication.

T: <u>Driving</u> or <u>operating</u> heavy machinery **is** to be avoided while on this medication.

Apostrophes

Apostrophes are used to show possession, indicate omitted letters or numbers, and occasionally to form plurals of single lowercase letters and numbers.

Eponyms

1. The stylistic trend is away from using the possessive form with eponyms. It is important to note, however, that use of the possessive form remains an acceptable alternative if dictated and/or if indicated as the preference by employer or client.

Apgar score	Alzheimer disease
Babinski sign	Down syndrome
Gram stain	Hodgkin lymphoma
McBurney point	Mohs technique
Janeway lesions	Osler nodes

2. The possessive form is preferred when the noun following the eponym is omitted although it is understood.

He was treated for a possible Wernicke's.
He has Alzheimer's but is otherwise in good health.

3. If *a, an,* or *the* precedes an eponym, do not use the possessive form.

She was placed in the Trendelenburg position.
The Bassini hernia repair was accomplished without difficulty.

4. Do not use an apostrophe to show possession in hyphenated eponyms.

Abbe-Estlander operation
Osgood-Schlatter disease
Jackson-Pratt drain

5. Do not use the possessive when referring to surgical instruments and medical devices.

Fogarty catheter (not Fogarty's catheter)
DeBakey clamp (not DeBakey's clamp)
St. Jude valve (not St. Jude's valve)

Missing elements

Use apostrophes to indicate missing letters or numbers. The use of contractions in medical reports is not recommended, except when quoting a patient.

Acceptable:
The patient described shortness of breath present since the '90s.
The patient complained, "I'm not passing any urine."

Not acceptable:
We won't know the results of the biopsy until Thursday.

Plurals

Do not use apostrophes to form the plurals of abbreviations or numbers, except to avoid confusion when lowercase letters or symbols are made plural.

serial 7's	x's and y's
+'s	4 x 4's
WBCs	ABGs
40s	1990s

Possession

1. Use an apostrophe to form the possessive of a unit of time. Add an apostrophe and *s* ('s) to singular nouns and after the *s* on plural nouns.

The uterus is 16 weeks' size.
1 hour's time
2 hours' time
3 days' time

2. Use an apostrophe to show possession with nouns.

the patient's chart
the recovery room's capacity
the RN's pen
the parents' concerns
the nurses' opinions
2 cents' worth

Articles: *A, An, The*

1. Articles *a, an,* and *the* are transcribed if dictated and may be supplied when not dictated. It is often very difficult to determine which of these words is being

dictated, or if they are being dictated at all. There are clues, however, to help you decide which one you hear. The words *a* or *an* are nonspecific. They will appear before a noun that is nonspecific. *The* is specific and will thus appear before a specific noun.

A rub was heard at the left base.
The child with measles had sat on the patient's bed and hugged her.

2. Use the article *a* before a consonant sound, the article *an* before a vowel sound. Use *a* or *an* before single letters, abbreviations, and numbers, depending on how they sound when spoken.

an MRI	a CAT scan
an introitus	an MI
a myocardial infarction	an attempt

Call Me *Madam*

Those 20 dwarfs turning handstands on the carpet of my mind must be medical transcriptionists. With the temperature at minus 29 degrees, I am getting a little bugsy myself and more than hyperalert at the computer.

Is the content of the medical dictation changing for the worse, or am I just suffering contact dermatitis from Tide in those new little boxes?

There is an increase in the inappropriate use of first names, not just in psychiatric summaries but in all specialties. A 71-year-old female enters the hospital for *rule out myocardial infarction* and the doctor tells us "Fiona" did this and that. If Fiona is from a nursing home, the chances increase dramatically that her surname will be amputated. The older a male patient becomes, the more likely is he to be called by his first name.

If a patient is admitted for drug or alcohol detoxification or any AIDS-related reason, the use of first names increases. I don't think it is a matter of confidentiality. I think it is a matter of doctors doing (pardon me, George) "the power thing."

For the past 30 years, I have been listening to the Ob/Gyn doctors, and one has to give them an A in consistency. They are still patronizing as heck, though they are much more democratic now and have progressed beyond the "little mothers." More women are practicing in obstetrics and gynecology and, unfortunately, have developed a style of "manly" dictation, i.e., using the patient's first name. All those nurse-midwives fought so hard in so many places for the right to be part of the hospital medical team. Then they dictate using the woman's first name, and oy, we are up to our ankles in girl stuff.

Am I the only sentinel? Are there other "first name police" out there? Weren't we trained never to transcribe the patient's name in the body of a report? Not for anyone, not even for babies and children. Is this a question of form, content, ethics, manners, or, heaven help us, total quality?

In the McDonaldization of American medical language as practiced in dictating summaries, there seems

to be less consideration, kindness, and, yes, morality when dealing with human suffering. What, in person, can be a ploy to ameliorate the dehumanizing technological aspect of medical care becomes, on paper, plain crass.

In routine long-term transcription for a sixtyish gentleman internist, I dutifully type his "chronic anxiety-depression syndrome" diagnosis for all his female patients over 40. Since the women never see the reports, I suppose they never know. The transcription supervisor told me he appeared on Valentine's Day morning and asked her why she wasn't wearing red. "I like to see all of my girls in red today."

Because what I am talking about is basic human dignity. Because when formal hospital documents become chatty and palsy-walsy and careless and sloppy, it worries me. And when a patient is bare-bottomed, poked, prodded, sedated, and confused, that is especially when he needs to be a *Mister*, not just *Joe*. A woman in diapers or bleeding through her clothes or being examined status post mastectomy needs to be a *Missus*, not just *Kathy*.

Last week I visited a friend who had cardiac surgery in a major Boston teaching hospital. He handed me his discharge summary. It was printed all in caps, with abbreviations from the diagnoses to the last sentence. "THE PT. WAS AD. TO THE HOS." The lengthy discharge diagnoses were all abbreviated. Hello, Joint Commission?

I called a woman in the biz who knows the area. She said the hospital was encouraging the residents to sit at the screen and peck out their summaries and paying them a couple of bucks to do it. "All they want is the record, Judith," she said. "Never mind anything else."

Next time you visit your doctor, see how the secretary addresses you. If it is by your first name, correct her. Then correct the doctor. It is a short hip-hop from name to attitude.

Judith Marshall
Medicate Me Again

Blood Pressure

The blood pressure reading contains two numbers separated by a slash mark or virgule (/). The dictator says "over" to indicate the slash. (Some ESL physicians may say "on" instead of "over.") The abbreviation for the unit of measure used with blood pressure is *mmHg* (millimeters of mercury). *Hg* is the chemical symbol for mercury. Transcribe *mmHg* when "millimeters of mercury" is dictated. If *BP* is dictated in a medical report, the translation *blood pressure* should be transcribed.

D: BP 120 over 80 millimeters of mercury.
T: Blood pressure 120/80 mmHg.

Brief Forms and Medical Slang

1. Brief forms are shortened forms of legitimate words that can be documented in a dictionary or have come into acceptance through usage. Brief forms can be confused with medical slang. A slang term is either not listed in a dictionary or is designated as slang. Sometimes it is difficult to differentiate between a slang word and a new term that may become standard usage with time. In the Quick-Reference Word List in the back of this book, slang terms are listed in quotation marks, indicating they must be expanded in medical reports ("lytes" = electrolytes).

2. Physicians commonly use medical slang when discussing a patient's condition, but that does not mean the same slang term is acceptable in the medical transcript. Avoid transcribing slang that disparages patients or staff. Physicians do not intend for offensive or off-color remarks to be entered into a patient's health record.

3. Medical slang should be avoided in medical documents for several reasons. A slang term may be obscure and might not clearly or accurately convey the intended meaning. Additionally, a slang term may be open to varied interpretations by different readers of the record, particularly obvious when a health record is subpoenaed for use in legal actions. It may be difficult to replace a slang term with an appropriate nonslang term. Flag the report if you cannot edit the term appropriately. In diagnoses and impressions, brief forms and abbreviations should be expanded.

Following are some terms that are currently deemed acceptable or equivocal and others that are unacceptable. Acceptable or equivocal means they are acceptable in some settings but not in others, or acceptable in some less formal reports like chart notes but not in others. Unacceptable are brief forms and medical slang that may be confused with similar terms and thus must be written out in medical transcription for

clarity. A good rule to remember is, "When in doubt, write it out."

Acceptable or equivocal brief forms

ab, Ab	abortion
bands	banded neutrophils
cardio	cardiology
chemo	chemotherapy
C-section	cesarean section
C-spine	cervical spine
basos	basophils
consult (n.)	consultation
eos	eosinophils
exam	examination
lab	laboratory
lymphs	lymphocytes
monos	monocytes
neuro	neurology, neurologic
NICU ("nick-yoo")	neonatal intensive care unit
PACU ("pack-yoo")	postanesthesia care unit
Pap smear	Papanicolaou smear
path	pathology
polys	polymorphonuclear leukocytes
postop	postoperative
preop	preoperative
prepped	prepared
rehab	rehabilitation
segs	segmented neutrophils
strep	streptococcal
temp	temperature
T-spine	thoracic spine

Unacceptable medical slang

aerosol pentam	aerosolized pentamidine
A fib	atrial fibrillation
alk phos	alkaline phosphatase
amp	ampule, ampicillin
appy	appendectomy
bicarb	bicarbonate
bili	bilirubin
BP	blood pressure
ca	carcinoma
cath, cath'd	catheter, catheterized
circ	circumflex artery
chole	cholecystectomy
coags	coagulation studies
crit	hematocrit
cysto	cystoscopy
DC, DC'd	discharge(d), discontinue(d)
diff	differential
dig ("dij," "didge")	digitalis, digoxin, digitoxin
echo	echocardiogram
fib	fibula, fibrillation
fib-flutter	fibrillation-flutter
H&H	hemoglobin and hematocrit

Unacceptable medical slang *(continued)*

H. flu	*H. (Haemophilus) influenzae*
kilo	kg (kilogram)
lap	laparotomy, laparoscopy
lap chole	laparoscopic cholecystectomy
lytes	electrolytes
med, meds	medication, medications
mets	metastases
multip	multipara
nitro	nitroglycerin
osteo	osteomyelitis
peds	pediatrics
pentam	pentamidine
postchemo	postchemotherapy
primip	primipara
procto	proctoscopy
psych	psychiatric
quads	quadriceps
Rx	prescription
sats	(oxygen) saturation
satting	saturating
SC, sq, subQ	subcutaneous
script	prescription
tab	tablet
tabby	therapeutic abortion
tach	tachycardia
tib-fib	tibia-fibula
tic	diverticulum
T max	maximum temperature
trep	treponema
trach	tracheostomy
trich	trichomonas
V fib	ventricular fibrillation
V tach	ventricular tachycardia
XRT	radiotherapy

Capitalization

Classifications and stages

Do not capitalize words that denote categories or classifications.

Bruce protocol
Child class C
class III cardiac failure
grade 1/6 murmur
stage I
TIMI grade 3 flow
type 2 diabetes
type IIb hyperlipidemia

Department names and specialties

1. Do not capitalize a term denoting a specialist, a specialty, or a department within a medical facility.

ophthalmology, ophthalmologist
physical therapy, physical therapist
emergency department
infectious diseases

2. Do capitalize department names and specialties if they are referred to as people or entities.

The patient will be seen by Pulmonology in the morning.
I have asked Neurology to see the patient prior to and after surgery.
Physical Therapy will plan a rehabilitation program for this patient after surgery.

Directions

Do not capitalize the first letter of points on a compass unless referring to geographical regions or for clarity.

The clinic is east of the hospital.
The patient is from the Southeast.
The patient is on 3 East.
He just moved to the West Coast.

Diseases and anatomical landmarks

Do not capitalize diseases or anatomic landmarks unless they are eponyms (named for a person).

chronic obstructive pulmonary disease
Alzheimer disease

Eponyms

1. Capitalize the person's name that is the basis of an eponym.

Gram stain
Lyme disease
Rovsing sign
Stargardt disease

2. Do not capitalize an eponym made into an adjective or verb.

cushingoid facies
gram-negative bacteria
malpighian bodies
parkinsonian
jacksonian seizure

Headings

Capitalize all letters in main headings, unless instructed otherwise. Only the initial letter of each word in a subheading is capitalized, except in the physical exam of an H&P, where the subheadings are listed vertically and in all capitals.

Capitalize the first word following a colon in a heading or subheading, if the narrative format is used. See **Formats** for more information on headings.

Race, ethnicity, skin color

Capitalize a person's race, ethnic or national origin, but not skin color. Hyphenating compound modifiers indicating national origin is no longer recommended.

Caucasian female	white female
African American male	black male
Asian female	Hispanic male

Titles and degrees

Capitalize titles such as *MD, DO, RN, CMT, CMA, RHIT,* and academic degrees such as *BA, MA, MEd, and PhD. Doctor* is correctly abbreviated as *Dr.* When transcribing a medical doctor's name, do not use both *Dr.* and *MD.* Abbreviations of degrees and professional ratings are often unpunctuated, but if periods are used, do not space between the letters.

MD, M.D.	PhD, Ph.D.
MA, M.A.	MEd, M.Ed.

Trade names

Capitalize trade names but not generic names or nouns associated with a trade name.

acetaminophen with codeine
Medtronic pacemaker
Tylenol with Codeine No. 3 tablets
Vicodin (hydrocodone; acetaminophen)

Classifications

Fractures

Fractures and other orthopedic maladies are often classified according to location, severity, and type. Roman numerals are most often used to designate *grade, stage,* or *type.* Capital letters may be used to indicate a substage.

A Salter-Harris type II fracture was evident on radiographs.
Diagnosis of Neer stage I shoulder impingement was subsequently made.
A grade I stress fracture was suspected although radiographs were negative.
Past history included a Mayo type II B comminuted fracture of her right elbow.

Gleason grade or score (prostate cancer)

1. The Gleason system is based exclusively on the architectural pattern of the glands of the prostate tumor. It evaluates how effectively the cells of any particular cancer are able to structure themselves into glands resembling those of the normal prostate. The ability of a tumor to mimic normal gland architecture is called its *differentiation,* and experience has shown that a tumor whose structure is nearly normal (well differentiated) will probably have a biological behavior relatively close to normal—that is, not very aggressively malignant.

2. Gleason grades go from very well differentiated (grade 1) to very poorly differentiated (grade 5). Of several biopsy specimens, the two highest scores are added together. The lowest possible Gleason score is $1 + 1 = 2$, where no specimen has a score higher than 1.

3. A very typical Gleason score is $2 + 3 = 5$, where the primary pattern has a Gleason grade of 2 and the secondary pattern has a grade of 3. The gravest diagnosis is $5 + 5 = 10$, where the primary and secondary patterns both have the most disordered Gleason grades of 5.

TNM classification of malignant tumors

1. Malignant tumors of the body are frequently classified according to the *TNM Classification of Malignant Tumors.* **T** represents the size of the tumor, **N** the clinical status of the nodes, and **M** the extent of metastasis.

T1	Direct extension of primary tumor.
T2	Direct extension of primary tumor to specific organs.
T3	Direct advanced extension of tumor, unresectable.
TX	Direct extension of tumor not assessed.
N0	Regional lymph nodes not involved.
N1	Regional lymph nodes involved.
NX	Regional lymph nodes not assessed.
M0	No distant metastases.
M1	Distant metastases present.
MX	Distant metastases not assessed.

stage I, T1-2, N0-M0 No extension or node involvement.
stage II, T3, N0, M0 Advanced extension, unresectable.
stage III T1-3, N1, M0 Node involvement.
stage IV, T1-3, N0-1, M1 Distant metastases present.

2. Substages *a* through *d* may be assigned, depending on the part of the body involved. TNM expressions are written with Arabic numerals with a space after each number.

Pathology report showed adenocarcinoma of the prostate, stage T2b N0 M0.

In this example, T2b N0 M0 means the tumor has invaded the deep muscle, but there are no involved lymph nodes or metastases.

3. Other staging indicators may occasionally be used along with TNM criteria to define cancers and assess stages. These are written in all capital letters with Arabic numerals.

grade (G)	G2
host performance (H)	H1
lymphatic invasion (L)	L2
residual tumor (R)	RX
scleral invasion (S)	S0
venous invasion (V)	V1

Colons

Headings

After a heading, use a colon followed by a space, if that is the selected format.

List or series

1. Use a colon after *as follows* or *the following* when it introduces a list or a series.

   His symptoms include all of the following: dyspnea on exertion, fatigue, and productive cough.

2. Do not use a colon after a verb or the words *such as* or *except*, even when they introduce a list.

   His symptoms include exertion, fatigue, and productive cough.
   He can eat just about anything except onions, bell peppers, and cucumbers.
   He was told to avoid activities such as running, climbing stairs, or mowing the lawn for the time being.

Ratios

Use a colon with numerals to express a ratio (a mathematical expression showing the relationship of one part to another).

   A/G ratio was 2:1.
   Albumin-globulin ratio was 2:1.
   I-to-E ratio was 1:2.
   1% lidocaine with 1:100,000 epinephrine
   Xylocaine, 8 cc of a 2% solution with epinephrine 1:40,000 solution was instilled.

   Note. Use a slash with letters, and a hyphen with words or phrases for the name of the laboratory test. Use a colon only in the numerical value (2:1).

Time

Use a colon to express hours and minutes. Do not use the colon and zeros if only the hour is dictated. Do not use a colon with military time.

   The patient was brought to the operating room at 2:20 a.m.
   9 o'clock, or 9 a.m.
   The procedure was begun at 1420 hours.

Note. Avoid redundant expressions like *12 noon, 12 midnight, a.m. in the morning.* Transcribe *noon, midnight,* and *a.m.*

Commas

1. The comma is probably the most misused punctuation mark in the written English language. Misuse includes inserting too many commas, too few, or using them inappropriately so that the meaning of a sentence is unclear or easily misconstrued. In medical transcription, this can have serious consequences by changing medical meaning.

2. In many short compound sentences with closely related independent clauses, it is acceptable to omit the comma before the conjunction; however, in the *MTF&P* transcripts the comma has been retained in most compound sentences for the sake of consistency.

3. In many nouns, adjectives, and phrases in a series, it is acceptable to omit the comma before the conjunction *and* or *or* as long as it does not change the meaning, but in the transcripts the comma has been retained for consistency and accuracy.

4. A comma after a single introductory adverb (*presently, postoperatively, hopefully, subsequently, similarly*) or short adverbial phrase is optional. Commas should be used after longer introductory phrases if the phrase is more than four words. If the introductory phrase contains a verb, it is a clause and requires a comma.

Absolute phrases

Use a comma before or after an absolute phrase—a noun or pronoun followed by a participle and possibly other words—when it appears at the beginning or end of a sentence.

   A DNR order having been signed, the patient was taken off life support.
   The patient was subsequently discharged, having received maximum benefit of hospitalization.

Adjectives following the noun

When even a single adjective follows a noun, as often happens in diagnoses, separate the noun and the adjective(s) with a comma.

   Questionable osteomyelitis, right calcaneus.
   Chronic otitis media, left ear.
   Left hemiparesis and hemiplegia, status post cerebrovascular accident (CVA).
   She did have a hemiarthroplasty, bipolar type, of the the left hip.

Adjectives in a series

1. Use a comma to separate adjectives in a series, but do not put a comma between the last adjective in a series and the noun that follows it.

   Fat pads were taken from the nasal, central, and lateral compartments of each lower lid.

2. Use a comma to separate paired coordinate adjectives that have no relationship to each other.

The patient had an enlarged, irregular uterus.

Tip: If you can substitute *and* for the comma or change the order of the adjectives, and the sentence sounds natural, it is usually safe to use the comma.

3. Do not use commas between cumulative adjectives, which are adjectives that build upon one another; that is, the first describes the second, the second describes the third, etc.

   bilateral lower extremity TED hose

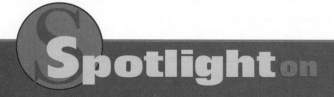

A Little Bit of Comma Sense

by Richard Lederer, Ph.D.

Are you confounded by commas, addled by apostrophes, and queasy about quotation marks? Do you believe that a bracket is just a support for a wall shelf, a dash is something you make for the bathroom, and a colon and semicolon are large and small intestines? If so, I'm pleased to tell you I'm about to be the father of a bouncing baby about mastering punctuation.

In *Comma Sense: A Fun-damental Guide to Punctuation* (St. Martin's Press), humorist John Shore and I present what we hope will be hilarious portraits of American icons and connect each one to a mark of punctuation. We hope that while you're laughing your head off over the weird but instructional examples, you'll master everything you need to know about punctuation through simple, clear, and right-on-the-mark rules.

Punctuation can make an enormous difference in meaning. Which dog has the upper paw?: "A clever dog knows its master." "A clever dog knows it's master." The second sentence, of course. Why do so many people insert a squiggle before the *s* in the possessive *its*?

Which speaker beheld a monster?: "I saw a man eating lobster." "I saw a man-eating lobster."

Note the effect of the missing apostrophe in this sentence: "The butler stood in the doorway and called the guests names." And in this classified ad: "WANTED: Guitar for college student to learn to play, classical non-electric, also piano to replace daughters lost in fire."

Note the startling result of the absence of hyphens in this headline: FATHER TO BE STABBED TO DEATH IN STREET.

Behold the effect of the missing serial comma (the one that should go before the "and") in this book dedication—"To my parents, the Pope and Mother Teresa." And in this sentence— "At summer camp I missed my dog, my little brother, the odor of my dad's pipe and my boyfriend."

Now have a look at the difference between these two love notes:

My Dear Pat,

The dinner we shared the other night—it was absolutely lovely! Not in my wildest dreams could I ever imagine anyone as perfect as you are. Could you—if only for a moment—think of our being together forever? What a cruel joke to have you come into my life only to leave again; it would be heaven denied. The possibility of seeing you again makes me giddy with joy. I face the time we are apart with great sadness.

John

P.S.: I would like to tell you that I love you. I can't stop thinking that you are one of the prettiest women on earth.

My Dear,

Pat the dinner we shared the other night. It was absolutely lovely—not! In my wildest dreams, could I ever imagine anyone? As perfect as you are, could you—if only for a moment— think? Of our being together forever: what a cruel joke! To have you come into my life only to leave again: it would be heaven! Denied the possibility of seeing you again makes me giddy. With joy I face the time we are apart.

With great "sadness,"

John

P.S. I would like to tell you that I love you. I can't. Stop thinking that you are one of the prettiest women on earth.

The power's in the punctuation, baby! The first letter is a clear (albeit clunky) profession of undying affection; the second is sure to sweep Pat onto her feet. The only thing separating one document from the other is, of course, punctuation, which can mean the difference between a second date and a restraining order.

Source: *Perspectives on the Medical Transcription Profession*

Explanation: In the above example, *bilateral* modifies *lower extremity* and the whole phrase modifies *TED hose* (a compound noun, not an adjective and noun).

Although the above example appears at first glance to be adjectives in a series, it is not. Cumulative adjectives generally follow a regular order as follows: Determiner (the articles *a, an, the,* numbers and other quantifiers such as *none* or *some,* and pronouns such as *those, these, my, your*), observation and subjective judgments (*size, shape, ugly, pretty, delicious, yucky, happy*), condition (*broken, sagging, wrinkled*), age (*old, young, new*), color (*red, blue*), nationality or origin (*American, Chinese*), religion (*Hindu, Christian, Jewish, Muslim*), qualifier (this last adjective is inseparable from the noun). This order may vary somewhat.

4. In most writing, it is considered bad form to use more than three or four adjectives in a row, but it happens quite often in medical transcription. Should the order of the dictated phrase vary, you would generally not edit to a different order but transcribe as dictated.

5. When the patient's race is given, consider it to be part of the noun and not an adjective.

> The patient is a frail, disoriented 70-year-old Caucasian female.

Adverbs in a series

Do not use a comma to separate an adverb from the adjective or other adverb it modifies. The adverbs are underlined.

> The patient had a <u>very</u> large, protruding, pendulous mass.
> The patient was <u>mildly</u> <u>hemodynamically</u> unstable while in the emergency department but stabilized on the floor.

Appositives

Use commas to set off an appositive—a noun or phrase situated next to or near a word that it expands upon or explains. While often nonessential, an appositive is sometimes essential, in which case no commas would be used.

> Marion Bartley, MD, was asked to come to the surgery suite to stent the ureters.
> After reviewing the patient's morning labs, including CBC, PT, and PTT, the procedure started.
> The patient had a very large mass, the size of an orange, filling most of the right atrium.

See **Essential elements** for appositives that should not be set off with commas.

Aside or afterthought

These terms are used here to identify late-coming explanations, usually adverbial phrases or clauses, and usually appearing at the end of a sentence.

> He subsequently was placed in rehabilitation where he improved, only to later show a decline in his walking.
> Femoral pulses were diminished in both right and the left, somewhat more on the left side.
> It was evident that the patient had a large prolapsing hemorrhoid, too large for rubber banding, and it was considered appropriate for a standard hemorrhoidectomy operation.

Note: In this last example, the phrase set off by commas appears at the end of an independent clause, although it is not at the end of the sentence.

Clauses in a series

Three or more independent clauses (complete sentences) that are clearly meant to be one sentence where the final two clauses are joined by a coordinating conjunction are punctuated with commas.

> The wound was irrigated and inspected, sutures were placed, and a bandage was applied.

Commas and compound sentences

1. Use a comma to separate two independent clauses (complete sentences) joined by a coordinating conjunction (*and, but, for, nor, or, so, yet*).

> The patient complains of difficulty finding the right word, but he denies any extremity weakness.
> The patient's condition improved, and he was transferred from ICU to a regular bed.
> The patient's cardiac catheterization revealed only moderate stenosis of the left circumflex, and we will treat him conservatively.

2. If the two independent clauses—each a complete sentence—are short (fewer than four or five words long) and closely related, a comma is optional.

> He had tried chemotherapy but it was not tolerated well.

Note: Compound coordinating conjunctions (*either . . . or*) do not require a comma to separate the clauses.

> Either the chemistry panel results are erroneous or this patient's electrolytes are completely off the scale.

3. Do not insert a comma before a coordinating conjunction like *but* that is not followed by both a subject and a complete verb (including helping verb).

Incorrect: Dermatitis apparently cleared after 34 days of ketoconazole and Augmentin, but recurred after 2 weeks off antibiotics.

Correct: Dermatitis apparently cleared after 34 days of ketoconazole and Augmentin but recurred after 2 weeks off antibiotics.

Incorrect: No adventitious lung sounds were noted, and no congestion identified.

Correct: No adventitious lung sounds were noted and no congestion identified.

Note: In this latter example, there is a subject and a verb after the conjunction, but the verb is incomplete (*was identified* would make it complete).

See **Clauses in a series** for punctuating more than two independent clauses. Other compound sentences require the use of a semicolon; see that section for rules and examples.

Commas in a series

Commas are used with nouns, adjectives, phrases, and clauses in a series according to the *a, b, and c rule* or the *a, b and c rule*. The use of the final comma before the words *and* or *or* in any list is optional if it does not distort medical meaning.

Essential elements

Do not use commas to set off elements that are grammatically essential to the sentence. In addition to the examples below, adjectival phrases beginning with *that* are not set off with commas. See **That** and **Which** for further explanation.

The patient whom you sent over to my office on Wednesday never showed up. (What patient? The patient whom you sent.)

The dog that bit the boy was tested for rabies. (Which dog? The dog that bit the boy.)

Insertions

1. Set off nonessential insertions with commas.

   The patient, surprisingly, recovered without intervention.

   Examination showed greater saphenous vein reflux at, at least, three or four calf sites.

   The patient, however, insisted on being discharged immediately.

2. If the rhythm or flow of the sentence is not significantly affected by the insertion, no comma is needed.

   He underwent subtotal resection of his acoustic neuroma but unfortunately also suffered injury to the brain stem and cerebellum.

   He subsequently was placed in rehabilitation where he improved.

Introductory remarks

1. Use a comma after an introductory clause (an expression that includes a verb), interjections, and the words *yes* or *no*. However, there is precedent in current usage for omitting the comma after introductory transitional words or phrases and other short introductory phrases of less than five words.

   When the patient arrived in the emergency department, he was already in extremis.

   Approximately a year and a half ago, she developed a persistent and intensely pruritic dermatitis.

   Neurologically, he is grossly intact regarding motor, sensory, and cerebellar function.

   Consequently, it was decided not to admit Mr. Smith at this time.

2. Commas are optional in the following sentences.

   As a result, we felt that the patient was not a candidate for cardiac bypass.

   As a result we felt that the patient was not a candidate for cardiac bypass.

   On palpation, there is some tenderness in the left inguinal area.

   On palpation there is some tenderness in the left inguinal area.

   Otherwise, he will return to see me in a month.

   Otherwise he will return to see me in a month.

Misplaced modifiers

Set off a modifying phrase that is separated from the word it modifies. If at the end of a sentence, precede it with a comma. For clarity, the sentence may sometimes be recast if editing is permitted by your employer or client.

This patient returned today with a spreading rash on her shoulders, upper chest, and back, which has been present for the last couple of months.

Nonessential elements

A nonessential element means that the word or phrase is not necessary to complete the thought. It is used here to include added or inserted elements such as appositives, absolute phrases, parenthetical expressions, asides, afterthoughts, interjections, and any other grammatically nonessential element. Another way to think of nonessential elements is as nonidentifying or nondefining. If a nonessential element is removed from a sentence, the sentence should still make complete sense.

Nouns in a series

Use a comma to separate nouns in a series.

They understood the options, benefits, risks, and complications and wished to proceed.

Parenthetical expressions

1. A parenthetical expression interrupts the flow of thought.

   The patient also has chief complaint of increased swelling of the lower abdominal girth, which is sort of vague, that has been somewhat more apparent in the last few weeks.

2. A parenthetical expression can also be enclosed in parentheses or set off by dashes if commas would be confusing.

   He was comfortable (according to him, for the first time in many weeks), and the pain could not be elicited despite stimulation of his right cheek, mandible, and gum trigger zone.

   He was comfortable—according to him, for the first time in many weeks—and the pain could not be elicited despite stimulation of his right cheek, mandible, and gum trigger zone.

Contractions

Contractions are not recommended in medical reports except when included in quotations, as in a patient's quoted statement. Do not use other dictated contractions unless acceptable to the facility. Do not use contractions when they are not dictated.

   Dictated and transcribed: The patient stated, "I can't walk 10 feet without getting short of breath."

   D: This was about a year ago, and he really didn't do too much in trying to improve this situation.

   T: This was about a year ago, and he really did not do too much in trying to improve this situation.

   D: She doesn't have any significant urgency.

   T: She does not have any significant urgency.

Dashes

Do not confuse a dash (—) with a hyphen (-) (see **Hyphens**). A hyphen differs in both use and appearance from a dash. Dashes are used to give greater emphasis, to explain a statement, to replace a comma or comma pair, or to set off a parenthetical statement. Do not space before or after a dash. Use the Help feature in your word processor to learn how to create a dash.

   The lungs reveal decreased breath sounds at the bases—right greater than left.

   FINAL DIAGNOSES
   1. Bilateral otitis media—under treatment.
   2. Sepsis suspected—ruled out.
   3. Rash—possible viral exanthem.

Editing *and Style*

In editing dictation, we do not go charging in, doctoring up reports in an aggressive way, in an intrusional way. It has to be done so subtly, so delicately, so carefully, that we get a favorable response from the dictator. . . .

We must be so involved with what we are transcribing that we know what is going on and can detect something that is dictated that does not make sense, that does not flow, that does not add up. We must listen with an educated ear, with an intelligent ear, so that we can produce an accurate, intelligent, clear document, always remembering the fine line between editing and tampering.

A blank is an honorable thing; it means you don't know. If you have tried everything you can try to fill in that blank and can't, leaving a blank is preferable to guessing. Guessing is bluffing. . . . A blank is entirely legal and entirely acceptable.

Medical transcriptionists don't dictate, physicians do. Don't type "The patient was draped in a sterile manner" when the surgeon dictates: "The patient was sterilely draped."

Vera Pyle
Current Medical Terminology

Dates

1. Dates in the demographic data can be either spelled out in upper and lowercase or written as numerals separated by virgules (slashes) or hyphens. Many institutions require that the year be four digits. Dictated and transcribed dates are written only as numerals.

May 25, 2007	25 May 2007
05/25/07	05/25/2007
05-25-07	05-25-2007

2. In the body of a report, set the year off with commas when it follows the month and day. Do not use punctuation when the day precedes the month or when only a month and year are given.

   Elective surgery was scheduled for March 30, 2007, but was canceled by the patient.
   The patient was admitted on 25 May 2007 and went to surgery the following day, on 26 May 2007.
   The patient had a hysterectomy in December 1999.

   Note: When the month is not given, it is acceptable to transcribe as dictated.

   He will see me on the 9th of next month.

Demographic Data

See **Format**.

Editing Dictation *on the Fly*

It really does not take much to tickle the funny bones of MTs who work with words all day long. The slip of a tongue ("the patient had a sinkable episode"), the unconscious transposition of a crucial consonant or vowel ("performed a slaplingotomy"), the inadvertent addition of a syllable or two ("patient was rotototated")—these simple faux pas have been known to trigger helpless mirth and frivolity in more than a few transcription pools or at-home offices.

Often it is not the words themselves (all perfectly valid, with easily understood meanings located in a dictionary), but the mental picture they conjure up that will start the giggling:

"The floor was full so patient was placed on telemetry." Try as I might, I cannot get past the picture of patients, packed in like sardines, lying head-to-toe all over the floor of a hospital ward, with one lone patient perched uncomfortably on top of a telemetry unit!

"The patient's dressing is falling apart, but is otherwise intact." I have to wonder if the Mummy has risen and is stalking about the waiting room trying to locate all the fragments of its dressing as they fall off on the floor.

"The patient was scoped and a very large rectal polyp was discovered in the office." Can't you just see the nurses and the physician jumping all over the office trying to trap that escaping polyp with a butterfly net?

An MT has no need of movies or television programs to provide mental stimulation and often colorful mental imagery:

"Patient is a 4-year-old male who voluntarily gave up his driver's license a few years ago."

"The patient's primary care provider recommended she be sent to a competent ophthalmologist, so she was inadvertently sent to me."

"The patient is pregnant and his wife is due in 6 weeks, so he is under some stress."

"Date of death 04/15/XXXX, the patient will be sent to an assisted-living facility for further rehabilitation."

"The patient's mother and sister have prostate cancer."

And, it never fails that on a day when one least suspects it, a dictator who is a frustrated creative writer will pepper his dictation with things like "Patient describes the diarrhea as being usually of a chocolate pudding consistency, but sometimes more watery, a bit like sauce or beef gravy, but never quite as thin as soup."

MTs are trained to transcribe many things in a "politically correct" manner. Perhaps my favorite of all descriptions for a deceased patient that follows the true precepts of "politically correct" is this sentence posted in an Internet message forum: "Patient failed to achieve wellness potential."

Some of the most creative mental pictures are provided by what is known as "doctorisms"—made-up words that may or may not exist in a dictionary but are perfectly valid for use in medical reports. An individual MT or patient may have never seen or heard them, but they are words that are commonly used, sometimes even in journal articles, that other dictators will understand without any problem at all:

"The patient almost syncopized in the restroom." This means the patient almost fainted, but it leaves one with visions of a patient unsuccessfully trying to get those feet moving in the same rhythm as the rest of the bathroom chorus line!

"The patient was primatized." I have to admit that at first I took this to mean that the patient, by some arcane sort of medical treatment, was converted into a primate, but I was indignantly informed that this meant the patient received a treatment of Primatene Mist.

Of course, it is not always the dictator who provides the occasion to see a report come back across our desks with great big red circles and exclamation points on it. It is just as likely to be the MT who hits that crucial wrong key or "hears" something that is a tad off: "Some of the glands exhibit secretary material"; ". . . performed a total abdominal hysterectomy and bilateral slaplingo-oophorectomy."

All in all, I tend to look at all this as *slaplingopathy*—the practice of slapping one's thigh and laughing uproariously. (Or would that be "ridiculopathy"?)

Renee Priest
Perspectives on the Medical Transcription Profession

Department Names as Entities

Sometimes dictators refer to departments and specialties as though they were individual people, that is, instead of a person's name. When this is done, it is appropriate to capitalize the department name or the specialty.

> Similar specimens were also sent to the CDC per request of Neurology.
> Infectious Disease was called in to monitor the patient's fever.
> Patient was seen by Pulmonary after he was extubated.

Diacritical Marks

1. Diacritical marks, such as acute (´) and grave (`) accents, umlauts (¨), and cedillas (ç), are optional in medical transcription and rarely used.

café au lait spots	cafe au lait spots
Laënnec cirrhosis	Laennec cirrhosis

2. The spelling of some words changes when the diacritical marks are not used.

Müller duct	Mueller duct
Grüntzig balloon	Gruentzig balloon

Editing

1. Every dictator has at one time or another misspoken and said something like, "The patient smokes two beers a day and drinks two packs," "Electrocautery was obtained with hemostasis," or referred to the surgery on the left leg in one paragraph and the right in the next (even though surgery was scheduled on only one leg). Dictating physicians are counting on the medical transcriptionist to be alert and, when necessary, to correct their mistakes.

2. On the job, your employer should make you aware of how much or how little editing is expected. Some employers insist on verbatim transcription—impossible to do because everyone makes unconscious edits, such as adding articles and correcting grammar. Others have very liberal editing policies and allow extensive recasting of sentences. Most are somewhere in the middle.

3. Editing is used minimally in the *MTF&P* transcripts and limited to only what is needed to correct obvious grammar, punctuation, and medical errors. When appropriate, footnotes suggest more extensive edits and/or flagging for clarification. The experienced medical transcriptionist, with a firm grasp of medical language and terminology and familiarity with the employer's or dictator's preferences, may edit in various ways throughout a report.

Additions and substitutions

Where warranted, the transcriptionist may add conjunctions (*and, but, for, or, nor*), prepositions (*of, to, in, on, with*), articles (*a, an, the*), pronouns (*he, she, it, you, we*) and nouns (*the patient, the procedure*) as the subject of a sentence, and verbs (especially helping verbs, such as *was, were, has,* or *had*) to complete a sentence. On the job, be sure to confirm with your supervisor if and when it is acceptable to do this. It is acceptable, however, to type as dictated, to preserve the style of the dictator. Examples of appropriate editing follow.

D: Noted some mild pedal edema.
T: She noted some mild pedal edema.
   or The patient noted some mild pedal edema.

D: He was seen in consultation for gastroenterology reasons, and felt that he had alcoholic liver disease.
T: He was seen in consultation for gastroenterology reasons, and it was felt that he had alcoholic liver disease.

D: Pelvic examination was compromised because of a tight vaginal introitus, unable to use a speculum.
T: Pelvic examination was compromised because of a tight vaginal introitus, and I was unable to use a speculum.

D: Her left foot was appreciably colder than the right foot, temperaturewise.
T: Her left foot was appreciably colder than the right foot.

D: Patient presents this date, a 2 to 3 week history of swelling of the left leg that started with soreness in the left ankle.
T: Patient presents this date with a 2- to 3-week history of swelling of the left leg that started with soreness in the left ankle.

D: We have worked her quads very good in therapy, and appear to be strengthening nicely.
T: We have worked her quadriceps very well in therapy, and they appear to be strengthening nicely.

D: Admitted and taken to surgery where an open reduction, plate fixation of the lateral malleolus carried out as well as the internal fixation of the posterior malleolus.
T: He was admitted and taken to surgery where an open reduction and plate fixation of the lateral malleolus were carried out as well as the internal fixation of the posterior malleolus.

D: A man, 68 years of age, sudden onset of cardiac asystole or ventricular fibrillation, no blood pressure, no pulse, and was coded at the scene, and then some semblance of rhythm was obtained, and it was felt that he either had ventricular tachycardia or supraventricular tachycardia.

T: This man, 68 years of age, had the sudden onset of cardiac asystole or ventricular fibrillation. He had no blood pressure, no pulse, and was coded at the scene. Then some semblance of rhythm was obtained, and it was felt that he either had ventricular tachycardia or supraventricular tachycardia.

Inconsistencies

1. Editing also includes watching for medical inconsistencies within a report, such as a hysterectomy reportedly done on a man, or different ages given for the same patient within one report, or a surgery that begins on the left leg and ends on the right. If an inconsistency cannot be resolved, the word or phrase in question should be flagged to the dictator's attention for clarification.

D: Laboratory data were entirely normal, including CBC revealing a hemoglobin of 32 and a hematocrit of 12, with a white blood count of 20,000 with a differential of 80 segs and 20 lymphs.

T: Laboratory data were entirely normal, including a CBC revealing a hemoglobin of 12 and a hematocrit of 32, with a white blood count of _____ (20,000) with a differential of 80 segs and 20 lymphs.

Rationale: A white blood count of 20,000 is elevated, and there is no indication in the rest of the report that note was taken of the elevated count. The hemoglobin and hematocrit were no doubt reversed.

Tense

1. In a History and Physical Examination (H&P) report, the chief complaint and history of present illness are usually dictated in the present tense, although the tense may vary when describing events that took place in the past. The past history is usually dictated in the past tense. The physical examination may be in the past or present tense, depending on the dictator's style. Consultations and chart notes generally follow the same patterns as an H&P report. In a discharge summary, the predominant tense is usually past tense. A dictator reading the history of present illness, however, may slip into the present tense if that is what was used in that report.

2. In all reports, tenses may change from present to past to future within a single sentence and be entirely appropriate. Be careful in editing verb tense. An appropriate edit might be to edit the physical examination or discharge summary to past tense if past tense is the predominant tense. Here are examples of appropriate edits for verb tense.

D: Hematocrit is 44; hemoglobin was 14.6.
T: Hematocrit was 44; hemoglobin was 14.6.

D: The sodium gradually decreased from 159 down to 135 by March 13, and the blood sugar decreasing from 166 to 97.
T: The sodium gradually decreased from 159 down to 135 by March 13, and the blood sugar decreased from 166 to 97.

3. Watch for the use of tenses like the "historical present" when making such edits, however.

The patient is a 29-year-old black female who was admitted for vague abdominal pain of 6 weeks' duration.

Explanation: The patient is still 29 years old; do not change the tense, even if the rest of the report is in past tense. The only time the past tense would be correct in such a construction is if the patient died in the hospital.

4. A common verb tense error is the use of helping verbs with the past tense form of a verb rather than with the past participle (*has drank* when it should be *has drunk*, for example). Related to this error, many transcriptionists hear *had had* and think it is a mistake. *Had had* is a perfectly acceptable construction and has a specific meaning. You should correct helping verb plus past tense to a helping verb plus past participle, but you should not change *had had*.

5. If a dictator consistently uses the present tense throughout a report, that's a pretty good clue that you should not edit to past tense.

Eponyms

1. The trend in medicine is to drop the possessive form of eponyms; however, the practice is not yet universally accepted. It is still acceptable to use the possessive form if dictated, or if it is an indicated preference of originator or employer. In the *MTF&P* transcripts, possessive forms of eponyms are retained if dictated, unless they are incorrect.

Lyme disease (no apostrophe *s*, even if dictated)

2. An eponym that is used as an adjective is usually capitalized; the noun which follows is not.

McBurney point	Tinel sign
Achilles tendon	Foley catheter

3. A word derived from an eponym is generally not capitalized.

ehrlichiosis (from Ehrlichia)
gasserian ganglion (from Gasser ganglion)

jacksonian seizure (from Jackson)
malpighian bodies
parkinsonian (from Parkinson disease)

4. Compound eponyms (two or more names) and eponyms preceded by *a*, *an*, or *the* should not be possessive.

Jackson-Pratt drain
the Ghon tubercle

Flagging Reports

1. When a medical transcriptionist or supervisor has unresolved questions about dictated words or phrases in a report, the report should be called to the attention of the dictator, or "flagged." The flag should clearly identify the report, the words or phrases in question and, if appropriate, include a phonetic rendering of what the word or phrase "sounds like."

D: The original hemoglobin was 22.1 and 66.9 secondary to the patient's severe dehydration.
T: The original hemoglobin was 22.1 and hematocrit 66.9 secondary to the patient's severe dehydration.

Even though it is clear from the context that the missing word is *hematocrit*, such an edit should be flagged to the dictator's attention, as should any edits that supply missing words or change medical content.

2. On the job, your employer or client will have specific instructions for how to create a flag. If your instructor allows you to use flags in your practice transcription, a blank line and a "sounds like" in parentheses following the blank should be sufficient.

Example: The patient was discharged on _____ ("Core Guard").

Footnotes

Footnotes are not typically used in medical transcription, but they are used in the *MTF&P* transcripts to show acceptable alternatives and provide additional information as a learning aid.

Format

Formats vary from facility to facility but are usually standardized within an individual facility. Standard formats are often turned into templates (see **Templates** below), into which the dictated report can be typed. The instructions described below are specifically for the *MTF&P Transcript Keys* and may or may not conform with what you encounter on the job. The style and order of formats on the job may also be different. The American Society

for Testing of Materials (ASTM) provides templates for histories and physicals and for discharge summaries.

Abbreviations in headings

Doctors may take shortcuts by dictating abbreviations for major report headings. Headings should always be spelled out in full, except for HEENT, which is an acceptable subheading in Review of Systems or in the Physical Examination.

HPI   HISTORY OF PRESENT ILLNESS
PE   PHYSICAL EXAMINATION
LAB   LABORATORY DATA
EXAM   EXAMINATION

Adding headings not dictated

If a physician dictates a narrative portion that typically belongs under a particular heading but fails to dictate the heading, the transcriptionist should insert the proper heading. Skill in adding appropriate headings and subheadings will come with knowledge and experience. (See Sample Reports in each chapter.) Do not turn a complete sentence into a fragment by lopping off part of it to use as a heading. However, if clipped sentences are dictated, they may be transcribed.

D: Heart has a regular rate and rhythm. Lungs are clear.
T: Heart: Heart has a regular rate and rhythm.
  Lungs: Lungs are clear.

Dictated and Transcribed: Heart: Regular rate and rhythm. Lungs clear.

Note: No colon is needed after *lungs* as the helping verb is understood; this is called a clipped sentence.

Demographics

1. Demographics refers to the information needed to identify the patient, dictator, date, and other information the facility deems essential. It can appear in a variety of forms. It may appear in a template or be applied automatically by the word processing software.

2. Demographics are displayed in many ways. It is important to note, however, that with the advent of the computerized patient record, demographic information may appear quite different, even foreign.

3. Following is an example of the demographic data block from a facility using computerized patient records. Some of the information required is self-evident, but each MT would have a printed form that would indicate what to insert in each field. All data is typed within the brackets. It is important that no spaces be added, that the case of letters be as on the template, and that all fields be completed. An uncompleted field would bounce the report back to

someone who would complete the data before it could be uploaded into the patient's computerized "chart." If the document needed to be printed, the codes would be stripped off, and only the pertinent data would appear on the printed document.

```
<TrID:mts>
<DMDNo:7054>
<DT:HP>
<Name:DOE,JANE>
<AMDNo:123456789>
<MRNo:M0101010101>
<BillNo:D000>
<32:>
<13:mm/dd/yyyy>
<31:mm/dd/yyyy>
<4:/yyyy>
<5:>
<15:8481>
```

Diagnosis/diagnoses

If a physician dictates the singular form *Diagnosis* and then lists several diagnoses, edit *Diagnosis* to the plural *Diagnoses*. If the dictator says "same" for the final diagnosis or postoperative diagnosis, referring to a previously dictated impression or diagnosis, copy the diagnosis in full.

Heading style

In the *MTF&P* transcripts, each major heading in an H&P, Consultation, Discharge Summary, and Operative Report should be on a line by itself, in all capital letters, and with no punctuation. The paragraph begins on the line immediately below the heading. Capitalize only the first letter of each word of a subheading, except for the physical examination in an H&P report; in that case, the subheadings are listed vertically with the subheading in all capitals. Follow the subheading with a colon. Follow with the related dictation on the same line, capitalizing the first word of the sentence. Do not underline headings even if the dictator instructs you to do so, unless it is the stated preference of the facility. Following the Allergies heading, some facilities require that the allergic medications also be placed in all capitals.

HISTORY AND PHYSICAL EXAMINATION

DATE OF ADMISSION
March 30, XXXX

CHIEF COMPLAINT
Nausea and vomiting.

HISTORY OF PRESENT ILLNESS
The patient was well until …

PAST MEDICAL HISTORY
Medical: Usual childhood diseases. Surgical: No prior surgeries.

ALLERGIES
PENICILLIN. No known allergies to other medications or food.

SOCIAL HISTORY
Does not smoke. Does not drink alcohol to excess.

REVIEW OF SYSTEMS
Neurological: The patient once had a grand mal seizure many years ago but had had no recurrence. Eyes: She denied diplopia, photophobia, or pain. Cardiorespiratory: She denied shortness of breath or cough. She denied history of asthma. She has only had occasional bouts of bronchitis. She has had no history of pneumonia, no history of heart disease, heart murmur, or rheumatic fever.
Gastrointestinal: No symptoms except those associated with the present illness. She denies hematemesis, ulcer disease, gallbladder or liver disease. She has had occasional loose stools for which she takes Imodium. Genitourinary: She denies frequency, hesitancy, dysuria, hematuria, or stone.
Obstetric/Gynecologic: She is para 0, gravida 0, and she has had a pelvic and Pap smear in August before coming to school. These were said to be normal. She has no history of sexually transmitted disease. Musculoskeletal: She denies joint pain, tenderness, or limitation of motion.

PHYSICAL EXAMINATION
GENERAL APPEARANCE: The patient was a well-developed, morbidly obese, pleasant white female who was alert and oriented x3.
VITAL SIGNS: Blood pressure 138/80, pulse 78 and regular, respirations 18 and regular and nonlabored.
HEENT: Normal.

et cetera

IMPRESSION
Nausea and vomiting.

PLAN
Admit for gastrointestinal workup.

Headings vary in phrasing

Just as formats vary, so does the way a heading is worded. Some facilities may use any wording dictated; others may prefer standardized wording, such as that promoted by ASTM standard E2184, Standard Specification for Healthcare Document Formats. For example, the Chief Complaint may also be called Reason for Admission. The History of Present Illness may be simply History, Present Illness, or Summary of Illness.

Narrative format

In a narrative paragraph, such as in chart notes, discharge summaries, and the physical exam portion of a consultation, rare headings may be followed by a colon with the subsequent word capitalized.

> PHYSICAL EXAMINATION: On exam today she is alert, in no distress. Vital signs are stable. She has been afebrile. HEENT: Head is normocephalic, conjunctivae pink. Oropharynx is clear. The neck is supple. There is good range of motion. No bruits are auscultated. There is mild tenderness only in the occipital region. There is not much spasm. She had good range of motion of the neck and the back. There is minimal spasm in the lumbar region. Also, straight leg raise test is negative. Lungs are clear to auscultation. Heart: Regular rate, no murmur.

Numbering diagnoses

1. Occasionally a dictator will begin to number the diagnoses and then give only one diagnosis. In that case, omit the number. Retaining the number gives the impression that there may be more diagnoses that were omitted.

2. In listing several diagnoses, dictators often lose track of the next number. They may inadvertently give the wrong number (which should be corrected by the transcriptionist) or delegate the numbering to the transcriptionist by saying "number next" to indicate the next diagnosis. The transcriptionist should supply numbers to a long list of diagnoses, even if the dictator fails to number them.

3. Numbered diagnoses should be presented in a vertical format on the left margin (not indented).

   1. Left knee medial collateral ligament tear.
   2. Anterior cruciate ligament tear.
   3. Possible meniscus tear.

Paragraphing

Paragraphing should be added to break up long reports or to set up a new heading and its accompanying paragraph. Be aware that when some physicians dictate "new line," they mean to begin a new paragraph. Dictators may also say "new paragraph" when a new paragraph is not necessary, for example, after every one or two sentences. It is sometimes acceptable to combine these paragraphs, but be certain a new paragraph is not needed.

Psychiatric diagnoses

See Chapter 15, Psychiatry, for a discussion of axes (multi-axial assessment as outlined in *DSM-IV*) and a sample report for information on how to format a psychiatric diagnosis.

Report logs

On the job, you may be required to keep report logs. Report logs record important data about the reports you have transcribed. A log may be generated electronically with the aid of macros, or you can keep a manual log to document your work.

Signature blocks

Every report has a signature of the dictator; it may be added electronically, be part of the template, or be added by the MT transcribing the report. Information included in the signature block includes the following: dictator's name, dictator's initials (usually in all capital letters) followed by a colon and the MT's initials (which are usually lowercase) or a number, and date (and often time and place) of dictation and transcription. The flush-left style is the most common style.

Templates

A template is a pattern or outline that contains format elements that are the same for every document. It is a time-saving device and adds uniformity and consistency to documents. A template may hold a variety of information, including a facility's letterhead and standard report headings. Sometimes multiple templates are merged within a single document, such as patient demographic data, signature lines, and even passages of text. We have not included templates for the *MTF&P* transcripts because formats vary considerably.

Genus and Species

1. Capitalize genus names and their abbreviated forms when they are accompanied by a species name. Lowercase species names.

   Clostridium difficile
   Escherichia coli
   Staphylococcus aureus

2. Lowercase genus names used in plural and adjectival forms and when used in the vernacular (when they stand alone without a species name).

   group B streptococcus
   mycoplasmal pneumonia
   salmonella outbreak
   staph infection
   staphylococcal infection
   strep throat

3. After the genus-species name has been written out in full in a transcript, it may thereafter be abbreviated, if dictated.

Clostridium difficile	C. difficile
Escherichia coli	E. coli
Staphylococcus aureus	S. aureus

4. Some references omit the period after the abbreviation, but it may be added for clarity.

5. Genus and species names are italicized in medical books and journals, but italics are not recommended in medical transcripts.

Grade, Stage, Type

The terms *grade*, *stage*, and *type* should not be capitalized. While the trend is toward the use of Arabic numerals with *grade* and *type*, Roman numerals are most often used with *stage*. Unfortunately, there are no *definitive* rules for using Arabic or Roman for any of these terms, and you should refer to your medical references for specific guidelines. See also **Classifications**.

> grade 2/6 systolic ejection murmur
> Crowe classification grade II
> FIGO stage IV ovarian carcinoma
> Gleason grade 2 +3 = 5
> stage 3 Garden fracture
> type 2 diabetes mellitus
> type IIb hyperlipidemia

Headings

See **Format**.

Hyphens

Many coined words commonly used in medical reports do not appear in dictionaries, and it is up to the transcriptionist to decide whether to hyphenate them for clarity. The trend in contemporary usage is to use fewer hyphens, especially in long-standing compounds after they become common (*weightbearing, nonweightbearing*). For example, no form of *weightbearing, weight-bearing, weight bearing, or non-weight-bearing* (terms commonly used in orthopedic reports) appears in English or medical dictionaries, with the exception of *The Oxford English Dictionary*, which hyphenates it as a noun and as an adjective.

Adverb-adjective combinations

1. Some adverb-adjective combinations are traditionally hyphenated when they appear before the noun and not hyphenated when following the noun.

> The patient is a well-developed, well-nourished 57-year-old white female appearing her stated age.
> The patient is well developed and well nourished.

2. Do not use a hyphen with compounds formed with adverbs ending in *-ly* plus a participle or adjective.

> poorly developed and poorly nourished patient
> highly complex symptoms

3. Do not use a hyphen when the word *very* precedes a compound adjective.

> The patient was a very well developed child for his age.

Ages

Hyphenate ages when they appear before the noun they modify. Do not hyphenate ages that appear after the noun they modify.

> The patient is a 36-year-old white male.
> The patient is 36 years old.

> This 22-year-old patient was admitted yesterday.
> The patient was 22 years old.

> *Exception*:
> The patient is a 36-year-old.
> (The noun is understood; thus, hyphens are needed.)

> *Tip*: When *years* is used instead of *year*, a hyphen is not used. Note, however, that some ESL dictators may dictate a phrase like "a 36-years-old patient," in which case you should edit *years* to *year* and include hyphens.

Clarity

1. Hyphens are not used with anatomic structures. In rare instances, a hyphen may be needed to clarify medical meaning.

> soft tissue mass
> small cell carcinoma
> small bowel obstruction *or* small-bowel obstruction

> *Explanation*: The latter is more controversial. It indicates an obstruction of the small bowel, not a small obstruction of the bowel. However, many believe that a hyphen is not needed in *small bowel obstruction* because *small bowel* is an anatomic structure and serves as a noun modifier just as *soft tissue* does in *soft tissue mass*. Also, they argue that anyone in medicine would know that bowel obstructions are not characterized as *small, medium, or large*.

2. Hyphens are not used with disease entities or anatomic structures.

> anterior superior iliac spine
> left lower extremity
> right lower quadrant
> chronic obstructive pulmonary disease
> left lower lobe pneumonia

3. The use of hyphens with *mid* varies. The word *mid* (meaning the middle position) may stand alone as an adjective or combined with a root word without a hyphen.

> mid (prefix or standalone word)

mid and left forefoot
mid and left lower lung
mid distal forearm
mid finger
midfoot
midline
mid-1980s

Compounds

1. Compound adjectives are routinely hyphenated when they precede the noun and not hyphenated when they follow the noun.

   This patient has snow-white hair but is only 46.
   The patient's hair was snow white.
   This is a 26-year-old patient.
   This patient is 26 years old. (Note the *s* on *years* when the phrase follows the verb.)

2. Compound color adjectives appear most often in pathology reports. They should be hyphenated: a red-brown lesion, a cherry-red nevus. Color compounds whose first element ends in *-ish* are hyphenated when they precede the noun but should not be hyphenated when they follow the noun. Degrees of color are not hyphenated.

   cherry-red nevus
   red-brown lesion
   reddish-brown piece of tissue
   a whitish-gray color
   tissue reddish brown in color
   dark brown to tan piece of tissue

3. Noun plus participle compounds used as adjectives or verbs are hyphenated.

   breast-fed
   skin-tested
   third-spacing

4. Some compounds are always hyphenated.

   up-to-date
   over-the-counter
   self-directed

5. In a complex modifying phrase that includes a prefix or suffix, hyphens are sometimes used to avoid ambiguity. An *en* dash (–), longer than a hyphen but shorter than an *em* (—) dash, may be used after the prefix.

   non–brain-injured patient
   non–insulin-dependent patient

Compound modifiers in a series

1. A suspensive hyphen may be used to connect a series of modifiers with the same base.

a 10- to 12-week history of symptoms
We used small-, medium-, and large-bowl curets.
The patient has 10- and 12-year-old brothers.

2. However, when the compounds are not normally hyphenated, repeat the root word each time.

   Dictated: The surgeon reported that the pre- and post-operative diagnoses were the same.
   Transcribed: The surgeon reported that the preoperative and postoperative diagnoses were the same.

Double letters

The use of a hyphen to separate two identical vowels or consonants when joining prefixes and combining forms is changing. The rule now is to use a hyphen when such a combination would place three vowels together or three identical consonants. Use a hyphen when necessary to aid pronunciation. Check a current dictionary to be certain a hyphen is necessary.

antiinflammatory	anti-inflammatory
aortobiiliac	aorto-bi-iliac
antiicteric	anti-icteric
intraaortic	intra-aortic
nonnegotiable	non-negotiable
salpingo-oophorectomy	
posttraumatic	
(post-traumatic also acceptable)	

Exceptions:
preexisting
reexamine

Numbers

1. Although the official SI method (International System of Measuring Units) recommends *no punctuation of any kind* be used with metric abbreviations, the insertion of hyphens in metric measurements used as adjectives is recommended in some books of style. This style reflects the compound adjective rule for words.

2. Others think that hyphens contribute nothing to clarity in metric measurements used as adjectives and follow the SI method of using no punctuation of any kind with metric abbreviations. In expressions such as 3.25 mm or 2 x 2 x 1.25 mm, hyphens seem particularly intrusive to some.

   Preferred: A 2-cm scar was noted.
   Acceptable: A 2 cm scar was noted.

   Preferred: The specimen was a 1 x 2 x 2-cm sample.
   Acceptable: The specimen was a 1 x 2 x 2 cm sample.

3. When an English unit of measure is used as a compound adjective, a hyphen is used.

   The patient sustained a 3-inch wound to his distal forearm.

Prefixes and suffixes

1. Most prefixes (*ante-, anti-, bi-, co-, contra-, de-, extra-, infra-, inter-, intra-, micro-, mid-, non-, over-, post-, pre-, pseudo-, re-, semi-, sub-, super-, supra-, trans-, tri-, un-, under-*) and suffixes (*-fold, -hood, -less, -like*) are attached to the root word without a hyphen unless a triple vowel or consonant combination will result or a pronunciation will be difficult.

   clockwise   predate
   incongruous   intracapsular

2. The prefixes *all-, ex-, self-,* and *vice-* and the suffix *-elect* retain the hyphen whether they precede or follow the nouns they modify.

   breast self-examination
   self-examination of the breast
   diagnosis is self-evident
   self-evident diagnosis

3. When *like* and *most* appear as suffixes, they are attached to the root word without a hyphen. If the root word ends with the same letter as the first letter of the suffix, hyphenate the word for clarity. If the root word has several syllables or pronunciation might be difficult, hyphenation is optional.

   anteriormost   anterior-most
   bandlike pain   barrel-like chest
   flulike illness   parrotlike
   shell-like growth   seizure-like

Ranges

Hyphens may be used in ranges that meet all the following conditions: The phrase must not contain the expression "from … to," "from … through," or "between … and"; the values must be positive numbers of less than four digits; and the values must not contain a decimal, other punctuation, or symbol. It is equally acceptable to use the words *to* or *through* as appropriate.

   4-6 weeks   4 to 6 weeks
   3-4 cm in length   3 to 4 cm in length
   days 1 through 10   days 1-10
   between 3 and 5 times   from days 1 through 21

Single letters

Do not use a hyphen to connect a single letter and noun combination. Use a hyphen to join a single letter and a noun, adjective, or participle modifying a noun.

   ST segment   *but* ST-segment elevation
   T wave   *but* T-wave abnormality
   T cells   *but* T-cell count

Numbers

1. Spell out numbers at the beginning of a sentence and numbers that might cause confusion. An article or other adjective may be placed in front of a number at the beginning of a sentence.

   One percent lidocaine was used.
   Lidocaine 1% was used.
   A 45-year-old white male . . .

2. Use numerals with units of age, distance, dosage, measure, time, and weight.

   He has had recurrent episodes of upper abdominal pain for 3 months.
   The incision was 7 cm in length.
   The patient runs 4 miles every day.
   He says the rash has been present for 5 days.
   The pain started 12 hours ago.
   Her weight was 155 pounds.
   The patient is to take metoprolol 50 mg 2 times daily.
   The patient's sister died at age 3.

3. Do not use two numerals in a row. Spell one out.

   The patient is taking Tylenol No. 3 two every 4 hours.
   Aldactone 25 mg, #60, one tab b.i.d.

4. Do not use numerals for pronouns. Spell out numbers at the beginning of a sentence. Numbers under *ten* may be written out if used in a non-numerical sense.

   One of the nodes was positive.
   The oncologist explained the ramifications to the two of them.
   Nine out of 11 nodes were positive.
   Four days have passed since her last visit.
   The only two structures identifiable were the parathyroid glands.
   Two clips were placed on the cystic duct, one on the gallbladder side.
   The patient's two brothers have heart disease.
   A 45-year-old white male who . . .
   This 13-year-old female was . . .

Ages

Use Arabic numerals for ages. Hyphenate the age when it appears before the noun it modifies. Do not hyphenate an age that appears after the noun it modifies. If a fraction is dictated, it may be written as a fraction.

   The patient is a 36-year-old white male.
   This is a 36-year-old who is 6 months' pregnant. (Noun implied.)
   The patient is 36 years old.
   The child is a 5½-year-old female. (also 5-1/2-year-old)

She is in her early 20s.
This is a 1-year 11-month-old toddler.
The patient is an 11½-year-old adolescent male.
(also 11-9/12-year-old)

Arabic numerals

Medical and technical reports often use Arabic numerals rather than words to express numbers with greater precision and accuracy. Numbers under ten need not be presented as numerals unless they are used with age, distance, dosage, time, units of measure, or weight. However, if the number is used as a pronoun or in a non-numerical sense, spell it out.

This patient is determined to be admitted one way or the other.
If one of the ED physicians is ill, the whole department is a mess.
I explained the procedure to the patient and his wife, and the two of them understood and agreed.

Cardinal numbers

Cardinal numbers indicate quantity: one (1), two (2), three (3), four (4), and so on. Ordinal numbers denote position in an ordered sequence: first (1st), second (2nd), third (3rd), fourth (4th), and so on.

Dates

Arabic numerals are used to express dates, and a comma pair is used to set off the year in the month/day/year format within a sentence. If the date is presented in the day/month/year format, do not use a comma pair to set off the year. Although the date *November 1* is pronounced *November first*, it is not acceptable to transcribe November 1st, 2006.

He was admitted on November 1, 2006, and discharged on November 5, 2006.
He was admitted on 1 November 2006 and discharged on 5 November 2006.

Degrees

1. Use degrees with temperatures and angles. The degree sign (°) is acceptable but is discouraged because it may not translate when transferred electronically.

Temperature 98.4   Temperature 98.4°
Temperature 98.4 degrees   a 35-degree angle
an angle of 35 degrees   an angle of 35°

2. If the physician dictates *Fahrenheit* or *Celsius* (previously known as *centigrade*), spell it out if you also spell out the word *degrees*. If you use the degree sign, you must abbreviate *Fahrenheit* as *F* and *Celsius* as *C*. Do not put a space between the numeral, the degree sign, and the letter *F* or *C*.

Temperature 98.4 degrees Fahrenheit
Temperature 98.4°F

Temperature 37.5 degrees Celsius
Temperature 37.5°C

3. If the word *degrees* is not dictated after temperature, it does not need to be added by the transcriptionist.

Temperature 98.6.

Metric units

1. Abbreviate metric and SI units of measure when preceded by a number. Abbreviations for metric and SI units of measure contain no periods and have the same form for both singular and plural.

cm	centimeter, centimeters
g	gram, grams
L	liter, liters
mg	milligram, milligrams
mL	milliliter, milliliters

Note. The internationally accepted abbreviations for *gram* and *milliliter* (*g* and *mL*, respectively) replace the older abbreviations *gm* and *ml*.

2. Metric numbers less than the number *one* should be preceded with a zero and a decimal point for clarity, even if the zero is not dictated.

0.5 mm in diameter
0.25% Marcaine

3. Do not add a zero to the right of the decimal unless the number is dictated. An additional zero implies a higher degree of accuracy of the measurement, e.g., 2 is not equivalent to 2.0.

4. In a series of metric measurements, the units of measure that accompany the numerals should be listed in a consistent fashion.

Dictated: 3.3 cm x 1 x 4
Transcribed: 3.3 x 1 x 4 cm

5. Do not repeat the unit of measure unless necessary to avoid confusion. Some pathologists are very particular in repeating the unit of measure (3 cm x 5 cm), in which case the transcriptionist would transcribe as dictated.

6. Metric fractions should also be transcribed in decimal format even if English fractions are dictated.

D: quarter percent Marcaine
T: 0.25% Marcaine

D: two and a half milligrams
T: 2.5 mg

Ordinal numbers

1. Ordinal numbers (often called *ordinals*) denote position in an ordered sequence: first (1st), second (2nd), third (3rd), fourth (4th), and so on. This is in contrast to cardinal numbers, which indicate quantity: one (1), two (2), three (3), four (4), and so on.

2. While it is acceptable to spell out ordinals (first, seventh), the use of numeric ordinals (1st, 7th) in medical transcription has become more accepted.

3. Ordinals written as numerics are frequently used to describe burn classifications (1st degree burn), editions of publications (2nd edition), specific times (the 9th of the month, the 21st century), specific anatomic structures (5th lumbar vertebra, 3rd rib, 6th cranial nerve) trimesters of pregnancy (3rd trimester), and so on.

4. Do not use a hyphen with numeric ordinals.

   D: On the inner aspect of the thigh is a third degree burn.

   T: On the inner aspect of the thigh is a 3rd degree burn (*not* 3rd-degree burn).

5. When in doubt whether to spell out an ordinal or use the numeral, determine whether the numeric ordinal or the spelled-out ordinal best communicates the idea. Clarity should take precedence.

   The patient is seen today for a deep puncture wound on the lateral aspect of the right forearm, stating that he won 2nd place in the men's bull-riding competition, but apparently the bull won 1st.

   The patient said that in the first place she had not taken her medication, and in the second place, the pharmacy had refused to refill it anyway.

English units of measure

1. Spell out English units of measure, even when preceded by a number, except in tables.

Singular, Plural	Table
1 inch, 3 inches	in.
1 foot, 5 feet	5 ft.
1 pound, 120 pounds	1 lb., 120 lbs.
1 ounce, 2 ounces	2 oz.

2. Do not use punctuation between feet and inches, pounds and ounces, hours and minutes when dictated in pairs.

   The patient is 5 feet 6 inches.
   The baby weighed 6 pounds 3 ounces.
   She exercised on the treadmill for 1 hour 10 minutes.

Hyphens

The insertion of hyphens with metric and SI units of measure used as adjectives is recommended but may be omitted if confusing rather than clarifying.

   Preferred: A 2.75-cm lesion was noted.
   Acceptable: A 2.75 cm lesion was noted.

Lists

1. The dictator may number the diagnoses in a long list to be presented vertically. Sometimes a dictator will give the first several numbers and then say "number next" rather than trying to remember the next number. The transcriptionist should enumerate a long list of diagnoses, even if numbers are not dictated. If there is only one diagnosis dictated, it should not be numbered. Do not enumerate diagnoses that are dictated in narrative form.

   DIAGNOSES
   1. Chronic intravenous drug user.
   2. Cellulitis, left arm.

2. Medications may be listed vertically if numbered and acceptable to the dictator or the facility.

   1. Lescol 2 mg at bedtime.
   2. DiaBeta 5 mg 1 q.a.m.
   3. Aspirin 325 mg 1 daily.
   4. Xanax 0.25 mg t.i.d. p.r.n.

Medications

Use numbers to express medication dosages and amounts.

   The patient received 1 g of Ancef during the procedure.
   The patient received Versed 5 mg IV just prior to the procedure.

Plurals

Use an apostrophe when pluralizing a single digit number but not numbers of two or more digits.

100s   4 x 4's

Ranges

Hyphens may be used in ranges that meet all the following conditions:

   The phrase must not contain the expressions "from … to," "from … through," or "between … and," and the values must be positive numbers of less than 4 digits and must not contain a decimal, other punctuation, or symbol. It is equally acceptable to use the words *to* or *through* as appropriate.

3-4 cm or 3 to 4 cm
days 1-5 or days 1 through 5

but

from days 1 through 21

between 30 and 40 mL

Roman numerals

Roman numerals are rarely used in technical medical reports except for established nomenclature as in cancer classifications or stages and EKG leads. Cranial nerves are traditionally represented with Roman numerals but are gaining greater acceptance in medical reports as Arabic numerals.

blood factors (e.g., factor VIII)

cancer stages I through IV

EKG leads I through III

ovarian carcinoma, FIGO stage II

cranial nerves II-XII *or* cranial nerves 2-12

Time

1. Use Arabic numerals with measurements of time, such as years, months, weeks, days, hours, minutes, and seconds. Use a colon to express hours and minutes, but do not use a colon or *a.m.* and *p.m.* with military time.

The patient was brought to surgery at 2:20 a.m.

Anesthesia was started at 1420.

6:15 a.m.	0615 hours
6:15 p.m.	1815 hours

2. Use *o'clock* only with whole numbers to indicate position or direction.

A 2 o'clock incision was made at the umbilicus.

The needle was inserted at the 4 o'clock position.

Verb forms

Always use a singular verb with units of measure.

Approximately 50 mL of fluid was aspirated from the peritoneal cavity.

Obstetrics Terms

1. Do not capitalize the terms *gravida* or *para*, but do capitalize their abbreviations (*G, P*). The brief form *ab* (abortion) may be lowercase or capitalized (Ab).

gravida 3, para 2, ab 1

2. G/TPAL is a more detailed system to keep track of each pregnancy and its outcome.

G	number of times pregnant
T	number of term births
P	number of premature births
A	number of abortions (spontaneous or induced)
L	number of living children

3. When *gravida* and *para* are abbreviated, use capitals.

G3, P3-0-0-3

Parentheses

1. Parentheses are used to set off supplemental material not closely related to the rest of the sentence, to clarify, or to distinguish data. If parentheses are dictated but the parenthetical material is closely related to the rest of the sentence, you may edit to commas.

He was comfortable (according to him, for the first time in many weeks), and the pain could not be elicited despite stimulation of his right cheek, mandible, and gum trigger zone.

The surgeon feels (and I strongly agree) that splenectomy is the course with the greatest potential for cure.

2. Parentheses are often used to separate normal laboratory values from the patient's values.

Uptake by the thyroid gland at 6 hours was 5.5% (normal 4-12%); 24-hour uptake was 14.0% (normal 7-24%).

Periods

Few physicians consistently dictate periods to denote the end of a sentence. Some dictate them sporadically, and still others never dictate them. The transcriptionist should be aware that the physician frequently loses track of what punctuation was dictated, and thus it is up to the transcriptionist to supply periods and other punctuation marks as appropriate.

Physicians educated in foreign countries may use the term *stop* or *full stop* to denote a period. Foreign accents may make punctuation difficult to understand. For example, physicians with a Middle Eastern accent may say "perr-ud" or "pedd-ud" instead of *period*.

Plurals

Medical words derived from Latin or Greek are pluralized according to guidelines in the recommended references. Some physicians may dictate Latin terms, applying English rules for forming plurals. The MT should follow the dictator's preference unless it is incorrect. For example, *diverticula* is the correct plural of *diverticulum*; it cannot end in *-ae* or *-i* even if dictated.

fistulas or fistulae	fossas or fossae
hernias or herniae	scleras or sclerae

Post, Status Post

1. When the prefix *post* (*after, behind, posterior*) is used as an adjective before a noun, it is connected to the root word without a hyphen, unless the root begins with a *t*, in which case the word may be closed or hyphenated.

   postacetabular
   postoperative course
   postsacral edema
   posttraumatic, post-traumatic

2. The word *post* in the phrase *status post* stands alone as a compound not connected to the noun it modifies. Status post is a Latin phrase meaning *state or condition after or following*. Sometimes *status* is omitted but is understood.

   The patient is status post closed fracture of the left leg.
   The patient is post complicated hysterectomy.

Pronouns

Which, Who, That

1. The pronoun *which* used as a relative pronoun (a noun substitute used to introduce clauses) refers to animals and things. *Which* is often used in nonessential clauses, which are set off by commas and are not necessary to the meaning of the sentence. In sentences where *which* introduces an essential clause, it is not preceded by a comma (see third example below).

   The patient has a large abdominal aortic aneurysm that is very large, which all his physicians and surgeon think should be repaired now.
   There could be a fracture involving the ischial or pubic rami, which are not visible at the present time.
   It was evident that the patient had a large prolapsing hemorrhoid which was too large for rubber banding.

2. The pronoun *who* (or *whom*) refers to people and sometimes animals.

   This is a 34-year-old woman who comes to the clinic today with a history of hypothyroidism.
   This is one of those patients, whom we classify as drug-dependent, who are always seeking Demerol in the ED.

3. The pronoun *that* can refer to any of the above. *That* is used almost exclusively to introduce essential clauses (clauses that are necessary for the understanding of the sentence and not set off by commas):

   The chamber that receives oxygenated blood from the lungs is the left atrium.

There are scattered hyperkeratotic lesions that the patient states are similar to the lesion resected on his right forearm.

Tip: A good test of some essential clauses is to leave out the relative pronoun, and if the sentence still makes sense, it is an essential clause.

There are scattered hyperkeratotic lesions the patient states are similar to the lesion resected on his right forearm.

4. *Who* and *whom* can be used in essential or nonessential clauses. *Which* and *that* can sometimes be interchanged, but *which* should not be used to refer to persons.

Objective Pronouns

1. Objective pronouns (*me, him, her, us, them, whom*) are used as objects of prepositions and verbs. They should not be used as subjects of a sentence or clause.

   Incorrect: This patient, *who* you referred to me 3 months ago for treatment of a nonhealing leg ulcer, is being released from my care.
   Correct: This patient, *whom* you referred to me 3 months ago for treatment of a nonhealing leg ulcer, is being released from my care. (*Whom* is the object of the verb *referred.*)

2. Too frequently, in an effort to sound exceedingly correct, people use subject pronouns as objects.

   D: I explained the risks, benefits, and complications of the procedure to *she* and her husband.
   T: I explained the risks, benefits, and complications to *her* and her husband. (*Her* is the object of the preposition *to.* "I explained the risks to . . . *she*" is obviously wrong.)

Reflexive Pronouns

Reflexive pronouns (*myself, yourself, himself, ourselves, themselves*) must reflect back to the noun or pronoun that is the subject of the sentence. Often, reflexive pronouns are used for emphasis.

   D: The patient was seen by *myself* in consultation.
   T: The patient was seen by *me* in consultation.
   (*By* is a preposition, so the objective pronoun *me* is required.)

Proofreading

1. Proofreading involves looking for mistakes of all types in the transcribed document and correcting them. The usual types of errors that occur include omitting important dictated words, selecting the wrong English or medical word, misspelling words, and

making typographical, grammatical, or punctuation errors. (See **How to Proofread**, Chapter 1, p. 31.)

2. Medical transcriptionists should conscientiously look up all unfamiliar words and spellings. They should proofread on the screen as they are transcribing. It is important to learn the skill of proofreading on screen and proofreading as you are transcribing because in the "real world" there is seldom time for a complete proofreading review of a report.

Question Marks

1. Medical transcriptionists should never, on their own initiative, insert a question mark within a document to denote a word they consider to be unclear or unknown. The appropriate way to flag a document for missing words is described under **Flagging Reports**.

2. On some occasions, a dictator may instruct the transcriptionist to insert a question mark into a document. If the physician is questioning a diagnosis, it is appropriate to enclose the question mark within parentheses. Sometimes the question mark may be dictated prior to the diagnosis.

    Dictated:
    DIAGNOSIS
    Carcinoma in situ, stage III, question mark.
    Transcribed:
    DIAGNOSIS
    Carcinoma in situ, stage III (?).

Quotation Marks

1. Quotation marks are used to denote the exact words of a patient as related by the dictator.

    Dictated: The patient states quote I feel lousy unquote.
    Transcribed: The patient states, "I feel lousy."

2. Physicians occasionally dictate quotation marks to set off unusual or slang terms. Quotation marks are also used to denote a word for special attention.

3. Always place commas and periods inside the quotation marks.

    The lesion did not appear "angry."

4. Semicolons and colons always go outside the quotation marks. Exclamation points and question marks go inside or outside the quotation marks depending on whether they are part of the quoted material or the sentence that incorporates the quote.

"Who are you?" asked the patient when I walked in.
Do you think the patient was being honest when he said, "I don't abuse drugs or alcohol"?

Ranges

See **Hyphens** and **Numbers**.

Ratios

See **Colons**.

Score

See **Classification, Grade, Stage, Type.**

Semicolons

1. Use a semicolon to separate two independent clauses that are closely related in meaning. A period is also acceptable, as each independent clause is a complete sentence.

    We could not see the left anterior descending; presumably it was intramyocardial.
    Cystoscopy was then performed; the findings were noted above.

2. Use a semicolon to punctuate two independent clauses joined by a conjunctive adverb or transitional phrase (*consequently, for example, furthermore, however, in addition, indeed, in fact, moreover, nevertheless, then, therefore, thus*). Place a semicolon before the conjunctive adverb or transitional phrase and a comma after it.

    We continued to dissect this; however, it became evident that the tumor was locally invasive into the trachea.
    The 2-cm nodule was easily palpated in the lower aspect of the upper lobe, and it was not on the surface; therefore, it was elected to do an excisional biopsy utilizing the TA-90 stapler.

    Note: In the last example there are three independent clauses, the first two joined by *and*, and the third joined by *therefore*.

3. Use a semicolon to separate a series of words, phrases, or clauses when separate internal elements are already separated by commas.

    The pericardium was opened vertically; T'd horizontally, superiorly, and inferiorly; and retraction sutures were placed in the pericardial edges.
    Procardia 10 mg 1 t.i.d.; nitroglycerin 0.4 mg p.r.n., to take one at onset of pain, a second one in 5 minutes, and a third 5 minutes later, and if no relief, go

immediately to the emergency department; and Coumadin 2.5 mg Mondays, Wednesdays, and Fridays and 5 mg on Tuesdays, Thursdays, and Saturdays.

Slang

See **Brief Forms and Medical Slang**.

Slash Mark

See **Symbols**.

Spelling and Usage

1. Some words have more than one acceptable spelling. When a term has an alternative spelling, it is customary to use the spelling accompanied by the definition. If both spellings are accompanied by definitions, either may be used. Some dictionaries, especially English dictionaries, may put two spellings separated by a comma as the main entry. In that case, the first spelling is preferred.

2. Preferred spellings may vary among English and medical reference books.

Preferred	Acceptable
anulus	annulus
calix	calyx
curet	curette
disk	disc
orthopedic	orthopaedic

3. Do not accept a dictator-spelled word. Verify the spelling in a reliable reference book.

4. Physicians frequently dictate combined forms of anatomical words and directions. When the physician's preference is not clear, it is acceptable to use either the combined form or the hyphenated form. Note that when the two hyphenated words are merged into a combined form, the spelling of the first word often changes.

Hyphenated Form	Combined Form
anterior-posterior	anteroposterior
metatarsal-phalangeal	metatarsophalangeal
posterior-lateral	posterolateral

5. Some medical words are spelled differently when their form changes.

inflamed	inflammation
tendon	tendinitis
Achilles tendon	tendo Achillis
fascia lata	tensor fasciae latae

6. **Ensure, insure**. While *ensure* and *insure* both mean "to make certain," American usage favors the spelling *ensure* for this meaning and *insure* for the meaning "guaranteeing persons or property against risk."

7. **Followup, follow up**. Use *followup* as a noun or adjective. (*Follow-up* is also acceptable and is preferred in some English dictionaries.) Note that the noun *followup* is often preceded by a preposition (*for, in, on, to*), and the adjective is followed by a noun (*visit, appointment*).

   Noun: She is scheduled for followup in 1 week.
   Adjective: Her followup visit is 1 week from today.
   Noun: She was lost to followup after her surgery.
      (*To* in this sentence is a preposition)

   Use *follow up* as a verb. Note that helping verbs (*was, has, will*) or the infinitive (*to*) are often used with the verb *follow up*.

   She will follow up with the therapist in 1 week.
   I asked the patient to follow up with me 3 days after surgery.

8. **Toward, towards**. The difference between these two words is dialectal. *Toward* is more common in American English; *towards* is the predominant form in British English. Both are correct.

9. **Tract, track, tracked**. Do not confuse *tract* and *track*. *Tract* is always a noun and means "a path" or "a system of organs that performs a specific function," such as the intestinal tract. While *track* can be a noun and also mean "path," as a verb it means "to follow a path or course."

   On anoscopy he was found to have external as well as internal hemorrhoids with no fistulous tract of the abscess cavity.
   We will track the patient's progress.

Subject-Verb Agreement

See **Agreement**.

Subscripts and Superscripts

1. Subscripts and superscripts are seldom used by transcriptionists in medical reports because they are not easily executed and may not transfer well electronically. Also, on printed reports it may be difficult for the reader to determine whether a number is a subscript or superscript for one line or a character on the line below or above it.

2. When a term that would ordinarily have a subscript is written with all characters on the baseline, no spaces or hyphens are used.

A2, P2 A_2, P_2
V1, V6 V_1, V_6
CO2 CO_2

3. The most common terms that have subscripts in medical transcripts include the following. It is recommended that the following be typed with all characters on the baseline.

blood gases	PCO2, PO2
chemical symbols	O2, CO2, H2O
EKG leads	V1, V2, V3, V4, V5, V6
heart sounds	S1, S2, S3, S4
thyroid tests	T3, T4
T1-weighted image	

4. The most common terms with superscripts in medical reports are elements such as those used in radiology and radiotherapy. When a term that would ordinarily have a superscript is written with all characters on the baseline, the superscript number that ordinarily precedes the element symbol now follows the symbol, and a space (not a hyphen) is used to separate the letters from the numerals.

technetium	^{99m}Tc sulfur colloid
technetium	Tc 99m sulfur colloid
gallium citrate ^{67}Ga	gallium citrate Ga 67
iodohippurate sodium ^{131}I	
iodohippurate sodium I 131	

5. A superscript is used occasionally in laboratory data as an exponent, i.e., to express a power of 10. These numbers should be transcribed as dictated. Do not place the exponent on the line with the numerical value or unit of measure.

D: The WBC count was ten to the fifth power.
T: The WBC count was 10^5.
    or The WBC count was 10 to the 5th.
    or The WBC count was 100,000.

D: Red blood cells were five times ten to the sixth power.
T: Red blood cells were 5 x 10^6.
    or Red blood cells were 5 x 10 to the 6th.
    or Red blood cells were 5,000,000.

D: The skin graft measured 15 centimeters squared.
T: The skin graft measured 15 cm^2.
    or The skin graft measured 15 sq cm.

Suture Sizes

Suture sizes range from 0 to 11-0 and from 1 to 7, with 11-0 the smallest and 7 the largest. Size 0 may be dictated as "one-oh," "number oh," or even "aught." A number sign (#) may or may not be dictated. As a general rule, transcribe as dictated. However, if a dictator consistently dictates "number" before most suture sizes but fails to do so in one or two instances, you may add the number sign for consistency. When the suture size is a single whole number, the number sign can be added for clarity.

D: oh Vicryl
T: 0 Vicryl or 1-0 Vicryl

D: Two oh Dexon
T: 2-0 Dexon

D: Number two oh Dexon
T: #2-0 Dexon

Symbols

1. In the transcription of medical reports, symbols are occasionally used to represent words.

2. The symbol *x* may be used to represent the dictated words *times* or *by* when followed by a numerical value. It is written as a lowercase letter. Do not substitute *x* for *times* when the word *for* can be used.

D: Bleeding times 3 days
T: Bleeding for 3 days

D: The ulcer is 2 by 4 cm in size.
T: The ulcer is 2 x 4 cm in size.

Note. Do not space between *x* and the numeral in the following examples.

D: Stools were negative for ova and parasites times 3.
T: Stools were negative for ova and parasites x3.

The patient was oriented x3.

3. The ampersand (*&*) is used to represent the word *and*. There is no space before or after the ampersand.

D: The patient underwent a D and C.
T: The patient underwent a D&C.

D: The lungs are clear to P and A.
T: The lungs are clear to P&A.

4. The **slash mark** or **virgule** (/)—sometimes referred to as a diagonal or stroke mark—is often used to represent the word *per*, especially in the expression of numerical values and units of measurement.

There were 2-4 wbc/hpf.
    (2 to 4 white blood cells per high power field)
She was placed on 1 mL/kg.
    (one milliliter per kilogram)

5. The slash mark is also used to represent the word *over*.

> Blood pressure is 140/84. (140 over 84)
> The patient's vision was 20/50. (20 over 50)

6. Other commonly used symbols are the plus or positive sign (+), the minus or negative sign (-), and the percent sign (%).

> The deep tendon reflexes are 2+ and equal for patellar and ankle jerks.
> FEV1 was 85% of predicted.

7. Do not use the plus or minus sign with blood types used as nouns.

> This is an O positive, Rh-negative pregnant lady, admitted in labor.

8. The symbols for foot (') and for inch (") are acceptable only in tables. Spell out the words in medical reports.

9. The **degree** symbol (°) may be used when the word *degrees* is dictated in temperatures and angles; however, the degree symbol may not transmit well electronically, and on the job the transcriptionist would ask the supervisor about the use of symbols.

Templates

See **Format**.

Tense

See **Format**.

That, Which

See **Pronouns:** *Which, Who, and That.*

Units of Measure

See **Numbers**.

Verbs

See **Agreement**.

Vertebrae

1. A total of 33 vertebrae are divided into five regions: cervical, thoracic, lumbar, sacral, and coccygeal).

2. Vertebrae are often expressed with capital letters (C, cervical; T, thoracic; L, lumbar; S, sacral) followed by Arabic numerals. There are seven cervical vertebrae (C1 through C7); twelve thoracic vertebrae (T1 through 12, also referred to as dorsal vertebrae; D1 through D12); five lumbar vertebrae (L1 through L5); five sacral vertebrae (S1 through S5); and four coccygeal vertebrae, known by lay persons as the tailbone.

2. A fairly common anatomical variant is sacralization of the fifth lumbar vertebra known as L6. Lumbarization of the first sacral vertebra is another anatomical variant.

3. Do not use a hyphen between the letter and the number of a specific vertebra, and do not use subscript or superscript numerals. Repeat the letter before each numbered vertebra in a list.

> L4
> T3
> D7
> C1
> S1
>
> Dictated: T2, 3, and 4
> Transcribed: T2, T3, and T4

4. Use a hyphen to express the space between two vertebrae (the intervertebral disk space). Repeat the same letter before the second vertebra in a disk space if it is dictated.

> C4-5 (or C4-C5 if dictated)
> T11-12 (or T11-T12 if dictated)
> L5-S1

Virgule

See **Symbols**.

Visual Acuity

Visual acuity is represented by a set of two numbers. The first number is usually 20, the number of feet away from the eye chart. The second number represents how the patient's vision compares to normal. The two numbers are separated by a virgule (slash mark). If a person has 20/20 (dictated "twenty twenty") vision, the patient can see at 20 feet what the average person sees at 20 feet. If the patient's vision is 20/40 (twenty forty), he or she can see at 20 feet what people with normal vision see at 40 feet. Twenty two hundred (20/200) and twenty four hundred (20/400) indicate that what people with normal vision see at 200 feet and 400 feet, respectively, the patient must be within 20 feet to see. Stereo acuity is tested with a four-dot test.

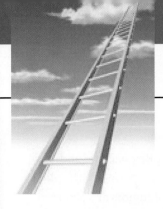

SkillsChallenge

Agreement of Subject and Verb

Instructions: Review the guidelines on correct subject-verb agreement in this chapter, and complete the following exercise. Circle either the singular or plural form of the verb or pronoun in the pairs in parentheses to demonstrate correct subject-verb agreement.

1. No evidence of congestive heart failure and edema (is, are) seen on chest x-ray.

2. The occlusions in the region of the left anterior descending artery (appears, appear) to be significant.

3. We have no way of telling what the exact relationship of his pathology to his symptoms (is, are).

4. There (is, are) minimal episodes of arrhythmia seen on the EKG.

5. No episodes of angina (was, were) noted by the patient.

6. The age and sex of a patient (cause, causes) variation in the normal range of laboratory values.

7. Finger-to-nose test and heel-to-shin test (is, are) normal.

8. Inspection of the upper extremities (show, shows) some scattered small abrasions over the dorsal aspects of the hands.

9. No evidence of mucosal ulcerations or polypoid filling defects (was, were) seen.

10. Some hypertrophy of the facet joints (is, are) noted at this level.

11. A moderate exudate of polymorphonuclear leukocytes (is, are) seen.

12. Acute blood clot and old organized and degenerate blood clot (is, are) observed.

13. His BUN was within normal limits, as (was, were) his sodium and potassium.

14. No fecalith or perforations (is, are) identified.

15. Cardiac and respiratory compensation (was, were) used.

16. The endocervical canals are patent, and each (connect, connects) with (its, their) respective (uterus, uteruses). (*Note:* The patient was didelphic.)

17. Examination of sections of both right and left lungs (show, shows) severe vascular congestion but (is, are) otherwise unremarkable.

18. Sections of the remaining breast tissue (show, shows) atrophy without evidence of additional tumor.

19. The wound was explored for foreign bodies, none of which (was, were) found.

20. The compression of the renal pelvis and deviation of the left upper ureter (is, are) essentially the same as seen on the intravenous pyelogram.

21. The nodules in the left lower lobe (has, have) not changed in size.

22. Approximately 10 cc of straw-colored fluid (was, were) obtained and sent for appropriate microbiologic studies.

23. We have no way of telling what the exact relationship of this mass to the subclavian vein and subclavian artery (is, are).

24. The sulci in the region of the temporo-occipital area on the right side (is, are) slightly effaced.

25. There (is, are) minimal degenerative change in the articular facets.

26. No definite adenopathy or mass (is, are) seen in the chest or around the chest wall or axilla.

27. Multinuclear giant cells and nuclear changes consistent with herpes or other viral infection (is, are) encountered.

28. There (is, are) minimal degenerative change in the articular facets.

29. No definite adenopathy or masses (is, are) seen in the chest or around the chest wall or axilla.

Apostrophes

Instructions: Insert apostrophes as appropriate in the following sentences.

1. Its too bad that the hospitals policy prohibits patients access to their own medical records.

2. Two sonograms were compatible with a fetus of 30 weeks gestation.

3. On x-ray examination, the femur showed a fracture in its most distal portion of approximately 2 weeks duration.

4. Dr. Howards consultation was received 2 days before the patients surgery was scheduled.

5. Although its clear that the genus has been identified, the species has not.

Brief Forms and Medical Slang

Instructions: In the following examples, decide which contain brief forms that do not need to be changed and which contain medical slang that must be translated. Make the appropriate translation.

1. LABORATORY DATA: Her crit was 35.

2. A procto was done to help identify the pathology on the right side of her anus.

3. Her Pap smear showed carcinoma in situ.

4. The patient was cath'd and the urine specimen showed 1+ bacteria.

5. LABORATORY FINDINGS: The patient had a white count of 12,500 with a diff of 68 segs, 1 band, 13 lymphs, 17 monos, and 1 eo.

Capitals

Instructions: Correct the capitalization errors in the following sentences.

1. She will be seen by our Orthopedic Consultant, DR. Ortega, tomorrow.

2. LABORATORY DATA: WHITE BLOOD COUNT 14,000.

3. The culture grew out staphylococcus aureus, sensitive to Ampicillin.

4. She has Cushing's Syndrome and has developed a Cushingoid facies.

5. Heart: Positive Grade 2/6 systolic murmur.

Colons

Instructions: Place colons in the following sentences where appropriate, then circle the colons.

1. PHYSICAL EXAMINATION: Heart Regular rate and rhythm.

2. Pathologically the following types of tumors are observed solitary and multiple polyps, adenomas, multiple polyposis, leiomyoma, neuroma.

3. PAST HISTORY Hospitalizations None. Surgery None. Serious medical illnesses None.

4. Differential diagnosis includes the following Hypersensitivity pneumonitis, mycoplasmal pneumonia.

5. Examination showed recurrence of the retinal detachment with an open retinal break at about the 530 position.

Commas

Instructions: Insert commas where appropriate in the following sentences, and circle the commas.

1. He is showing more comedo formation and a higher proportion of pustular lesions than before and he now has a scattering of cysts over his upper back.

2. He was started on treatment with ephedrine Periactin and Sinequan and his hives are almost but not completely gone.

3. It is suspected that the cyst will recur and if it does the cyst will be excised.

4. The patient had a total protein of 5.4 albumin level was 3.2 chloride was 106 and a total bilirubin was 1.2.

5. He is to take prednisone 40 mg q.a.m. for 3 days 20 mg for 3 days 10 mg for 3 days 5 mg for 3 days 2.5 mg for 4 days and then off.

6. He will be seen by social services rehabilitative medicine and by his private cardiologist.

7. His angina however will continue until he undergoes a bypass procedure in the near future.

8. This patient as far as I can see is ready for rehabilitation.

9. She was discharged on Cardizem diuretics nitroglycerin and Atromid-S.

10. The improvement if any is very slight.

11. Her CPK levels however continued to remain within the normal range.

12. He has been instructed in the use of a low-salt diet; however it is doubtful that he will comply.

13. Her symptoms included dyspnea on exertion diaphoresis and a crushing chest pain.

14. The patient is a 72-year-old Asian female with no complaints of angina today.

15. Her hypertension is controlled with Dyazide and seems to be relatively stable.

16. The surgery was completed without complication and the patient was taken to the recovery room in satisfactory and stable condition.

17. She is scheduled for coronary artery bypass graft on September 15 2007 and she will be admitted for preoperative testing on the preceding day.

Editing

Instructions: The transcriptionist has a responsibility to make editing changes that will enhance but not alter medical meaning. Type your answers to the following.

1. List three ways in which medical transcriptionists are expected to perform editing functions.

2. List two minor editing changes routinely made but not affecting medical meaning.

3. List five examples of inconsistencies or discrepancies that would require calling the dictator's attention to a transcribed report.

4. List three of the most common errors in transcribed reports.

Eponyms

Instructions: Circle the correct eponym in the following sentences.

1. The patient experienced a (Jacksonian, jacksonian) seizure last week.

2. X-ray examination revealed (Osgood-Schlatter, Osgood-Schlatter's) disease.

3. We then inserted a (Rush's, Rush) rod into the tibia.

4. The abdomen was opened through a (Bevan, Bevan's) incision.

5. A (Jackson-Pratt, Jackson-Pratt's) drain was inserted for drainage.

Format

Instructions: Answer *True* or *False* to the following statements.

___ 1. Many medical facilities have instituted standard format outlines (templates) for each type of report dictated.

___ 2. If important headings are not dictated, the transcriptionist should supply them.

___ 3. Transcriptionists should type abbreviated major report headings (such as HPI) as dictated when physicians take shortcuts in dictation.

___ 4. Transcriptionists should always type the diagnoses in paragraph form even if the physician says to list and number diagnoses vertically.

___ 5. Paragraphing may be added by the transcriptionist to break up long reports appropriately.

Hyphens

Instructions: Supply hyphens as needed in the following sentences.

1. This well developed and well nourished 13 month old boy was referred to the pediatric clinic for follow up.

2. She complains of a continual stabbing like pain over a 3 week period.

3. This 25 year old woman was admitted with a history of pain in the shoulder over the last 24 hour period.

4. The x ray demonstrates an intra articular fracture.

5. The patient's pain medication was self administered as needed.

Numbers

Instructions: Find and correct the errors involving numbers and units of measure.

1. Laboratory data showed a total bilirubin of .5 mg.

2. She is 5.5 feet tall and weighs 160.5 pounds.

3. A 2 cms nodule is noted in the left lower lung.

4. There is another mole several mm away from the malignancy that we will need to check periodically.

5. The patient's blood pressure is 160 over 82 millimeters of mercury.

Punctuation Marks

Instructions: Correctly punctuate the following sentences, supplying dashes, parentheses, periods, quotation marks, and slashes when needed.

1. Three weeks ago the following diagnoses hepatic insufficiency with cirrhosis secondary to alcohol abuse, prostatic hypertrophy, chronic obstructive lung disease, and hiatal hernia were made

2. The patient's confabulation indicated to me that 1 he had little insight into his situation and 2 his judgment was grossly impaired

3. The patient's blood pressure was 142 90.

4. The patient will continue on Vicodin tabs 1 or 2 for pain qid prn and return to see me in 3 weeks sooner if pain does not remit.

5. Patient presents with the chief complaint I have a sore on my right hip.

Semicolons

Instructions: Supply semicolons as needed in the following sentences.

1. His respirations remain labored however he continues to produce copious amounts of sputum.

2. Cross-clamp time was 1 hour and 18 minutes cardiopulmonary bypass time 2 hours and 10 minutes lowest esophageal temperature was 24°C.

3. Left ureteral stricture was dilated there were no stones apparent.

4. I have examined her underwear today they are of a heavy stretch type, they contain 12% spandex, and portions of her bra panels contain 16% spandex.

5. Her medications include Medrol 4 mg 1 tablet daily, Lasix 20 mg daily, Micro-K 10 mEq daily, #28, as well as Zantac 150 mg p.o. b.i.d., #14, doxycycline 100 mg p.o. daily for 14 days, verapamil 80 mg, #30, and Proventil inhaler 2 puffs q.i.d., 2 inhalers, 6 refills.

Soundalikes

Instructions: Circle the correct soundalike from the words in parentheses.

1. Moderate exercise would certainly (complement, compliment) the patient's post-CABG therapy.

2. The patient had a (discrete, discreet) mass in her left breast.

3. She was unwilling to sign the contract as a matter of (principal, principle).

4. To (affect, effect) a cure requires compliance from the patient.

5. There are multiple side (affects, effects) to this treatment.

6. If the trauma (affects, effects) the emotions, then the reactions, the attitude, and the patient's performance will suffer.

7. During the hospitalization, the patient's (affect, effect) became more appropriate.

8. We could not (elicit, illicit) a response from the patient who reportedly took an (elicit, illicit) drug.

9. The (pallet, palate) was noted to have a high arch.

10. The indication for C-section is failure of (descent, dissent).

Spelling and Usage

Instructions: Circle words that are spelled incorrectly and correct them.

1. He has had recurence of the catching feeling when he trys to breath, usualy at night.

2. The following dictations are breif examples of dictated labortory test results.

3. His speech is slured, and he has some tingleing and weakness in the right arm.

4. He has moderate weekness of the extremities both distaly and symetricaly.

Part Two

The Practice of Medical Transcription

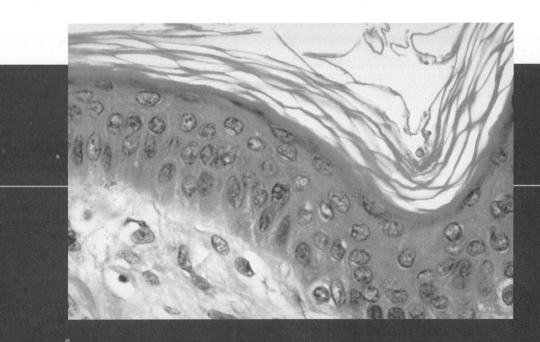

Dermatology

Chapter Outline

Learning Objectives

- Describe the structure and function of the skin.
- Spell and define common dermatologic terms.
- Identify types of questions a physician might ask a patient about the skin in a review of systems.
- Describe common features a physician looks for on examination of the skin.
- Identify common diseases of the skin. Describe their typical cause, course, and treatment options.
- Identify and define diagnostic and surgical procedures of the skin.

- List common dermatologic laboratory tests and procedures.
- Identify and describe common dermatologic drugs and their uses.
- Demonstrate knowledge of anatomical, medical, pharmacological, adjectival, and soundalike terms by correctly completing the exercises in this chapter.

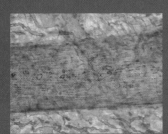
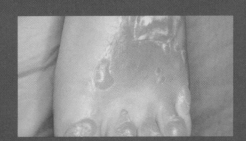
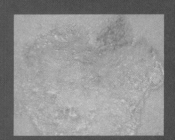

Transcribing Dermatology Dictation

Anatomy in Brief

The skin, the largest organ, and the most accessible for diagnosis and treatment, consists of two layers: the outer epidermis and the inner dermis or true skin.

The **epidermis** is a thin sheet of squamous (flat) epithelial cells, several layers thick, which are constantly renewed as the deepest layer grows steadily outward to replace surface cells (see Figure 4-1). Most of the cells of the epidermis are keratinocytes, containing a horny material, keratin, that provides mechanical toughness. A few are pigment cells, containing melanin, which imparts to the skin its characteristic color, varying according to race, familial characteristics, age, sun exposure, and other factors. Pigment distribution is more intense in certain areas, such as around the nipples and in the anogenital region. At bodily orifices, the epidermis undergoes a transition to mucous membrane.

The **dermis** is a tough layer of connective tissue containing blood vessels, sensory nerves, hair follicles, and sebaceous and sweat glands. Hair protects the body surface and provides thermal insulation. Each hair follicle is accompanied by a sebaceous gland, which produces oil (sebum) that is discharged on the skin surface and exerts protective and moisture-retaining effects. Sweat glands secrete sweat, which helps in temperature regulation.

Terminology Review

abscess   A localized zone of inflammation due to staphylococcal infection, in which pus forms in a tissue space walled off from surrounding tissues by fibrin, coagulated tissue fluids, and eventually fibrous tissue.

alopecia   Local or widespread loss of scalp hair.

avulsion   The ripping or tearing away of a part.

blepharitis   Inflammation of one or both eyelids.

bulla (pl. *bullae*)   A blister; a fluid-filled epidermal sac larger than a vesicle.

carbuncle   A spreading lesion made up of furuncles communicating by subcutaneous passages.

cellulitis   A type of infection occurring in soft tissues, including the skin, whose cardinal features are diffuse and spreading tissue swelling, redness, pain, and fever; often caused by streptococci.

cicatrix (scar)   A zone of fibrous tissue occurring at the site of a healed injury or inflammatory or destructive lesion extending into the dermis.

crust   A hard, friable, irregular layer of dried blood, serum, pus, tissue debris, or any combination of these adherent to the surface of injured or inflamed skin; a scab.

cryoprobe   A cryosurgical instrument containing a circulating refrigerant, which can be rapidly chilled so as to deliver subfreezing temperature to tissues.

dermatitis   Inflammation of the skin.

dermatosis   A general term for any abnormal condition of the skin, but usually excluding inflammatory conditions, which are called dermatitis.

dermatographism   The property of abnormally sensitive skin by which strokes or writing with a pointed object are reproduced on the skin surface as raised red lines.

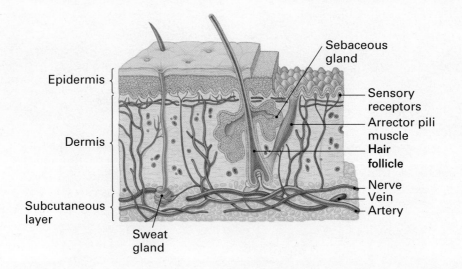

Figure 4-1
Skin Structure

discoid   Consisting of small, flat plaques.

erosion   A surface defect in the epidermis produced by rubbing or scratching.

eschar   The crust that forms on a burn.

exacerbation   An increase in the severity of a disease, particularly when occurring after a period of improvement (remission).

excoriation   Abrasion of the epidermal surface by scratching.

fissure   A linear defect or crack in the continuity of the epidermis.

friable   Crumbly; fragmenting or bleeding easily on touch or manipulation; said usually of diseased tissue.

furuncle   A deep, solitary abscess.

hypertrophic   Overgrown, usually as a result of increase in the size of cells.

keloid   A firm, nodular, irregular, often pigmented mass of fibrous tissue representing a hypertrophic scar.

lichenification   Thickening, coarsening, and pigment change of skin due to chronic irritation, usually scratching.

macule   A flat patch or mark differing in color from surrounding skin.

malar   Pertaining to or situated on the cheeks.

nevus   (1) A pigmented lesion of the skin. (2) A skin lesion present since birth (birthmark).

occult   Hidden; not obvious, but sometimes able to be inferred from indirect evidence.

papule   A small elevated zone of skin.

pit   A small depression in the skin resulting from local atrophy or scarring after trauma or inflammation.

plantar (*not* planter)   Pertaining to the sole of the foot.

pruritus, **pruritic**   Itching.

pyoderma   General term for any purulent (pus-forming) infection of the skin.

rhinophyma   Enlargement and deformity of the external nose, usually as a result of rosacea.

scab   See *crust*.

scale   A flake of epidermis shed from the skin surface.

scar   See *cicatrix*.

telangiectatic   Pertaining to telangiectasia; a permanent dilatation of small blood vessels (capillaries, arterioles, venules), visible through a skin or mucous surface.

ulcer   A cutaneous defect extending into the dermis.

vector   An animal (for example, a rat) that transmits a pathogenic organism from one host to another.

vesicle   A small thin-walled sac containing clear fluid.

wheal (weal, welt)   The characteristic lesion of hives. A small zone of edema in skin, which may be red or white; wheals are typically multiple and appear and disappear abruptly.

Lay and Medical Terms

athlete's foot	tinea pedis
baldness	alopecia
bruise	contusion
blackhead	comedo
blister	vesicle
hives	urticaria (or wheals)
wrinkles	rhytides
zit	(acne) pustule

Medical Readings

History and Physical Examination

Review of Systems. Skin. The patient is questioned about prior diagnosis of severe or chronic cutaneous disease and any treatments used for them in the past or at present. The more common skin complaints include local or general eruptions or rashes, itching, dryness or scaling, pigment changes, and solid tumors of various kinds. Disorders of the hair (abnormal appearance of the hair, excessive hair, hair loss) and nails (deformity, discoloration) are also part of the dermatologic history.

The physician questions the patient about the duration of the problem; whether it comes and goes, remains unchanged, or is gradually getting better or worse; whether it is spreading from one area to others; whether the patient can suggest any reason for the problem; and whether anything seems to make the problem better or worse.

Physical Examination. Cutaneous diagnosis depends on a consideration of many factors: the type, number, grouping, and location of lesions; combinations of features occurring together; signs of evolutionary change, secondary infection, or the effects of treatment; and the presence of associated symptoms such as fever, headache, or pain in the joints or abdomen. While many skin problems (acne, warts, poison ivy, ringworm) arise in the skin and stay there, many others (hives, the eruptions of chickenpox and lupus erythematosus) are signs of systemic disease.

In assessing the skin, the physician ensures adequate exposure of the surface by removing clothing, dressings, bandages, and ointments and by using bright natural or artificial light and, as needed, a magnifying lens.

Examination of the skin is not carried out by inspection alone. The examiner palpates any area of skin that appears abnormal and observes its temperature, texture, tenseness or laxness, moistness or dryness, and also looks for tenderness and crepitation.

Turgor is the degree to which tissue spaces, particularly in the skin and subcutaneous tissues, are filled with extracellular fluid. When a zone of normally lax skin, such as on the abdomen, is gently picked up between thumb and finger and then released, it should flatten out again immediately. Failure to do so (tenting) indicates poor skin turgor, a sign of significant dehydration.

In evaluating skin color, the examiner considers the intensity and distribution of normal pigment (melanin) and any abnormal coloration, including cyanosis (blueness), erythema (redness), jaundice (yellowness), and bronzing. Localized or generalized loss of pigment is also noted, as well as any tattoos and surgical or traumatic scars. When local or diffuse redness is present, a diascope can be used to distinguish capillary dilatation from other causes. A diascope is a small flat piece of clear glass or plastic, which is pressed firmly against the reddened skin. Blanching (fading of redness) on pressure indicates that redness is probably due to dilatation of skin capillaries. Redness that is due to hemorrhage or abnormal pigmentation will not fade on pressure.

Common Diseases

Atopic Dermatitis (Eczema). A chronic pruritic condition of the skin.

Cause: Unknown. Most patients have a personal or family history of allergy. May be exacerbated by irritants, emotional stress.

History: Recurrent itching, particularly affecting the back of the neck and the antecubital and popliteal areas, usually causing constant scratching.

Physical Examination: Patches of redness, sometimes with weeping, scaling, or vesiculation. Excoriations and lichenification from scratching. Sometimes evidence of secondary infection.

Diagnostic Tests: Scratch tests and RAST may be positive for many allergens.

Course: Chronic, with remissions and exacerbations. Secondary infection may result from scratching, and very chronic lesions may progress to fibrosis or pigmentation.

Treatment: Avoidance of known allergens, irritants, strong soaps, excessive wetting of skin and excessive bathing. Moisturizers to restore texture of skin, and topical adrenocortical steroids to reduce itching and inflammation.

Contact Dermatitis. Dermatitis resulting from contact with an irritant or allergen (Figure 4-2).

Cause: Numerous substances, including industrial chemicals, cosmetics, toiletries, and household products, can cause either an irritant or allergic-type of contact dermatitis. Irritant contact dermatitis results from direct chemical attack on the skin and typically produces symptoms within minutes of exposure. Allergic contact dermatitis occurs only in sensitized persons, and there may be a latent period of 2-5 days between exposure and appearance of symptoms.

History: Itching, burning, stinging, with variable amounts of swelling, redness, and other physical signs, on parts of the skin that have been exposed to the causative agent.

Physical Examination: Redness, swelling, vesicles or bullae, weeping, crusting. Signs of damage from scratching or of secondary infection may be present.

Course: Secondary infection may occur.

Treatment: Avoidance of the cause, soothing applications, topical or even systemic adrenocortical steroids.

Impetigo. A spreading bacterial infection of the skin causing itching and crusted sores (Figure 4-3).

Cause: Staphylococci, sometimes streptococci. Infection may begin in a trivial cut or abrasion. Impetiginization refers to the development of impetigo in an area of skin already damaged by a noninfectious dermatitis. Scratching and poor personal hygiene, particularly among children, lead to rapid spread of lesions and often transmission to household contacts, schoolmates, or playmates.

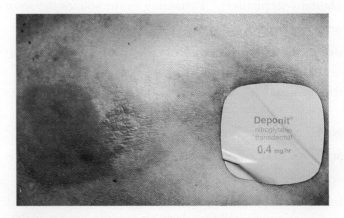

Figure 4-2
Contact Dermatitis from Latex Allergy

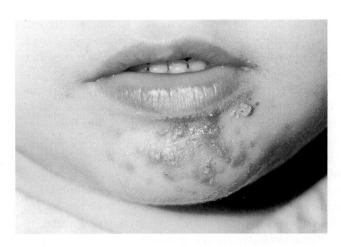

Figure 4-3
Impetigo

History: Itching and crusted sores, especially on the face.

Physical Examination: Macules, vesicles, bullae, pustules, and copious gummy purulent exudate forming honey-colored crusts on an erythematous base. In severe infection there may be fever.

Diagnostic Tests: Smear and culture can identify the causative bacteria.

Course: Without treatment, increasing spread often occurs. Systemic effects (toxemia, dehydration) may occur in children, particularly those already debilitated by disease or malnutrition. A severe form of impetigo known as ecthyma may leave scars.

Treatment: Strict attention to personal hygiene; isolation may be appropriate. For most cases of impetigo, the antibiotic mupirocin applied as an ointment is curative. In the presence of extensive disease, fever, or toxemia, antibiotics are administered systemically.

Tinea Corporis (Tinea Circinata, Ringworm of the Body). Superficial fungal infection of the skin.

Cause: Fungi of the genera *Epidermophyton*, *Microsporum*, and *Trichophyton*. Transmission from infected persons or animals sometimes occurs. Moisture and friction favor invasion of skin.

History: One or more slowly expanding round or oval patches of red, scaly skin, usually on exposed surfaces, with a variable amount of itching. There may be a history of recent new exposure to domestic animals or to persons with similar lesions.

Physical Examination: Lesions are pink, red, or tan, round or oval and sharply circumscribed, and covered with fine scales. The outer border of a lesion is raised slightly, and with continuing expansion of the margin, the skin near the center of the lesion gradually clears and assumes a normal appearance.

Diagnostic Tests: Scrapings of scales heated with potassium hydroxide (KOH) often show fungal material on microscopic examination. Culture on Sabouraud's medium may be required to confirm the presence of fungi. Examination with Wood light shows characteristic fluorescence only when infection is due to species of *Microsporum*.

Course: Tinea may become chronic and widespread, with extension to scalp, hair, and nails. Secondary bacterial infection may complicate diagnosis and treatment. In some persons an autoimmune phenomenon called a **dermatophytid** or **id reaction** may cause eruption of vesicular lesions on areas not infected with fungus, particularly on the hands.

Treatment: Numerous antifungal medicines are effective in topical form. Topical adrenocortical steroids may also be used if inflammation and itching are severe. Systemic antifungal treatment may be needed when infection is severe or resistant to topical treatment.

Other Superficial Fungal Infections of the Skin.
The fungal organisms responsible for tinea corporis can also cause more localized infections. In **tinea capitis** (ringworm of the scalp), infected hairs break off at the scalp surface, leaving patchy areas that appear bald, often with black dots representing the roots of broken-off hairs. Mild itching and scaling may occur. Treatment is with oral antifungals such as griseofulvin and selenium sulfide shampoo. **Kerion** is a complication, with boggy edema and exudation of pus though hair follicle openings.

Tinea pedis (athlete's foot) causes erythema, itching, scaling, fissuring, maceration, and vesicle formation of varying degree, particularly between the toes. **Tinea cruris** (jock itch) is a similar infection of the groin. **Tinea versicolor**, caused by *Malassezia furfur*, consists of variable numbers of white to tan macules with very fine scales. Patches are lighter than surrounding tanned skin, but darker than surrounding untanned skin, hence the name *versicolor* "changing colors." Tinea pedis, tinea cruris, and tinea versicolor usually respond to topical antifungals.

Tinea unguium (onychomycosis) is probably the most important chronic nail disease. Fungal infection of fingernails and toenails causes discoloration, deformity, splitting, crumbling of nails, and separation from nail beds, generally without other symptoms. Oral antifungal treatment, usually for several months, is standard. Topical methods and even avulsion of infected nails are sometimes used.

Candidiasis (or candidosis; infection of skin and mucous membranes with the yeastlike fungus *Candida albicans*) causes shiny, sharply delineated patches of intense erythema with itching or burning. Infection is more common in diabetics and typically occurs on areas where two skin surfaces are in apposition, with trapping of moisture: under the breasts, in the anogenital area, and in skin folds of obese persons. Diagnosis is confirmed by microscopic examination for hyphae or culture. Infections in the mouth (called thrush) and the vagina are treated with either topical or systemic antifungals.

Herpes Simplex. Local viral infection of skin or mucous membranes, causing vesicular lesions, typically recurrent (Figure 4-4).

Cause: Herpesvirus type 1 (oral, labial, facial herpes) and type 2 (genital herpes). Transmission is by direct contact with an infected person, not necessarily with visible lesions. Genital herpes is a sexually transmitted disease. The virus may lie dormant for months or years before causing symptoms. Viral activation, with ensuing skin eruption, may be triggered by physical or emotional stress, fever or respiratory infection (hence the lay terms "cold sore" and "fever blister"), sun exposure, and menstruation.

History: Clusters of small, painful vesicles about the nose or lips or on the genitals. These often recur in the same place, at greater or lesser intervals, in response to triggering factors mentioned above, or for no apparent reason. Vesicles may ulcerate. Women with genital herpes may have severe pain on urination. The first episode of infection is typically the most severe.

Physical Examination: A cluster of 4-6 small vesicles or ulcers on an erythematous, edematous base. With a first infection there is often fever and regional lymph-

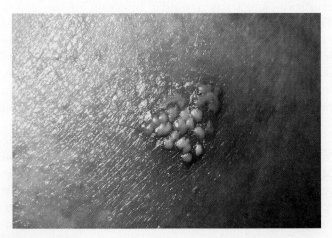

Figure 4-4
Herpes Simplex

adenitis. Secondary infection may cause pustule formation, crusting, and even impetigo (discussed above).

Diagnostic Tests: Viral culture yields proof of herpes infection.

Course: An episode of infection typically runs its course in about a week. Secondary bacterial infection may lead to exacerbation of symptoms. Intrauterine infection is associated with abortion or fetal damage. A child delivered through an infected birth canal may acquire localized or widespread neonatal infection, typically severe. Ocular infection with herpes simplex virus causes herpetic (dendritic) keratitis, a severe ulcerative disorder of the cornea that can lead to visual impairment.

Treatment: Analgesics and topical applications to control pain. Topical or (preferably) systemic treatment with antiviral drugs (acyclovir, penciclovir, valacyclovir).

Warts (Verrucae). Virally induced coarse papules of the skin and mucous membranes.

Cause: Human papillomavirus (HPV), of which about 80 types have been identified by immunologic means. Most types preferentially affect particular areas (plantar warts on soles of the feet, genital warts on the external genitalia or uterine cervix). Transmission is by direct contact. Genital warts are transmitted sexually. Scratching and picking at lesions causes **autoinoculation** (implantation of infective viral material at new sites, with spread of lesions).

History: One or more papules on skin surface, or on anogenital mucosa. Mild itching may occur, and occasionally bleeding.

Physical Examination: One or more coarsely textured papules, varying from flat (on the sole of the foot or the face) to elevated (on the hands or the genitals). Typical genital warts are narrow-based, raised, and tend to come to a point; lesions of this type are called **condylomata acuminata** (singular, **condyloma acuminatum**). There may be evidence of excoriation or damage from scratching, picking, or crude attempts at removal. Secondary infection may occur.

Diagnostic Tests: Suspicious lesions treated with dilute acetic acid become chalky gray or white (acetowhitening) if they are warts. Diagnosis is usually clinically evident, but biopsy can provide histologic confirmation. Wart virus cannot be cultured. Cervical infection produces characteristic changes on Pap smear, but the Pap smear is not an adequate screening test for HPV infection. DNA typing of HPV present on the cervix can identify types associated with risk of malignant change (see below).

Course: Without treatment most HPV infections resolve within 18-36 months, but meanwhile the condition may have been transmitted to others. Cervical infection with certain types of HPV is the leading cause of cervical carcinoma, usually after a latent period of more than 10 years.

Treatment: Depending on the site of infection, surgical excision, electrocautery, laser ablation, and **cryotherapy** (freezing with liquid nitrogen or a cryoprobe) are currently the most popular methods. Others include destruction with caustic chemicals such as salicylic acid, bichloracetic acid, and podofilox, application of the immune response modifier imiquimod, and injection of interferon directly into lesions.

Acne Vulgaris. A chronic eruption of comedones, papules, pustules, and cysts occurring primarily in adolescence.

Causes. The ultimate cause is unknown. There may be a genetic predisposition (identical twins are equally affected). The disease tends to be worse in males but does not occur in castrated males. It comes on about the time of puberty and typically resolves within 5-8 years, but may persist into the middle and late 20s or beyond. Acne or acneform lesions develop in Cushing syndrome, including the type induced by treatment with adrenocortical steroids; in women with hyperandrogenism of any cause; and in persons exposed to certain chemicals (chloracne, due to industrial exposure to chlorine; iodism, due to medicinal administration of iodide). Acne typically gets worse during times of emotional stress.

The lesions of acne develop in oil (sebaceous) glands, apparently as a result of heightened sebum production that leads to retention of sebum and plugging of gland ducts. Plugged, enlarged glands are called **comedones** (singular, **comedo**). These are colloquially called *whiteheads* when closed, and *blackheads* when the gland orifices are open, exposing sebum plugs, which darken as a result of chemical changes (not dirt). Very large comedones form cysts. Retained sebum is broken down by bacteria (*Propionibacterium acnes*) or spontaneous chemical changes to form fatty acids, which cause local inflammation and induce a foreign body reaction. Surface bacteria (staphylococci) invade inflamed tissue to produce pustules. Symptoms are aggravated by application of greasy or oily cosmetics and by repetitive picking or squeezing of lesions. Healing of pustules may be protracted and may leave pits or scars.

History: Appearance of lesions varying in type (blackheads, whiteheads, papules, pustules, cysts), number, distribution, and severity on the face, upper back, and chest; rarely elsewhere.

Physical Examination: Essentially as above.

Diagnostic Tests: Culture may be useful to identify unusual organisms causing secondary infection. Other laboratory studies may disclose underlying or contributing causes.

Course: Eventually, spontaneous remission occurs. This can take years, however, and in the meantime the patient may suffer severe emotional distress. The course of cystic acne may be especially protracted, and any severe case of acne is likely to leave some scarring.

Treatment: Vigorous skin hygiene with greaseless soaps and cleansers is the foundation of treatment. Topical drugs include benzoyl peroxide, azelaic acid, retinoids (adapalene, tazarotene, tretinoin), and antibiotics (clindamycin, erythromycin). Antibiotics such as tetracycline, minocycline, and erythromycin may also be administered orally for long periods. Expression of sebum from comedones with a comedo extractor by a physician may reduce symptoms. Injection of adrenocortical steroid into lesions may also help by lessening local inflammation. In women, cyclical hormone therapy with an oral contraceptive containing norgestimate and ethinyl estradiol often provides long-term control. Isotretinoin taken orally for 4-6 months induces lengthy, usually permanent resolution of acne, but it is reserved for severe cases because of side effects (peeling of lips in 90%; elevation of blood cholesterol in 15%; abnormal liver function tests; grave risk of fetal damage if taken by a pregnant patient).

Rosacea (Acne Rosacea). A reddish facial eruption occurring in the middle-aged and elderly.

Cause: Unknown. Occurs more commonly in persons with migraine headaches. Responds to antibiotic treatment. A rash similar to rosacea sometimes results from prolonged application of potent topical adrenocorticosteroids to the face.

History: Burning and flushing of the face, with patchy or diffuse rosy tint, papules, and sometimes pustules or excessive sebum production.

Physical Examination: As noted above. The cheeks, nose, and chin show a faint to bright inflammatory blush. Papules, pustules, **telangiectases** (visible patches of dilated skin vessels), and oiliness are usually present to some degree. Inflammation of the eyelids and even the cornea may occur. In some patients marked hyperplasia of the tissues of the nose (rhinophyma) eventually develops.

Course: Rosacea is highly chronic, but treatment provides a fair degree of control.

Treatment: Topical metronidazole or other antibiotics provide improvement in symptoms. Oral antibiotics and topical corticosteroids may be required. Lasers can obliterate telangiectases. For severe rhinophyma, plastic surgery is required.

Urticaria (Hives). An acute, often transitory eruption of intensely itchy papules or wheals.

Cause: Urticaria is caused by a release of histamine from mast cells in the dermis, with resultant local edema, capillary dilatation, and stimulation of nerve endings. Many factors can incite this reaction: allergies to food (shellfish, strawberries), medicines (aspirin, penicillin), insect bites or stings (bee stings), nonallergic sensitivity to medicines (atropine, codeine), parasitic infestation, sunlight, cold, heat (cholinergic urticaria), and even, in susceptible individuals, simple stroking of the skin (dermographism).

History: Sudden onset of a localized or generalized eruption of intensely itchy wheals or papules, which may be transitory.

Physical Examination: Wheals (raised white or red papules) surrounded by erythema. Wheals may be round or scalloped and confluent. Signs of scratching may be evident.

Diagnostic Tests: Blood studies and allergic screening may indicate the underlying cause, but usually do not.

Course: Urticaria often occurs in attacks at intervals of a few hours, but typically resolves within 1-2 weeks unless continued exposure to the causative agent occurs. Urticaria persisting beyond one month may point to occult infection or malignancy. Complications: Secondary infection due to scratching.

Treatment: Severe urticaria responds to intramuscular epinephrine. Antihistamines such as diphenhydramine or hydroxyzine may be given orally or by injection to control an acute attack. Regular use of antihistamines prevents or mitigates further attacks. The nonsedating antihistamines fexofenadine and loratadine may be useful prophylactically, even though they are ineffective in other forms of pruritus. Doxepin, a tricyclic antidepressant, is also effective either orally or topically. In severe cases, topical and systemic corticosteroids may be used.

Psoriasis. A chronic skin disorder characterized by scaly plaques (Figure 4-5).

Cause: Increased proliferation of epidermal cells. Evidently an autoimmune disorder, to which some persons are genetically predisposed.

History: Plaques of scaly thickening of the skin, particularly the scalp, knees, and elbows, with moderate itching. Nails and joints may also be affected.

Physical Examination: Reddish-purple thickened plaques of skin covered with silvery, firmly adherent scales. Pitting or stippling of nails and inflammation of joints, particularly the distal interphalangeal joints, may also be noted. In guttate psoriasis the plaques are small and numerous. **Koebner phenomenon** (formation of lesions at sites of trauma) may be noted.

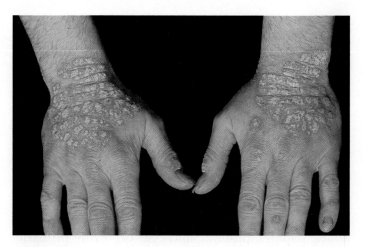

Figure 4-5
Psoriasis

Diagnostic Tests: Skin biopsy (usually unnecessary) shows characteristic changes in the epidermis.

Treatment: Topical steroids, calcipotriene, tar ointments; tar shampoos to the scalp. UVB (ultraviolet B); PUVA (psoralen + ultraviolet A). Oral methotrexate, etretinate, cyclosporine.

Pityriasis Rosea. A mild, benign, self-limited scaly eruption.

Cause: Possibly viral. More common in spring and fall. The male to female attack ratio is 2:3. Person-to-person transmission has not been demonstrated.

History: Appearance of a solitary scaly patch (herald patch) on the skin, followed in 1-2 weeks by a generalized eruption of similar but smaller lesions. Itching is mild or absent.

Physical Examination: A widespread eruption of oval fawn-colored macules with fine scales on the trunk and proximal extremities. The hands, face, and feet are typically spared. Trunk lesions follow a segmental distribution, especially on the back, giving a "Christmas tree" appearance.

Diagnostic Tests: Because pityriasis simulates secondary syphilis, a serologic test for syphilis is often done to rule out that possibility.

Course: Lesions disappear spontaneously in about 6 weeks.

Treatment: Ultraviolet treatments, oral erythromycin, and topical or oral steroids may hasten clearing, but treatment is seldom needed since itching is mild, affected body parts can easily be covered by clothing, and spontaneous resolution within weeks is virtually certain.

Basal Cell Carcinoma. A slowly growing, waxy or pearly papule with telangiectatic vessels, appearing usually on parts of the body exposed to sunlight, particularly

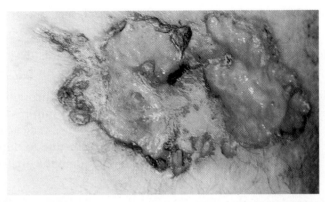

Figure 4-6
Basal Cell Carcinoma

the face (Figure 4-6). Most appear in the middle-aged or elderly. Ulceration and widespread erosion may occur if treatment is delayed, but metastasis is rare. Treatment is by surgical excision, including Mohs chemosurgery and cryotherapy.

Squamous Cell Carcinoma. A hard red nodule appearing on sun-exposed skin, usually in a middle-aged or elderly person. The lesion may develop in a preexisting actinic keratosis and may rapidly ulcerate. Metastasis is uncommon. Treatment is by excision.

Melanoma. A pigmented malignancy of the skin (Figure 4-7) that develops in persons of all ages, progresses rapidly, metastasizes widely, and is fatal without treatment. Among malignancies melanoma ranks ninth in incidence, and incidence is increasing. At least some cases are due to sun exposure. It is estimated that, for a person under age 30, visiting a tanning parlor 10 or more times a year increases the risk of melanoma sevenfold. The risk is also higher in persons of white race, persons with many pigmented nevi, and persons with a family history or prior personal history of melanoma.

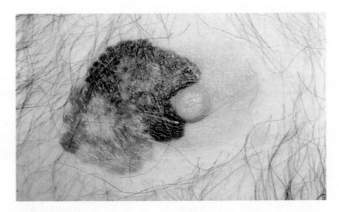

Figure 4-7
Melanoma

Melanoma can arise anew or develop from a previously benign pigmented nevus. Features of a pigmented lesion that suggest malignancy are irregularity of shape or border, uneven distribution of pigment, pink, blue, or black color, bleeding or ulceration, and rapid enlargement.

Treatment is by excision. Prognosis depends on the thickness of the tumor (Breslow classification) or the depth of invasion (Clark classification). In metastatic disease, radiation and chemotherapy may prolong survival.

Thermal Burns. Thermal burns are caused by contact of skin or mucous membrane with hot objects, liquids, or vapors. The amount of injury depends on the degree of heat and the extent and duration of contact. High heat induces an intense inflammatory reaction with leakage of fluid into tissues. It also coagulates protein and destroys tissues by vaporization or carbonization.

Skin burns are classified as **first degree** (redness of the surface without blistering), **second degree** (redness and blistering), and **third degree** (redness, blistering, and charring) (Figure 4-8). First and second degree

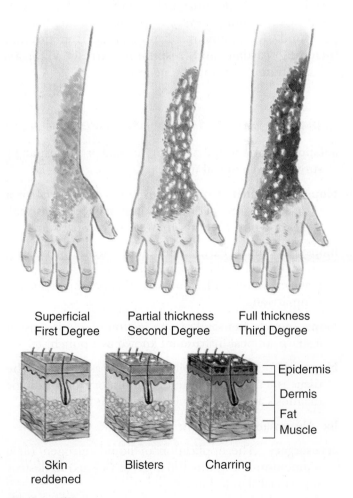

Figure 4-8
Burns

burns normally heal without scarring unless they become infected. In third degree burns, the nature and depth of injury usually lead to scarring. Deep burns can destroy tissues below skin level: subcutaneous fat, muscles, nerves, tendons, and even bone.

Extensive burns, even when only first degree, typically cause severe biochemical imbalance, due to sequestration of fluid in the burned area with proportionate reduction of blood volume. Dehydration, shock, toxemia, and severe local or systemic infection may complicate any severe burn.

Treatment is aimed at correcting fluid and electrolyte imbalances, relieving pain, and preventing or treating infection. Third degree burns often require grafting.

Cold Injury. The harmful local effects of intense cold (frostbite) are similar to those of heat: local inflammation, often with blistering and tissue destruction. Treatment is similar to that for burns. Exposure to atmospheric cold, or prolonged immersion in cold water, can induce systemic hypothermia, a drop in the rectal (core) temperature below 35°C. The basic treatment is rewarming. Severe hypothermia can lead to profound derangement of physiologic functioning, including cardiac and respiratory arrest. Vigorous resuscitation efforts may be necessary.

Diagnostic and Surgical Procedures

ablation Total removal of a part, normal or abnormal, by surgical or chemical means.

biopsy, excisional Complete excision or removal of a skin lesion. In addition, some adjacent normal-appearing tissue is also removed for comparison.

biopsy, incisional Partial removal of a lesion by making an incision into the lesion and removing a section of it as well as some adjacent normal-appearing tissue for comparison.

biopsy, punch Removal of one section of a lesion using a sharp surgical instrument known as a punch.

biopsy, skin Removal of all or part of a skin lesion. The tissue is sent to the pathology laboratory for histologic diagnosis and to determine whether it is malignant.

bx Abbreviation for *biopsy.*

cryosurgery The application of liquid nitrogen (at a temperature of minus 196 degrees Celsius) to destroy superficial skin lesions.

cryotherapy Local treatment of neoplasms or other lesions by freezing.

debridement Successive scraping away of dead skin down to viable tissue that bleeds, especially for burns.

diascopy Inspection of red or purplish lesions through a transparent plastic or glass plate, which compresses the skin. If the color is due to dilated blood vessels, it blanches (fades) with compression; color due to deposition of pigment, including blood pigment, in tissues is not altered by surface pressure.

electrodesiccation See *fulguration.*

fulguration The application of an electrical current to destroy superficial skin lesions.

graft A section of skin transplanted to an area of the body.

intradermal test The injection into the intradermal layer of the skin of a chemical or other type of substance known to produce an allergic reaction in sensitive individuals. This creates a wheal which is outlined with a pen and/or measured. The area is examined again in 30 minutes. A reddened, enlarged area at the site of the injection indicates a positive allergic reaction to that chemical or allergen.

patch test The application to the skin of a piece of filter paper containing a chemical or other type of substance known to produce an allergic reaction in sensitive individuals. Many patches are taped to the skin and labeled. After 24-48 hours the skin underneath is examined. Reddened, raised areas of skin indicate a positive allergic reaction to that chemical or allergen.

plastic surgery Surgery concerned with the restoration, reconstruction, correction, or improvement in the shape and appearance of body structures that are defective, damaged, or misshapen by injury, disease, growth, development, or aging.

scratch test The application, to a superficial scratch made in the skin, of a chemical or other type of substance known to produce an allergic reaction in sensitive individuals. Many scratches are made in the skin, and the area is examined again in 30 minutes. Reddened, raised areas of skin indicate a positive allergic reaction.

Wood light An ultraviolet lamp with a filter that selects wavelengths under which certain funguses infecting skin or hair fluoresce brightly.

Laboratory Procedures

blood studies May identify underlying, perhaps systemic, conditions or provide additional information about the skin disorder.

culture Exudate, pus, crusts, or scrapings for bacteria, fungi, or viruses.

microscopic examination of scrapings from the skin To identify fungal material, the mites of scabies, and distinctive kinds of scales; skin scrapings are usually treated with potassium hydroxide (KOH) and heat, which partially or completely dissolve human tissue but leave fungal elements unchanged.

Pharmacology

Because of the superficial nature and location of most dermatologic diseases, they respond well to topical drug therapy. Mild cases of skin diseases such as acne, psoriasis, poison ivy, contact dermatitis, superficial infections, herpes simplex infections, lice, and diaper rash can be successfully treated with topical agents. However, systemic drugs may be necessary when dermatologic problems become widespread or particularly severe.

Acne drugs. Acne vulgaris is the most common form of acne, usually seen in adolescence. Topical creams, lotions, liquids, and gels are used to remove oil and dead skin (keratolytic action), to close the pores (astringent action), to inhibit the growth of skin bacteria (antiseptic action), and to kill skin bacteria (antibiotic action).

Topical prescription antibiotics may be used to treat more serious cases of acne vulgaris.

> azelaic acid (Azelex, Finevin)
> chlortetracycline (Aureomycin)
> clindamycin (Cleocin T, C/T/S)
> erythromycin (A/T/S, Emgel, EryDerm, Erygel, Staticin, T-Stat)
> meclocycline (Meclan)
> tetracycline (Achromycin, Panmycin, Sumycin, Tetracyn, Tetralan)

Tetracycline may be prescribed orally for systemic treatment of acne vulgaris, and severe cystic acne that is unresponsive to antibiotic treatment may be treated topically with a form of vitamin A such as tretinoin (Retin-A) or systemically with isotretinoin (Accutane). These drugs cause epithelial cells to multiply more rapidly. This rapid turnover prevents pores from becoming clogged and infected and decreases cyst formation.

Psoriasis drugs. Psoriasis is treated with coal tar lotions, gels, shampoos, and bath liquids to decrease the rate of epidermal cell production, correct abnormalities of the keratinocytes, cleanse away dead skin (keratolytic action), and decrease itching (antipruritic action).

> Aqua Tar
> Balnetar
> Denorex, Extra Strength Denorex
> Estar
> Neutrogena T/Derm, Neutrogena T/Gel
> Tegrin for Psoriasis, Tegrin Medicated, Tegrin Medicated for Psoriasis
> Zetar

The red, scaly patches of psoriasis are caused by abnormal keratinocytes within the skin. Synthetic vitamin D-type drugs such as calcipotriene (Dovonex) are applied topically to activate vitamin D receptors in the keratinocytes and slow the abnormal cell growth.

Psoralens for psoriasis. Severe, disabling psoriasis may also be treated by exposure to ultraviolet light in combination with a drug that sensitizes the skin to the effects of ultraviolet light. Drugs such as methoxsalen (Oxsoralen-Ultra, 8-MOP) are collectively known as **psoralens**. This combined treatment damages cell DNA and decreases the rate of cell division. The combination therapy of methoxsalen and ultraviolet light is known as **PUVA** (psoralen/ultraviolet wavelength A).

Topical corticosteroids, both over-the-counter and prescription, are used to relieve contact dermatitis, poison ivy, and insect bites. They are also used to treat psoriasis, seborrhea, and eczema.

Topical corticosteroids come in several strengths and in several forms (ointment, gel, lotion, cream, and aerosol). Some common over-the-counter and prescription topical corticosteroid drugs are:

> alclometasone (Aclovate)
> amcinonide (Cyclocort)
> betamethasone (Alphatrex, Betatrex, Diprolene, Diprolene AF, Diprosone, Luxiq, Maxivate, Psorion, Teladar)
> clobetasol (Cormax, Olux, Temovate)
> clocortolone (Cloderm)
> desonide (DesOwen, Tridesilon)
> desoximetasone (Topicort, Topicort LP)
> dexamethasone (Decadron, Decaspray)
> diflorasone (Florone, Florone E, Maxiflor, Psorcon E)

fluocinolone (Derma-Smoothe/FS, Flurosyn, Synalar, Synalar-HP)
flurandrenolide (Cordran, Cordran SP)
fluticasone (Cutivate)
halcinonide (Halog, Halog-E)
halobetasol (Ultravate)
hydrocortisone (Cortaid Intensive Therapy, Cortaid with Aloe, Cort-Dome, Cortizone-5, Cortizone-10, Dermacort, Dermolate, Hycort, Hytone, Lanacort 5, Lanacort 10, Locoid, Maximum Strength Bactine, Maximum Strength Caldecort, Maximum Strength Cortaid, Maximum Strength KeriCort-10, Pandel, Scalpicin, T/Scalp, Westcort)
mometasone (Elocon)
prednicarbate (Dermatop)
triamcinolone (Aristocort, Aristocort A, Flutex, Kenalog, Kenalog-H)

Topical antibiotics are used to treat minor, superficial bacterial skin infections. They act to inhibit the growth of or kill bacteria by blocking their ability to maintain a cell wall. Topical antibiotics are manufactured as gels, lotions, creams, ointments, and sprays.

bacitracin (Baciguent)
gentamicin (Garamycin)
mupirocin (Bactroban, Bactroban Nasal)
neomycin (Myciguent)

Drugs for fungus and yeast infections. Fungal infections such as ringworm (tinea corporis), athlete's foot (tinea pedis), jock itch (tinea cruris), and fungal infections of the nail (onychomycosis) can be effectively treated with topical antifungal drugs. These drugs alter the cell wall of the fungus and disrupt enzyme activity, resulting in cell death. These drugs are manufactured in cream, ointment, lotion, and shampoo forms.

Over-the-counter topical antifungal drugs include Desenex, miconazole (Micatin, Monistat-Derm), and tolnaftate (Aftate, Tinactin). Prescription drugs for fungus infections include:

butenafine (Mentax)
ciclopirox (Loprox, Penlac Nail Lacquer)
clioquinol
clotrimazole (Cruex, Desenex, Lotrimin, Lotrimin AF 1%)
econazole (Spectazole)
haloprogin (Halotex)

ketoconazole (Nizoral, Nizoral A-D)
miconazole (Lotrimin AF 2%, Micatin, Monistat-Derm, Prescription Strength Desenex, Ting)
naftifine (Naftin)
nystatin (Mycostatin, Nilstat)
oxiconazole (Oxistat)
sulconazole (Exelderm)
terbinafine (Lamisil AT, Lamisil DermGel)
tolnaftate (Absorbine Athlete's Foot Cream, Absorbine Footcare, Aftate for Athlete's Foot, Aftate for Jock Itch, Tinactin, Tinactin for Jock Itch)
triacetin (Fungoid, Fungoid Creme, Fungoid Tincture)

Severe topical fungal skin infections may be treated with oral drugs such as griseofulvin, itraconazole, ketoconazole, and terbinafine. Yeast infections of the skin, caused by *Candida albicans*, are treated with topical drugs such as miconazole (Monistat-Derm) and ketoconazole (Nizoral), such as those used for fungi.

Drugs used to treat itching. Topical corticosteroids inhibit inflammation and itching, and antihistamines inhibit inflammation, redness, and itching caused by allergic reaction and the release of histamine. As a group, these drugs are also known as *antipruritics*. (*Pruritus* means *itching*.) These combination drugs are applied topically:

Bactine Antiseptic Anesthetic (benzalkonium, lidocaine)
benzocaine (Americaine Anesthetic, Bicozene, Dermoplast, Lanacane, Solarcaine, Solarcaine Medicated First Aid)
Caladryl (calamine, diphenhydramine)
Caladryl Clear (diphenhydramine, zinc oxide)
Calamycin (benzocaine, calamine, pyrilamine, zinc oxide)
Cetacaine (benzocaine, butamben, tetracaine)
EMLA (lidocaine, prilocaine)
lidocaine (Solarcaine Aloe Extra Burn Relief, Unguentine Plus, Xylocaine, Zilactin-L)
Medi-Quik (benzalkonium, lidocaine)
Ziradryl (diphenhydramine, zinc oxide)

For severe itching, these antihistamines may be given orally:

cyproheptadine (Periactin)
diphenhydramine (Benadryl)
hydroxyzine (Atarax, Vistaril)

TRANSCRIPTION**TIPS**

1. The term *Mohs* (rhymes with *toes*) *surgery* or *Mohs chemosurgery* is often encountered in dermatology dictation. If the possessive form of the eponym is preferred, the apostrophe should be placed at the end of the word *(Mohs')*. The technique is named for Dr. Frederic Mohs, an American surgeon.

2. There is no official brief form for the terms *subcutaneous* or *subcuticular*. If the brief form *subcu* is dictated, it may be translated if the correct term is known; otherwise, *subcu* should be transcribed as dictated. Do not use a brief form unless it is dictated.

3. Similar medical terms in English may be derived from different Latin and Greek roots. Both word roots, the Latin *cutaneo-* (cutaneous, subcutaneous) and the Greek *dermato-* (dermatitis, dermatologist) refer to *skin*. The Latin word for skin is *cutis*, the Greek *derma*. The Greek root *onycho-* (onychomycosis) and the Latin root *unguo-* (subungual) both mean *nail*.

4. The noun *callus* describes a local growth of hard, horny epithelium, as in "There is a callus on the palm of his hand from using a heavy hammer." The less-used synonym for *callus* is *callosity*. (Callus also forms at the site of a healing bony fracture and is eventually replaced with hard bone.) The site of a callus is often said to be *callused*: "There is a callused area on the palm of his hand." The adjective *callous*, meaning "hard, tough," usually refers to an uncaring, insensitive personality rather than to physical toughness. Note that there is no such word as *calloused*.

5. The term *pruritus* (from the Latin *prurire, to itch*) is often misspelled because of the mistaken impression that it ends in the suffix *-itis* (inflammation of). *Psoriasis* and *psoriatic* are hard to spell and even more difficult to locate in a medical dictionary because of their initial silent *p*. Memorize these and other hard-to-spell dermatologic terms.

callus/callous	psoriasis, psoriatic
eczema	verrucous
onychomycosis	xanthoma

6. Note these uniquely spelled dermatology drugs.

    gentamicin (the generic name ends in *-micin*)
    Garamycin (the trade name ends in *-mycin*)
    interferon alfa-2b
    pHisoHex (unusual for its lowercase initial letter and internal capitalization, patterned after *pH*, which indicates acid/alkaline parameters)

Spotlight on

Dermatology Dictation

by John H. Dirckx, M.D.

The long-established lay term **ringworm** causes much misunderstanding and consternation. Skin diseases known by this name are not due to worms, and physicians never thought they were. The word *ring* in *ringworm* refers to the circular shape of the lesions, with central clearing. *Worm* is just a metaphorical allusion to the "moth-eaten" appearance of skin infected by various superficial fungi. Clothes-eating moth larvae are incorrectly called worms. *Tinea*, the Latin term for ringworm, also means "moth."

The genus name *Pthirus* was derived incorrectly from *phtheir*, the Greek word for "louse." Although writers and editors constantly "correct" the spelling to *Phthirus*, the "wrong" spelling **Pthirus** is officially "right." The next time you use the expression "lousy" or "nit-picking" in a metaphorical sense, stop and think what you are saying.

When the rash of **zoster** appears on the trunk of the body, it is so distinctive that the diagnosis can hardly be missed. Even many laypersons can accurately recognize it. When fully developed, the cutaneous eruption looks like a belt or sash running around half of the body. *Zoster* is a Greek word for "belt." Another is *zone*, which in its latinized form *zona* was formerly used as a name for this condition. The lay English term *shingles* is a corruption of Latin *cingulum*, which also means "belt, girdle."

Source: *Human Diseases*

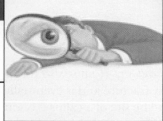

Proofreading Skills

Instructions: In the paragraphs below, circle the errors. Identify misspelled and missing medical and English words and write the correct words in the numbered spaces opposite the text.

1	This 17-month-old infant was healthy until a bout 8	1	about
2	days ago, when his mother observed severe	2	
3	erythematous blotches over his face and neck.	3	
4	particularly about the mouth. The mother then used	4	
5	an oil or salve of some type, which seemingly	5	
6	exacerbated they lesions. During the next 3-4 days	6	
7	these developed into crusted ulcers. In addition, the	7	
8	child became fretful and refused his diet. The mohter	8	
9	thought he might have been a bit febrile.	9	
10		10	
11	He was seen by Dr, Monash at Pediatrics East on	11	
12	Tuesday September 21 and a diagnosis of impetigo was	12	
13	made. He was begun on Bactroban ointment and oral	13	
14	Ceclor however the lesions progressed and the patient's	14	
15	general condition deteriorated. His temperture went	15	
16	up, and he refused solid food and began vomiting last	16	
17	p.m. He hsa been on no medicine except as	17	
18	mentioned.	18	
19		19	
20	There is no history of cronic or infectious disease	20	
21	feeding problems or failure to thrive. Family	21	
22	dermatologic history is significant in that two maternal	22	
23	uncles have psoriasis.	23	
24		24	
25	The child's development appears normal for his age.	25	
26	He looks toxic, being both lethargic and iritable.	26	
27	Temperature 101.6°. (This temp is rectal.) The whole	27	
28	skin surface displays erythematous blanching on	28	
29	pressure. There are numerous bullae, some of which	29	
30	contain clear to cloudy fluid and others frank pus.	30	
31	Many lesions consist of ruptured bullae with abundant	31	
32	crust made up of epidermal debris combined with	32	
33	seropurulent exudate.	33	
34		34	
35	There is no scleral icterus or nuchal ridigity and I	35	
36	observed no respiratory findings. Abdomen is soft and	36	
37	there are no masses. I feel he is somewhat dehydrated	37	
38	but this is difficult to assess fully.	38	
39		39	
40	DIAGNOSTIC IMPRESSION	40	
41	Bullous impetigo with septicemia. Rule out Ritter's	41	
42	disease, pemphigus, and immune deficiency.	42	

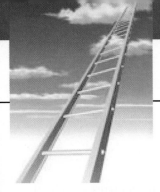

SkillsChallenge

Medical Terminology Matching Exercise

This matching exercise will test your knowledge of the root words, anatomic structures, symptoms, and disease processes encountered in dermatology.

Instructions: Match the definitions in Column A with the terms in Column B.

Column A	Column B
1. ___ skin growth caused by a virus	**A.** wart
2. ___ itching	**B.** pruritus
3. ___ fungal infection of the skin	**C.** tinea
4. ___ noninfectious disease of scaly patches	**D.** psoriasis
5. ___ infectious disease caused by mites	**E.** sebum
6. ___ pigment-containing tissue cells that determine skin color	**F.** adipose tissue
	G. wheal
7. ___ most superficial layer of skin	**H.** alopecia
8. ___ fat	**I.** keloid
9. ___ oil secreted by skin glands	**J.** melanocyte
10. ___ benign tumor of subcutaneous fat	**K.** pustule
11. ___ fungal infection of the nails	**L.** scabies
12. ___ malignant skin growths seen in AIDS	**M.** lipoma
13. ___ produced by an allergic reaction	**N.** epidermis
14. ___ skin lesion filled with clear fluid	**O.** onychomycosis
15. ___ abscess containing pus	**P.** vesicle
16. ___ red, flat skin lesion	**Q.** comedo
17. ___ hair loss	**R.** Kaposi sarcoma
18. ___ tiny skin hemorrhages	**S.** macule
19. ___ blackhead	**T.** petechiae
20. ___ enlarged scar tissue	

Adjectives Exercise

Adjectives are formed from nouns by adding adjectival suffixes such as *-ac, -al, -ar, -ary, -eal, -iac, -ic, -ical, -oid, -ous, -tic,* and *-tous*. In addition, some adjectives have a different form entirely from the noun which may be either Latin or Greek in origin.

Instructions: Write the adjectival form of the following dermatology words. Consult a medical dictionary to select the correct adjectival ending as necessary.

1. epidermis   <u>epidermal, epidermoid</u>
2. epithelium   _____
3. integument   _____
4. erythema   _____
5. seborrhea   _____
6. xanthoma   _____
7. macule   _____
8. cyst   _____
9. papule   _____
10. vesicle   _____
11. eczema   _____
12. psoriasis   _____
13. callus   _____

Plurals Exercise

Instructions: Write the plural form of the following nouns. Consult a medical dictionary to determine the correct plural.

1. acuminatum   <u>acuminata</u>
2. bulla   _____
3. comedo   _____
4. condyloma   _____
5. hypha   _____
6. petechia   _____
7. scapula   _____
8. telangiectasis   _____
9. verruca   _____
10. staphylococcus   _____

Soundalikes Exercise

Instructions: Circle the correct term from the soundalikes in parentheses in the following sentences.

1. Stomatitis and (abscess, aphthous) ulcers made it almost impossible for the patient to eat.

2. After observing the silvery gray, scaling patches on the patient's skin, the dermatologist diagnosed (cirrhosis, psoriasis).

3. The patient had an allergic rash of unknown origin which was diagnosed as (atopic, trophic, ectopic) dermatitis.

4. The bedridden patient had a chronic, weeping (atopic, trophic, ectopic) ulcer on his ischial (eminence, imminence).

5. The patient had an obvious bee sting which was surrounded by an inflamed halo of (edema, erythema, arrhythmia).

6. From ankles to knees, the patient had a weeping, brawny (edema, erythema, arrhythmia).

7. Both great toenails were deformed by (fundal, fungal) growths.

8. Because the patient had a solitary boil or (carbuncle, caruncle, furuncle) on her left buttock, she could not sit.

9. Without treatment, the physician feared that the solitary boil would expand, creating a cluster of boils or (carbuncle, caruncle, furuncle) cluster.

10. The patient had violaceous papules with a fine, shiny, scaly appearance that resembled (lichen, liken) planus.

11. The flat molelike lesion had a (melenic, melanotic) appearance.

12. The dermatologist removed the numerous small (palpations, palpitations, papillations) from around the patient's neck because they were constantly irritated by her necklaces.

13. The patient complained of an intense (parietes, pruritus) associated with the poison ivy rash.

14. The (varicose, verrucous) warts were benign, and no treatment was needed.

15. The child's feet and ankles were covered with numerous small (vesicals, vesicles) from the red ant bites.

Dictation Exercises

Instructions: Prior to transcribing the dermatology dictations, complete these activities.

1. **Using Chapter 3, Style Guide**

   a. What do you do when the doctor dictates a decimal such as "point 1"?
   b. The doctor begins dictating the diagnosis with "number one" but dictates only one diagnosis. How should you handle this?
   c. The doctor dictates a diagnosis but after the first diagnosis says "number two" and goes on to dictate several more diagnoses, numbering each one except the first one. How do you handle this?
   d. The doctor dictates some measurements but fails to dictate the unit to go with the numbers. What should you do?
   e. How would you make references to time possessive; for example, how would you correctly transcribe "3 days time"?
   f. Read the sections on using Roman and Arabic numbers. Give examples of which to use when.
   g. How do you transcribe ordinal numbers?
   h. What is the proper way to transcribe eponyms?
   i. How do you transcribe "times" followed by a number?
   j. What does the Style Guide says about clipped sentences and verbatim transcription?
   k. How to you punctuate coordinate adjectives?
   l. Perhaps the most common situation in which subject-verb agreement errors occur is in sentences beginning with *there*. Read the section in Chapter 3, Style Guide, called "Sentences beginning with *there*" under the Agreement of Subject and Verb section.
   m. When, according to the Style Guide, do you expand brief forms?
   n. How do you handle sentences that begin with numbers?
   o. What is the correct way to transcribe ratios?
   p. Consult the Style Guide for information on suture sizes and how to transcribe them. Give examples.

2. **Problem Solving**

This activity is to help you prepare ahead of time for some of the problems you'll encounter in the dictations. Some of these items may not have a definitive answer but are intended to simply get you thinking about how to handle a variety of situations that are common in transcription. If nothing else, they will help you recognize a problem when you encounter it in the dictations.

a. In a report, the doctor dictates a word that you cannot verify in a dictionary. It may be a mispronunciation, a coined word, slang, or a nonword. What do you do?

b. Some options might be to spell the word the way it sounds, flag it (leave a blank and put a "sounds like" in parentheses after the blank), or simply leave a blank. Justify your choice. Is there a time when you might do one thing and another time something else?

3. **Preparatory Research**

Any information requested in these questions not readily available in your textbook (including the appendix) or required references can easily be found using Internet search engines such as Google or on-line medical dictionaries.

a. Do a Google search for wound dressings and bandages. Bookmark the pages that seem to have the best lists. Give some examples of wound dressings and bandages.

b. Look up the word *clavus*. Write out the definition. What is the plural spelling of this term? What is the etymology (origin) of the term?

c. What is the Mohs technique? What kinds of conditions are treated with Mohs?

d. To prepare for transcribing an operative report on basal cell carcinoma of the ear, review the external anatomy of the ear, including structural anatomy and positional terms.

Sample dermatology reports appear on the following pages, illustrating a variety of reports. Fictional names are provided for illustration of proper format, and no resemblance to actual persons is intended. Sample transcripts were prepared according to the *AAMT Book of Style*, where possible.

Letter

June 28, XXXX

Blue Cross Insurance
2334 Wilshire Blvd.
Los Angeles, CA 95634

Re: William Rubin

Gentlemen:

The patient returned to our office and had 17 intracutaneous tests to reaffirm that he was allergic or not allergic to some additional allergens. We also performed a set of allergy tests by the epicutaneous method. We discussed giving allergy injections for those allergens which were unavoidable. I then gave him his first allergy shot, divided up into his left and right arms.

I felt that I had communicated why he was going to be getting allergy injections and why we were going to try to improve his chronic sinusitis problem. The next day the patient stopped payment for his $276 charge.

I think that, as a practicing allergist who is board-certified, I personally provided an adequate examination as well as adequate allergy testing, both epicutaneous and intracutaneous, as well as consultation services. He was also given his first allergy injection, and he was made fully aware of all the problems related to injections.

I hope that this establishes some additional information concerning this problem.

Sincerely yours,

Nathan E. Day, MD

NED:hpi

JESSUP, JENNIFER
#123456
Admitted 1/24/XXXX
ROSALIND SKINNER, MD

HISTORY
This 17-year-old was admitted via the emergency department. She gives a history of shooting crank. Since that time the left antecubital space has been infected.

PAST HISTORY
The patient has been shooting for at least a year. She denies use of drugs other than crank. The patient has a 2-year-old child and a 3-week-old child and has been in the hospital only for that. Denies accidents, injuries, and other infections.

SOCIAL HISTORY
The patient is a 17-year-old IV drug user.

PHYSICAL EXAMINATION
VITAL SIGNS: Temperature 102.2 degrees. Pulse 112. Respirations 20. Blood pressure 104/60.
GENERAL: Well-developed, well-nourished, English-speaking Caucasian 17-year-old female.
EENT: No gross abnormalities. Pupils constricted. Fair dental repair.
NECK: Supple, no palpable nodes.
CHEST: Lungs are clear.
HEART: Heart regular, not enlarged, no murmurs.
BREASTS: Breasts normal.
ABDOMEN: Soft. No palpable masses.
PELVIC AND RECTAL: Not done.
EXTREMITIES: Examination of the left antecubital space reveals there is a generalized area of tender cellulitis with a moderate amount of swelling on the left as compared with the right.

X-RAYS
No x-rays are available for review.

DIAGNOSES
1. Chronic intravenous drug user.
2. Cellulitis, left arm.

PLAN
The patient should be admitted to the hospital for IV antibiotics and possible opening of the wound.

ROSALIND SKINNER, MD

RS:hpi
d: 1/24/XXXX
t: 1/24/XXXX

WERNIG, INGE
#987654321
Admitted: 6/1/XXXX
Discharged: 6/10/XXXX

ADMISSION DIAGNOSES
1. Left lower leg cellulitis.
2. Left lower leg ulceration.
3. Diabetes mellitus.
4. Possible psoriasis.

DISCHARGE DIAGNOSES
1. Left lower leg cellulitis.
2. Left lower leg ulceration.
3. Diabetes mellitus.
4. Lichen simplex chronicus.

BRIEF HISTORY
This is a 48-year-old white female with obesity and diabetes who has had a smoldering left lower extremity cellulitis for the past 2-3 months. It is possibly related to her pruritus and psoriasis. She has been treated in the past with Coumadin and IV antibiotics. On the day of admission she presented to my office with worsening of the cellulitis and a new 2-cm ulceration, and was admitted for IV antibiotics and further evaluation.

EXTREMITIES
Extremities revealed bilateral edema 1 to 2+ to the knees, with erythema and diffuse excoriations with erythema from the ankle to the midshin area on the left lower extremity. She had a 2 x 2 cm superficial ulcer on the lateral aspect of the ankle.

LABORATORY
Labs on admission revealed sodium was 138. Electrolytes were normal. BUN and creatinine were normal. The creatinine was 1.4, which is probably acceptable for this obese woman. PT was slightly elevated at 15.6, PTT was normal. A subsequent chemistry panel was essentially normal. CBC revealed a white blood cell count of 6,000, hemoglobin 12, hematocrit 35, with 345,000 platelets and a normal smear.

HOSPITAL COURSE
The patient was seen in consultation by the dermatologist, who confirmed my diagnosis of cellulitis. She was placed on IV Kefzol for 48 hours with marked improvement in her cellulitis. Her skin condition was consistent with lichen simplex chronicus, and she was begun on Topicort cream b.i.d. Her Coumadin was not continued, as she had no venogram or Doppler evidence of deep venous thrombosis in the past. As well, she seems to feel that the Coumadin made her rash worse.

DISCHARGE MEDICATIONS
Glyburide 2.5 mg daily, Keflex 500 mg p.o. q.i.d., Lasix 20 mg daily, Mellaril 50 mg nightly, Topicort cream to affected areas b.i.d., and normal saline and dressing changes for wound care.

NATHAN E. DAY, MD

NED:hpi
d: 6/10/XXXX
t: 6/11/XXXX

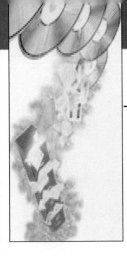

Transcription Practice

Key Words

The following terms appear in the dermatology dictations. Before beginning the medical transcription practice for Chapter 4, look up each term below in a medical or English dictionary and write out a short definition.

After completing all the readings and exercises in Chapter 4, transcribe the dermatology dictations. Use both medical and English dictionaries and your Quick-Reference Word List in the Appendix as resource materials for finding words. Proofread your transcribed documents carefully, listening to the dictation while you read your transcripts.

Transcribe (*not* retype) the same reports again without referring to your previous transcription attempt. Initially, you may need to transcribe some reports more than twice before you can produce an error-free document. Your ultimate goal is to produce an error-free document the first time.

acne vulgaris
aseptic debridement
basal cell carcinoma
Botox injection
conchal bowl block
debridement
dermatitis
epithelization or
    epithelialization
excision of basal cell
    carcinoma
facial spasm

helix
hemifacial spasm
human bite
impetigo
lap pad
onychomycosis
open wound of lower
    extremity
perichondrium
12 o'clock position
ulcer of leg

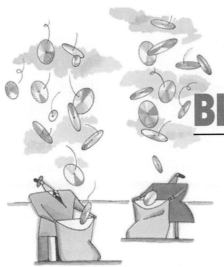

BLOOPERS

Incorrect	*Correct*
Six pricks on the chin.	Cicatrix on the chin.
Kwell lotion was applied gaily during her hospital stay.	Kwell lotion was applied daily during her hospital stay.
Keratosis removed from forearm by defecation.	Keratosis removed from forearm by desiccation.
He has an ulceration on his left lower third leg.	He has an ulceration on the lower third of his left leg.

Otorhinolaryngology

Chapter Outline

Learning Objectives

- Describe the structure and function of the ears, nose, and throat.
- Spell and define common otorhinolaryngology terms.
- Identify types of questions a physician might ask a patient about the ears, nose, and throat during the review of systems.
- Describe common features a physician looks for on examination of the ears, nose, and throat.
- Identify common diseases of the ears, nose, and throat. Describe their typical cause, course, and treatment options.
- Identify and define diagnostic and surgical procedures of the ears, nose, and throat.
- List common otorhinolaryngology laboratory tests and procedures.
- Identify and describe common otorhinolaryngology drugs and their uses.
- Demonstrate knowledge of anatomical, medical, pharmacological, adjectival, and soundalike terms by accurately completing the exercises in this chapter.

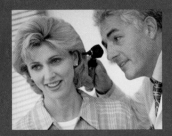
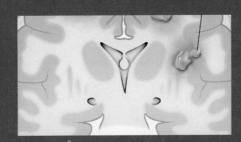
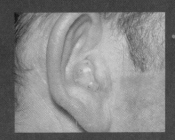

Transcribing Otorhinolaryngology Dictation

The ears, nose, and throat (ENT) are adjacent to one another anatomically, similar in histologic structure, and subject to many of the same diseases. Diseases, injuries, and abnormalities of the ears, nose, and throat are the special field of the otorhinolaryngologist.

Anatomy in Brief

Each ear has three parts (see Figure 5-1):

1. The **outer ear**, consisting of the **pinna** (the cartilaginous appendage on either side of the head, which collects sound waves like a funnel) and the **external auditory meatus** (a tube that conducts sound waves from the pinna to the middle ear). The meatus is lined with skin that secretes **cerumen** (earwax), a mildly antimicrobial substance that traps dust and other particulate foreign material.

2. The **middle ear**, a cavity in the temporal bone separated from the external auditory meatus by the **tympanic membrane**, which vibrates in response to sound waves and imparts the vibration to a series of very small bones (**malleus**, **incus**, and **stapes**), which in turn transmit them to the inner ear.

3. The **inner ear**, consisting of the **cochlea** (an organ shaped like a snail shell, in which sound vibrations are converted to nerve impulses to be sent through the eighth cranial, or **vestibulocochlear**, **nerve**) and the vestibular system, the organ of balance (containing minute position sensors in a fluid medium, which send information about head position to the balance center in the brain, also through the eighth cranial nerve).

The middle ear communicates with the pharynx by a minute passage called the **auditory (eustachian)** tube, which serves to equalize air pressure between the middle ear and the atmosphere. It also communicates with epithelium-lined air cells within the skull, called **mastoid air cells.**

The external nose (see Figure 5-2) is supported by a framework of cartilage and covered by skin. The **nostrils** (anterior **nares**) open into paired passages lined with **mucous membrane**, which is rich in serous and mucous glands and blood vessels. The lining membrane of these passages is closely attached to convoluted ridges of bone

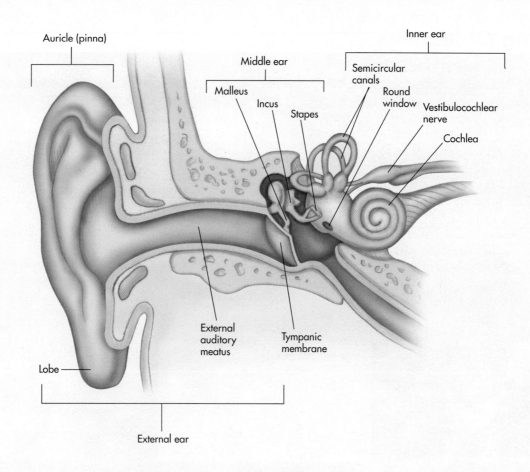

Figure 5-1
The Ear

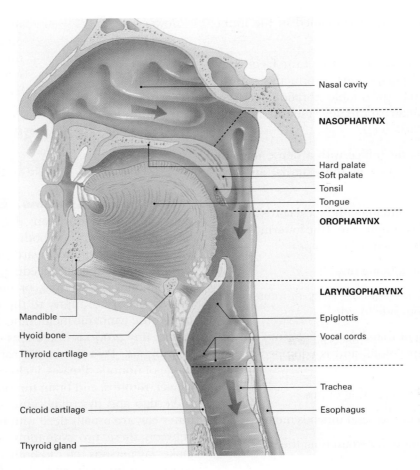

Figure 5-2
Nasopharynx, Oropharynx, and Laryngopharynx

called **turbinates** (three on each side), which increase the surface area of membrane that is exposed to inspired air. Adjacent to the nasal passages, and communicating with them by narrow orifices, are the **paranasal sinuses**. These are cavities within the bones of the skull, somewhat variable in size and shape, and lined with mucosa like that of the nose. The nasal passages end at the **choanae**, or posterior nares, where they enter the **nasopharynx**, the uppermost part of the pharyngeal cavity. The nasal passages warm and moisturize inspired air, and particulate matter in the air is trapped in the mucus film lining them.

The throat, or **pharynx**, is a cavity lined with mucous membrane that conducts air from the nose and mouth into the trachea, and food and drink from the mouth into the esophagus. It consists of three portions: the **nasopharynx,** on a level with the nasal passages and communicating with them; the oropharynx, on a level with the mouth and communicating with it; and the **hypopharynx** or **laryngopharynx,** which lies below the **oropharynx** and gives entry to the esophagus and the larynx.

The **tonsils** and **adenoids** are masses of lymphoid tissue surrounding the zone between the mouth and the oropharynx. At the boundary between the oropharynx and the hypopharynx lies the **epiglottis**, a flexible valve that closes the respiratory passage during swallowing of food or drink.

The lining of the pharynx secretes **mucus**, which keeps the surface moist, traps inhaled particles, and supplements the saliva as a lubricant for food. **Lymph glands** in the front and back of the neck receive lymphatic drainage from the throat and adjacent structures.

Terminology Review

aneurysm   Abnormal dilatation of a blood vessel.

bulla (pl. **bullae**)   A blister or bleb.

decibel   A measure of the loudness of sound; one tenth of a *bel* (named for Alexander Graham Bell).

endolymph   The fluid medium contained in the inner ear.

Hz   Abbreviation for *hertz*, a measure of the frequency of a vibration, particularly one producing sound; equivalent to one cycle (or double vibration) per second. The normal human ear can detect sounds ranging in pitch from 20 to 20,000 Hz.

impaction   Plugging of an orifice with a dense mass of some material, as cerumen in the external auditory meatus.

larynx   The voice box, containing the vocal cords and situated between the laryngopharynx (the lowermost part of the throat) and the trachea (windpipe).

malaise   A vague sense of being unwell.

nystagmus   Rhythmic, involuntary, jerky movements of both eyes, usually from side to side.

otoscope   An instrument that directs a light into the ear through a conical speculum, and is equipped with a magnifying lens.

purulent   Containing or consisting of pus.

rhinitis   Inflammation of the nasal mucous membrane.

rhinoscope   An instrument for examining the interior of the nose.

serous gland   One producing a thin, watery secretion, not containing mucus.

speculum   An instrument for inspecting a body cavity or orifice, often equipped with a light source, a magnifying lens, or both.

stenosis   Abnormal narrowing of a passage or vessel.

TMJ   Temporomandibular joint.

topical   Referring to a medicine applied directly to skin or mucous membrane.

Valsalva maneuver   Attempt at forced expiration, with the lips and nostrils closed; this drives air into the auditory tubes unless they are obstructed.

vasoconstrictor   A medicine that constricts blood vessels, either when applied topically or through systemic action.

Lay and Medical Terms

dizziness	vertigo
eardrum	tympanic membrane
earwax	cerumen
hammer, anvil, stirrup	malleus, incus, stapes
lower jaw	mandible
nosebleed	epistaxis
ringing in the ears	tinnitus
upper jaw	maxilla

Medical Readings

History and Physical Examination

Review of Systems. Ears. The physician inquires about the duration, degree, and pitch range of hearing loss in one or both ears; ringing, popping, or other abnormal sounds heard by the patient; pain, pressure, itching, swelling, bleeding, or discharge; history of occupational, avocational, or military exposure to loud noises; history of injury to the ear, particularly perforation of the tympanic membrane; recent air travel or scuba diving; any previous operations on the ear; and use of a hearing aid. Pain felt in the ear can result from a wide range of nonotic diseases, including pharyngitis, laryngeal cancer, mumps, and brain tumor.

Vertigo and dysequilibrium, suggesting disease of the inner ear, are usually dealt with here also. The distinction between these two symptoms is sometimes difficult to make; lay persons refer to both as "dizziness." Vertigo is a constant or intermittent feeling that one is spinning ("like I just got off a merry-go-round"). In contrast, dysequilibrium means difficulty maintaining one's balance when standing or walking.

Nose. The nasal history includes mention of any acute or chronic pain, swelling, obstruction, or discharge affecting the nose; sneezing, nosebleeds, or frequent colds; seasonal or occasional allergies; sinus infections; disturbance of the sense of smell; history of fracture or other injuries; submucous resection for deviated septum, removal of polyps, cautery for nosebleeds, or other surgical procedure; and regular or long-term use of decongestants or antihistamines for nasal symptoms, particularly inhalers, drops, or sprays.

Throat. The throat includes not only the pharynx, the common channel shared by the respiratory and digestive tracts, but also the larynx. Important historical points include sore throat (the most common presenting symptom in many outpatient practices), postnasal drip, choking, and difficulty swallowing; atypical throat pain, which may be due to foreign body, abscess, tumor, or neurologic disease; hoarseness or other change in the voice; and history of tonsillectomy or other throat operation. Pain, swelling, or mass in the neck is included here for convenience.

Physical Examination. The amount, distribution, texture, and color of scalp hair are observed, as well as the pattern of any hair loss. The scalp is inspected for scaling, dermatitis, signs of acute or past trauma, and other lesions. Any tremors or involuntary movements of the head are noted.

Facial configuration and symmetry can be distorted by various congenital syndromes. Paralysis due to peripheral neuropathy (Bell palsy) or stroke can also cause facial asymmetry as a result of impaired mobility of one part of the face. The examiner may instruct the patient to perform various movements, such as wrinkling the forehead, showing the teeth, and pursing the lips to whistle, in order to test for facial muscle weakness or paralysis.

Pain in the lower jaw or difficulty in chewing or speaking will prompt an assessment of the mandible, the temporomandibular joints, and the muscles of mastication for mobility, spasm, swelling, crepitus, or tenderness.

Any swellings or masses are palpated for size, shape, consistency, mobility, pulsatility, and tenderness. Additionally, the entire neck is felt for enlarged lymph nodes, which may appear in any of several locations. Each anatomic group of nodes "drains" (receives lymphatic channels from) a specific region of the head, face, neck, or thorax.

The thyroid gland is felt and its size and consistency assessed. For this examination the physician may stand behind and ask the patient to swallow in order to move the gland up and down under the palpating fingers. The larynx and the uppermost part of the trachea are also felt and any lesions or lateral deviation noted.

Common Diseases

Otitis Externa (Swimmer's Ear). Infection of the external auditory meatus.

Causes: Infection with bacteria (*Proteus, Pseudomonas*) and sometimes fungi (*Aspergillus*). Predisposing causes include water exposure (swimming, showering), excessive cerumen, mechanical trauma (probing with paper clip), foreign body (cotton, pencil eraser), diabetes mellitus, and immune compromise.

History: Earache, itching in the external auditory meatus, purulent discharge. Hearing loss if the meatus is occluded by swelling or exudate.

Physical Examination: Redness and swelling of the meatus, sometimes with complete occlusion; purulent exudate, perhaps with excessive cerumen or foreign body visible. Tenderness on manipulation of the pinna.

Course: Generally benign, but in diabetes mellitus and AIDS an external ear infection may resist conservative treatment and become chronic, perhaps invading the skull or brain, with resulting neurologic damage.

Treatment: After gentle cleansing and removal of any foreign material, cerumen, or exudate, topical antibiotics (ear drops), often with hydrocortisone to combat local inflammation, are instilled several times a day. Sometimes a gauze wick is inserted to facilitate penetration of ear drops when edema of the meatus is extreme. In invasive infections, intravenous antibiotics and even surgery may be required.

Otitis Media. Bacterial infection of the middle ear and adjoining mastoid air cells.

Cause: Infection by *Streptococcus pneumoniae, Haemophilus influenzae, Streptococcus pyogenes*, and other bacteria. Otitis media commonly occurs as a sequel to a viral upper respiratory infection. Obstruction of the auditory tube by edema leads to pressure changes within the middle ear and secretion of mucus and serous fluid, which becomes infected by bacteria already present in the tissues. Otitis media is often bilateral. It is commoner in infants and small children than in adolescents and adults, accounting for one third of all pediatric office visits.

History: Pain and pressure in one or both ears, hearing loss, sometimes fever.

Physical Examination: Redness of the tympanic membrane, sometimes with formation of bullae. Immobility of the tympanic membrane, reflecting malfunction of the auditory tube. Occasionally bulging of the membrane. If spontaneous rupture occurs, blood or purulent exudate in the external auditory meatus.

Course: It is estimated that 20-80% of all cases of otitis media will resolve spontaneously without treatment. When there is fever or severe pain, antibiotic treatment is usually prescribed because of the risk of serious complications in a few patients. Neglect of the infection, its failure to respond to standard initial treatment, or a series of recurrent infections can lead to chronic otitis media, typically due to different organisms (*Proteus, Pseudomonas*, staphylococci) than acute infection.

Complications of chronic otitis media include spontaneous rupture of the tympanic membrane, with chronic purulent drainage; destruction of the bones within the middle ear that transmit sound; invasion of mastoid air cells (**mastoiditis**), skull bones, and even the central nervous system by infection; formation of **cholesteatoma**, a benign but locally invasive growth of the tympanic membrane caused by prolonged negative pressure (partial vacuum) in the middle ear. Chronic otitis media can lead to permanent conductive hearing loss and, in small children, speech defects because of inability to hear speech sounds properly.

Treatment: In the absence of fever and severe pain in patients over age two, analgesics and observation are preferred to antibiotic treatment. For selected patients, systemic antibiotics (amoxicillin with or without clavulanic acid, erythromycin, trimethoprim-sulfamethoxazole), decongestants, analgesics. If tympanic membrane rupture threatens, **myringotomy** (surgical puncture of the membrane, with release of pus). In children with recurrent or refractory infections, polyethylene tubes may be placed in the tympanic membrane(s) to aerate the middle ear(s) and allow for escape of purulent secretion. Cholesteatoma and mastoiditis are treated surgically. Chronic perforation of the tympanic membrane requires surgical repair (**tympanoplasty**).

Vertigo. A sense of motion (spinning, falling, floor tipping) when no such motion is occurring.

Causes: Labyrinthitis, often following respiratory infection and hence often called viral. Degenerative changes in the balance-sensing mechanism of the inner ear. Increased pressure within the endolymphatic sac (Ménière disease). Vascular or neoplastic disease of the inner ear or temporal lobe of the cerebral cortex. Diplopia, head injury, multiple sclerosis, drugs, alcohol.

History: A feeling of spinning or falling to one side, or a sense that the floor is tipping or rotating, coming on suddenly, often with head movement, and lasting seconds, minutes, hours, days, weeks, or months. When severe, vertigo may make it impossible for the patient to stand or walk and may be accompanied by nausea and vomiting. There may also be tinnitus and hearing loss.

Physical Examination: May be essentially normal. The **Romberg test** (patient standing with eyes closed) may indicate inability to maintain equilibrium. Eyes may show nystagmus.

Treatment: May be limited to treatment of the underlying cause. In **Ménière disease**, salt restriction and diuretic therapy may help by reducing the pressure of the endolymph. Medicines such as meclizine and dimenhydrinate may diminish or abolish vertigo temporarily. In some cases of positional vertigo, head manipulation can reduce symptoms by promoting reorientation of the balance mechanism.

Hearing Loss. Reduction, often permanent, in the acuity of hearing in one or both ears. Hearing loss is divided into three types depending on the location of the abnormality.

Conductive hearing loss: Disease or abnormality in the outer or middle ear: cerumen impaction, otitis media with effusion, hardening of the tympanic membrane (otosclerosis), injury or disease of the ossicles.

Sensory hearing loss: Disease of the cochlea: acoustic trauma, ototoxicity (aminoglycosides, loop diuretics, cisplatin), aging.

Neural: Eighth nerve lesions; cerebrovascular disease. Hearing loss is assessed by audiometry and the Weber and Rinne tests.

Treatment is that of the underlying cause, if possible. Generally no treatment is effective.

Coryza (Common Cold). A common, mild rhinitis caused by viruses.

Causes: Any of numerous viruses spread readily from person to person. Risk of catching colds may be heightened by exposure to severe winter weather (especially whole-body chilling), drying of indoor air by heating systems, or crowding indoors during the winter.

History: Headache, nasal stuffiness, runny nose, sneezing, throat irritation, malaise. Occasionally fever, chills, anorexia, and muscle aching.

Physical Examination: Erythema and edema of nasal mucosa. Temperature may be slightly elevated.

Course: Generally self-limited. Sometimes complicated by sinusitis, otitis media, pharyngitis, bronchitis.

Treatment: Purely symptomatic. Oral decongestants are moderately effective. Aspirin, acetaminophen, or ibuprofen relieve discomfort. Rest, fluids. Antihistamines do not decongest, antibiotics do not kill cold viruses, and nasal decongestant sprays cause rebound congestion worse than the disease.

Allergic Rhinitis (Hay Fever). A recurrent, often seasonal inflammation of the nasal mucous membrane caused by allergy to inhaled materials.

Causes: Sensitivity to pollens, grasses, mold spores, dust mites, animal dander, second-hand cigarette smoke, and other inhalant allergens.

History: Recurrent or constant nasal congestion and irritation, with copious watery discharge, itching, sneezing (often many times in a row), and itching and watering of the eyes. Symptoms may occur consistently at certain seasons (spring, fall) or, especially when due to house dust, may be perennial.

Physical Examination: Watery, red eyes. Pale or bluish, markedly swollen nasal mucosa. **Polyps** (massive overgrowths of chronically inflamed mucosa) may be present.

Diagnostic Tests: Nasal smear shows eosinophils. Skin testing or RAST (radioallergosorbent testing) can identify causative allergens.

Treatment: Decongestants, antihistamines, nasal corticosteroid spray. Avoidance of known allergens when possible. Use of air filters as appropriate. Continued administration of desensitizing antigens often markedly reduces symptoms.

Epistaxis (Nosebleed). Bleeding from the nose may be due to nasal trauma, irritation of the mucosa by dust or dry air, upper respiratory infection or allergic rhinitis, or coagulation defect.

Treatment of acute nosebleed is by application of direct pressure and, if necessary, topical vasoconstrictor. If bleeding persists or recurs, cautery with silver nitrate or anterior nasal packing may be necessary.

Rarely, bleeding comes from the posterior nares (usually in middle-aged or elderly patients with hypertension or arteriosclerosis) and requires a posterior nasal pack.

Prevention of further nosebleeds may include use of lubricating applications to the mucosa, humidification of air, and avoidance of dusts and other irritants.

Sinusitis. Infection of one or more paranasal sinuses.

Cause: Usually occurs as a complication of viral or allergic rhinitis. Swelling of the nasal mucosa leads to blockage of the sinus openings, with accumulation of purulent secretion within the sinuses affected. Attacks may occur repeatedly in some persons, and sinusitis may become chronic.

History: Pressure or pain in one or more sinus cavities, often aggravated by bending forward. Pain may be manifested as a severe headache or may radiate into the teeth. Purulent nasal or postnasal discharge may be present. Occasionally fever, chills, and malaise.

Physical Examination: Edema and erythema of nasal mucosa. Purulent discharge in nasal passages or oropharynx (postnasal drip).

Diagnostic Tests: In chronic sinusitis, x-ray or other diagnostic imaging shows thickening of sinus membranes and often presence of fluid within cavities.

Treatment: Decongestant, analgesic. A short course of nasal decongestant spray may help to open and drain sinuses. Control of allergic component if present. When symptoms (severe, persistent pain) or clinical picture (fever, bloody discharge) suggests bacterial infection, an oral antibiotic (amoxicillin, trimethoprim-sulfamethoxazole) is prescribed. Chronic sinusitis may respond to prolonged antibiotic therapy (ciprofloxacin). Surgical procedures can be used to correct anatomic lesions predisposing to sinusitis, or to improve drainage of a chronically infected sinus.

Acute Pharyngitis (Sore Throat). Acute inflammation of the throat due to infection.

Cause: Usually viruses, including the Epstein-Barr virus, which causes infectious mononucleosis. Occasionally bacteria such as *Streptococcus pneumoniae* and Group A beta-hemolytic *Streptococcus pyogenes* ("strep throat"), or fungi such as *Candida*. Infection with cold viruses may predispose to bacterial infection. Sore throat is more prevalent in cold weather.

History: Pain, irritation, or a sense of fullness or swelling in the throat, accentuated by swallowing and often radiating to the ears. Fever, painful glandular swelling in the neck.

Physical Examination: May be essentially normal. Fever is often present. Edema and erythema of the oropharynx, often involving the tonsils, soft palate, and uvula, occur in most bacterial and many viral throat infections. Severe infections, including streptococcal pharyngitis (strep throat) and infectious mononucleosis, cause formation of white or gray exudate (consisting of dead tissue, white blood cells, and bacteria) on pharyngeal walls and especially on the tonsils.

A firmly adherent exudate is characteristic of *Candida* infection (**thrush**). The presence of vesicles or ulcers suggests viral infection (herpes simplex virus, **coxsackievirus**). Severe pain and swelling may cause a hollow or "hot potato" voice, and may make swallowing virtually impossible, so that the patient drools to avoid swallowing saliva, and becomes dehydrated from lack of fluid intake. Extreme swelling may compromise the airway. Cervical lymph glands may be swollen and tender. Some strains of beta-hemolytic streptococci cause a widespread red rash (**scarlet fever**, **scarlatina**).

Diagnostic Tests: Throat culture or **strep screen** may identify the causative organism. Blood studies (white blood cell count and differential, ASO titer, heterophile antibodies) help to diagnose strep throat and infectious mononucleosis. Smears or scrapings of exudate can confirm presence of *Candida*.

Course: Viral sore throat runs its course within a week or two. Occasionally it becomes complicated by streptococcal infection, which may lead to acute rheumatic fever. It may also progress to otitis media, acute or chronic tonsillitis, or lower respiratory infection. **Peritonsillar abscess** (quinsy) is a severe bacterial infection developing above and behind one tonsil and causing extreme pain and swelling, with deviation of the uvula away from the affected side.

Treatment: Acute viral pharyngitis requires no treatment except analgesics, gargles, soothing lozenges, and perhaps a soft diet. If streptococcal infection is diagnosed, a 10-day course of an antibiotic known to be able to eradicate streptococci (such as penicillin V, erythromycin, or cephalexin) is mandatory. Candidal oropharyngitis (thrush) is treated with topical antifungal medicine. The treatment of peritonsillar abscess is surgical drainage.

Diagnostic and Surgical Procedures

audiography A precise measurement of the faintest loudness (in decibels) that the subject can hear, each ear tested separately at each of several pitches (for example, 250, 500, 1000, 2000, 3000, 4000, 6000, and 8000 Hz); this can be performed by a trained technician with carefully calibrated testing equipment, or by automated machinery activated by the subject.

biopsy The removal, for pathological examination, of masses or lesions suspected of being malignant.

insertion of collar button (ventilation) tubes Surgical placement of tiny tubes in the eardrum to prevent chronic ear infections.

inspection of the throat With a focused light, often with the aid of a tongue depressor (tongue blade) to press the tongue out of the field of vision.

otoscopy Inspection of the external auditory meatus and tympanic membrane with an otoscope; mobility of the tympanic membrane can be assessed when the

Spotlight on

Who Nose?

by Susan M. Turley

If Bo knows football and baseball, then it might be correct to say that I now know noses. Recently I had the chance to see surgery from the other side—the patient's side.

After many years of extreme nasal stuffiness, I gathered my courage and decided to have a surgical correction or, as my mother-in-law so aptly put it, "go under the knife."

I mentioned my decision to my internist who specializes in natural medicine. With a shocked expression on his face, he described the surgery as "having a bulldozer up your nose." My feelings of courage began to evaporate. He insisted I cancel my upcoming appointment with the plastic surgeon. I solemnly considered that perhaps he was right, until, moving on to another of my medical problems, I asked him what he advised his patients to do for PMS. "Have a hysterectomy," he said with a perfectly straight face. "What?" I yelled. "You don't want me to have a simple nasal surgery but you recommend a hysterectomy for PMS!" He wasn't smiling. Obviously he had a hidden agenda. I kept my appointment with the plastic surgeon.

The plastic surgeon confirmed that my turbinates were grossly hypertrophied and were the cause of my inability to breathe. After we agreed that a turbinectomy would be beneficial, he then asked delicately if I had considered having any plastic surgery at the same time. Ever considered plastic surgery? Just since the day I was born! He gently asked what would I like to have done. "Hey," I said, "I have a list!"

We started with number one on the list: a nose job. It was painful hearing him brutally describe the unacceptable aspects of my nose—bulbous tip, uneven width, drooping tip, drooping underside, excessive length—even though I had seen all these problems myself in the mirror.

Then there were finances to consider. My insurance would pay for the functional nasal surgery (turbinectomy and cartilage graft) but not for any cosmetic surgery. I would be responsible for the surgeon's fee, hospital's fee, and anesthesiologist's fee that pertained to the cosmetic part of the surgery. I was surprised to learn that the total cost of the cosmetic surgery could vary greatly (as much as $3000), depending on the hospital I selected. Naturally I chose the cheapest hospital where, my surgeon assured me, the care was excellent.

The surgeon's secretary informed me that his fee needed to be paid IN FULL 10 days IN ADVANCE. That was a shock. I guess too many cosmetic surgery patients had stiffed him and walked away from their bills with their beautiful new noses in the air. At least that was what I liked to think. The alternative—that the bills were not paid because the patients were undergoing psychiatric treatment for a permanently botched-up nose—was too painful to contemplate.

On the morning of surgery, I found myself first paying the hospital's bill in full with my VISA card. I then undressed and was put in a recovery room bed where I could either watch TV or read. I chose to read; the nurse handed me a *Newsweek* in which the confidence-inspiring cover story was about doctors with AIDS. The anesthesiologist came in and started an IV in my right hand. He left before I could remind him that I was supposed to pay him in full before my surgery. I had no doubts, though, that he would return, and he did. With my right hand, I then laboriously wrote out a check to him for $700. Question: Did the first patient to undergo a rhinoplasty coin the phrase "paying through the nose"?

subject swallows or performs the Valsalva maneuver (or when, in children, the examiner blows a puff of air into the ear).

palpation of cervical lymph glands and of masses, swellings, or other structures within the throat.

pneumotympanometry Assessment of the mobility of the tympanic membrane by applying pressure to its outer surface with a device fitting tightly in the external meatus.

posterior rhinoscopy Inspection of posterior nares with angled mirror placed in the oropharynx.

rhinoplasty Surgical correction of nasal deformities for functional or cosmetic purposes ("nose job").

Rinne test The sound of a vibrating tuning fork positioned so that the tines are near the pinna (**air conduction**) should be heard by the subject even after the sound sensed when the shank of the tuning fork is placed on the mastoid process behind the ear (**bone conduction**) can no longer be heard. When bone conduction is heard longer than air conduction in an ear with reduced hearing, the hearing loss is due to obstruction of the meatus or disease of the middle ear.

I reminded the anesthesiologist that the last time I had had general anesthesia (about eight years ago), I had been given Pentothal and asked to count backwards from 100. When I stopped counting I assumed I was asleep and so did the anesthesiologist who proceeded to intubate me. Not being fully asleep, however, I had to violently resist the urge to throw up. After surgery, two anesthesiologists came to my room and sheepishly asked me if I thought everything had gone well with my surgery. I told them what had happened and they apologized profusely, all the while throwing knowing looks at each other. This experience, I explained to the anesthesiologist, I had no wish to repeat. He assured me that that type of unfortunate accident was never supposed to happen. He hastily told me that he would be sure to give me an amnestic agent before the induction agent so that I would not remember anything.

After the anesthesiologist left, the plastic surgeon arrived to mark my nose and cheeks with a skin marking pen. I gave my checkbook (thank goodness, no one else needed to be paid) and glasses to the nurse and was wheeled into the operating room.

The temperature in surgery was no warmer than 50 degrees, it seemed. Even the nurses were complaining of the cold. They gave me lots of warm blankets, though, and I was comfortable. Someone said, "How are you doing?" "Who, me?" I answered. Without my glasses I couldn't tell if the staff was talking to me or just chitchatting among themselves. "Me? I feel fine." That was all she wrote, as they say. I never felt drowsy; I never even knew when I fell asleep. That's what I call a smooth induction.

The next thing I knew I was in the recovery room. Disembodied voices kept calling my name and saying the surgery went fine. A nurse asked me how much pain I was having, and I said my nose felt like when I slammed my hand in the car door. She promptly provided a shot of Demerol and Compazine. (I had dry heaves for what seemed like hours.) I was very chilly, and the nurses wrapped warm blankets around me, even putting them on my head so that I could pretend I was hibernating in a warm cave.

When my husband and son were allowed into the recovery room to see me, they maintained a respectful distance, not quite sure how to react to my extensively bruised face. From my eyebrows down to my cheekbones, the skin was pitch black, as if some prankster had poured indelible black ink all over my face. Later at home, my husband regained his sense of humor and cheerfully told well-wishers on the phone that I looked as if I had gone several rounds with Mike Tyson. Actually I thought I looked WORSE than that. But within five days, the bruising was barely noticeable.

The week following surgery had its own set of annoying problems. My glasses did not sit right over the nasal splint and, with my eyelids still swollen, it was nearly impossible to enjoy the new Tom Clancy book I had purchased especially for the occasion. My nose was filled with packing so that I mouth-breathed, snored, and coughed without getting much sleep for nearly a week. One small blessing was that some nasal packing now used is absorbable and does not need to be painfully pulled out of the nose.

As the swelling went down and the nasal splint came off, I began breathing more fully than I had in years, and I really liked my new nose. Would I do it again? Sure. By the way, where is that list?

Source: *Perspectives on the Medical Transcription Profession*

tonsillectomy and adenoidectomy (T&A) Surgical removal of the palatine tonsils and adenoids in the throat due to recurrent episodes of infection and chronic hypertrophy.

tympanocentesis Puncture of the tympanic membrane and withdrawal of fluid from the middle ear for examination, including culture.

Weber test A vibrating tuning fork placed against a bony surface of the head at the midline sends vibrations through the bones of the skull. These should be heard equally in the two ears. If there is hearing loss due to blockage of the external auditory meatus or to injury or disease of the middle ear, the tone of the fork will be heard louder in the affected ear. In hearing loss due to damage to the inner ear or acoustic nerve, however, the tone will be heard louder in the more normal ear.

x-ray To identify foreign bodies, masses, or abnormalities of the airway due to injury or disease.

Laboratory Procedures

ASO titer A test to detect and measure antistreptolysin O in serum. This antibody is present during and shortly after streptococcal infections. The value is measured in Todd units.

nasal smear Examination of a stained smear of scrapings from the nasal mucosa for evidence of infection (neutrophilic leukocytes) or allergy (eosinophilic leukocytes).

strep screen Faster than culture, but detecting only beta-hemolytic streptococci. "Strep" is an acceptable brief form for streptococcus.

throat culture To identify bacterial pathogens.

Pharmacology

Decongestants act as vasoconstrictors to reduce blood flow to edematous tissues in the nose, sinuses, and pharynx. They produce vasoconstriction by stimulating alpha receptors in the smooth muscle around the blood vessels. Decongestants decrease the swelling of mucous membranes, alleviate nasal stuffiness, allow secretions to drain, and help to unclog the eustachian tubes. Decongestants are commonly prescribed for colds and allergies. They can be administered topically as nose drops or nasal sprays, or can be taken orally. Decongestants are often combined with antihistamines in cold remedies.

> desoxyephedrine (Vicks Inhaler)
> oxymetazoline (Afrin, Dristan, Duration, Sinex)

> phenylephrine (Neo-Synephrine, Nostril)
> pseudoephedrine (Drixoral, Sudafed)
> tetrahydrozoline
> xylometazoline (Otrivin)

Antihistamines exert their therapeutic effect by blocking **histamine H_1 receptors** in the nose and throat. Histamine is released by the antibody-antigen complex that occurs during allergic reactions. Histamine causes vasodilation, which causes blood vessels and tissues to become engorged, swollen, and red. Histamine also irritates these tissues directly, causing pain and itching. Antihistamines block the action of histamine at the H_1 receptors. Antihistamines dry up secretions, shrink edematous mucous membranes, and decrease itching and redness. A significant side effect of early antihistamines was drowsiness; however, newer antihistamines have a different chemical structure that does not produce drowsiness.

> azatadine (Optimine)
> brompheniramine (Dimetane)
> cetirizine (Zyrtec)
> chlorpheniramine (Chlor-Trimeton)
> clemastine (Tavist)
> dexchlorpheniramine (Polaramine)
> diphenhydramine (Benadryl)
> fexofenadine (Allegra)
> loratadine (Claritin)
> phenindamine (Nolahist)
> promethazine (Phenergan)

Mast cell inhibitors act to stabilize the membrane of mast cells and prevent them from releasing histamine. This prevents edema of the nasal passages in patients with allergic rhinitis. Example is cromolyn (Nasalcrom).

Corticosteroids act by inhibiting the body's inflammatory response by decreasing vasodilation and edema of the mucous membranes. Corticosteroids have no antihistamine effect. Corticosteroids have no effect on the common cold. They are administered intranasally to treat allergic and nonallergic rhinitis. Corticosteroids for the nose include:

> beclomethasone (Beconase, Vancenase)
> budesonide (Rhinocort, Rhinocort Aqua)
> flunisolide (Nasalide)
> fluticasone (Flonase)
> mometasone (Nasonex)
> triamcinolone (Nasacort, Tri-Nasal)

Corticosteroids can be applied topically as a paste to treat mouth ulcers and inflammation. Example is triamcinolone (Kenalog in Orabase).

Antibiotics are not effective in treating the common cold which is caused by a virus; however, they are prescribed for infections caused by bacteria, particularly streptococci. Antibiotic solutions may be prescribed for topical application in the ears to treat external otitis media and other infections.

> chloramphenicol (Chloromycetin Otic)

Corticosteroids and antibiotics are often combined in a single solution for topical application in the ear.

Antitussive drugs decrease coughing by suppressing the cough center in the brain or anesthetizing the stretch receptors in the respiratory tract. Their main purpose is to stop nonproductive dry coughs. They are not prescribed for a productive cough that generates sputum because it is important for the patient to cough up this sputum. Some antitussives are narcotics, such as codeine and hydrocodone; these are prescription schedule drugs. Over-the-counter antitussives contain the non-narcotic dextromethorphan or diphenhydramine.

> benzonatate (Tessalon Perles)
> codeine
> dextromethorphan (Benylin DM, Pertussin ES,
>   Robitussin, Sucrets, Vicks Formula 44D)
> diphenhydramine (Benylin Cough)
> hydrocodone (Hycodan)

Expectorants reduce the viscosity or thickness of sputum so that patients can more easily cough it up. Expectorants are prescribed only for productive coughs.

> guaifenesin (Humibid L.A., Robitussin)
> terpin hydrate

Antifungal and antiyeast drugs. Yeasts, which are closely related to fungi, grow easily in the warm, dark environment of the mouth, particularly in immunocompromised patients. *Candida albicans* yeast infections are alternatively known as oral candidiasis, moniliasis, or thrush. Antifungal drugs are applied topically as a solution (the patient is told to "swish and swallow") or supplied as a troche (to suck on as a lozenge). Nizoral is also available as an oral tablet that acts systemically.

> clotrimazole (Mycelex)
> nystatin (Mycostatin, Nilstat)

Combination ENT drugs. A number of trade name drugs contain various combinations of decongestants, antihistamines, antitussives, expectorants, and the pain relievers acetaminophen or ibuprofen.

TRANSCRIPTION TIPS

1. Don't confuse the soundalike prefixes *oro-* (mouth) and *auri-* (ear).

2. Both the Latin *auri-* (aural) and the Greek *oto-* (otic) mean *ear*.

3. *AD, AS, AU* (right ear, left ear, and each ear) are traditional abbreviations that are on the list of error-prone abbreviations list. Although physicians continue to dictate these abbreviations, JCAHO directs that they be expanded in medical transcripts to avoid confusion with similar abbreviations. Thus, even if dictators use these abbreviations, medical transcriptionists should translate them and place the abbreviation in parentheses following the translation.

4. Both the Latin *myringo-* and the Greek *tympano-* refer to the *eardrum* or *tympanic membrane*.

5. Do not confuse the *malleus* (a bone of the middle ear) and the *malleolus* (a bone in the ankle).

6. The term *auricle* refers to the protruding flap of the external ear, also known as the *pinna*. However, *auricle* also refers to an ear-shaped appendage on each cardiac atrium. The use of *auricle* as a synonym for *atrium*, though long out of date, still appears in some reference books.

7. When the term *mental* is used in ENT dictation, it refers to the *mentum*, or *chin*, *not* to thought processes.

8. The term *alveolar* in ENT dictation refers to a bony ridge in the oral cavity, *not* to the alveoli of the lungs.

9. Do not mistake *serous* (as in otitis media) for *serious*, especially in dictation by ESL physicians.

10. *Nares* is the plural form of the medical term for nostrils. *Naris* is the singular, not *nare*, as sometimes dictated.

11. Do not confuse *Contac* (medication) with *contact*, the English word.

11. Do not confuse *Dimetane* and *Dimetapp*.

12. Note unusual internal capitalization of the following: NasalCrom, NyQuil, PediaCare

13. Do not confuse *pseudo-* (pseudoephedrine) with *suda-* (Sudafed).

14. Note the spelling of Tessalon Perles (*not* pearls).

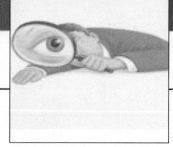

Proofreading Skills

Instructions: In the paragraphs below, circle the errors. Identify misspelled and missing medical and English words and write the correct words in the numbered spaces opposite the text.

1. This 17 year old female was seen in consultation
2. with her mother regarding problems referable to
3. her nose, The patient has had progressive problems
4. of congestoin and sniffing with difficulty moving air
5. through her nose and sinsation of pressure. She is a
6. "mouth brether" and has a history of allergy to
7. polens and dust. The patient feels these problems
8. are becoming more severe. Her complaints are fairly
9. consistant.
10.
11. EXAMINATION: She presents with edema of her
12. nasal mucosa, incraese in the size of the turbinates,
13. deviation of the nasal septum, and a rather
14. narrowed nasal airweigh.
15.
16. DIAGNOSIS
17. 1. Probable allergic rinitis with hypertrophy of the
18.   turbinates.
19. 2. Deviated nasal septum.
20. 3. Narrow inadequate nasal airway.
21.
22. COMMENTS
23. 1. I have discused with this patient and with her
24.   mother the surgical approach to improving her
25.   nasal airway with septoplasty, possible submucous
26.   resection of deviated portions of the septum, and
27.   possible reduction of the inferior turbenates. At
28.   the same time, I would be performing a
29.   rinoplasty procedure to smooth out the dorsal
30.   nose.
31. 2. Because of the history of allergies to pollens dust
32.   and environmental pollutants it is quite possible
33.   the patient will continue to have some snifing and
34.   consequently the degree of improvement of her
35.   nasal airway with surgery cannot be precisely
36.   determined.

1 <u>17-year-old</u>
2 _____
3 _____
4 _____
5 _____
6 _____
7 _____
8 _____
9 _____
10 _____
11 _____
12 _____
13 _____
14 _____
15 _____
16 _____
17 _____
18 _____
19 _____
20 _____
21 _____
22 _____
23 _____
24 _____
25 _____
26 _____
27 _____
28 _____
29 _____
30 _____
31 _____
32 _____
33 _____
34 _____
35 _____
36 _____

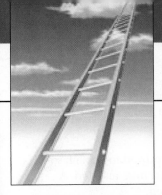

SkillsChallenge

Abbreviations Exercise

Common abbreviations may be transcribed as dictated in the body of a report. Uncommon abbreviations must be spelled out, with the abbreviations appearing in parentheses after the translation. All abbreviations (except for a few laboratory test names such as *VDRL*) must be spelled out in the Diagnosis or Impression section of any report.

Instructions. Define the following ENT (ear, nose, and throat) abbreviations. Then memorize both the abbreviations and the definitions to increase your speed and accuracy in transcribing ENT dictation.

AD _____

AS _____

AU _____

EAC _____

ENT _____

HEENT _____

PE tube _____

PND _____

T&A _____

TM _____

TMJ _____

Medical Terminology Matching Exercise

Complete the following matching exercise to test your knowledge of the word roots, anatomic structures, symptoms, and disease processes encountered in the medical specialty of otorhinolaryngology.

Instructions: Match the definitions in Column A with their terms in Column B.

Column A

1. ___ wax
2. ___ dizziness from sense of motion
3. ___ auricle, or outer ear
4. ___ hearing
5. ___ where sounds are translated to nerve impulses
6. ___ ringing in the ears
7. ___ nosebleed
8. ___ eardrum
9. ___ ear

Column B

A. tinnitus
B. pinna
C. myringo-
D. cochlea
E. cerumen
F. oto-
G. epistaxis
H. vertigo
I. audio-

Abbreviations and Symbols Exercise

1. What is the difference between an abbreviation and an acronym? What is an initialism? Give examples.

_____
_____
_____
_____
_____
_____

2. Why would you *not* translate such abbreviations as *VDRL*, *SGOT*, *tPA*, and *DPT* shot? (Before answering, find out what each abbreviation means.)

_____
_____
_____
_____
_____
_____

3. Abbreviations are rarely appropriate in which parts of a report?

_____
_____
_____
_____

4. Translate the following abbreviations. Under what circumstances would you *not* translate the abbreviations? Under what circumstances would you *always* translate the abbreviations?

ABGs _____
CHF _____
COPD _____
EKG _____
MRI _____
PID _____
q.3 h. _____
t.i.d. _____

5. What are the abbreviations for the following?

four times a day _____
at hour of sleep _____
urinary tract infection _____
millimeters of mercury _____
certified medical transcriptionist _____
doctor of medicine _____

6. Correct abbreviation errors in the following sentences. Translate any abbreviations which you feel are inappropriate.

A 0.5-cm incision was made, but it proved too small, so a 1-in incision was made and the chest tube inserted. A total of 300 mL of fluid was obtained.

_____
_____
_____

Final Diagnosis: CHF with right pleural effusion, 300 mL of fluid removed.

_____
_____

Disposition: Patient placed on digitalis 0.25 mg bid, hold IV D5W until the am.

_____
_____

Dictation Exercises

Prior to transcribing the dictations, complete these activities.

1. **Using Chapter 3, Style Guide**

   a. When do you capitalize a word referring to a person's race?
   b. What is the proper style for compound designations of national origin?
   c. How do you present the singular possessive and plural possessive for units of time? Give an example for each.
   d. When is it acceptable to transcribe contractions?
   e. How do you transcribe fractions used with English units of measure (like pounds and inches)? How do you transcribe fractions used with metric units of measure (like milligrams and centimeters)?
   f. It's common for diagnoses to be dictated in a non-standard order, with noun first and any relevant adjectives following. How would the following sentence be punctuated? Otitis media chronic unresponsive to treatment.
   g. What is the proper way to transcribe hours and minutes? How do you transcribe the time if only the hour is dictated?
   h. When do you capitalize department names?
   i. When in a report is it appropriate to use quotation marks?
   j. Read the section on Brief Forms and Medical Slang in the Style Guide. List the slang term(s) that refer to units of measure and the correct way to transcribe slang.

k. When, according to the Style Guide, do you expand brief forms?

l. The doctor dictates a dosage of medicine, but does not dictate the unit of measure; what do you do?

m. For local anesthesia, Xylocaine and epinephrine are used in a ratio of one to the other. How do you transcribe this ratio?

n. Give examples of the proper use of *followup* and *follow up*?

2. **Problem Solving**

This activity is to help you prepare ahead of time for some of the problems you'll encounter in the dictations. Some of these items may not have a definitive answer but are intended to simply get you thinking about how to handle a variety of situations that are common in transcription. If nothing else, they will help you recognize a problem when you encounter it in the dictations.

a. The doctor dictates something that sounds like "see-pap." From the context of the report, you can guess that it has something to do with sleep apnea. How do you research this?

b. How would you handle dictation in which drug dosages were dictated without the units of measure? Example, Cipro 250 b.i.d.

c. Physicians occasionally interject words into a report that are *not* meant to be transcribed. The most obvious interjection is the dictation of punctuation, which can sometimes be interpreted as a medical or non-medical word. What are some of the other things physicians might say or dictate that are not meant to be transcribed?

3. **Preparatory Research**

Any information requested in these questions not readily available in your textbook (including the Appendix) or required references can easily be found using Internet search engines such as Google or online medical dictionaries.

a. Look up *perfuse* and *profuse*. These two words are frequently confused. Define them.

b. What is *sleep apnea*? What causes it? What are the symptoms? How is it treated?

c. What does *epistaxis* mean?

d. What is the singular and plural anatomical term for *nostril*?

e. Definite *dysphasia* and *dysphagia*. Which is more likely to accompany a sore throat?

f. Review anatomy of the ear. List the three main parts of the ear.

g. Review anatomy of the mouth and throat. What is the little appendage of tissue that hangs in the back of the throat called? What is the roof of the mouth called?

h. Look up *myringotomy*. What is done in this procedure?

i. What is the medical term for *tooth decay*?

j. Define or explain *pulse oximetry*.

k. What is an *exudate*?

l. What is a *differential diagnosis* (as opposed to a *final diagnosis*)?.

m. What is a *Battle sign*?

n. When a patient is in an auto accident, what does the EMS typically do if they suspect that the patient has a neck injury? What if they suspect a back injury?

o. What does *icteric* mean? What prefix would you add to *icteric* to mean *not icteric*?

p. What is the medical word for *earwax*?

q. Look up the correct spelling and definition for a word that sounds like "plej-et."

r. Review the anatomy of the inner ear and surrounding structures. Summarize.

s. What is an *ossicle*? What would be the adjectival form of this word?

t. Define *perforation*.

u. Define *scutum*.

v. Do a Google search for *mastoidectomy*. Check out sites with lots of pictures and ear anatomy. Summarize your findings.

Sample Reports

Sample otorhinolaryngology reports appear on the following pages, illustrating a variety of reports. Fictional names are provided for illustration of proper format, and no resemblance to actual persons is intended. Sample transcripts were prepared according to the *AAMT Book of Style*, where possible.

Chart Note

TWITCHELL, DAVID
Age 65
June 1, XXXX

The patient comes in stating he has some irritation in his right ear. He does wear an ITE hearing aid on that side. He also has what he terms a smell hallucination, in that there is kind of a musty smell in his nose when he inhales and exhales. He has been using some Ocean nasal spray from time to time.

PHYSICAL EXAMINATION
EARS: Right ear: External canal is slightly irritated at the outer third, but the inner two thirds is okay. Tympanic membrane is intact and not inflamed. Left ear is clear. There is no cerumen in either side.
NOSE: Airway is quite adequate. Septum slightly deviated to the right. No evidence of polyps or abnormal discharge.
THROAT: Normal mucous membrane. No evidence of inflammation.
NECK: No adenopathy.

IMPRESSION
Mild right external otitis.

DISPOSITION
Recommended 0.5% hydrocortisone cream in the outer ear and a couple drops of alcohol in the ear at night before he goes to bed to try to keep the canal dry. Nasal irrigation using a normal saline solution. He was asked to return if symptoms progress, and we will go ahead and get a sinus view.

OF:hpi

Letter

January 21, XXXX

Marisa Godwin, MD
2562 County Road
Dayton, OH 45429

Re: Angelica Huston

Dear Dr. Godwin:

This 21-year-old woman stated that she has been having some problems with a "swollen gland on the right side." She saw you about a week and a half ago, and you ruled out the presence of a stone within the saliva gland. She states the swelling "tends to go up and down."

Her general health is described as good, but she does have asthma. She is presently taking Motrin and albuterol inhaler.

Physical exam: Ears: Canals are clear. Tympanic membranes normal. Nose: Airway adequate. No discharge. Throat: Normal mucous membrane. No postnasal drainage. Her right submandibular gland is slightly enlarged but soft and nontender.

Under the operating microscope, I was able to dilate Wharton's duct on the right, and after dilatation the gland resumed its normal size. There was no evidence of a purulent discharge or calculi. Hopefully, this will do the trick.

I explained to her that we can only treat this symptomatically or excise the gland, and I suggested that symptomatic treatment for a while is indicated.

Thank you for the referral. If I can be of any further assistance, please let me know.

Best regards,

Stephen Schutte, MD

SS:hpi

Operation Report

LOOPER, HARRY
#090988

Date of Operation: 7/25/XXXX

PREOPERATIVE DIAGNOSIS
Chronic adenotonsillitis.

POSTOPERATIVE DIAGNOSIS
Chronic adenotonsillitis.

OPERATION
Adenotonsillectomy.

DESCRIPTION OF PROCEDURE
The patient was brought to the operating room and general endotracheal anesthesia induced by Anesthesia without difficulty. The patient was placed in the Rose position, and the McIvor mouth gag was inserted in the routine fashion.

A red rubber catheter was passed transnasally, and the adenoid bed was inspected with a mirror. Using the adenoid curets, the adenoid bed was then curetted. Adenoid packs were placed and attention turned to the right tonsil.

The right tonsil was grasped with a tonsil tenaculum, and using the electrocautery, a mucosal incision was created. Using scissors and a combination of sharp and blunt dissection, the tonsillar capsule was entered. The electrocautery was then used to free the mucosal and fibrotic attachments of the right tonsil. The right tonsil was then snared without difficulty, and tonsil packs were placed. An identical procedure was carried out on the left side. The tonsillar beds were then dried up using the suction cautery. The adenoid bed was then inspected, and the suction cautery was used on the adenoid bed as well until cessation of any further bleeding.

The wounds were inspected. There was no further bleeding. The hypopharynx was carefully suctioned, the mouth gag was removed, and the procedure was deemed complete. The patient was transferred to the recovery room with all vital signs being stable.

MARIAH STEWART, MD

MS:hpi

D: 7/25/XXXX
T: 7/26/XXXX

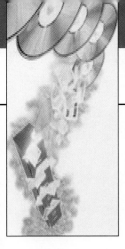

Transcription Practice

Key Terms

The following terms appear in the otorhino-laryngology dictations. Before beginning the medical transcription practice for Chapter 5, look up each term below in a medical or English dictionary and write out a short definition.

CPAP
closed reduction of nasal
   fracture
congestion
epistaxis
facial trauma
fascial graft
incus reposition
lymphadenopathy
mastoidectomy

open reduction of nasal
   fracture
otitis media
periapical abscess
strep pharyngitis
tympanic membrane
   perforation
tympanoplasty
viral syndrome

After completing all the readings and exercises in Chapter 5, transcribe otorhinolaryngology dictation. Proofread your transcribed documents carefully, listening to the dictation while you read your transcripts.

Transcribe (*not* retype) the same reports again without referring to your previous transcription attempt. Initially, you may need to transcribe some reports more than twice before you can produce an error-free document. Your ultimate goal is to produce an error-free document the first time.

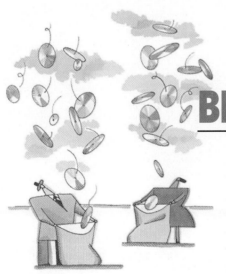

BLOOPERS

Incorrect	Correct
All fangs not inflamed.	Oropharynx not inflamed.
Prognathism prevented proper masturbation.	Prognathism prevented proper mastication.
He has flapping of the left side of his face.	He has flattening of the left side of his face.
The pair of nasal sinuses were involved.	The paranasal sinuses were involved.
Head point sinuses.	Ethmoid sinuses.
Gross hearing appears to be attacked.	Gross hearing appears to be intact.
Finger in the nose testing was done well.	Finger-to-nose testing was done well.

Ophthalmology

Learning Objectives

- Describe the structure and function of the eyes.
- Spell and define common ophthalmology terms.
- Identify types of questions a physician might ask about the eyes during the review of systems.
- Describe common features a physician looks for on examination of the eyes.
- Identify common diseases of the eyes. Describe their typical cause, course, and treatment options.
- Identify and define diagnostic and surgical procedures of the eyes.
- List common ophthalmic laboratory tests and procedures.
- Identify and describe common ophthalmic drugs and their uses.
- Demonstrate knowledge of anatomical, medical, pharmacological, adjectival, and soundalike terms by accurately completing the exercises in this chapter.

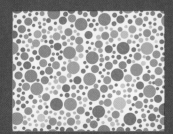
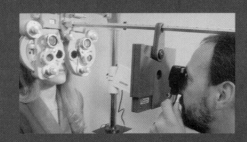
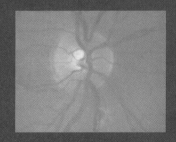

Transcribing Ophthalmology Dictation

Ophthalmology is the branch of medicine that is devoted to the prevention, diagnosis, and treatment of eye diseases.

Anatomy in Brief

Each **eye** (see Figure 6-1) is a roughly spherical structure protected on all sides except the front by the bones and soft tissues of the orbit. Blood vessels and nerves enter at the back of the eye. The **eyeball** (bulb, globe) consists of three concentric layers: the outer **sclera**, a tough coat of connective tissue; the pigment layer or **uveal tract**, a delicate, spongy, vascular membrane of pigmented cells; and the innermost layer, the light-sensitive **retina**.

Anteriorly the sclera is modified to form the transparent **cornea**, through which light rays enter the eye. The uveal tract consists of three parts: the **iris**, which regulates the amount of light entering the eye; the **ciliary body**, which adjusts the focus of the eye; and the **choroid**, which underlies the retina. The retina is a layer of specialized nerve cells that are stimulated by light rays within the visible range. Nerve fibers of these cells unite to form the **optic nerve**.

The **ocular fundus** is the rear wall of the eye as viewed through the pupil with an **ophthalmoscope** (discussed below). The fundus consists of the retina and its arteries and veins and the **disk** (optic nerve head). The disk appears as a round, ivory-colored plaque raised somewhat from the surrounding retina and having a shallow central depression, the **cup**. The disk lies on the nasal side of the fundus, not at its center. The central portion of the retina, concerned with central vision and hence the most sensitive, appears as a faint yellow spot, the **macula lutea**. The retinal vessels (branching arteries, each closely accompanied by a vein) emerge from the center of the disk.

The optic nerve passes back through an aperture in the orbit and crosses the optic nerve of the opposite eye, with which it exchanges some fibers. Behind the crossing, the newly assorted bundles of fibers, called the **optic tracts**, carry visual impulses into the brain.

On their way to the retina, light rays pass through both the cornea and the lens, a transparent structure suspended just behind the cornea. The shape of the lens can be altered by the pull of muscles originating in the ciliary body, and this alteration adjusts the focal distance of the eye. The iris, the colored part of the eye, lies between the cornea and the lens, and controls the amount of light entering the eye by changing the diameter of the **pupil**, the black-appearing round aperture in the middle of the iris.

The part of the eye lying anterior to the lens contains a watery fluid, the **aqueous humor**, which is produced by the ciliary body and drains into small veins in the anterior chamber at the "drainage angle" (the slight angle between cornea and sclera). The space occupied by the aqueous

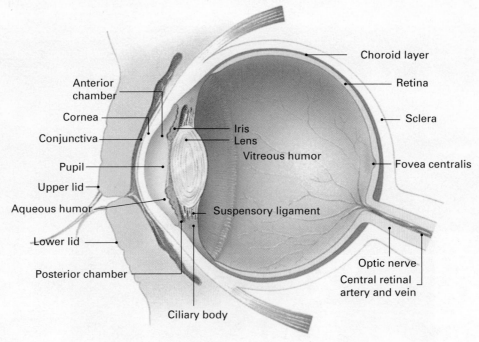

Figure 6-1
Anatomy of the Eye

humor is divided into the **anterior chamber** (between cornea and iris) and the **posterior chamber** (between iris and lens). Behind the lens, the cavity of the eye is filled with a somewhat denser fluid, the **vitreous humor**. Both humors are refractive media, participating in the transmission and refraction of light rays.

The **eyelids** are folds of skin, supplied with oil and sebaceous glands and lash follicles, that shut out light and provide a watertight seal over the eyes. The medial or nasal junction or angle between upper and lower lids is called the **inner canthus**; the lateral or temporal angle is called the **outer canthus**. The visible part of the sclera is covered by a delicate vascular membrane, the **conjunctiva (bulbar conjunctiva)**, which is continuous with the lining of the inner surfaces of the eyelids (**palpebral conjunctiva**). The conjunctiva does not extend over the cornea.

A **lacrimal gland** is situated near the front of each **orbit**, above and lateral to the eyeball. This gland produces **tears**, which moisten, lubricate, and cleanse the eyeball.

Tears flow downward and medially to drain by way of the **lacrimal puncta** (minute openings at the inner canthus) and nasolacrimal ducts into the nose.

Each eye is equipped with six **extraocular muscles**, which produce eye movement and control the direction of gaze (Figure 6-2). Three **cranial nerves** (III, oculomotor; IV, trochlear; and VI, abducens) supply these six muscles. In addition, the oculomotor nerve sends motor branches to the upper eyelid, the ciliary body (focus), and the iris (light/dark adaptation). Coordination of the movements and position of the two eyes and fusion of

their images into a single three-dimensional one takes place in the brain.

Terminology Review

Argyll Robertson pupil A pupil that constricts when the subject focuses on a near object, but not when the eye is stimulated with light; due to central nervous system disease, most often syphilis.

AV (arteriovenous) nicking Tapering of a venule where an arteriole crosses it.

blepharospasm Spasm of the eyelids, usually due to local irritation, photophobia, or both.

chemosis Marked watery edema and bulging of the conjunctiva.

coloboma (iridis) A congenital defect in the iris, in which a wedge-shaped segment is absent, giving a keyhole appearance to the pupil; similar defects are created by certain types of ocular surgery.

cupping of the disk The normal optic nerve head has a slight central depression (physiologic cupping). Increase in the depth of the cup occurs with increased intraocular pressure (glaucoma) or atrophy of the optic nerve.

diplopia Double vision; seeing two overlapping two-dimensional images instead of one three-dimensional

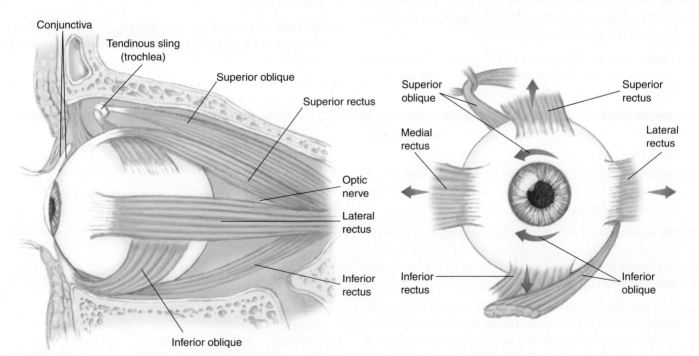

Figure 6-2
Eye Muscles, Left Eye, Lateral and Anterior Views

image; may result from injury or disease of one or both eyes or from failure of fusion of images in the cerebral cortex, due to alcohol, drugs, fever, infection, neoplasm, or trauma.

ectropion Eversion (turning outward) and drooping of the lower eyelid, exposing the conjunctival surface and allowing overflow of tears.

entropion Inward turning of the margin of the lower eyelid, often so that the lower lashes touch the eyeball.

epiphora Chronic overflow of tears from the lower eyelid onto the cheek; may be due to blockage of the nasolacrimal duct or to deformity of the lower lid (ectropion).

exophthalmos Abnormal bulging of the eye between the lids; may be due to local disease (orbital cellulitis or neoplasm) or (when bilateral) to systemic disease (Graves disease).

fundus The rear of the interior of the eye, consisting of the retina, its blood vessels, and the optic nerve head.

glaucoma Any of several related disorders in which sustained elevation of increased intraocular pressure can lead to irreversible impairment of vision.

hyphema Presence of blood in the anterior chamber.

hypopyon Presence of pus in the anterior chamber.

lacrimation (tearing) Increased flow of tears.

miosis Sustained constriction of the pupil, which may be due to ocular or nervous system disease or to the effect of drugs (pilocarpine, morphine).

mydriasis Sustained dilatation of the pupil, which may be due to ocular or nervous system disease or to the effect of drugs (atropine, cyclopentolate).

nyctalopia Marked reduction of visual acuity at night (that is, under conditions of near-darkness). Also called *night blindness.*

nystagmus A rhythmic back-and-forth movement of the eyes usually due to congenital abnormality or central nervous system disease.

ocular discharge A serous, mucous, or purulent material formed on conjunctival surfaces, often gluing the eyelids together and producing crusting of the eyelashes; usually due to infection or allergy.

pain in the eye May be a superficial irritation or scratchy feeling on the cornea or sclera (as from an abrasion or ulcer) or a deep, throbbing pain within the eyeball (as in acute glaucoma).

papilledema Swelling of the optic disk, as observed with an ophthalmoscope; usually due to increased intracranial pressure (**"choked disk"**) (caused by intracranial hemorrhage, neoplasm, or disturbance of cerebrospinal fluid circulation) or intrinsic eye disease (**optic neuritis**). The disk appears edematous and perhaps injected, and the retinal vessels as they emerge from the swollen disk appear to be kinked (**"stepping" of vessels**).

photophobia Aversion to bright light, which causes a sense of pain in the eye, usually because of irritability or spasm of the iris.

physiologic cupping The slight central depression normally seen in the optic nerve head.

ptosis Drooping of an upper eyelid that cannot be fully corrected by voluntary effort.

redness of the eye Due either to local inflammation and hyperemia of the conjunctiva or to hemorrhage in the sclera.

retinitis Inflammation of the retina, the light-sensitive membrane at the back of the eyeball.

scotoma A blind spot; a gap in the visual field of one or both eyes in which objects cannot be seen. A scotoma that appears identical in each eye is always due to a disease or condition of the central nervous system (for example, migraine headache). A scotoma may appear as a black hole or may show flashes or swirls of white or colored light.

strabismus A general term for any condition in which the direction of gaze is different in the two eyes, as noted by an observer.

trichiasis A growing inward of some eyelash hairs, with resultant irritation of the eye.

visual field defect See *scotoma.*

xerophthalmia Abnormal dryness of the eye, usually due to decreased flow of tears.

Lay and Medical Terms

blindness	amaurosis
crossed eyes	esotropia
double vision	diplopia
farsightedness	hyperopia
lazy eye	amblyopia
nearsightedness	myopia
wall-eye	exotropia
white of the eye	sclera (pl. sclerae)

Medical Readings

History and Physical Examination

Review of Systems. A thorough review of ocular history elicits information about past or present symptoms such as blurring of vision, double vision, partial or complete loss of vision, difficulty of near adaptation; seeing spots or flashes; seeing halos or rings around lights; undue visual impairment with reduced illumination; pain in, on, or behind the eyeball; redness, discharge, watering, abnormal sensitivity to light; swelling, drooping, itching, or crusting of lids; and full details about the use of glasses or contact lenses and the date of the most recent eye exam. Eye symptoms can indicate neurologic or systemic rather than purely local disease, as in the case of loss of vision due to a brain tumor or retinopathy due to diabetes.

Physical Examination. Normally the patient sits upright for the eye examination, if possible. The orbital margins are inspected for swelling or ecchymosis, and may be palpated for tenderness if any clue to recent trauma is noted. The lids are observed for evidence of deformity, swelling, discoloration, masses, crusting, or disorders of the tear glands and ducts. Bulging or protrusion of one or both eyes (exophthalmos) can result from hyperthyroidism or orbital disease.

The **anterior segment** of the eye—the part in front of the pupil—is easily studied with the help of a hand lamp. The physician looks for opacities in the cornea and anterior chamber, abnormalities of the iris, and irregularities in the shape of the pupil, incidentally observing whether the pupil constricts when light is shone directly into the eye. This procedure also serves as a test for photophobia (abnormal sensitivity to light).

A check of the accommodation reflex may also be made by asking the patient to look at a near object and noting whether the pupils constrict. Astigmatism, a warping of the cornea out of its expected spherical form, can sometimes be detected by noting distortion in the reflection of some regularly shaped object on the cornea, but is more precisely determined by vision testing with refracting lenses designed for the purpose which only an ophthalmologist would normally have on hand. The location of a lesion of the cornea or iris is indicated by the hour position to which it would be nearest if the eye were a clock dial (e.g., 5 o'clock).

Abnormalities of the white of the eye can be due to discoloration or disease of the **sclera** or of the overlying **conjunctiva**, usually the latter. Mild or early jaundice is typically more evident in the sclerae than in the skin. Conjunctival swelling and discharge or lacrimation (excessive tearing) are noted, as well as the degree and distribution of any redness. Very thin sclerae, such as occur in some connective tissue disorders, appear blue.

Imbalance of the **extraocular muscles** may or may not be readily apparent. Imbalances are called tropias when the eyes cannot be made to look in the same direction, phorias when there is a tendency to deviation that the patient habitually controls so as not to see double.

The **visual field** of an eye is that part of the space before it that it can see while held motionless. Abnormalities of visual field, which can be caused by retinal or neural disease or injury, represent partial loss of vision in the form of blind spots (scotomata) or narrowed range of vision. Visual fields can be roughly tested by the confrontation method. The subject is instructed to gaze at the examiner's nose while first one eye and then the other is covered. The examiner moves a finger or a light from the side and then from above and below into the subject's range of vision, and the subject reports when the object first becomes visible. If the examiner in turn gazes at the subject's nose (and if the examiner's own visual fields are normal), both should see the object at the same time. More elaborate equipment is needed for more precise mapping of visual fields.

The **optic fundus** is the portion of the interior of the eye that can be seen by an examiner looking through the pupil with an ophthalmoscope, a handheld instrument with a light source and a set of magnifying lenses that can be quickly changed.

The principal features of the fundus are the retina, the optic disk or nerve head, and branches of the central retinal artery and vein. Retinal and optic nerve disease as well as the effects of systemic conditions such as diabetes, arteriosclerosis, and hypertension, are readily observed in the fundus.

Vision testing is usually performed with the familiar **Snellen eye chart** (Figure 6-3) for far vision and a set of Jaeger test types for near vision. The subject reads the lowest (smallest) letters that are legible on the wall chart at a distance of 20 feet, and this performance is expressed as a fraction of normal. Thus 20/20 vision indicates normal far visual acuity, while 20/40 means that the subject can see no letters at 20 feet smaller than those that a normal person can see at 40 feet. Firm palpation of the eyeball through the closed lids (moderately uncomfortable and slightly dangerous) can reveal undue hardness, such as occurs in acute and chronic glaucoma. In some settings, **tonometry** is a routine part of the examination of persons over 40.

Vision Charts

Vision (Distance and Near). Vision testing is usually performed with standard charts containing letters or words of various sizes. The eyes are tested both separately and together. For children and illiterates, charts with pictures or symbols are used.

For the assessment of distant vision, the subject is placed 20 feet from the Snellen chart (Figure 6-3), and visual acuity is recorded as the smallest line of type in which the subject can read more than half the letters correctly. Each line is designated by the distance at which a person with normal vision can read it. Thus, 20/20 ("twenty twenty") vision is normal, while 20/80 ("twenty eighty") vision means that the subject must be as close as 20 feet to read a type size that a person with normal distant vision can read at 80 feet.

Remember that the first number will always be "20" followed by a second, usually the same or larger, number. Once this is clear, there is no danger the transcriptionist will erroneously type "2200" or "22-100" when the physician dictates, "The patient had vision in the right eye of twenty two hundred."

For **near vision** testing, lines or paragraphs are printed in various sizes of type (Jaeger test types) on a card that can be held in the hand. Testing may involve finding the smallest print that the subject can read at a standard distance, or finding the range of distances through which the subject can read a particular size of type.

Visual field testing is used to map areas of impaired or absent vision due to retinal disease or other ocular or neurologic abnormality. An Amsler grid consists of a network of lines, usually white on black, around a central point at which the subject is instructed to gaze while the examiner moves a small object through various parts of the visual field to detect defects.

Perimetry is an assessment of peripheral vision, performed by testing the subject's ability to discern moving objects or flashing lights at the extreme periphery of the visual fields.

Tests for color blindness employ printed figures made up of variously sized dots in various colors and shades (Figure 6-4). Persons with normal color vision perceive numbers against a background of differently colored dots, but color-blind persons see only a random scattering of dots.

Refraction. Refraction is the use of an instrument containing lenses of various powers to measure deficiencies of near and distant vision more precisely than is possible with vision charts alone. This procedure enables the examiner to determine the strength of the corrective lens that must be prescribed to correct nearsightedness (myopia) or farsightedness (hyperopia).

By testing cylindrical lenses of various strengths at various angles, the examiner can also measure astigmatism (distortion of images by warping of the cornea out of the normal spherical shape) and prescribe appropriate correction. Refraction refers to the sum total of "refractometry," or measuring the refractive error of the eye. It is the essential component needed prior to prescribing spectacles.

> "The refractive error in the right eye was a -0.50 + 1.00 axis 113 with a reading add of 2.25 which gave a J1 reading."

The previous sentence describes the geometric calculations needed to establish the index of refraction for the manufacture of spectacles particular to the patient's needs. "Reading add" refers to the total dioptric power added to a distance prescription to supplement accommodation for reading.

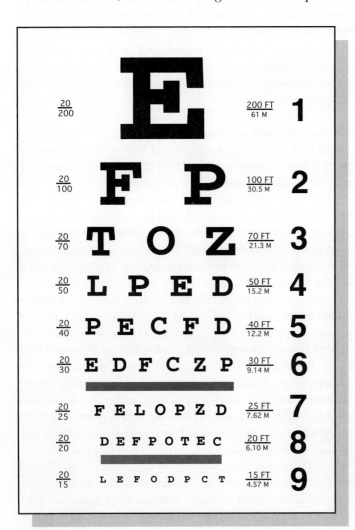

Figure 6-3
Snellen Eye Chart

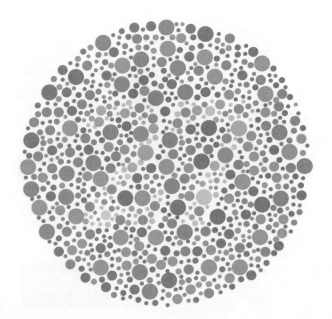

Figure 6-4
Color Vision Chart

Abbreviations. OD, OS, OU—simple, basic abbreviations for *oculus dexter* "right eye," *oculus sinister* "left eye," and *oculus uterque* "each eye." Although physicians continue to dictate the abbreviations, JCAHO directs that they be expanded in medical reports to avoid confusion with similar abbreviations. The abbreviation for "millimeters of mercury," used by ophthalmologists to describe the intraocular pressure, is "mmHg."

Common Diseases

Conjunctivitis. Inflammation of the conjunctiva.
Causes: Infection, allergy, injury (including injuries due to chemicals, heat, or other radiant energy), or other process affecting the anterior part of the eye. Infection may be due to viruses (particularly certain adenovirus types) or bacteria (including chlamydia and gonococcus). Transmission is generally by hand contact. Neonatal conjunctivitis is acquired from an infected birth canal.
History: Soreness, itching, or irritation of one or both eyes, with redness of the conjunctiva; inability to tolerate contact lenses. Depending on cause and severity, lacrimation or mucopurulent discharge that crusts the lashes and glues the eyelids together, swelling of the eyelids, blurring of vision, or photophobia may also occur.
Physical Examination: Patchy or diffuse injection of the conjunctiva, sometimes with coarsely granular appearance ("**cobblestoning**," typical of some allergic conjunctivitis). Lid edema, blepharospasm, lacrimation, ocular discharge, photophobia, chemosis (typically allergic), and sometimes blepharitis, keratitis, or enlargement of preauricular lymph nodes (nodes in front of the ear). Slit lamp examination precisely locates areas of inflammation.
Diagnostic Tests: Microscopic examination of conjunctival scrapings can identify infection due to chlamydia. Culture is necessary to confirm gonococcal conjunctivitis.
Course: Most conjunctivitis is benign and self-limited. Untreated gonococcal conjunctivitis can spread to the cornea, causing perforation and blindness. Chlamydial conjunctivitis is of two kinds. *Chlamydia trachomatis* types A-C cause **trachoma**, a severe conjunctivitis with keratitis, often leading to lid deformity and blindness. Types D-K cause a milder infection, **inclusion conjunctivitis**, which typically resolves without sequelae. Seasonal or perennial allergic conjunctivitis is typically recurrent or chronic during times of exposure to allergens.
Treatment: Allergic conjunctivitis is treated with topical vasoconstrictors, mast cell stabilizers (cromolyn, lodoxamide), and corticosteroids. Systemic antihistamines and steroids may be required. Bacterial infection is treated with topical sulfonamide or antibiotic drops. Both forms of chlamydial conjunctivitis respond to systemic tetracycline, doxycycline, or erythromycin. Gonococcal conjunctivitis is treated with systemic ceftriaxone.

Acute Epidemic Conjunctivitis (Pinkeye). Infection of the conjunctiva, usually caused by viruses but occasionally by bacteria including gonococcus and chlamydia.
Viral conjunctivitis often occurs in association with a viral upper respiratory infection. Symptoms include irritation, mild itching, or foreign body sensation in one or both eyes; hyperemia of the conjunctivae over the white of the eye and on the inner surfaces of the lids; and a mucopurulent discharge that may blur vision, crust the eyelashes, and glue the lids shut during sleep.
Acute infectious conjunctivitis is highly contagious and is usually spread by hand contact. Most viral conjunctivitis is benign and self-limited. However, laboratory studies to identify the pathogen are unreliable, and most physicians choose to treat acute conjunctivitis with a topical sulfonamide or antibiotic. Careful handwashing is important in preventing spread of infection to others.

Hordeolum (Stye). An acute staphylococcal abscess, typically small, that forms near the margin of an upper or lower eyelid. Treatment is with warm compresses and topical sulfonamide or antibiotic. Incision and drainage may be necessary.

Chalazion. A chronic, nontender fibrotic nodule in an eyelid, resulting from nonresolution of a stye that has developed in a conjunctival gland. The lesion may grow large and become cosmetically objectionable. Treatment is incision and curettage.

Keratitis. Inflammation of the cornea.

Causes: Keratitis may result from injury (chemical, abrasion, erosion, puncture, contact lens wear), infection (bacterial, viral, fungal, or protozoan), or systemic disease. Bacteria causing keratitis include pneumococcus, staphylococcus, *Pseudomonas*, and *Moraxella*. Syphilitic and tuberculous keratitis (due to systemic infection) also occur. Viral keratitis may be due to herpes simplex virus or varicella-zoster virus. Keratitis in contact lens wearers may be due to the protozoan parasite *Acanthamoeba*.

History: Pain in the eye, aggravated by opening and closing the lid; lacrimation, photophobia, visual blurring. There may be a history of corneal trauma (fingernail scratch, cigarette ash, airborne foreign body) or of systemic infection (tuberculosis, syphilis).

Physical Examination: Conjunctival injection, particularly near to the corneal rim. Photophobia, lacrimation, watery or purulent discharge. Fluorescein staining of the cornea followed by examination with cobalt blue light shows ulceration or other epithelial defects.

Diagnostic Tests: Microscopic examination or culture of scrapings from the cornea may indicate a causative organism.

Course: Certain infections (herpes simplex virus, *Acanthamoeba*) cause progressive and severe damage if untreated, with visual loss due to corneal scarring. Thinning and bulging (descemetocele) of an inflamed zone of cornea may also occur. Corneal infection can extend to the sclera, iris, or optic nerve.

Treatment: Specific antimicrobial treatment, if available, is mandatory. Topical antibiotics usually suffice in bacterial keratitis. Viral infections are treated with topical idoxuridine or trifluridine and systemic acyclovir. Topical steroids are used in selected cases.

Open Angle Glaucoma. The most common type of glaucoma (an ocular condition in which the pressure of the aqueous humor is abnormally high), consisting of a persistent elevation of intraocular pressure (Figure 6-5).

Cause: Unknown; apparently related to decreased reabsorption of aqueous humor from the anterior chamber of the eye. However, the drainage angle is not demonstrably narrowed, hence the name (contrast the next condition). Both eyes are about equally affected, and the condition runs in families.

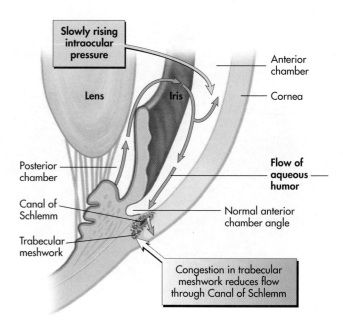

**Figure 6-5
Open Angle Glaucoma**

History: Gradual loss of peripheral vision. Appearance of halos around lights, especially at night, when intraocular tension is very high.

Physical Examination: Increased cupping of the optic disk (increased cup-to-disk ratio).

Diagnostic Tests: Intraocular tension, as determined by tonometry, is elevated (normal 10-21 mmHg). Visual fields are diminished.

Course: Optic atrophy, with partial to complete loss of vision within 15-20 years if untreated.

Treatment: Long-term treatment with miotics: beta-adrenergic blocking agents (timolol, levobunolol, metipranolol, epinephrine, and pilocarpine). Laser trabeculectomy surgery may be undertaken in refractory cases to improve drainage.

Narrow Angle Glaucoma. Acute onset of unilateral ocular pain and visual loss due to sudden obstruction of the outflow of aqueous humor (Figure 6-6).

Cause: *Predisposing*: A narrow anterior chamber angle (more common in the elderly, in persons with hypermetropia, and in Asians). *Precipitating*: Prolonged dilatation of the pupil, such as occurs in a darkened theater or after administration of certain drugs (anticholinergic medicines orally, mydriatic drops for eye examination).

History: Sudden onset of pain in one eye, with blurring of vision, halos around lights; often nausea, vomiting, and abdominal pain.

Physical Examination: Redness of the eye, steamy cornea, dilated nonreactive pupil.

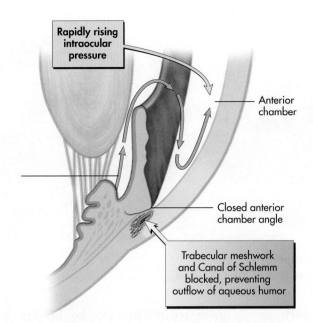

Figure 6-6
Narrow Angle Glaucoma

Diagnostic Tests: Tonometry shows markedly elevated intraocular pressure.

Course: Severe and permanent visual loss occurs if acute glaucoma is not promptly treated.

Treatment: Intravenous acetazolamide and mannitol are administered to reduce intraocular pressure.

Laser **iridectomy** (destruction of a wedge of iris) permits drainage of the anterior chamber. The unaffected eye is usually operated on prophylactically as well.

Cataract. An ocular lens that has become cloudy or opaque because of intrinsic physical or chemical change (Figure 6-7).

Causes: Largely unknown. Infantile cataracts occur after maternal rubella or when the child has galactosemia.

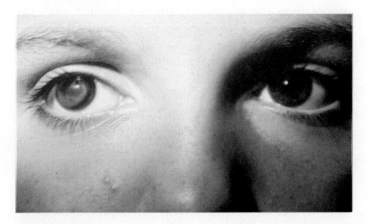

Figure 6-7
Cataract of Right Eye

Cataract can occur in various systemic diseases (diabetes mellitus, hypoparathyroidism) or as a complication of other ocular disease (uveitis, glaucoma) or injury (penetrating injury of the lens, ionizing radiation). The most common type is **senile cataract**, occurring as part of aging, with onset after age 50. The risk is increased by cigarette smoking.

History: Gradual painless loss of vision, not improved by glasses, and seeing rings or halos around lights at night.

Physical Examination: Inspection confirms the presence of partial or complete opacity of one or both lenses. A fully developed cataract, with severe impairment of vision, is called "ripe." Slit lamp examination gives more precise information about the type, extent, and location of lenticular opacity.

Course: Without treatment the entire lens eventually becomes opaque and vision is lost. Surgery restores vision at any stage by removing the lens.

Treatment: Surgical removal of the opaque lens by a variety of techniques, leaving the posterior capsule of the lens intact. Fragmentation with ultrasound (**phacoemulsification**) is the standard procedure. A synthetic lens is usually implanted at the time of cataract extraction.

Retinopathy. A general term for degenerative disorders of the retina, usually accompanied by loss of vision and often due to systemic disease. Two types will be discussed here: hypertensive retinopathy and diabetic retinopathy.

Hypertensive Retinopathy. Degenerative retinal changes due to impairment of blood supply to the retina and choroid in persons with severe hypertension, with variable degrees of visual loss. Chronic hypertension accelerates the development of arteriosclerosis, and many of the physical findings are due to vascular changes. The **Keith-Wagener-Barker** classification is often used to grade funduscopic observations:

Grade I—focal or diffuse narrowing of retinal arterioles, with reduction of the arteriole-venule ratio (**AV ratio**; normally 4:5) to 3:4 or 1:2; narrowed arterioles may be described as having a **copper-wire** or **silver-wire** appearance.

Grade II—further narrowing of arterioles, with reduction of the AV ratio to 1:2 or 1:3; crossing phenomena or AV nicking (tapering of a venule where an arteriole crosses it).

Grade III—all of the above, with "flame" (flame-shaped) hemorrhages and **cotton wool spots** (exudates); these are fluffy opaque zones of degenerative change following microscopic infarction and hemorrhage in the retina.

Grade IV—all of the above, with papilledema. Close observation of the changes of hypertensive retinopathy is of value in judging hypertensive vascular damage elsewhere in the body. There is no treatment.

Diabetic Retinopathy. Degenerative vascular changes in the retina occurring in diabetes mellitus, particularly in poorly controlled diabetes; the principal cause of legal blindness before age 65. Two forms are recognized. In **proliferative retinopathy** there is formation of new blood vessels (**neovascularization**) in the retina, with visual loss and a risk of vitreous hemorrhage and retinal tears. The condition is detected by fluorescein angiography and treated by laser photocoagulation (occasionally, surgery).

In **nonproliferative retinopathy**, changes are limited to venous dilatation, **microaneurysms** (appearing as tiny red spots adjacent to vessels), retinal hemorrhages and **hard** (sharp-bordered) **exudates**, and retinal edema. As retinal edema resolves, it may leave folds or tucks in the retina, which appear as whitish streaks, often arranged in fanlike configurations. A complete encirclement of the macula by radially disposed streaks constitutes a macular "star figure." Visual impairment correlates poorly with extent of disease. Laser coagulation is the usual treatment. Maintaining good control of diabetes reduces the risk of severe retinopathy.

Strabismus. A disorder of ocular motility in which the two eyes do not look in exactly the same direction (Figure 6-8), and cerebral fusion of their images into a three-dimensional one cannot occur.

Heterophoria is a transient deviation of one eye from the normal position with respect to the other. It may occur as a slight congenital weakness or imbalance of ocular muscles that is symptomatic only in the presence of fatigue. Other causes include fever, alcohol and drug use. Inward deviation of one eye is called **esophoria**, outward deviation is called **exophoria**, and normal positioning of both eyes is called orthophoria. **Heterotropia** is a persistent deviation of one or both eyes, due to congenital ocular muscle weakness or imbalance. If one eye is consistently affected, central suppression of its image eventually occurs, with resulting **amblyopia** (dulling of vision that cannot be corrected with a lens). Treatment of heterotropia must be carried out before amblyopia has developed. Treatment consists of prismatic lenses that permit images to fuse, occlusion of one eye to preserve the vision of the other, exercises to improve strength and coordination of ocular muscles, and surgery to bring the eyes into line.

Paralytic strabismus results from paralysis of one or more eye muscles due to congenital abnormality, trauma, infection, multiple sclerosis, herpes zoster, neoplasm, or

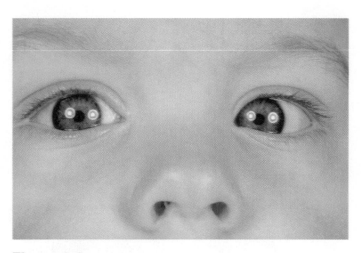

Figure 6-8
Strabismus in Young Child

hemorrhage. Surgical treatment may be helpful in selected cases.

Nystagmus is involuntary rhythmic movements of the eyes, typically bilateral, due to congenital abnormality, multiple sclerosis, or central nervous system tumor, infection, or hemorrhage, or intoxication (chronic alcoholism). Transitory nystagmus occurs after riding on a merry-go-round or in the presence of vertigo. There is no treatment for nystagmus other than removing the cause, if it can be detected.

Visual Impairment

Emmetropia: Normal vision.

Hyperopia (farsightedness): The focus of light rays passing into the eyes lies behind the retina, due to a congenitally short anteroposterior diameter of the eyeball. Treatment is with corrective lenses.

Myopia (nearsightedness): The focus of light rays passing into the eye lies in front of, rather than on, the retina, because of a congenitally long anteroposterior diameter of the eyeball. This condition, much commoner than the preceding, shows a familial tendency and when severe it predisposes to glaucoma. Treatment is with corrective lenses.

Astigmatism: The image falling on the retina is distorted because the curvature of the cornea is not the same in all axes (that is, the cornea is not spherical). Correction is with lenses having a cylindrical curvature to neutralize the effect of corneal distortion.

Presbyopia: Loss of normal accommodation with aging, due to diminished elasticity of the eyes, with inability to focus on objects or print near to the eye. Treatment is with corrective lenses for reading. Persons with myopia as well as presbyopia require bifocals or even trifocals (often with no-line progressive lenses) to provide a choice of focal distances.

Diagnostic and Surgical Procedures

Amsler grid See *visual field testing.*

cataract extraction Surgical removal of the clouded lens of the eye, often with placement of an artificial intraocular lens.

color blindness test Usually these are printed figures made up of variously sized dots in various colors and shades. Persons with normal color vision perceive numbers against a background of differently colored dots. Color-blind persons see only a scattering of dots.

electroretinography Instrumental determination of changes in electrical potential of the retina in response to light stimuli; identifies visual abnormalities due to retinal disease.

fluorescein dye May be applied to the cornea and conjunctiva, and the surface of the eye examined with a cobalt blue light, to detect injuries, ulcerations, or foreign bodies. See also *retinal arteriography.*

funduscopic examination Inspection of the fundus (the rear of the interior of the eye, consisting of the retina, its blood vessels, and the optic nerve head). The examination is performed with an **ophthalmoscope**, an instrument with a light source and a set of changeable lenses to enable the examiner to focus on the fundus regardless of refractive errors in the subject's lens. Possible findings with the ophthalmoscope include swelling or cupping of the disk, vascular and other abnormalities associated with retinopathy, and retinal detachment.

LASIK (laser in situ keratomileusis) A corneal procedure for vision correction. A flap of anterior corneal stroma is dissected, the deeper layers are partially ablated with the laser, and the hinged superficial flap is then replaced.

orbital imaging X-rays or MRI of the skull with emphasis on the orbit(s) to identify orbital or intraocular foreign body.

perimetry A means of assessing peripheral vision by testing the subject's ability to discern moving objects or flashing lights at the extreme periphery of the visual fields.

phacoemulsification Fragmentation of the lens of the eye with ultrasound.

PRK (photorefractive keratectomy) A vision correction procedure using computer-guided excimer laser ablation to reprofile the anterior corneal curvature. Also, **T-PRK** (tracker-assisted photorefractive keratectomy).

Seeing *Is Believing*

For 45 years I had worn glasses with Coke-bottle lenses for severe myopia and astigmatism, yet my vision had never been corrected to 20/20 with glasses, and I had never been able to wear contact lenses. Imagine my delight now to be able to drive, watch television and movies, and perform the usual activities of daily living *without corrective lenses.* It's a medical miracle!

My right eye required a correction of -3.75 diopters, my left eye a correction of -6.25 diopters, with a reading add of 2.50 for each eye. Besides that, I needed a cylindrical correction (for astigmatism) of -4.75 in the right eye and -1.75 in the left eye. Thus, I had a LASIK (laser in situ keratomileusis) procedure on both eyes in 1996. Almost immediately my far vision was good, whereas my refraction error was off the charts before surgery (counting fingers, only). I now need eyeglasses only for reading and computing.

My experience with LASIK was totally positive. A lid speculum was inserted to hold the eyelids open during the procedure, and the surgeon warned me in advance that the speculum insertion might be difficult and thus painful because I have small eyes. When the lid speculum was inserted, I felt a pinching or burning pain for a few seconds at the outer edge of the right eyelid, but I was able to endure it easily, knowing it would last only a few seconds. Fortified with preop Valium and numbing eye drops, I concentrated on relaxing and following instructions to look at the flashing red light in the center.

The LASIK procedure is colloquially referred to as "flap and zap." The surgeon incises a thin layer of corneal epithelium, creating a flap with a hinge and temporarily folding it to one side. The cornea is then reshaped with the excimer laser. After the laser treatment, the flap of tissue is repositioned over the cornea, and it re-adheres or self-bonds tightly without sutures. Hence, the reshaped cornea is protected by the flap during the healing process and generally does not require protective contact lenses for several days. However, my doctor placed a protective lens over my left eye and removed it the next day.

Immediately I could see better. At first, my far vision was good but my near vision was terrible. Over-the-counter reading glasses (2.50 times magnification) helped me read menus and instructions for applying prescribed antibiotic and anti-inflammatory eye drops for the first few days. *Improved* vision was my realistic goal, not perfect correction, so I was very pleased with my results. Within three weeks postop my far vision had improved to 20/40 and then to 20/30 within six weeks.

Computerized laser eye surgery was an excellent investment for me and achieved significant improvement in my vision. And now, seeing is believing!

Sally C. Pitman
Perspectives on the Medical Transcription Profession

refraction Determination of near and distant vision more precisely than is possible with vision charts. The instrument used enables the examiner to try a large number of lenses of standard magnification so as to determine the refractive error of each eye and hence the strength of the corrective lens that must be prescribed to correct the error. The instrument is also used in detecting and measuring astigmatism.

retinal arteriography Imaging of the retinal arteries with fluorescein injected into an arm vein.

pneumatic retinopexy Fixation of the retina in its proper position with the injection of a bubble of gas into the interior of the eye in the vitreous cavity. With proper postoperative positioning, the retina can be pushed back into proper position and then the gas will spontaneously disappear in a few weeks. Gases used in this procedure may be either perfluoropropane or sulfur hexafluoride.

slit lamp examination A low-power microscope with built-in illumination projected through a narrow slit. This instrument enables the physician to view a magnified cross-sectional image of the anterior structures of the eye: cornea, anterior chamber, iris, and lens. Significant abnormal findings on slit lamp examination include **flare and cells** (diminished clarity of the aqueous humor due to protein leakage from the iris; swirls of inflammatory cells in the anterior chamber due to inflammation); and **keratic precipitates** (KPs) (whitish deposits of inflammatory cells on the posterior surface of the cornea).

Snellen chart See *vision testing*.

tonometry Determination of the pressure of the aqueous humor, to detect glaucoma. Tonometers of various types are used.

vision testing Usually performed with standard charts containing letters or words of various sizes. For assessment of *distant vision*, the Snellen chart is placed 20 feet from the subject, and visual acuity is recorded as the smallest line of type in which the subject can read more than half the letters correctly. Each line is designated by the distance at which a person with normal vision can read it. Thus, 20/20 vision is normal, while 20/80 vision means that the subject must be as close as 20 feet to read a type size that a normal person can read at 80 feet. For *near vision testing*, lines or paragraphs are printed in various sizes of type on a card that can be held in the hand. Testing may involve finding the smallest print that the subject can read at a standard distance, or finding the range of distances through which the subject can read a particular size of type. The eyes are tested both separately and together. For children and illiterates, charts with pictures or symbols are used.

visual field testing Use of a black felt sheet or screen mounted on a wall to map areas of impaired or absent vision. An Amsler grid consists of a network of lines, usually white on black, around a central point at which the subject is instructed to gaze while the examiner moves a small object through various parts of the visual field to detect defects.

Laboratory Procedures

blood glucose May be ordered if arteriovenous nicking of the eye vessels occurs, to rule out diabetes mellitus.

cytomegalovirus (CMV) A herpesvirus that is often not symptomatic but can cause infections, and particularly virulent in persons with AIDS, resulting in CMV retinitis.

thyroid panel May be ordered if bulging eyes are noted, to rule out thyroid disease.

Pharmacology

Ophthalmic drugs may be applied topically to treat superficial infections or inflammations of the cornea and surrounding tissues, treat allergy symptoms in the eye, treat glaucoma, or produce anesthesia or mydriasis to facilitate examination of the eye. Some ophthalmic drugs are taken systemically for severe infection or inflammation in the interior of the eye. All drugs intended for topical application in the eye are specially formulated in solution that is physiologically similar to fluids in the eye so as not to damage the delicate eye tissues.

Antibiotic drugs. These drugs are used to treat superficial bacterial infections of the cornea, conjunctiva, eyelids, and tear ducts.

Antibiotics are not effective against viral infections. Ophthalmic antibiotics are dispensed as ointments or solutions.

    bacitracin
    chloramphenicol (Chloromycetin, Chloroptic)
    ciprofloxacin (Ciloxan)
    erythromycin (Ilotycin)
    gentamicin (Garamycin, Genoptic, Gentacidin, Gentak)
    levofloxacin (Quixin)
    norfloxacin (Chibroxin)
    ofloxacin (Ocuflox)
    tobramycin (Tobrex)

Anti-infective drugs effective in treating fungal infections of the eye include natamycin (Natacyn).

Sulfonamides. Sulfonamide ophthalmic drugs are not classified as antibiotics, but they do inhibit the growth of bacteria and are used to treat infections in the eye. Examples include sulfacetamide (Bleph-10, Cetamide, Ocusulf, Sulamyd) and sulfisoxazole (Gantrisin).

Corticosteroids are used topically in the eye to treat the inflammation that results from trauma, surgery, contact with chemicals, or allergies.

dexamethasone (Decadron, Maxidex)
fluorometholone (Flarex, Fluor-Op, FML, FML Forte)
loteprednol (Alrex, Lotemax)
prednisolone (Econopred, Inflamase Forte, Pred Forte, Pred Mild)
rimexolone (Vexol)

Antiviral drugs act by inhibiting viral DNA reproduction. Topical antiviral drugs for the eye that are effective against herpes simplex virus (HSV) include:

trifluridine (Viroptic)
vidarabine (Vira-A)

Systemic antiviral drugs that are effective against cytomegalovirus (CMV) retinitis, a disease most often seen in AIDS patients, include:

cidofovir (Vistide)
ganciclovir (Cytovene, Vitrasert)
valganciclovir (Valcyte)
foscarnet (Foscavir)

Nonsteroidal anti-inflammatories are used topically to treat inflammation that results from surgery or allergic reactions.

diclofenac (Voltaren)
ketorolac (Acular)

Antihistamines and mast cell inhibitors. Topical antihistamines relieve the symptoms of allergic conjunctivitis. These symptoms are caused by histamine released by the antibody-antigen complex that forms during allergic reactions. Histamine causes vasodilatation, which causes blood vessels and tissues to become engorged, swollen, and red. Histamine also irritates these tissues directly, causing pain and itching. Antihistamines exert their therapeutic effect by blocking **histamine (H$_1$) receptors** in the eye.

azelastine (Optivar)
emedastine (Emadine)
levocabastine (Livostin)
olopatadine (Patanol)

Topical mast cell inhibitors act to stabilize the cell membranes of mast cells and prevent them from releasing histamine. This prevents redness and vasodilation in the eye.

cromolyn (Crolom, Opticrom)
lodoxamide (Alomide)

Drugs for glaucoma. Drugs for glaucoma act either by decreasing the amount of aqueous humor circulating in the anterior and posterior chambers (to decrease the intraocular pressure) or by constricting the pupil (miosis) to open the angle of contact between the iris and the trabecular meshwork (to allow the aqueous humor to flow freely).

Direct-acting miotics cause pupillary constriction by stimulating the iris muscle around the pupil to contract and produce miosis. These were the first drugs developed for glaucoma and are used less often now. These drugs are administered topically as eye drops.

carbachol (Carboptic, Isopto Carbachol)
phenylephrine (Mydfrin, Neo-Synephrine)
pilocarpine (Akarpine, Isopto Carpine, Pilocar, Pilopine HS)

These drugs inhibit cholinesterase, an enzyme that normally destroys acetylcholine. As excess acetylcholine accumulates, it causes miosis.

demecarium (Humorsol)
echothiophate iodide (Phospholine Iodide)

Carbonic anhydrase inhibitors decrease the production of aqueous humor by blocking the enzyme carbonic anhydrase, which is active in the production of aqueous humor.

acetazolamide (Diamox, Diamox Sequels)
brinzolamide (Azopt)
dichlorphenamide (Daranide)
dorzolamide (Trusopt)
methazolamide (Neptazane)

(continued on page 174)

Spotlight on

The Ophthalmology Medical Transcriptionist

by Mary Ann D'Onofrio

Physicians in private practice know the value of written communication and its place in the successful operation of their offices. For the general practitioner with only a small correspondence need, the office secretary/receptionist usually is quite capable of handling it. Medical correspondence for the specialist is quite another matter, however.

For the specialist, the dictated letter provides the documentation that often verifies or clarifies points discussed in person or via the phone with referring physicians. Documenting when and why a particular medical opinion was given is a legal record. It may verify for a community or governmental agency the need a patient has for services from that agency.

An accurately transcribed, attractive letter sent in a timely manner is a vital component of the physician's practice. The letter reflects the knowledge and judgment of the physician and, by inference, the quality of the staff. Having the right person available to carry out this task is the physician's prescription for success in maintaining communications with a vast array of people.

In the medical specialist's office practice, who is responsible for this very important correspondence? An ophthalmologist, for example, with a freestanding surgicenter as part of the practice, may employ up to a dozen people, including an office/business manager, billing clerk/bookkeeper, a reception staff, nurses and/or surgical assistants. None of these people generally have the time or training to handle the specialist's technical correspondence. These physicians need a professional familiar with the specialized material reflected in their medical correspondence. In short, they need a medical transcriptionist or a medical secretary with a strong background in medical transcription.

Medical specialists use technical language specific to their practice. For the ophthalmologist, this could include disease processes from anopsia to xerophthalmia, Adie-Holmes syndrome to Vogt-Koyanagi syndrome, Ault line to von Graefe sign. It might include a physical exam describing spots from Bitot to Roth, procedures from aqueous aspiration to Ziegler cautery, special medications from acetazolamide to Zolyse, or lenses from achromatic to X chrome. Technical language, indeed. The trained medical transcriptionist knows what it means and how to spell it.

Medical transcriptionists come with a variety of talents and experience. Knowing what is required in each job setting is the key to success. Which transcriptionist or medical secretary will get that job in the specialist's office? It all depends on what skills are required, and who is best equipped to do the job. The following scenario featuring two applicants illustrates these points.

An applicant currently taking a medical terminology course tries out for the job. She has been a secretary before and has good typing speed and produces letters that look good; however, her knowledge of medical terminology is still in its formative stages. She knows basic structures and diseases of the eye, but she lacks knowledge of a whole array of ophthalmic eponyms and pharmacologic terms. There are suture materials, types and manufacturers of intraocular lenses and instruments she has never heard of, and she lacks knowledge of the special language needed to describe refraction of the eye. She spends more time researching than transcribing. She is asked to reapply when her skills are improved, as the office cannot afford a full-time employee who produces so little.

Another applicant is interviewed and hired. She has been a medical transcriptionist in a small hospital and has transcribed many kinds of reports, including ophthalmology. Eponyms, surgical procedures, and ancillary terms, as well as a good grasp of pharmaceutical terms, are part of her background. When she took a general typing course, she received instruction in the art of correspondence and techniques for typing letters in a variety of styles. She has not used this skill in some time and has spent extra time at home brushing up on her little-used secretarial skills before applying for the job. She is soon producing excellent-looking and accurate correspondence for her ophthalmologist employer. She also suggests reference books for the office library which will assist in transcription.

Depending upon the practice and the office needs, a medical secretary or medical assistant with strong medical transcription skills may be the right choice for the office setting. If the practice is small she may have both front and back office duties. In a surgeon's office where I was employed, our staff of two handled reception, billing and bookkeeping, medical correspondence, and coding for insurance claims. At the same time we were also preparing examination trays, prepping patients, assisting with endoscopic procedures, and preparing specimens for laboratory analysis. A medical transcriptionist may be taught the back office skills on the job if the office staff is small, yet the need for a variety of skills, including medical transcription, is vital to office function.

Not all specialists want or need in-office professionals to transcribe the physician's dictation. When the volume does not justify using an employee, the next logical choice is to have the dictation transcribed by an off-site transcription service which employs transcriptionists with a variety of skills, or the self-employed transcriptionist with skills in the area needed.

Whether working in the physician's office or in a private service office, this particular aspect of medical transcription is personally and financially rewarding. Preparing correspondence often involves all the skills of medical transcription found in hospital transcription: knowledge of laboratory values, pharmacology, operative terms, disease processes, radiologic noninvasive procedures, and more. Wages or fees should be comparable to those paid a hospital medical transcriptionist.

The special language skills, along with general secretarial letter preparation skills, are a winning combination for the medical transcriptionist or medical secretary to enhance the image of any medical specialist's office. These skills are the medical transcriptionist's prescription for success.

Source: *Perspectives on the Medical Transcription Profession*

Beta-blockers block the production of aqueous humor to decrease intraocular pressure. They have no effect on pupil size and therefore do not cause the blurred vision or night blindness associated with other miotics that constrict and fix the pupil. These drugs are administered topically as eye drops.

>   betaxolol (Betoptic, Betoptic S)
>   carteolol (Ocupress)
>   dapiprazole (Rev-Eyes)
>   levobetaxolol (Betaxon)
>   levobunolol (Betagan Liquifilm)
>   metipranolol (OptiPranolol)
>   timolol (Betimol, Timoptic)

Alpha/beta receptor agonists activate both alpha and beta receptors in the eye. This increases the flow of aqueous humor present while decreasing the overall production of aqueous humor.

>   apraclonidine (Iopidine)
>   brimonidine (Alphagan, Alphagan P)
>   dipivefrin (Propine)
>   epinephrine (Epifrin, Glaucon)
>   epinephryl (Epinal)

Prostaglandin F agonists mimic the action of naturally occurring prostaglandin F by combining with its receptors to increase the flow of aqueous humor. Example is latanoprost (Xalantan).

Mydriatic drugs are used to dilate the pupil (mydriasis) and paralyze the muscles of accommodation (cycloplegia) of the iris. They block the action of acetylcholine, which normally tends to constrict the pupil. Mydriatic drugs are used to prepare the eye for internal examination and to treat inflammatory conditions of the iris and uveal tract.

>   atropine (Atropine Care, Atropisol,
>   Isopto Atropine)
>   cyclopentolate (Cyclogyl, Pentolair)
>   homatropine (Isopto Homatropine)
>   hydroxyamphetamine (Paredrine)
>   phenylephrine (Neo-Synephrine, Mydfrin)
>   scopolamine (Isopto Hyoscine)
>   tropicamide (Mydriacyl)

TRANSCRIPTION TIPS

1. Visual acuity at a distance is always expressed in two numbers which should be transcribed separated by a virgule (slash). The first number will always be 20 (for the 20 feet between the vision chart and the patient). A dictated value that sounds like "twenty two hundred" or "twenty over two hundred" is correctly transcribed as 20/200. The phrase "twenty two hundred minus 2" is transcribed 20/200-2.

2. The abbreviation *PERLA* (pupils equal, reactive to light and accommodation) or *PERRLA* (pupils equal, round, and reactive to light and accommodation) may be dictated as "per-la" rather than spelled out letter by letter.

3. *Disk* (with a *k*) is the preferred spelling for an anatomical structure such as the optic disk (a circular or rounded plate). The spelling *disk* (from the Greek *diskos*) is preferred over *disc* (from Latin *discus*), although *disc* is also used and is preferred by some ophthalmologists.

4. Memorize these difficult-to-spell ophthalmology terms:

   accommodation   ophthalmology
   fluorescein   pterygium (silent *p*)
   ptosis (silent *p*)   funduscopy (not *-oscopy*)

5. When the dictator is reporting on examination of *both* eyes, use the plural form of the anatomical structures.

   Scler*ae* and conjunctiv*ae* are normal.

6. Do not confuse the terms *recession* and *resection*.

7. The ending *-olol* is common to generic names of beta-blocking drugs.

8. *Capsulorhexis* with one *r* or *capsulorrhexis* with two? The jury is still out. Although the doubled *r* follows traditional spelling practice for words from Greek, the simpler spelling is currently far more popular in print and on the Internet.

9. Physicians routinely dictate abbreviations *OD* (*oculus dexter*, right eye), *OS* (*oculus sinister*, left eye), and *OU* (*oculus uterque*, each eye). JCAHO directs that the abbreviations be expanded in medical reports to avoid confusion with similar abbreviations.

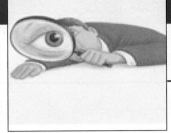

Proofreading Skills

Instructions: In the paragraphs below, circle the errors. Identify misspelled and missing medical and English words and punctuation errors. Write the correct words and punctuation marks in the numbered spaces opposite the text.

1. SOAP NOTE
2.
3. S: This 36 year old man presents with the complaint
4.   of tearing and irritation of the left eye for about 48
5.   hours. She has a thick mucous discharge which
6.   sticks the lids togehter overnight. Vision seems okay
7.   except for some bluring by mucus. He denies
8.   trauma or prior occular pathology. He denies any
9.   symptom of URI or alergy and does not wear
10.   contact lenses or glasses. She denies photofobia. He
11.   has not been around anyone with pinkeye.
12.
13. O: The conjunctiva of the left eye is diffusely hyperemic
14.   and there is moderate chemosis and lid edema.
15.   Traces of a mucopurulent dischrge are evident on
16.   the lid margins and lashes. EXam with Pontocaine
17.   and florescein reveal no corneal abrasion or
18.   ulcertion. No foreign bodies is noted on the
19.   palpable conjunctiva or on the globe. Pupil is round
20.   and reactive. The occular fundus is entirely normal.
21.   Slit lamp exam shows no pathology in the cornea
22.   anterior chamber or lens. Tonometry is defurred.
23.   Far point vision testing with the smelling chart is
24.   twenty twenty in each eye.
25.
26. A. Acute bacterial conjunctivitis left eye.
27.
28. P. 1. Sulamyd opthalmic solution 2 drops left eye q.i.d.
29.   2. Treat right eye also at first sign of symptoms their.
30.   3. Cold compresses left eye ad lib. for comfort.
31.   4. Careful handwashing and avoiding close
32.   personal contact for 24 to 48 hours.

1 _____
2 _____
3 _36-year-old_____
4 _____
5 _____
6 _____
7 _____
8 _____
9 _____
10 _____
11 _____
12 _____
13 _____
14 _____
15 _____
16 _____
17 _____
18 _____
19 _____
20 _____
21 _____
22 _____
23 _____
24 _____
25 _____
26 _____
27 _____
28 _____
29 _____
30 _____
31 _____
32 _____

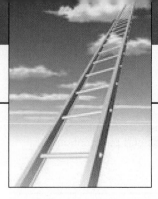

SkillsChallenge

Medical Terminology Matching Exercise

Instructions: Match the definitions in Column A with the terms in Column B.

Column A	Column B
1. ___ nearsightedness	**A.** strabismus
2. ___ clouding of the lens	**B.** oculo-
3. ___ increased intraocular pressure	**C.** cataract
4. ___ deviation of one or both eyes	**D.** lacrimo-
5. ___ lens	**E.** myopia
6. ___ tears	**F.** palpebro-
7. ___ decrease in visual acuity due to age	**G.** glaucoma
8. ___ eye	**H.** presbyopia
9. ___ eyelid	**I.** phako-

Soundalikes Exercise

Instructions: Circle the correct term from the soundalikes in parentheses in the following sentences.

1. Diagnosis: (Anisocoria, Anisophoria), left pupil being 1 mm, right being 1.5 mm.

2. On examination of the retina, the (aura, ora) was normal.

3. The patient had a (choreal, chorial, corneal) abrasion from the metal shaving that lodged in his eye.

4. Healon was (installed, instilled) into the eye, followed by a patch and shield.

5. (Intraocular, Intralocular) lens was (installed, instilled) after the native lens was removed.

6. The patient complained of unequal vision, with the plane of (cite, sight, site) in the left eye lower than the right, most likely due to (anisocoria, anisophoria).

Abbreviations Exercise

Common abbreviations may be transcribed as dictated in the body of a report. Uncommon abbreviations must be spelled out, with the abbreviations appearing in parentheses after the translation. All abbreviations (except laboratory test names) must be spelled out in the Diagnosis or Impression section of any report.

Instructions: Define the following ophthalmology abbreviations. Then memorize both abbreviations and definitions to increase your speed and accuracy in transcribing dictation from ophthalmology.

AV nicking _____

AV ratio _____

CMV _____

EOM _____

EOMI _____

IOL _____

KPs _____

mmHG _____

OD _____

OS _____

OU _____

PEARLA _____

PERRLA _____

Dictation Exercises

Prior to transcribing the dictations, complete these activities.

1. **Using Chapter 3, Style Guide**

   a. What is the proper way to transcribe decimal numbers less than one? For example, how do you correctly transcribe "point 12" and "point 5"?
   b. What are the abbreviations for *left eye* and *right eye*, and how do you transcribe them?
   c. How do you transcribe visual acuity? For example, if the dictator says a person has "twenty twenty visual acuity," how do you transcribe it? How would you transcribe "twenty four hundred" visual acuity?
   d. How should the numerals in percentages be transcribed? For example, if "half percent Marcaine" is dictated, how would you transcribe it?
   e. Review the style for transcribing suture sizes. Give examples.

2. **Problem Solving**
   This activity is to help you prepare ahead of time for some of the problems you'll encounter in the dictations. Some of these items may not have a definitive answer but are intended to simply get you thinking about how to handle a variety of situations that are common in transcription. If nothing else, they will help you recognize a problem when you encounter it in the dictations.

   a. Many people misspell *funduscopic*. Think of a mnemonic device to help you remember the spelling.
   b. At the beginning of a report, you hear an abbreviation that has many different translations. There are no nearby context clues to help you with the translation, but you've been instructed to expand abbreviations in the body of the report. How would you handle this?
   c. The dictator uses an abbreviation to refer to what you're pretty sure is a drug because of the context of the report. It's one of those abbreviations where some of the letters sound like other letters (*b* or *v*, for example). You need to confirm the abbreviation and find the expansion. How do you research a drug name you cannot understand?
   d. The dictator mispronounces a word and you cannot verify the term. You think you've found the correct word, but it doesn't match the pronunciation. What do you do?

3. **Preparatory Research**
   Any information requested in these questions not readily available in your textbook (including the Appendix) or required references can easily be found using Internet search engines such as Google or on-line medical dictionaries.

   a. Familiarize yourself with the funduscopic exam procedure. Summarize.
   b. Research the types of anesthesia that may be used in ophthalmological surgery. Name them.
   c. What type of surgery is performed to treat glaucoma? How does this surgery help to control glaucoma?
   d. On the Internet, find lists of instruments used in cataract and glaucoma surgery. Give examples.
   e. Look up *egress*. What does it mean?
   f. What type of surgery is performed to treat cataracts?
   g. What types of systemic conditions might be associated with abnormal ANCA, CBC, treponema, and Lyme titers?

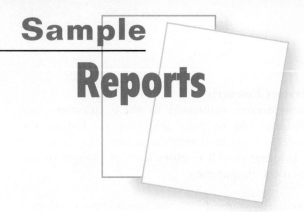

Sample Reports

Sample ophthalmology reports appear on the following pages, illustrating a variety of reports. Fictional names are provided for illustration of proper format, and no resemblance to actual persons is intended. Sample transcripts were prepared according to the *AAMT Book of Style*, where possible.

Chart Note

JOSE CANUSI
Age 62
October 25, XXXX

In May the patient had a diagnosis of cataracts and elevated intraocular pressures which were 24 mmHg, right eye, and 23 mmHg, left eye. He has undergone bilateral cataract operations, and he also has keratitis sicca with a Schirmer test of 3 mm, each eye. He had bilateral cataract surgery with a good visual result of 20/40, right eye, and 20/25, left eye.

The refractive error in the right eye was a -0.50 + 1.00 axis 113 with a reading add of 2.25, which gave a J1 reading. His intraocular pressures were controlled on Pilocar 4% and Betoptic eye drops. He was switched to Phospholine Iodide 0.125% b.i.d. in the left eye. His intraocular pressure on this examination was 15 mmHg, right eye, and 20 mmHg, left eye. His optic disks showed a 0.3 cup of each disk, and the peripheral retinas were within normal limits.

In addition, the patient has a small chalazion, right upper eyelid. It is recommended that he begin hot moist soaks t.i.d. to the right eyelid, as well as Tobrex ointment to the right upper eyelid b.i.d.

DIAGNOSIS
1. Pseudophakia, each eye.
2. Bilateral open angle glaucoma.
3. Keratitis sicca.
4. Chalazion, right upper eyelid.

It is recommended that he return in 3 weeks for a followup evaluation. If the chalazion does not improve or increases in size, he may need incision and drainage in the office.

OUS:hpi

Letter

May 17, XXXX

Thomas Oliphant, MD
2020 Lupus Way, Suite 20
Sewell, NY 12840

Re: Anna Lokotui

Dear Dr. Oliphant:

The patient was seen in February of this year and followed with a diagnosis of aphakia, left eye, and early nuclear cataract, right eye, as well as narrow angle glaucoma suspected in the right eye. She was placed on Pilocar 1% q.i.d., right eye. Gonioscopy showed a grade III angle superiorly using Scheie classification, with a grade II pigmentation. Her intraocular pressures were slightly elevated, and she was placed on Pilocar 1% b.i.d. In April she underwent YAG laser peripheral iridotomy, right eye, for narrow angle glaucoma, with subsequent widening of the peripheral iridotomy.

Her cataract progressed, and her visual acuity more recently has been 20/50 in the right eye. She has always had visual acuity in the left eye of counting fingers on the basis of the aphakia and a pupillary membrane with updrawn pupil. Her optic disks have had a cup-to-disk ratio of 0.34 in each eye, and the peripheral retinas have been within normal limits.

Recently she complained of redness and discomfort in both eyes on the basis of a moderate degree of superficial punctate keratitis and was placed on Lacri-Lube ointment at frequent intervals. Her intraocular pressure was 28 mmHg in the right eye and 20 mmHG in the left eye. Therefore, she was begun on Betoptic b.i.d. and epinephrine at h.s. to the right eye. Because of her superficial punctate and some allergic conjunctivitis, she was switched to Celluvisc q. 2 hours and cold compresses and was continued on her glaucoma drops.

IMPRESSION
1. Cataract, right eye.
2. Status post YAG peripheral iridotomy, right eye (OD), for narrow angle glaucoma.
3. Glaucoma suspected, each eye (OU).
4. Aphakia with pupillary membrane and updrawn pupil, left eye (OS).
5. Keratitis with ocular surface disease.

Thank you for the consultation on this patient. If I can be of any further help, please do not hesitate to contact me.

Best regards,

Bruce Seymour, MD

BS:hpi

Operative Report

SNOW, BRENDA
#121496

DATE OF OPERATION
June 21, XXXX

PREOPERATIVE DIAGNOSIS
Cataract of right eye.

SURGICAL PROCEDURE
Extracapsular cataract extraction with lens implant of right eye.

PROCEDURE
The patient was placed in the supine position on the operating room table after having received preoperative sedation and dilating drops to the right eye. An O'Brien akinesia of the right eye was done using 4 mL of a mixture containing two thirds Marcaine 0.75% and one third Xylocaine 2% plain with Wydase. A retrobulbar block was given through the lower lid temporally using 3 mL of the same. Light digital pressure was applied for a few minutes, and satisfactory anesthesia was achieved. The right eye and face were prepped with 0.5% Betadine solution and draped in a sterile fashion.

A lid speculum was inserted into the right eye and 4-0 silk traction sutures passed through the superior and inferior rectus muscles. The Zeiss operating microscope was swung into position. A conjunctival peritomy was opened over the superior 140 degrees at the limbus and episcleral bleeders cauterized. A groove was made in the surgical limbus with a #64 Beaver blade and a 7-0 silk suture passed at 12 o'clock. The anterior chamber was entered at 11 o'clock with a razor blade knife and an irrigating cystitome used to do a 360 degrees anterior capsulotomy. Dissection was completed with corneoscleral scissors, and the lens nucleus was expressed. The 7-0 silk suture was tied and cut, and an additional 8-0 Vicryl was placed 3.5 mm on either side of the silk. The Cavitron AIS irrigating-aspirating needle was placed into the anterior chamber, and using balanced salt solution (BSS) for irrigation, the lens cortex was removed and the posterior capsule remained intact. The posterior capsule was polished and the capsular bag filled with Amvisc. The 7-0 silk sutures were removed.

An Iolab intraocular lens, model G157E, power +24.0 diopters, control #011288G157E5902, was inspected under the microscope and appeared to be grossly free of defects. It was grasped with angulated McPherson forceps and placed into the capsular bag. The implant was rotated to the 3 to 9 o'clock position with a Sinskey hook. The Amvisc was replaced with balanced salt solution (BSS) and the pupil constricted with Miochol. The incision was closed securely with nine additional 10-0 nylon sutures. The conjunctiva was drawn over the suture line and coapted at 3 and 9 o'clock with bipolar cautery. Garamycin 20 mg and 20 mg of Kenalog were injected subconjunctivally below, and a patch and Fox shield were put in place. Prior to the patch, a drop of Timoptic was placed on the cornea. The patient tolerated the procedure well and returned to the outpatient surgery area in good condition.

STELLA CHOW, MD

SC:hpi
D&T: 6/21/XXXX

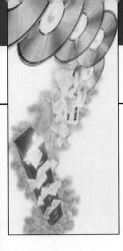

Transcription Practice

Key Words

The following terms appear in the ophthalmology dictations. Before beginning the medical transcription practice for Chapter 6, become familiar with the terminology below by looking up each word in a medical or English dictionary. Write out a short definition of each term.

cataract extraction
cholesterol emboli in eyes
conjunctivitis
diplopia
glaucoma
immunoglobulin
IVIG
macular dystrophy
open angle glaucoma

peripheral iridectomy
phacoemulsification
pinkeye
scleritis
Stargardt disease
subconjunctival
   hemorrhage
trabeculectomy

After completing all the readings and exercises in Chapter 6, transcribe the ophthalmology dictation. Proofread your transcribed documents carefully, listening to the dictation while you read your transcripts.

Transcribe (*not* retype) the same reports again without referring to your previous transcription attempt. Initially, you may need to transcribe some reports more than twice before you can produce an error-free document. Your ultimate goal is to produce an error-free document the first time.

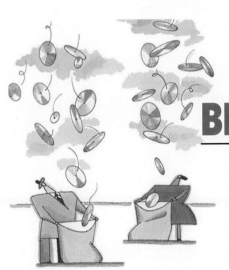

BLOOPERS

Incorrect	Correct
Papal edema.	Papilledema.
Frequent changing of menses without benefit.	Frequent changing of lenses without benefit.

Pulmonary Medicine

Chapter Outline

Learning Objectives

- Describe the structure and function of the pulmonary system.
- Spell and define common pulmonary terms.
- Identify types of questions a physician might ask a patient about the respiratory system during the review of systems.
- Describe common features a physician looks for on examination of the lungs.
- Identify common diseases of the pulmonary system. Describe their typical cause, course, and treatment options.
- Identify and define diagnostic and surgical procedures of the pulmonary system.
- List common pulmonary laboratory tests and procedures.
- Identify and describe common pulmonary drugs and their uses.
- Demonstrate knowledge of anatomical, medical, pharmacological, adjectival, and soundalike terms by accurately completing the exercises in this chapter.

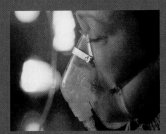
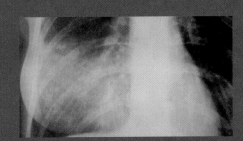
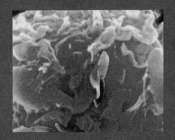

Transcribing Pulmonary Medicine Dictation

The pulmonary, or respiratory, system (Figure 7-1) comprises all the organs and tissues that serve to deliver oxygen to circulating blood and to remove carbon dioxide from it. The respiratory system consists of the nose, mouth, pharynx, larynx, trachea, bronchi, lungs, pleura, diaphragm, and chest wall (ribs and muscles).

Anatomy in Brief

Inspiration occurs when the diaphragm moves downward and the chest wall moves outward. This creates a slight vacuum within the chest cavity, causing the lungs to expand and draw air inward through the airway (mouth and nose, throat, trachea, and bronchi) into the lung tissue proper. At the end of inspiration, the diaphragm and chest wall relax, so that the lungs passively contract and expel air. This is known as **expiration**. During both phases of respiration, blood in pulmonary vessels takes up **oxygen** from the inspired air and releases **carbon dioxide** into the air that is about to be exhaled. Respiration is under involuntary control from a center in the brain stem. Respiratory rate varies with changes in the oxygen and carbon dioxide levels in the blood as well as in the composition and **pH** (alkalinity vs. acidity) of the serum.

The airway is lined by mucous membrane, which contains glands producing both mucous and serous secretions. The walls of the trachea and bronchi are reinforced by partial rings of cartilage, which prevent their collapse under negative pressure.

Lung tissue proper consists of numerous microscopic air sacs or **alveoli** (singular, **alveolus**), through whose extremely thin epithelial walls the respiratory gases can readily diffuse between the air within them and the blood in adjacent pulmonary vasculature. The lungs are protected by a delicate serous membrane called the **pleura**. The **visceral** layer of the pleura is closely applied to the surfaces of the lungs; the **parietal** layer lines the chest cavity. Normally the two layers are in contact, with a minute amount of serous fluid between them to serve as a lubricant as the lungs move with respect to the chest wall during respiration.

Terminology Review

accessory muscles of respiration Neck and upper chest muscles not needed for normal breathing.

atelectasis Collapse of lung tissue.

auscultation Listening to the chest, particularly breath sounds, with the use of a stethoscope.

basilar Pertaining to the bases (lowermost parts) of the lungs.

bronchiectasis Abnormal, irreversible dilatation of bronchi, related to chronic infection.

cough May be variously described as brassy, bubbling, croupy, hacking, harsh, hollow, loose, metallic, nonproductive, productive, rasping, rattling, or wracking.

cyanosis Bluish color of skin, particularly lips and nail beds, due to presence of excess unoxygenated blood in the circulation.

cuffing, peribronchial Thickening of bronchial walls as seen on chest x-ray.

digital clubbing Enlargement of fingertips with elevation of proximal parts of nails, due to chronic pulmonary disease.

dullness to percussion Muffling on percussion due to consolidation of lung tissue by infection or neoplasm, or to fluid in the pleural space.

dyspnea Shortness of breath.

hemoptysis Coughing up blood from respiratory passages.

hyperresonance Accentuated breath sounds on auscultation due to a cavity within lung tissue or air in the pleural space.

infiltrate Diffusion of inflammatory fluid or exudate into air cavities of the lung, or their walls, producing cloudiness of lung tissue on chest x-ray.

intercostal retractions Sucking in of muscles between ribs on inspiration.

PCP Abbreviation for *Pneumocystis* pneumonia, due to *Pneumocystis jiroveci* (formerly *P. carinii*).

pleura A delicate serous membrane protecting the lungs.

pleural friction rub A creaking, grating, or rubbing sound caused by friction between inflamed pleural surfaces during breathing.

pleuritic pain Sharply localized stabbing pain in the chest that is aggravated by taking a deep breath, and virtually abolished by breathholding. It typically results from irritation of the pleura due to pleurisy, pneumonia, pulmonary infarction, or chest wall injury.

production of sputum Phlegm from the respiratory passages. Can be watery, viscous, or purulent.

rale An irregular discontinuous sound, like bubbling fluid, crackling paper, or popping corn. Rales are heard on auscultation of the lungs and are due to passage of air through fluid—mucus, pus, edema fluid, or blood—or to the sudden expansion of small air passages that have been plugged or sealed by mucus.

respiratory distress Indicated by increased effort to breathe, pursing of lips, and use of accessory muscles of respiration.

rhonchi (singular, **rhonchus**) Whistling or honking sounds resulting from passage of air through a respiratory passage narrowed by bronchospasm (in asthma), swelling, thickened secretions, or tumor. Rhonchi vary widely in pitch and intensity; in asthma, rhonchi of many different pitches may be heard together ("**musical chest**").

shortness of breath Feeling out of breath; breathlessness; difficulty catching one's breath.

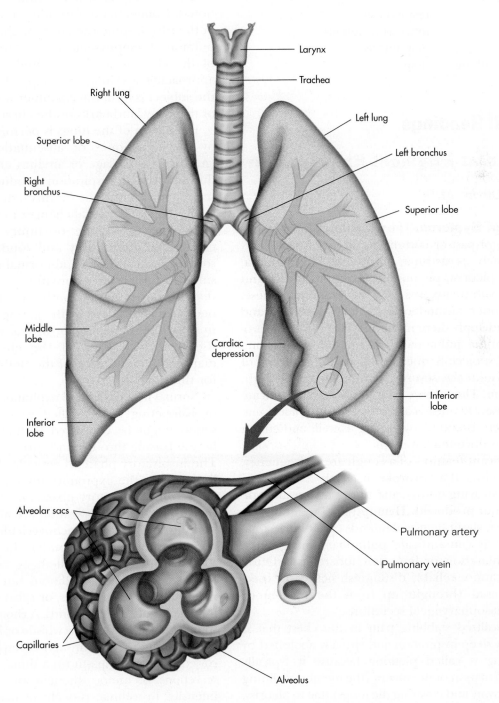

Figure 7-1
The Respiratory Tract

sputum May be variously described as blood-streaked, bloody, clear, foul-tasting, frothy, gelatinous, green, purulent, putrid, ropy, rusty, viscid, viscous, watery, or yellow.

tachypnea Increased respiratory rate.

wheezing Whistling sound made in breathing.

Lay and Medical Terms

breaths	respirations
phlegm	mucous secretions
sweating	diaphoresis
trouble breathing	dyspnea

Medical Readings

History and Physical Examination

by John H. Dirckx, M.D.

Review of Systems. The respiratory history begins with a survey of past or current diagnoses of respiratory problems such as asthma, bronchitis, pneumonia, emphysema, pleurisy, pneumothorax, tuberculosis, and lung cancer, with treatments prescribed for any of these. Lay persons often misunderstand the terms **asthma** and **bronchitis** and apply them indiscriminately and inappropriately to various pulmonary and nonpulmonary complaints. The subject is questioned about shortness of breath (intermittency, severity, inciting factors), cough, and chest pain. These three symptoms can also indicate cardiac disease. Dyspnea is a cardinal feature of asthma. Generally there is audible wheezing as well, and cough which may produce thick sputum.

The significant features of a cough are its frequency, character, factors that provoke it (such as cold air, smoke, dust, or lying down), and the character and volume of sputum produced. **Hemoptysis** (coughing up blood) of even slight degree demands careful investigation because it can indicate pulmonary malignancy, pulmonary infarction, or, less often, tuberculosis. Often the subject cannot reliably distinguish between expectorated material (brought up from the trachea or lungs) and nasopharyngeal secretions.

Sharply localized stabbing pain in the chest that is aggravated by deep inspiration and virtually abolished by breath-holding is called **pleuritic** because it typically results from irritation of the **pleura** (the membrane lining the thoracic cavity and covering the lungs) due to pleurisy, pneumonia, pulmonary infarction, or chest wall injury.

The lungs themselves contain no pain-sensitive nerves. If the smoking history and details of any known respiratory allergies have not previously been recorded, they may be brought in here.

Physical Examination. The physician observes the configuration of the chest walls, breathing movements, the skin, and the breasts as well as the internal organs of the thorax.

The development and symmetry of the thorax are noted. Congenital deformities and injuries or diseases of the ribs or spine can alter the shape of the thorax. In pulmonary emphysema the anteroposterior diameter of the chest is often increased so that the rib cage approaches a cylindrical shape (**barrel chest**). Unless the subject is thin, the examiner will need to find some of the bony landmarks of the chest wall by palpation.

Evaluation of the lungs is performed almost entirely by the techniques of auscultation and percussion (**A&P**). The passage of air into and out of the lungs during normal respiration produces a characteristic sequence of sounds heard through the chest wall with a stethoscope. Structural changes in the breathing apparatus due to disease or injury cause predictable changes in the quality and loudness of the breath sounds and can induce abnormal sounds as well. The subject is instructed to breathe somewhat more deeply than normal with the mouth open (so as to avoid extraneous sounds caused by the passage of air through the nose) while the examiner listens at specific places on the front and back of the chest. Ordinarily the diaphragm chest piece of the stethoscope is preferred for this purpose.

Normal inspiration and expiration yield a faint sighing or whispering sound called vesicular breathing. This sound might be compared to that of a steady, gentle breeze passing through and stirring the leaves of a tree. The inspiratory phase of vesicular breathing is slightly longer than the expiratory phase, and slightly louder. In fact, the expiratory phase may be inaudible. When the two phases of respiration are about equal in intensity, one speaks of **bronchovesicular breathing**. When the expiratory phase is louder, the term **bronchial** (or tubular) **breathing** is applied.

Certain abnormal conditions can superimpose **abnormal sounds** (rhonchi, rales, or rubs) on the basic inspiratory-expiratory breath sounds. A **rhonchus** is a continuous sound such as is made by a whistle or horn. Rhonchi result from passage of air through a respiratory passage narrowed by bronchospasm (in asthma), swelling, thickened secretions, or tumor. Rhonchi vary widely in pitch and intensity. In asthma, rhonchi of many different pitches may be heard together ("musical chest").

A **rale** is an irregular, discontinuous sound, like bubbling fluid, crackling paper, or popping corn. Rales are due to passage of air through fluid—mucus, pus, edema fluid, or blood—or to the sudden expansion of small air passages that have been plugged or sealed by mucus. Asking a subject with rales or rhonchi to cough and then listening again to the breath sounds may supply helpful information about the character or severity of the underlying disorder. The examiner carefully notes in what part of the chest and at what part of the breathing cycle rhonchi or rales are heard or are loudest.

Reduction or absence of breath sounds over a part of the chest wall can result from any of several conditions—collapse of lung tissue (**atelectasis**), consolidation of lung tissue due to pneumonia, presence in the pleural space of air (**pneumothorax**), blood (**hemothorax**), pus (**empyema**), or fluid (**hydrothorax, pleural effusion**), and tumor. Some of these can be differentiated by determining how well the sound of the subject's voice passes through the involved area. When the subject says "ee," the examiner hears "ee" through normal lung, "ay" through consolidated lung or air in the pleural space. Enhancement of sound transmission by consolidated lung is called bronchophony. Whispered pectoriloquy means that even whispered words are clearly heard through the stethoscope.

In another test using the subject's voice, the examiner places the flat of the hand over various parts of the chest while the subject repeatedly says "bananas," "ninety-nine," or some other word or phrase yielding similar resonance and overtones. The vibration felt by the examiner, known as vocal fremitus, is enhanced by consolidation of lung, damped by intervening air or fluid.

Percussion of the chest, though a valuable diagnostic procedure, has been largely supplanted by x-rays. This procedure is based on the fact that structural alterations within the thorax change the behavior of sound waves that are produced when the chest wall is tapped. In the standard technique, called mediate percussion, the examiner places the palm of one hand with outspread fingers against the subject's chest and taps the back of the middle finger smartly with the flexed tip of the other middle finger.

The percussion note over normal lung tissue is described as resonant. In atelectasis, consolidation, or pleural effusion the note is dull or even flat; in pneumothorax or emphysema it may be hyperresonant or even tympanitic (drumlike). Percussion can be used to find the levels of the right and left hemidiaphragms in inspiration and expiration and to trace the left border of an enlarged heart.

As a rough test for obstructive pulmonary disease, the examiner may instruct the patient to blow out a match held several inches from the mouth without pursing the lips.

Common Diseases

Acute Bronchitis. Acute, self-limited inflammation of the bronchial passages.

Cause: Usually viral in origin, as a complication of an upper respiratory infection. Sometimes due to bacterial secondary infection. Can also be due to irritation by smoke or dust.

History: Cough, usually productive, occurring as a complication of a respiratory infection. When severe it may be accompanied by fever, shortness of breath, and wheezing.

It's Breathtaking!

Asthma is a common disease worldwide. In the United States it is responsible for 14.5 million outpatient visits and 5000 deaths yearly. Asthma is the most common chronic respiratory disease of children, accounting for 25% of elementary school absenteeism and for more emergency pediatric consultations than any other condition. The prevalence rate of asthma in prepubertal children is nearly twice that in adolescents and adults. (To put it differently, about half of children with asthma "outgrow" it as they get older.)

In childhood, the prevalence of asthma in boys is twice that in girls, whereas no sex difference is noted in adults. Geographic variations in the prevalence of asthma are striking: from 2-3% of the population in Eastern Europe and India to 20% in Great Britain and Australia. The roles of genetics, environment, and socioeconomic level in these variations have yet to be explored fully.

Certainly there are significant racial differences in the mortality of asthma. Age-adjusted mortality for African Americans during 1993-1995 was 38.5 per 1 million population, as compared with 15.1 for Caucasians. Mortality is also higher among Hispanics of Puerto Rican origin than those of Cuban or Mexican origin.

Between 1980 and 1994 the prevalence of asthma in this country rose about 75% (from 3.1% to 5.4%), with by far the greatest increase (160%) occurring in children under five. Similar increases have been documented throughout the world. Although the mortality of asthma in the United States also increased more than twofold between 1977 and 1989, mortality statistics have stabilized during the past decade.

John H. Dirckx, M.D.
Perspectives on the Medical Transcription Profession

Cough may be worsened by the recumbent position and may keep the patient awake at night.

Physical Examination: Often no physical findings other than frequent or spasmodic coughing. The breath sounds may be bronchial, or rhonchi may be heard, chiefly on inspiration.

Diagnostic Tests: Blood studies are normal. Smear and culture of sputum may indicate bacterial infection but usually do not. Chest x-ray may show increased bronchial markings.

Course: Cough may continue for weeks or months, but resolution is eventually complete. Cough may result in rib fracture or other complications. Bronchitis lasting for three months and occurring in two successive years is termed chronic bronchitis.

Treatment: Largely symptomatic, with hydration, expectorants, and cough suppressants, at least for nighttime use. Many patients experience improvement when taking bronchodilator drugs either orally or by inhaler. Most patients are treated with antibiotics (clarithromycin, trimethoprim-sulfamethoxazole, tetracyclines), even though the vast majority of cases of bronchitis are due to viral infection.

Chronic Bronchitis.
Chronic productive cough lasting for at least three months in each of two successive years. Chronic bronchitis is one form of **chronic obstructive pulmonary disease**, the other being **emphysema**. The two forms may be combined in varying proportions.

Cause: Most cases occur in smokers. Air pollution, allergy, and infection may play a part in some cases. Obesity is a risk factor.

History: Severe persistent cough with copious production of bronchial mucus, particularly on arising in the morning.

Physical Examination: Wheezes and inspiratory rhonchi on auscultation of the chest. When bronchitis is severe, cyanosis may be noted.

Diagnostic Tests: The hematocrit may be slightly elevated, reflecting **polycythemia** (increase in number of circulating red blood cells) in response to diminished oxygen exchange in the lungs. Arterial blood shows reduction of oxygen and increase of carbon dioxide. Chest x-ray shows increased bronchopulmonary markings. Electrocardiogram may show right axis deviation and P pulmonale.

Course: Progressive deterioration of pulmonary function and heightened susceptibility to bacterial infection.

Treatment: Cessation of smoking and avoidance of respiratory irritants and infections are essential. Bronchodilators orally or by inhaler may improve bronchial air flow. Ipratropium by inhaler is particularly effective. Hydration, exercise, and postural drainage may assist in freeing the tract of secretions. When hypoxia is severe, home oxygen may be useful.

Asthma (Reactive Airways Disease, RAD).
A chronic or recurrent inflammatory disease of the trachea and bronchi characterized by recurrent narrowing of air passages with wheezing and shortness of breath (Figure 7-2).

Cause: Abnormal sensitivity of respiratory passages to a wide variety of triggering factors: emotional stress, airborne irritants (dust, cigarette smoke) and allergens (pollen, animal dander, dust mite protein), physical exertion (exercise-induced asthma), respiratory infection, and drugs (aspirin, beta-blockers). Asthma affects about 5% of the population; there may be a genetic predisposition.

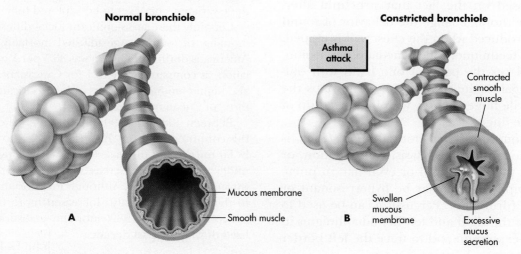

Figure 7-2
Asthma Attack: A) Normal Bronchiole; B) In Asthma Attack

History: Paroxysms of wheezing, dyspnea, cough, and tightness in the chest. Severe asthma may result in physical exhaustion and symptoms of **hypoxia** (deficiency of oxygen in circulating blood).

Physical Examination: Tachypnea; labored, noisy respirations with prolongation of the expiratory phase. **Sibilant** (whistling) or **sonorous** (humming) rhonchi may be heard throughout the chest, particularly on expiration. In severe asthma, retraction of intercostal muscles may be noted on inspiration. The chest may be hyperresonant to percussion, and cyanosis may indicate hypoxia.

Diagnostic Tests: Pulmonary function tests indicate significant reduction in measures of air flow, particularly FEV_1 (forced expiratory volume in the first second of exhalation). When the diagnosis is in doubt, a provocative test (challenge of an asymptomatic patient with methacholine or histamine) will lead to reduction in air flow. During an asthmatic attack, administration of bronchodilator by injection or inhalation leads to marked improvement in air flow measurements. In severe asthma, the blood level of oxygen may be reduced. The eosinophil count may be increased in allergic asthma, and eosinophils may be detected in sputum. Chest x-ray may show hyperinflation of the thorax.

Course: Many cases of childhood asthma are "outgrown." Asthma may persist and progress throughout life, depending on its underlying cause and triggering factors. Infection, cor pulmonale, and acute respiratory distress syndrome are possible complications.

Treatment: Avoidance of known inciting factors; smoking cessation. For intermittent symptoms and exercise-induced asthma, aerosolized bronchodilator administered by inhalation usually suffices to control symptoms. More severe or chronic disease is better treated with aerosolized corticosteroid, with bronchodilator treatment during exacerbations. The patient may be instructed to adjust the dosage of these agents on the basis of measurements made with a simple portable peak flow meter. Other treatments include oral theophylline, mast-cell stabilizers (cromolyn, nedocromil), leukotriene antagonists (montelukast, zafirlukast), and the atropine-like drug ipratropium. In severe refractory asthma (**status asthmaticus**), oxygen is administered by inhalation and bronchodilators and corticosteroids are administered by injection.

Pneumonia (Pneumonitis). Inflammation of lung tissue, usually due to infection.

Cause: Infection by a variety of microorganisms, including *Streptococcus pneumoniae* (pneumococcus), *Klebsiella pneumoniae*, *Mycoplasma pneumoniae*, *Chlamydia pneumoniae*, *Legionella pneumophila*, *Staphylococcus aureus*, *Pneumocystis jiroveci*, and various viruses. Symptoms, signs, and clinical course depend on the infecting agent.

Predisposing causes are debility, impaired immunity, cigarette smoking, chronic pulmonary or bronchial disease, and advanced age. Pneumonia often occurs as a complication or extension of upper respiratory infection.

History: Fever, chills, cough, purulent or bloody sputum, **pleuritic chest pain** (stabbing, sharply localized pain with respiratory movements), dyspnea, myalgia, malaise.

Physical Examination: Most patients have fever. The pulse and respiratory rate may be markedly increased. Examination of the lungs reveals rales or evidence of **consolidation** (reduced or absent breath sounds, flat percussion note). In mycoplasmal or viral pneumonia, physical findings may be minimal.

Diagnostic Tests: The white blood count may be elevated. Examination of stained sputum shows white blood cells and the infecting organism, if bacterial. Sputum culture yields growth of bacterial agents. Bronchoscopy and bronchoalveolar washings may be necessary to obtain satisfactory sputum for examination. Chest x-ray shows evidence of pulmonary infiltrates or consolidation, atelectasis, pleural effusion.

Course: Some pneumonias, including most viral and mycoplasmal infections, resolve spontaneously. Lobar pneumonia due to *Streptococcus pneumoniae*, staphylococcal pneumonia, and (in immunocompromised hosts) *Pneumocystis jiroveci* pneumonia frequently progresses to a fatal termination, even with treatment. Pneumonia ranks sixth as a cause of death in the U.S.

Complications: Pleural effusion, empyema, septicemia, endocarditis, arthritis, respiratory failure.

Treatment: Oral antibiotics may suffice in mild disease. Penicillins, cephalosporins, and erythromycin are the agents usually chosen. In more severe disease, hospitalization, intravenous antibiotics, and oxygen by inhalation may be necessary.

Influenza is an acute respiratory infection caused by any of several related viruses.

Onset is abrupt, with fever, chills, myalgia, and cough. Inflammation of lower respiratory mucosa often progresses to pneumonitis, and bacterial superinfection is common. The disease is highly contagious and may occur in epidemics in late fall, winter, and early spring.

Influenza causes about 50,000 deaths annually in the U.S., most of them in the elderly. Vaccination confers effective protection and is recommended for all persons over 50 and for those with diabetes mellitus, immunodeficiency, and cardiac or pulmonary disease. However, vaccines must be reformulated annually because of spontaneous alteration in viral antigenic makeup.

For exposed persons who have not been immunized, prophylaxis with amantadine, rimantadine, oseltamivir, or zanamivir can prevent illness. Treatment of established infection with these agents slightly reduces the duration of clinical symptoms. Therapy otherwise is symptomatic.

Pulmonary Tuberculosis

Cause: Infection of lungs and other tissues and organs by *Mycobacterium tuberculosis*. Person-to-person spread by respiratory droplets is the usual route of infection. Primary infection may be asymptomatic but leaves a focus of infective organisms in the lung and induces a state of hypersensitivity to the infecting organism. Postprimary infection, which may result from breakdown of a primary focus or from a new dose of organisms from without, typically leads to significant and chronic clinical disease. The infection can also be transmitted by unpasteurized milk from infected cows. Other species, notably those of the *M. avium intracellulare* complex (MAI, MAC) may also cause tuberculosis, typically acquired through the gastrointestinal tract. Persons with AIDS are at particular risk of tuberculosis, including MAI tuberculosis.

History: Cough, purulent or bloody sputum, fever, night sweats, weakness, anorexia, weight loss.

Physical Examination: Fever, cachexia (wasting), evidence of rales, consolidation, or cavitation in the lungs.

Diagnostic Tests: The tuberculin skin test is positive. Sputum contains acid-fast organisms, and sputum culture is positive for *M. tuberculosis*. Chest x-ray may show a calcified primary focus, hilar lymphadenopathy, upper lobe infiltrates, pleural effusion, or cavitation.

Course: Prognosis with treatment is good. Complications include **phthisis** (wasting) and hemorrhage.

Treatment: Simultaneous treatment with three or four drugs (isoniazid, rifampin, pyrazinamide, streptomycin, ethambutol) for a protracted period is the standard.

Emphysema. An abnormal and irreversible enlargement of air spaces in lung tissue due to breakdown of walls of air sacs.

Cause: Cigarette smoking is a principal cause. Some cases are due to infection, allergy, or respiratory irritants. In some patients, emphysema is linked to an inherited deficiency of alpha$_1$-antitrypsin in respiratory epithelium and other tissues.

History: The onset is usually after age 50. Shortness of breath, growing progressively worse, is the dominant symptom. Some patients experience weakness and weight loss.

Physical Examination: Tachypnea and dyspnea may be evident, with activity of the accessory respiratory muscles and pursed lips. The anteroposterior diameter of the chest is increased (**barrel chest**). There is hyperresonance of the thorax on percussion, and the breath sounds are reduced on auscultation. Weakness and wasting of the muscles of the extremities are often noted.

Diagnostic Tests: Chest x-ray typically shows hyperinflation of the chest cavity (low diaphragm, heart in vertical position) and **hyperlucency** (reduced resistance to passage of x-rays) of lung tissue. X-ray may also show **bullae** or **blebs** (air-filled cavities). Blood gas studies are usually normal but may show diminished partial pressure of oxygen. Pulmonary function tests show increased total lung capacity but reduced vital capacity and rate of air exchange.

Course: Recurrent respiratory infections, congestive heart failure (right ventricular failure, cor pulmonale), progressive respiratory failure.

Treatment: Smoking cessation, bronchodilators, oxygen inhalation, antibiotics as needed, physical therapy. For cardiac failure, sodium restriction and diuretics.

Pulmonary Embolism and Infarction. Obstruction of parts of the pulmonary arterial circulation by one or more emboli.

Cause: Thromboemboli from the deep veins of the lower extremities or pelvis passing through the right ventricle are the principal cause. Emboli may also consist of tumor material, amniotic fluid, fat, air, or injected foreign material. Predisposing causes of pulmonary thromboembolism include prolonged immobilization, surgery, childbirth, injury to venous endothelium, hypercoagulable state (cancer, oral contraceptives), congestive heart failure, obesity, and advanced age. Trapping of an embolus in a pulmonary artery results in both reflex vasoconstriction with extensive compromise of pulmonary circulation and reflex bronchoconstriction with impairment of pulmonary gas exchange.

History: Sudden onset of dyspnea, chest pain, anxiety, diaphoresis, collapse. If infarction occurs, chest pain may be pleuritic and there may be hemoptysis.

Physical Examination: Tachycardia, tachypnea, crackling rales or wheezes, pleural friction rub, cyanosis, fever.

Diagnostic Tests: The arterial oxygen tension is diminished. The electrocardiogram may show right axis deviation or right heart strain. Chest x-ray in acute pulmonary embolism may show an infiltrate or atelectasis. If infarction occurs, a wedge-shaped zone of opacification may be apparent. A **ventilation-perfusion scan** (radionuclide scan) shows areas of lung tissue that are normally ventilated (normal air flow) but not normally perfused (impeded blood flow). Pulmonary angiogram confirms and localizes pulmonary arterial obstruction. The source of the embolus may be discovered by venography, ultrasonography, impedance plethysmography, or other diagnostic modality.

Course: About 10% of patients die within the first hour, and the overall mortality rate is about 30%. Fatal outcome is usually due to right ventricular failure or cardiogenic shock.

Treatment: Vigorous supportive efforts, including oxygen and treatment for shock and cardiac failure. Thrombolytic therapy with streptokinase, urokinase, or **tissue plasminogen activator** (tPA) is often successful in dissolving the embolus. Intravenous heparin and oral warfarin are administered to prevent further thrombosis of deep veins. Passage of further emboli through the inferior vena cava may be prevented by surgical plication, ligation, or insertion of a filter. Prevention of pulmonary embolism includes use of compressive stockings in surgical and other bedfast patients, early ambulation after surgery, and use of low-dose heparin in selected medical and surgical patients.

Pleural Effusion.
Presence of fluid in the pleural space as a result of local or systemic disease.

Causes: **Pleural transudates** (fluid relatively low in protein) occur in congestive heart failure, cirrhosis with ascites, nephrotic syndrome, myxedema, and obstructive disorders of the pulmonary circulation (superior vena cava obstruction, pulmonary embolism, constrictive pericarditis). **Pleural exudates** (fluid higher in protein and also containing LDH) are due to pneumonia and other pulmonary or pleural infections including tuberculosis, malignant disease, and uremia.

History: There may be no symptoms. With large effusions, dyspnea. With local inflammation, pleuritic chest pain.

Physical Examination: Reduced breath sounds, dullness to percussion, reduced **tactile fremitus** (transmission of vocal vibrations to the examiner's hand on the chest wall) over the effusion. In the presence of pleural inflammation, a pleural friction rub may be heard.

Diagnostic Tests: Chest x-ray, particularly **lateral decubitus films** (taken with patient lying on side), shows the effusion. Fluid obtained by **thoracentesis** (needle puncture of chest wall with aspiration of fluid by syringe) is examined for protein and LDH (lactic dehydrogenase) to distinguish between transudate and exudate, and for white blood cells, pathogenic microorganisms, and malignant cells to establish an underlying cause for the effusion. Pleural biopsy, closed (needle) or open, may be required for definitive diagnosis.

Treatment: Correction of the cause of effusion, if possible.

Spontaneous Pneumothorax.
Sudden leakage of air from a lung into the pleural space (Figure 7-3).

Cause: Rupture of a bleb or bulla, which may be solitary or part of a generalized process. The condition is commoner in males and in smokers.

History: Sudden onset of chest pain and dyspnea, which may occur at rest or during sleep.

Physical Examination: Tachycardia; reduced breath sounds, hyperresonance, and reduced tactile fremitus over the pneumothorax.

Diagnostic Tests: Chest x-ray (inspiratory and expiratory films) shows pneumothorax.

Course: A small pneumothorax resolves spontaneously. Larger ones may severely compromise cardiopulmonary dynamics. The recurrence rate is 50%.

Treatment: Thoracostomy tube connected to a water seal bottle and suction, to withdraw air from the pleural space. **Thoracotomy** (open surgery) may be required for a continuing leak or for recurrent pneumothorax.

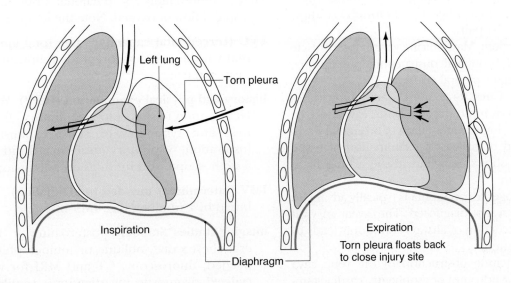

Figure 7-3
Sucking Chest Wound (Pneumothorax)

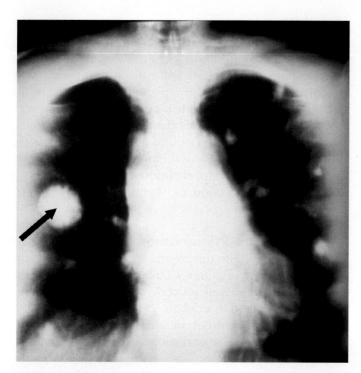

Figure 7-4
X-ray of Chest with Lung Cancer

Bronchogenic Carcinoma. A malignant tumor of the lung arising from bronchial epithelium (Figure 7-4). Bronchogenic carcinoma ranks first as a cause of cancer death in both men and women in the United States.

Causes: Cigarette smoking is by far the most common cause of bronchogenic carcinoma. Inhalation of industrial carcinogens, particularly asbestos, and exposure to ionizing radiation or radon are other known causes.

History: Gradual onset of cough (or change in a chronic cough), dyspnea, wheezing, hemoptysis, anorexia, weight loss, chest pain.

Physical Examination: May indicate weight loss, muscle wasting, or signs of bronchial obstruction, pneumonia, atelectasis, cavitation, or pleural effusion.

Diagnostic Tests: Chest x-ray or CT scan demonstrates a solitary nodule, mass infiltrate, atelectasis, cavitation, or pleural effusion. Cytologic examination of bronchial washings or pleural fluid or histologic examination of tissue obtained by biopsy shows malignant tissue arising from bronchial epithelium.

Course: Bronchogenic carcinoma is typically advanced and inoperable when first diagnosed. The 5-year survival rate is 10-15%. Obstruction of airways commonly leads to atelectasis and pneumonia.

Complications include obstruction of the vena cava (superior vena cava syndrome) or esophagus, cardiac tamponade or arrhythmia, neurologic disorders (phrenic nerve palsy, Pancoast syndrome due to involvement of the brachial plexus), and paraneoplastic syndromes (Cushing syndrome, hypercalcemia) due to production of hormone-like agents by tumor cells.

Treatment: Surgery, radiation, and chemotherapy.

Diagnostic and Surgical Procedures

bronchoalveolar lavage (BAL) Obtaining of material from lung tissue by washing.

bronchoscopy Inspection of the interior of the trachea and main bronchi with a fiberoptic instrument. Specimens and biopsies can be taken through the instrument.

cardiopulmonary resuscitation (CPR) The use of external compression of the heart coupled with breathing techniques to revive a victim whose heart and respirations have stopped.

chest x-ray (CXR) X-rays of the chest are taken to assess the clarity of the lung fields. Milky or opaque shadows in the lung fields can denote edema or mucus secretions. An anterior-posterior (anteroposterior) (AP) film shows the lungs as the x-rays pass from the front of the body (anterior) to the back (posterior). A posterior-anterior (posteroanterior) (PA) film shows the lungs as the x-rays pass from the back of the body to the front.

FEV_1 (forced expiratory volume in one second) The amount of air that can be forcefully exhaled in one second following maximum inspiration.

FiO_2 Abbreviation for fractional inspired oxygen or inspired flow of oxygen. Note the lowercase *i*.

FVC (forced vital capacity) The total amount of air that can be exhaled forcefully following maximum inspiration.

history and physical examination (H&P) With particular attention to skin color, respiratory effort, the fullness and symmetry of chest expansion during inspiration, respiratory noises heard with or without a stethoscope, and findings on percussion.

IMV (intermittent mandatory ventilation) Usually followed by a number, e.g., IMV of 5.

imaging studies Standard posteroanterior (PA) and lateral chest x-rays, oblique or tomographic studies as needed; fluoroscopy; CT and MRI for various specialized diagnostic investigations; **ventilation-perfusion scan** (comparison of distribution of inspired radioactively tagged gas with distribution of injected radioactively tagged albumin, particularly useful in the diagnosis of pulmonary embolism).

Mantoux test Skin test for tuberculosis (TB). A needle is inserted intradermally, and a small amount of purified protein derivative (PPD) from the bacterium *Mycobacterium tuberculosis* is inserted under the skin. A Mantoux test is a definitive test and is usually done to confirm a previously positive tine test. A positive reaction means the patient has or has had tuberculosis.

O$_2$ saturation The amount of oxygen being carried by the hemoglobin, compared to the amount that could be carried, and expressed as a percent (100% being total saturation).

pH A measure of the acidity or alkalinity of a substance. A pH of 7.0 indicates neutrality. Numbers above 7.0 indicate alkalinity, numbers below indicate acidity. The *p* is always a lowercase letter. When the term *pH* begins a sentence, insert the word *The* before it.

pleural or lung biopsy Either by percutaneous (needle) or open procedure.

PPD test See *Mantoux test, tine test.*

pulmonary function tests (PFTs) To measure the rate and volume of gas exchange in the respiratory system by means of finely calibrated instruments.

sputum examination For pathogenic organisms (by smear and culture), neoplastic cells, or other abnormal findings.

tine test Skin test for tuberculosis. A multiple-puncture device is used to pierce the skin and insert a small amount of purified protein derivative (PPD) from the bacterium *Mycobacterium tuberculosis*. A positive reaction is confirmed by doing a Mantoux test. The four small blades used to puncture the skin are called tines because they resemble the tips or tines of a fork.

ventilation-perfusion (V-P) scan A nuclear scan so named because it studies both airflow (ventilation) and blood flow (perfusion) in the lungs. The initials V-Q are used in mathematical equations that calculate airflow and blood flow. The purpose of this test is to look for evidence of a blood clot in the lungs, called a pulmonary embolus, that lowers oxygen levels, causes shortness of breath, and sometimes is fatal.

Laboratory Procedures

ABGs Arterial blood gases.

acid-fast stain A staining procedure in which sputum, tissue, or other material is exposed to fluorochrome dye and then washed with acid-alcohol. Organisms of the genus *Mycobacterium* and some others retain the dye and are said to be acid-fast.

agglutinins, cold Antibodies formed by persons with mycoplasmal pneumonia, which cause red blood cells to clump when chilled but not at room or body temperature.

agglutinins, febrile A group of antibody tests, each for a specific febrile (fever-causing) infectious disease, used as a screening procedure in patients with fever of unknown origin (FUO).

arterial blood gases (ABGs) So-called because they are usually measured in a specimen of blood drawn from an artery. See *blood gases.*

blood gases Oxygen and carbon dioxide, the principal gases dissolved in the blood. Sometimes called arterial blood gases because they are usually measured in a specimen of blood drawn from an artery. Blood gas measurements include partial pressures of oxygen (pO_2) and of carbon dioxide (pCO_2) and oxygen saturation. From these data and the serum pH, it is possible to calculate the bicarbonate level. Alternatively, the base excess may be reported as the variation from a neutral blood pH.

electrolytes, sweat Sodium and chloride ions in the sweat, increased in persons with cystic fibrosis.

Pharmacology

Respiratory diseases such as asthma (reversible obstructive airways disease), bronchitis, chronic obstructive pulmonary disease (COPD), and emphysema require medication to treat chronic symptoms as well as prevent acute attacks. Aside from the antibiotics used to treat respiratory infections, there are several classes of drugs prescribed to treat pulmonary diseases and to treat patients on ventilators, as well as to help patients stop smoking.

Bronchodilators relax the smooth muscle that surrounds the bronchi, thereby increasing air flow. This dilatation of the bronchi is due either to stimulation of beta$_2$ receptors in the smooth muscle of the bronchi, to the release of epinephrine which itself stimulates beta$_2$

receptors, or to inhibition of acetylcholine at cholinergic receptor sites in smooth muscle.

Bronchodilators are given orally as a tablet or liquid, via nebulizer as a liquid that is made into a fine mist, intravenously, or as a solution or powder released from an aerosol canister through a dispenser with a special mouthpiece. The **metered-dose inhaler** (MDI) automatically injects a premeasured dose into the lungs as the patient inhales through the mouth. The dosage for MDIs is given as a number of metered sprays or **puffs**. Bronchodilators can also be given as a capsule that releases a microfine powder for inhalation when used with a Rotahaler inhalation device. Bronchodilators administered through inhalers include:

albuterol (Proventil, Ventolin)
aminophylline (Phyllocontin)
bitolterol (Tornalate)
epinephrine (Ana-Guard, AsthmaHaler Mist,
    microNefrin, Primatene Mist)
fenoterol (Berotec)
ipratropium (Atrovent)
isoproterenol (Isuprel)
metaproterenol (Alupent)
pirbuterol (Maxair Autohaler)
salmeterol (Serevent)
terbutaline (Brethaire, Brethine, Bricanyl)
theophylline (Accurbron, Bronkodyl,
    Elixophyllin, Quibron-T Dividose, Respbid,
    Slo-bid Gyrocaps, Slo-Phyllin Gyrocaps,
    Sustaire, Theobid Duracaps, Theolair,
    T-Phyl, Uni-Dur, Uniphyl)

Leukotriene receptor antagonists. Leukotriene is produced in the body in response to inhaled antigens and causes airway edema, bronchial constriction, and inflammation. Leukotriene receptor antagonists block the action of leukotriene at the receptor level.

montelukast (Singulair)
zafirlukast (Accolate)
zileuton (Zyflo)

Corticosteroids (hydrocortisone and cortisone) are produced naturally by the adrenal glands. They suppress the inflammatory response of the immune system. Corticosteroids reduce inflammation and tissue edema associated with asthma and other chronic lung diseases and prevent acute attacks. They do not produce bronchodilation; they are always used in conjunction with bronchodilators. They are administered prophylactically because they are not effective during acute attacks of bronchospasm. These drugs are given by inhaler, and dosage is prescribed in numbers of puffs.

beclomethasone (Beclovent, Vanceril)
budesonide (Pulmicort Turbuhaler)
flunisolide (AeroBid)
fluticasone (Flovent, Flovent Diskus,
    Flovent Rotadisk)
triamcinolone (Azmacort)

Mast cell inhibitors stabilize the cell membranes of mast cells and prevent them from releasing histamine during the immune system's response to an antigen. This prevents bronchospasm in patients with bronchial asthma due to allergies. Mast cell stabilizers are not bronchodilators so they are not effective in treating acute asthma attacks but only in preventing attacks.

Note: Cromolyn is given by nebulizer or by a special device called a Spinhaler turbo-inhaler that punctures the capsule and allows the powdered drug within to be inhaled.

cromolyn (Intal)
nedocromil (Tilade)

Antituberculosis drugs. Tuberculosis (TB) is caused by *Mycobacterium tuberculosis*, a gram-positive bacterium that is resistant to antibiotics that are usually effective against gram-positive bacteria. Treatment with a combination of antituberculosis drugs is necessary.

aminosalicylic acid (Paser Granules)
aminosidine (Gabbromicina)
capreomycin (Capastat)
cycloserine (Seromycin Pulvules)
ethambutol (Myambutol)
ethionamide (Trecator-SC)
isoniazid (INH, Nydrazid)
rifampin (Rifadin, Rimactane)
rifapentine (Priftin)
streptomycin

Combination drugs to treat tuberculosis include Rifamate (isoniazid, rifampin) and Rifater (isoniazid, rifampin, pyrazinamide).

Drugs used to treat AIDS patients. *Pneumocystis* pneumonia (PCP) is the most common serious complication in AIDS patients and eventually affects about three fourths of all AIDS patients. *Pneumocystis jiroveci* (formerly called *P. carinii*) is a protozoan that seldom causes symptoms in healthy individuals.

atovaquone (Mepron)
Bactrim (trimethoprim and sulfamethoxazole)
clindamycin (Cleocin)
dapsone
pentamidine (NebuPent, Pentam 300)
primaquine

Septra (trimethoprim and sulfamethoxazole)
tobramycin
trimethoprim
trimetrexate (NeuTrexin)

Drugs used to treat AIDS wasting syndrome by stimulating the appetite of AIDS patients include:

Cachexon (glutathione)
cyproheptadine (Periactin)
dihydrotestosterone (Androgel-DHT)
dronabinol (Marinol)
marijuana
megestrol (Megace)
oxandrolone (Oxandrin)
sermorelin (Geref)
somatropin (BioTropin, Serostim)
testosterone (AndroGel, Theraderm Testosterone
   Transdermal System)
thalidomide (Thalomid)

Mycobacterium avium-intracellulare complex (MAC) infection is a common late-stage complication of AIDS. Drugs used to treat MAC infection include:

aminosidine (Gabbromicina)
clarithromycin (Biaxin, Biaxin XL)
gentamicin, liposomal (Maitec)
piritrexim
rifabutin (Mycobutin)
rifalazil
rifapentine (Priftin)
streptomycin

Drugs used for respiratory syncytial virus infection (RSV) include ribavirin (Virazole) and RSV immunoglobulin (RespiGam).

Surfactants. Natural surfactants derived from ground-up cows' lungs are used to supplement low levels of natural surfactant in the lungs of premature infants suffering from infant respiratory distress syndrome (IRDS), also known as hyaline membrane disease. Surfactant maintains surface tension to prevent the lungs from collapsing with each breath. Surfactants are administered via endotracheal tube. Examples are beractant (Survanta), colfosceril palmitate (Exosurf), Curosurf, and Infasurf.

TRANSCRIPTION TIPS

1. Memorize these difficult-to-spell pulmonary terms:

   asthma, asthmatic (*asth-* pronounced *az-*)
   larynx (*not* lar-nyx)
   pharynx (*not* phar-nyx)
   phlegm (starts with *ph*, *g* is silent—"flem")
   pneumonia (silent *p*)
   xiphoid (the initial *x* is pronounced *z*)

2. The respiratory term *alveolar* refers to the alveoli in the lungs. *Alveolar* is also used to describe a ridge in the oral cavity and may be heard in dental dictation or other dictation relating to the nose, mouth, and throat.

3. Note the correct format for transcribing these terms related to smoking history: . . . a *50-pack-year* history of smoking (meaning a pack a day for 50 years, or 2 packs a day for 25 years, etc.)

4. Translate the slang term *trach* (tracheostomy) when heard in dictation.

5. The unusual phrase *pulmonary toilet* refers to various measures such as postural drainage, percussion, and hydration that are used to clear secretions from the respiratory tract.

6. Do not confuse *perfusion* (the amount of blood reaching a tissue) and *profusion* (present in abundance).

7. Note the unusual spellings of some pulmonary medications:

   *Azma*cort is used to treat *asthma.*
   Bronkaid (bronchodilator) (spelled with a *k*,
      not *ch*)
   Pulmicort Turbuhaler (*not* pulmo, *not* turbo)

8. Note the unusual internal capitalization of some pulmonary medications.

   AeroBid
   microNefrin

Spotlight on

Confessions of an Addict

by Judith Marshall

I grew up in Cleveland under the shadow of the great steel mills. I thought the color of the sky was orange and the natural quality of air was acrid. I would wake up and hear the birds coughing. I thought all mothers and fathers, aunts and uncles, and grandparents came with cigarettes in their mouths and lived in a cloud of smoke. At age 14 I got a work permit and somehow it seemed natural that I began smoking in the basement of a hospital, desperately trying to appear sophisticated and grown up.

Over 30 years ago I began my smoking career and, oh, how I loved it. Cigarettes were my best friend, my pal, my lover, my source of strength, my comfort, delight, reward, and badge of elegance. Cigarettes were then socially acceptable and medically benign.

Smoking and medical transcription were natural together. As soon as I could bounce a *Dorland's* on my knee, I realized that I was born to smoke and to transcribe, preferably at the same time. I perfected a system of drinking coffee in the morning and cola in the afternoons along with the two packs (and later three) of cigarettes a day. My system was so full of caffeine and nicotine it was no wonder I typed two thousand words a minute.

I blamed my near-constant headaches on the dumb doctors who didn't know how to dictate. The cough and shortness of breath were more insidious in onset, and I found I could blame those on something other than cigarettes as well. All of us working in the hospital basement smoked all day long and so did the doctors. The dictation room was like Brigadoon, wafting in and out of a fog.

Each new voice on the tape called for another cigarette. Each tape completed, another cigarette. Every break in the cafeteria demanded a cigarette. There were ashes in my typewriter, in my hair, and in my shoes. I remember a little soft brush I kept in my desk so I could whisk the work before I turned it in.

My excuse was that I smoked to keep my weight down. Then one day I took a cigarette, sat in front of a mirror, and smoked it. In the mirror I saw A FAT SMOKER.

Then began the desperate search for a painless way to quit. I began asking doctors how they quit smoking. The younger ones had never started, they were quick to tell me. The older ones stressed a beatific attitude I came to despise. "Oh," they said nonchalantly, "I just threw them out the car window one day and

that was that, fifteen years ago." Litterbugs! The weaker of that group took up gumballs, chocolates, mints, or chewing gum. The stronger took up scalpels. I don't trust anyone who is not addicted to something.

Hypnotism appealed to me, but its fascination was short-lived. It frightened me more than cigarettes. I was positive that once I went under, other more virulent habits would surface—I would begin eating chalk or running amok wearing banana leaves (and probably rolling them up and smoking them as well).

The bookstore was no help. There were hundreds of books on dieting but none on how to quit smoking. I discovered the powerful tobacco industry had its tendrils everywhere. I turned to popular magazines. They just made me want to smoke more. All those slender, beige, beautiful people. They were rich, well-dressed, laughing, carefree people partying on rooftops on a gorgeous summer evening. No one looked over 30.

I couldn't relate to the strong and handsome cowboys or sailors, but I did begin to collect other ads. I bought white satin pajamas and a white satin dog. I wanted that satin moment. I wanted to go a long way, baby. I wanted flowers decorating my cigarettes and a butterfly tattoo on my ankle. My favorite was the

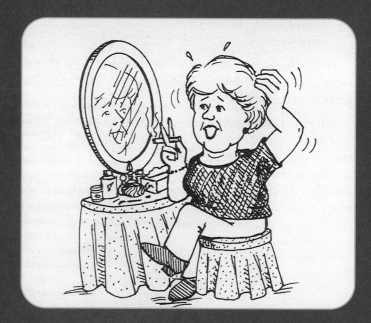

Source: Judith Marshall, *Medicate Me*, illustrated by Cindy Stevens

ballerina ad. She was young, slim, beautiful, and slightly damp from all those pliés. She was relaxing in the dance studio, lighting up. The message was that she could function and exercise without trouble breathing.

I went to work out at the gym and it was Cardiac City. Obviously it was my fault, not the cigarettes.

Remarkable creature that I am, I can play bingo, crochet, talk, and smoke, simultaneously. So I began to choose the workplace with an eye towards the comfort and ease with which I could smoke. I shifted from hospital to doctor's office to transcription service in a ceaseless hunt for the ashtray.

I began to scour the charts looking for patients with lung cancer who had never smoked. This gave me immeasurable feelings of security. Conversely, I delighted in patients whose summaries indicated that they lived to an old age despite 80 pack years. I mentally logged this as more proof that I too could escape. Everyone has an Uncle Joe who beats the odds, smokes four packs a day, drinks a fifth of bourbon a day, and lives to 95. It helps us rationalize our habits. From my vantage point in transcription I adopted literally hundreds of Uncle Joes. It was very consoling.

Professional meetings were more appealing to me if they were dinner or luncheon meetings. I could smoke with impunity in the restaurant. And the Scotch with the cigarettes wasn't bad, either. My major concern while flying out to the national meeting in Denver in 1982 was whether the altitude would affect my smoking habit and make it less enjoyable. (It certainly did.) I was furious at that meeting because some of the morning session rooms did not have coffee, only ice water. Only a smoker can appreciate how welcome hot coffee is with a cigarette in the morning and how repulsive ice water.

What new trade would I have to learn if I quit smoking? I was positive I could not transcribe without smoking. I became angry with doctors. I wanted answers from them. "The patient was placed on a 1200-calorie ADA diet, advised to exercise and quit smoking." Pompous, unfeeling clucks. What did they know about it? I could hear the disgust in the doctors' voices as they related in the course of the discharge summary that the patient, having sustained a moderate myocardial infarction and having undergone CABG, resumed smoking upon discharge.

The answer never did come from the doctors. The postman delivered it. In the summer of 1983 an innocent-appearing postcard addressed to Occupant fluttered into my mailbox. It promised a free introductory stop-smoking session. It promised to unhook me forever from the habit of coffee-cola-cigarettes,

practically painlessly. I told the counselor that if they could do all of that, I was the Queen of Romania.

Everyone calls me Your Majesty now. I quit smoking July 29, 1983. After five weeks of participation in a group, doing all my homework, using a method of gradual withdrawal and behavior modification, I graduated.

On a steaming hot Friday I put out that last cigarette and, like any rational intelligent adult, headed for the kitchen. I defrosted everything in the freezer and as soon as it was cooked, I ate it. Then I began working on the larger freezer in the basement. If I had had a microwave oven instead of having to wait, I would have cleaned out our entire year's supply of codfish balls. Finally I asked my husband to chain me inside the car, pack a suitcase for the dogs, and drive us to the Maine coast so I could sit on the rocks and breathe (without smoking or eating). I calmed down.

Our stop-smoking program recommended saving the money spent on cigarettes and putting it in a glass jar, then buying oneself a present. So far we have a new complete set of English bone china. Next is a trip to England!

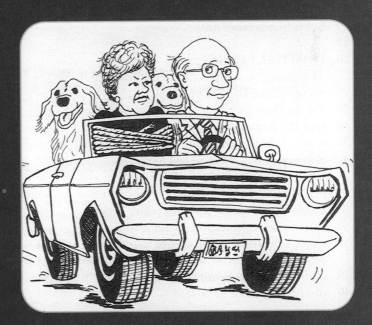

Source: Judith Marshall, *Medicate Me*, illustrated by Cindy Stevens

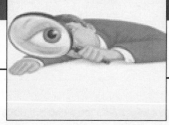

Proofreading Skills

Instructions: In the paragraphs below, circle the errors. Identify misspelled and missing medical and English words and punctuation errors. Write the correct words and punctuation marks in the numbered spaces opposite the text.

1. DISCHARGE DIAGNOSES
2. 1. Right lower lobe pneumonia.
3. 2. Chronic obstructive pulmonary disease (COPD).
4. 3. History of CHF.
5. 4. Atrial arrhythmia.
6.
7. ADMITTING HISTORY AND PHYSICAL
8. FINDINGS
9. The patient is an 82-year-old Hispanic male who had
10. increasing shortness of breath and weekness and
11. weight loss and anorexia for two or three days prior
12. to admission. There had been evidently no change
13. in her medications. Phisical exam revealed temp to
14. be 100°, pulse was 88. Coronary: Regular rate and
15. rhythm. Lungs clear. Extremties without edema.
16.
17. LABORATORY ON ADMISSION
18. CBC white count 19,800 with 73 polys 15 bands
19. 12 lymphs. Hematocrit 39.8. Electrolytes were within
20. normal limits. Chest x-ray showed some bluring of
21. the right costophrenic angle consistant with a right
22. lower lobe pneumonia. Further lab showed a
23. digoxin level of 1.2, theophylline level of 30.4,
24. quinidine level of 6.0.
25.
26. HOSPITAL COURSE
27. The patient was admitted to the medical floor. The
28. theophylline was witheld until levels dropped into
29. the therapeutic range. Quinidine was discontinued,
30. and the patient was changed to verapamil. He was
31. noted to have occasional PVCs and PACs
32. Subsequently he was noted to occasionally have
33. multifocal atrial tachycardia with aberrancy versus
34. occasional PVCs. LDH isoenzymes failed to show any
35. evidence of myocardial infarction. Serial
36. cardiograms showed no acute changes. Follow-up
37. chest x-ray the day before discharge failed to show
38. any improvement from admission, but the patient's
39. clinical status had improved to the point that
40. dischrge was felt to be safe.

1 _____
2 _____
3 _____
4 _____
5 _____
6 _____
7 _____
8 _____
9 _____
10 _____
11 _____
12 _____
13 _____
14 _____
15 _____
16 _____
17 _____
18 _____
19 _____
20 _____
21 _____
22 _____
23 _____
24 _____
25 _____
26 _____
27 _____
28 _____
29 _____
30 _____
31 _____
32 _____
33 _____
34 _____
35 _____
36 _____
37 _____
38 _____
39 _____
40 _____

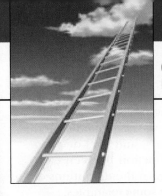

SkillsChallenge

Medical Terminology Matching Exercise

Instructions: Match the definitions in Column A with the terms in Column B.

Column A

1. _____ smallest branches of bronchi
2. _____ crackling sounds on inspiration
3. _____ diaphragm
4. _____ uppermost area of lung
5. _____ depression on side of lung where blood vessels enter
6. _____ mucus coughed up
7. _____ genetic disorder causing thick mucus secretions
8. _____ bluish discoloration of skin
9. _____ breathing
10. _____ collapsed lung
11. _____ membrane around lungs
12. _____ air sac where gas exchange takes place
13. _____ closes opening to larynx
14. _____ spasm of bronchi
15. _____ division of lung

Column B

A. cyanosis
B. epiglottis
C. bronchioles
D. asthma
E. alveolus
F. -pnea
G. pleura
H. lobe
I. atelectasis
J. hilum
K. phreno-
L. apex
M. cystic fibrosis
N. rales
O. sputum

Abbreviations Exercise

Instructions: Define the following pulmonary medicine abbreviations and memorize both abbreviations and definitions to increase your speed and accuracy in transcribing pulmonary medicine dictation.

A&P _____
ABGs _____
AP _____
COPD _____
CPR _____
CXR _____
DOE _____
ET tube _____
FEV$_1$ _____
FUO _____

FVC _____
LLL _____
LUL _____
MAC _____
MAI _____
PA _____
PFTs _____
PPD _____
RAD _____
RDS _____
RLL _____
RUL _____
SOB _____
TB _____
URI _____
V-P scan _____

Adjectives Exercise

Adjectives are formed from nouns by adding adjectival suffixes such as *-ac, -al, -ar, -ary, -eal, -ed, -ent, -iac, -ial, -ic, -ical, -ive, -lar, -oid, -ous, -tic,* and *-tous.* In addition, some adjectives have a different form entirely from the noun, which may be either Latin or Greek in origin.

Instructions: Test your knowledge of adjectives by writing the adjectival form of the following pulmonary medicine words. Consult a medical dictionary to select the correct adjectival ending as necessary.

1. lung _____
2. bronchus _____
3. hilum _____
4. alveolus _____
5. diaphragm _____
6. pleura _____
7. cyanosis _____
8. trachea _____
9. dyspnea _____
10. emphysema _____

Dictation Exercises

Instructions: Prior to transcribing the pulmonary medicine dictations, complete these activities.

1. **Using Chapter 3, Style Guide**

   a. When, according to the Style Guide, do you expand brief forms?

   b. What is the correct abbreviation for milliequivalents?

   c. What is the correct way to transcribe plural numbers?

   d. When is it appropriate to write out (rather than abbreviate) *milligrams, milliliters, centimeters,* and other metric units of measure?

   e. How do you transcribe the dictated phrase "times two days"?

   f. Review the proper way to transcribe eponyms.

   g. Review the hyphens section, particularly the style concerning prefixes used with phrases (e.g. non-insulin-dependent diabetes mellitus).

   h. Review the list of acceptable brief forms. Give examples.

   i. What should you do when the abbreviation *DC* or *DC'd* is dictated?

2. **Problem Solving**

   This activity is to help you prepare ahead of time for some of the problems you'll encounter in the dictations. Some of these items may not have a definitive answer but are intended to simply get you thinking about how to handle a variety of situations that are common in transcription. If nothing else, they will help you recognize a problem when you encounter it in the dictations.

   a. Sometimes, the sound at the end of one word comes out sounding like the beginning of the next word. Similarly, articles in front of a noun can sound like part of the noun. The dictator gives a medication that sounds like it starts with an *a;* however, you cannot find anything that sounds like the drug in question beginning with *a.* What might be happening here in terms of the way you are hearing the dictation?

   b. Both medical and English homophones (or sound-alikes) are frequent stumbling blocks for students. Find lists of common English words, like *course* and *coarse* (perhaps on the Internet), and start devising mnemonics for making a distinction between each pair or triad. You'll need to learn the definitions of the homophones as well. Give some examples.

   c. The patient's glucose is out of control, and the endocrinologist puts him on a drug that sounds like "NBH," "NVH," or "NPH." How do you determine which of these similar-sound abbreviations is the drug used?

   d. The doctor dictates a drug dosage without the accompanying unit of measure. What should you do?

3. **Preparatory Research**

   Any information requested in these questions not readily available in your textbook (including the Appendix) or required references can easily be found using Internet search engines such as Google or on-line medical dictionaries.

   a. Look up *labile.* What does it mean?

   b. What is the abbreviation (chemical formula) for *potassium chloride?*

   c. There are four heart sounds addressed in one of the reports in this chapter. How should they be transcribed?

   d. What is a *gallop sound* (referred to in the heart examination)? Can you find an audio file on the Internet illustrating the heart sounds?

   e. How is the word *rales* pronounced? What does it mean?

   f. What is a *systolic ejection murmur?*

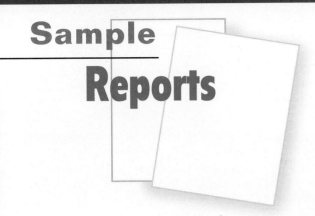

Sample Reports

Sample pulmonary medicine reports appear on the following pages, illustrating a variety of reports. Fictional names are provided for illustration of proper format, and no resemblance to actual persons is intended. Sample transcripts were prepared according to the *AAMT Book of Style*, where possible.

Pulmonary Medicine Consultation

SINGH, PRAKASH
#101091
Date: 01/02/XXXX
Attending: Theodore Liou, MD

This is a 32-year-old East Indian male, lifelong nonsmoker, referred to me. He complains of a less than 2-week history of dry cough associated with dull substernal discomfort and dyspnea, particularly on exertion. Otherwise, he has been remarkably free of any other associated symptoms. In particular, he denies any preceding cold or flu or allergic exposure. He denies any associated fevers, chills, night sweats, or weight loss.

He admits to having childhood asthma, but felt he grew out of this by the time he was a teenager. He has traveled extensively throughout the U.S., including travel to the California deserts and Central Valley. He has not had pneumonia vaccine. He had a TB skin test 10 years ago and a flu vaccine 3 years ago.

PAST MEDICAL HISTORY
Past medical history is remarkably negative.

PHYSICAL EXAMINATION
Blood pressure 140/80, pulse 85, respiratory rate 22, temperature 99.3. Chest exam is completely normal, with no rales, wheezes, rhonchi, or rubs. Even on forced exhalation there was no cough or prolongation. Cardiac exam showed a regular rate and rhythm with no murmur or gallop.

LABORATORY DATA
PA chest x-ray is striking for a new interstitial infiltrate seen in both midlung zones with some shagging of the cardiac borders, indicating involvement of the lingula and right middle lobe. Surprisingly, the lowest part of the lung fields and the apices appear to be spared.

Spirometry before and after bronchodilator performed in my office shows a vital capacity of 3.79 or 69% after an 11% improvement with bronchodilator. The FEV1 achieves 3.24 liters or 72% of predicted after 12% improvement with bronchodilator. The FEV1/FVC ratio was mildly increased at 85 instead of predicted 82.

(continued)

SINGH, PRAKASH
#101091
Date: 01/02/XXXX

ASSESSMENT AND PLAN
Differential diagnosis includes the following:
1. Hypersensitivity pneumonia.
2. Mycoplasmal pneumonia.
3. Less likely candidates appear to be Wegener's granulomatosis, Goodpasture's syndrome, sarcoidosis, alveolar proteinosis, and allergic bronchopulmonary aspergillosis.

RECOMMENDATIONS
1. CBC with differential, chem-20, Wintrobe sed rate, angiotensin-converting enzyme, urinalysis, and mycoplasma titers.
2. Full pulmonary function tests within 2 weeks.
3. Vibramycin 100 mg daily for 14 days.

If he still has significant symptoms and restrictions on PFTs within 2 weeks, he will have to be evaluated for one of the more chronic diagnoses, which may ultimately require open lung biopsy. Otherwise, we should hope that within 2 weeks the patient will be improved and his x-ray will have cleared.

RICHARD GOTTLIEB, MD

RG:hpi
D&T: 01/02/XXXX

Chart Note

CLARKSON, HOLLY
12/12/XXXX

Symptoms of recurrent episodes of coughing and wheezing. She has never had a hospitalization, but her major symptom of asthma requires daily therapy with inhaled bronchodilator. She is much better using a Pulmo-Aide with inhalations of Alupent and atropine and Intal than she is in using the handheld nebulizers. The medication as delivered by the Pulmo-Aide is much more effective because of a better delivery system. I had prescribed this some time ago and believe that she will continue to need this on a permanent basis.

RICHARD GOTTLIEB, MD

RG:hpi

Chart Note

DUVERNEY, PATRICIA
12/12/XXXX

The patient was seen in my office for skin testing, and all of her skin tests have turned out to be negative. It is my impression, therefore, that she has intrinsic asthma. I have seen her for several visits. Since her last visit to my office, I attempted to get her off steroids, but she prefers the use of long-term, every-other-day prednisone in an attempt to decrease her costs for other medications. She understands all of the risks of steroids, and I am reluctantly agreeable to go along with this. At the present time she is taking Theolair 125 mg per day, albuterol inhaler, prednisone 10 mg every other day, Azmacort, and Vancenase, and I have recently added Robitussin-DM.

ALI AHMED, MD

AA:hpi

Emergency Department Report

TAKAHASHI, JOY
#082741
06/25/XXXX
Attending: Hiyas Fonte, MD

HISTORY OF PRESENT ILLNESS
The patient is a 1-year-old female who has been congested for several days. The child has sounded hoarse, has had a croupy cough, and was seen by Dr. Blank 2 days ago. Since that time she has been on Alupent breathing treatments via machine, amoxicillin, Ventolin Diskus, cough syrup, and Slo-bid 100 mg b.i.d., but is not improving. Today the child is not taking food or fluids, has been unable to rest, and has been struggling in her respiration.

PHYSICAL EXAMINATION
GENERAL; Exam showed an alert child in moderate respiratory distress.
VITAL SIGNS: Respiratory rate was 40, pulse 120, temperature 99.6.
HEENT: Within normal limits.
NECK: Positive for mild to moderate stridor.
CHEST: Chest showed a diffuse inspiratory and expiratory wheezing. No rales were noted.
HEART: Regular rhythm, without murmur, gallop, or rub.
ABDOMEN: Soft, nontender. Bowel sounds normal.
EXTREMITIES: Within normal limits.

In viewing the chest wall, the patient had subcostal and intercostal retractions. The child was sent for a PA and lateral chest x-ray to rule out pneumonia. No pneumonia was seen on the films. It was agreed to admit the patient to the pediatric unit for placement in a croup tent with respiratory therapy treatments q.3 h. The child was placed on Decadron besides the amoxicillin and continuation of Slo-bid.

EMERGENCY DEPARTMENT DIAGNOSIS
1. Acute laryngotracheal bronchitis.
2. Bronchial asthma.

ELIZABETH GRAUL, MD

EG:hpi
d&t: 6/25/XXXX

Operative Report

BERGQUIST, BARRY
Date: 01/02/XXXX

PROCEDURE
Fiberoptic bronchoscopy

BRONCHOSCOPIST
Rodney Kwun, MD

INDICATIONS
Worsening pulmonary infiltrates in a febrile patient, unknown etiology. Rule out resistant nosocomial pneumonia.

PREMEDICATION
Versed 1 mg IV.

ANESTHESIA
1% topical Xylocaine, total of 30 cc.

INSTRUMENT
Olympus BFP10 bronchoscope.

PROCEDURE
After informed consent was obtained from the patient's mother and appropriate premedication, the bronchoscope was inserted directly through the tracheostomy tube while the patient continued to receive oxygen supplementation. The lower trachea and tracheobronchial tree were then fully examined in this fashion. There was very severe, intense tracheobronchitis noted, with very friable mucosa. Patchy areas of denudation of the mucosa were also noted, particularly along the right lateral wall. The main carina was sharp and in the midline. The right and left bronchial trees showed the same diffuse erythematous changes but no purulence and no endobronchial abnormalities. Bronchial washings were obtained from throughout the tracheobronchial tree and submitted for Gram stain, routine acid-fast bacilli, fungal smears and cultures, and cytologic review. The instrument was then removed and the procedure terminated. No complications were encountered.

DIAGNOSTIC IMPRESSION
Severe tracheobronchitis.

RODNEY KWUN, MD

RK:hpi
D: 01/02/XXXX
T: 01/02/XXXX

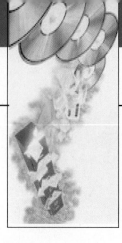

Transcription Practice

Key Words

The following terms appear in the pulmonary medicine dictations. Before beginning the medical transcription practice for Chapter 7, look up each term below in a medical or English dictionary and write out a short definition.

asthma
bronchoscopy
carcinoma of lung
cerebral aneurysm
COPD
dyspnea
dyspnea on exertion
gastroscopy
interstitial lung disease
labile hypertension

metastatic carcinoma
    of lung
non-small cell carcinoma
pneumothorax
shortness of breath
thoracotomy
tracheobronchitis
tracheostomy
URI

After completing all the readings and exercises in Chapter 7, transcribe the pulmonary medicine dictation. Proofread your transcribed documents carefully, listening to the dictation while you read your transcripts.

Transcribe (*not* retype) the same reports again without referring to your previous transcription attempt. Initially, you may need to transcribe some reports more than twice before you can produce an error-free document. Your ultimate goal is to produce an error-free document the first time.

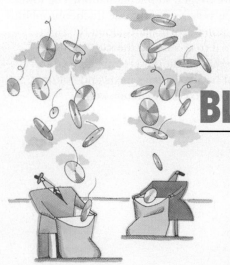

BLOOPERS

Incorrect	Correct
The patient complains of perineal asthma.	The patient complains of perennial asthma.
Atelectasis due to inspissated bugs.	Atelectasis due to inspissated plugs
Pain in the chest aggravated by defreezing.	Pain in the chest aggravated by deep breathing
He had a lot of waterbowl wheezing.	He had a lot of audible wheezing.

Cardiology and Hematology

Chapter Outline

Learning Objectives

- Describe the structure and function of the cardiovascular system.
- Spell and define common cardiovascular terms.
- Identify types of questions a physician might ask a patient about the cardiovascular system in the review of systems.
- Describe common features a physician looks for on examination of the heart and vessels.
- Identify common diseases of the cardiovascular system. Describe their typical cause, course, and treatment options.
- Identify and define diagnostic and surgical procedures of the cardiovascular system.

- List common cardiovascular laboratory tests and procedures.
- Identify and describe common cardiovascular drugs and their uses.
- Describe blood cells and their functions and identify common blood disorders.
- List basic laboratory tests used to to study blood cells and the coagulation process.
- Demonstrate knowledge of anatomical, medical pharmacological, adjectival, and soundalike terms by accurately completing the exercises in this chapter.

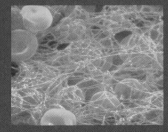
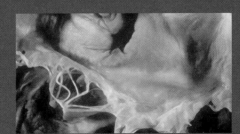
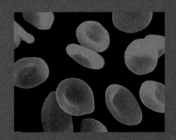

Transcribing Cardiology Dictation

The **cardiovascular** or **circulatory system** consists of the heart and the blood vessels (arteries, capillaries, veins) (see Figures 8-1 and 8-2). The purpose of the system is to provide rapid delivery to the tissues of oxygen from the lungs; nutrients, minerals, vitamins, and water from the digestive system; hormones from glands; and white blood cells from bone marrow and lymphoid tissue, while removing waste products and delivering them to the lungs (carbon dioxide), liver (broken-down red blood cells), and kidney (surplus water, nitrogenous wastes) for excretion.

Anatomy in Brief

The heart is a pump—actually two synchronized pumps, each handling a different segment of the circulating blood at any given moment. The **right atrium** (antechamber) and the **right ventricle** receive venous blood from the systemic circulation and pump it into the lungs for gas exchange. The **left atrium** and **left ventricle** receive freshly oxygenated blood from the lungs and pump it through the arteries into the systemic circulation.

The contraction of a heart chamber is called **systole**; relaxation and refilling is called **diastole**. Valves in the heart (one for each of the four chambers) prevent backflow of blood from a chamber during systole. The heart is encased in a protective sac called the **pericardium**.

The names of the coronary arteries and branches are frequently mentioned in angiographic and surgical reports. The major vessels are the left main coronary artery, the left anterior descending (LAD) coronary artery, the right coronary artery (RCA), and the circumflex coronary artery. Names of branches of these take on additional terms, such as the left anterior descending diagonal (LADD). Other vessels to remember are the circumflex marginal, distal branches, and the posterior descendings. The major conduits are the aorta and pulmonary artery. The valves are aortic, mitral, pulmonary, and tricuspid.

Terminology Review

anemia Deficiency of red blood cells.

arrhythmia Irregular rhythm of the heartbeat, with or without an abnormally slow or fast rate.

ascites Swelling of the abdomen due to effusion of fluid into the peritoneal cavity.

auscultation of the heart The physician notes the quality and loudness of heart sounds heard through a stethoscope at the four valve areas.

bradyarrhythmia A pulse that is both irregular and abnormally slow.

bradycardia Abnormal slowness of the heartbeat (pulse less than 60/min).

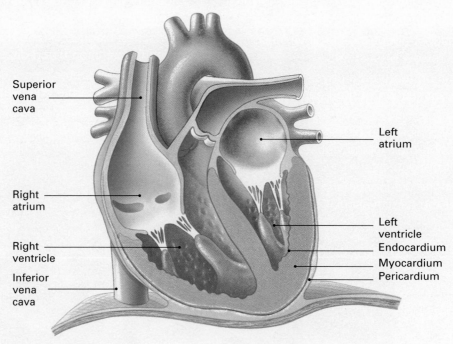

Figure 8-1
The Heart; Anterior View of Heart Chambers

MAJOR ARTERIES

MAJOR VEINS

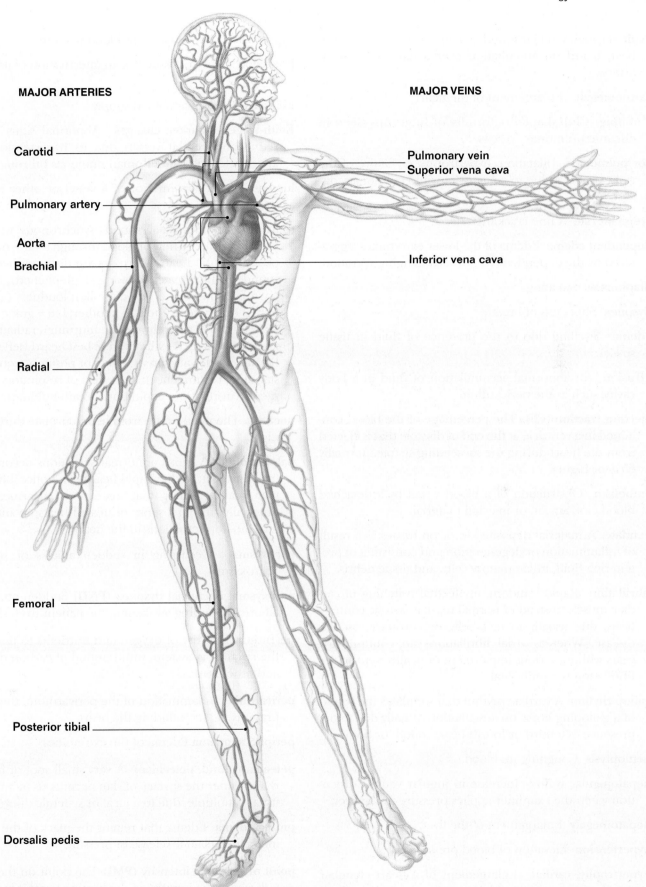

Carotid

Pulmonary artery

Aorta

Brachial

Radial

Femoral

Posterior tibial

Dorsalis pedis

Pulmonary vein
Superior vena cava

Inferior vena cava

Figure 8-2
The Circulatory System

bruit A rough vascular sound, synchronous with the heartbeat, heard on auscultation over a narrowing in an artery.

cardiomegaly Enlargement of the heart.

clubbing Club-shaped deformity of fingertips, seen in chronic pulmonary disease.

cor pulmonale Dilatation, hypertrophy, or failure of the right ventricle due to acute or chronic pulmonary disease.

crepitant rale A fine crackling rale.

dependent edema Edema of the lower extremities, aggravated by the dependent (downward hanging) position.

diaphoresis Sweating.

dyspnea Shortness of breath.

edema Swelling due to the presence of fluid in tissue spaces.

effusion An abnormal accumulation of fluid in a body cavity, such as the pericardium.

ejection fraction (EF) The percentage of the blood contained in a ventricle at the end of diastole that is ejected from the heart during the succeeding systole, normally 65% or higher.

embolism Obstruction of a blood vessel by a detached blood clot, air, fat, or injected material.

exudate A material deposited in or on tissues as a result of inflammation or degeneration and consisting of protein-rich fluid, inflammatory cells, and tissue debris.

fibrillation Rapid, random, ineffectual twitching of cardiac muscle, instead of normal regular systolic contractions, due usually to metabolic or coronary vascular disease. Whereas atrial fibrillation can continue for years without serious impairment of health, ventricular fibrillation is rapidly fatal.

gallop rhythm A cardiac rhythm that simulates the sound of a galloping horse on auscultation, usually due to the presence of a third or fourth heart sound, or both.

hemoptysis Coughing up blood.

hepatojugular reflux Increase in jugular venous distention when the examiner applies pressure to the liver.

hepatomegaly Enlargement of the liver.

hypertension Elevation of blood pressure.

hypertrophy, cardiac Enlargement of a heart chamber due to increase in the thickness of its muscular wall.

hypotension Abnormally low blood pressure.

infarction Death of tissue due to interruption of its blood supply.

ischemia Inadequate blood supply.

Keith-Wagener-Barker changes Abnormal signs in the retina and retinal vessels due to hypertension and arteriosclerosis, using Roman numerals I through IV.

lumen The hollow interior of a vessel or other tubular structure.

murmur An abnormal sound, synchronous with the heartbeat, due to flow of blood through a valve or other passage in the heart. Murmurs are distinguished as to sound quality (harsh, blowing, high-pitched); timing (systolic, mid-systolic, late diastolic); loudness (grade 1 to 6 in one system, 1 to 4 in another; 1/6 = grade 1 on a scale of 1 to 6, a barely audible murmur); radiation (to apex, carotids, left axilla); where best heard (left sternal border, aortic valve area); effect of position (squatting, standing, recumbency); and effect of respiratory movements (inspiration, expiration, breath-holding).

nocturia The need to rise from bed to urinate during the night.

palpitation(s) Various abnormal sensations accompanying heartbeat; unduly rapid heartbeat; noticeably irregular beat; a feeling that some or all heartbeats are unusually strong; a sense of missed beats; or intermittent flip-flop sensations in the heart.

paroxysmal Occurring in sudden attacks or seizures (paroxysms).

paroxysmal nocturnal dyspnea (PND) Sudden attacks of labored breathing awakening the patient from sleep.

perfusion Delivery of oxygen and nutrients to tissues by the circulatory system, with removal of carbon dioxide and other wastes.

pericarditis Inflammation of the pericardium, the membranous sac surrounding the heart.

peripheral edema Edema of the extremities.

petechia (plural, **petechiae**) A very small spot of hemorrhage under the surface of skin or mucous membrane, usually multiple, due to a local or systemic disorder.

pitting edema Edema that retains the mark of the examiner's fingers after release of pressure.

point of maximal intensity (PMI) The point on the chest wall where the impulse of the beating heart is most distinctly felt by the examiner's fingers.

precordial In front of the heart.

pulse The heartbeat, and by extension the rate of heartbeat, as measured at the wrist (radial pulse), the cardiac apex (apical pulse), or elsewhere.

rale A crackling or bubbling sound heard on auscultation of the breath sounds, usually due to fluid in small respiratory passages.

rhonchus (plural, rhonchi) A whistling or humming sound caused by passage of air through narrowed parts of the respiratory tract.

shock (precordial) An abnormally strong thrust applied to the chest wall by the beating heart, as detected by the examiner's fingers.

splitting Separation of the first or second heart sound, or both, into two distinctly audible components.

stigma (plural, **stigmata**) A structural or functional peculiarity or abnormality that is characteristic of an inherited or acquired condition, and may be useful in its diagnosis.

syncope Sudden loss of consciousness; fainting.

tachyarrhythmia A pulse that is both irregular and abnormally rapid.

tachycardia Rapid heart rate (over 100/min).

thrill An abnormal sensation felt by the examiner over the heart when blood jets through an anomalous or narrowed orifice.

(tunica) intima The innermost layer or lining of an artery.

vascular Pertaining to one or more blood vessels.

vasculitis Inflammation of blood vessels.

Lay and Medical Terms

heart attack	myocardial infarction
high blood pressure	hypertension
hardening of the arteries	arteriosclerosis, atherosclerosis
chest pain (of cardiac origin)	angina pectoris

Medical Readings

History and Physical Examination

by John H. Dirckx, M.D.

Review of Systems. The cardiovascular history begins with a review of past diagnoses of congenital or acquired heart murmurs, rheumatic fever, enlarged heart, coronary artery disease, heart attack, high blood pressure, varicose veins, thrombophlebitis, and treatments, past or present, prescribed for any of these. Note is made of the results of past diagnostic studies such as electrocardiograms, echocardiograms, stress testing, cardiac catheterization, and angiography, and of any surgical procedures, such as pacemaker implantation, valve repair or replacement, and coronary artery bypass graft.

Because coronary artery disease is a major cause of disability and death, any complaint of **chest pain** must be carefully evaluated to determine whether it represents angina pectoris, the cardinal symptom of coronary disease. A full description of chest pain includes its character, intensity, location, extent, radiation, duration, and frequency of occurrence; the effect of position, movement, breathing, and swallowing; associated symptoms such as shortness of breath, sweating, and palpitations; the effect of resting or taking medicines such as antacids or nitroglycerin; and triggering factors such as physical exertion, smoking, eating, strong emotion, or exposure to cold.

When shortness of breath is due to **cardiac failure**, it is typically less oppressive in the upright position (orthopnea) and may occur in attacks that awaken the patient during the night (paroxysmal nocturnal dyspnea, PND). Orthopnea is graded by the number of pillows needed to avoid respiratory distress (e.g., three-pillow orthopnea). Wheezing, coughing, and exertional dyspnea are common to cardiac and noncardiac disorders.

Physical Examination. Auscultation of the heart provides more information than any other procedure. Stethoscopes used for cardiac auscultation have two chest pieces: a narrow cone-shaped "bell" for lower pitched sounds, and a wide, flat diaphragm for higher pitched sounds. The examiner changes back and forth from one to the other as needed during the examination. The stethoscope is applied to the chest in specific areas according to a basic routine but may be varied as circumstances dictate.

Four areas of the anterior chest are designated according to the **valves** whose sounds are best heard there: the **mitral** area, the **pulmonic** area, the **aortic** area, and the **tricuspid** area (see Figure 8-3). The subject may need to

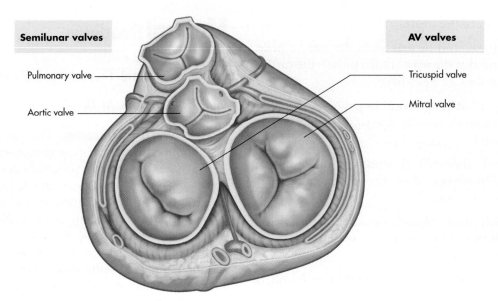

Semilunar valves		AV valves

Pulmonary valve

Aortic valve

Tricuspid valve

Mitral valve

Figure 8-3
The Valves of the Heart, in Closed Position Viewed from the Top

change position, such as by leaning forward or lying on the left side, to enable the examiner to evaluate heart sounds adequately. The physician also listens for abnormal sounds: **murmurs** caused by abnormal flow of blood through a valve or other orifice; **clicks or snaps**, caused by abnormal valve function; **rubs**, creaking or grating sounds caused by friction between the beating heart and an inflamed pericardium; **bruits**, caused by passage of blood through a narrowed artery; and others.

The normally beating heart produces two **sounds** in alternation, traditionally represented as *lup-dup*. The first heart sound, or S1, which is louder, deeper in pitch, and longer, results from contraction of the ventricles and closure of the mitral and tricuspid valves. For practical purposes it is considered synchronous with the beginning of systole, or ventricular contraction. The second heart sound, S2, results from closure of the aortic and pulmonic valves just after systole ends. S2 is taken as the beginning of diastole, or ventricular relaxation and refilling.

The first and second heart sounds heard at specific valve areas are sometimes so designated: A1, the first heart sound at the aortic valve area; P2, the second heart sound heard at the pulmonic valve area; and so on.

Cardiac **murmurs** are produced by turbulence in the flow of blood passing forward through a stenotic valve, leaking back through an incompetent valve, or crossing from a place of higher pressure to a place of lower pressure through an abnormal orifice, such as an interventricular septal defect. The diagnostician characterizes a murmur by recording its location (the point on the chest wall where it is heard best); its radiation or transmission (for example, to the carotid arteries or left

axilla); its character, intensity (graded on a scale of 1 to 6; less often, 1 to 4), and duration; and its timing within the cardiac cycle. Valvular clicks and snaps are similarly characterized.

A Doctor's View

Cardiology and Cardiovascular Surgery

by Michael J. O'Donnell, M.D.

Cardiology and cardiovascular surgery are both concerned with the diagnosis and treatment of diseases of the heart, great vessels, and peripheral circulation. The difference between cardiologists and cardiovascular surgeons lies in the methods used to treat these diseases.

The cardiologist is, by training, an internist who specializes in the diagnosis and medical treatment of cardiovascular disease. The cardiac surgeon specializes in the surgical treatment of cardiovascular disease. In no other area of medicine does an internist work so closely with a surgeon as in the management of cardiovascular disease.

Cardiologists must rely on their cardiovascular surgeon colleagues when surgical intervention is needed in the treatment of their patients. Similarly, cardiovascular surgeons rely on their cardiologist colleagues for the majority of their case referrals. The cardiologist and cardiovascular surgeon collaborate during a surgical procedure if the patient develops hemodynamic instability or refractory cardiac arrhythmia, and also during the postoperative period in the routine management of the cardiac surgery patient. Thus there is considerable overlap between the two specialties.

Cardiac Catheterization. This is an invasive technique (Figure 8.4) that requires the introduction of a diagnostic catheter through a peripheral vessel, under fluoroscopic guidance, into the various cardiac chambers.

By this means, pressure readings can be taken directly from a variety of sites. Placement of the catheter in the coronary ostia (openings) and injection of contrast medium permits radiographic visualization and recording of the coronary blood flow on motion picture film (coronary cineangiography).

The purpose of all of these cardiac diagnostic studies is to strive to treat the patient medically. In about half of the patients, however, an invasive therapy will be indicated. This may include coronary artery angioplasty, balloon valvuloplasty, or cardiac surgery either with coronary artery bypass grafting or repair or replacement of a valve.

Cardiovascular Surgery. The simplest cardiovascular surgical procedure is carotid endarterectomy. This involves opening up a segment of the internal carotid artery that has become obstructed by atherosclerotic disease, causing intermittent neurologic problems. In this procedure, the diseased portion of the artery is exposed via a surgical incision in the lateral aspect of the neck. Once the carotid artery is exposed, it is clamped above and below the obstruction. Then an incision is made into the vessel and the atherosclerotic material is peeled away.

The incision in the vessel is sutured, the clamps are removed, and the skin is sewn closed. During this procedure, the patient is under general anesthesia but does not require the use of a heart-lung bypass machine.

The most difficult kind of cardiac surgery is repair of congenital heart defects in the infant. The surgery is technically difficult, as extensive cardiac remodeling must often be done to correct these complex abnormalities. The best example of an involved procedure in regular use would be the Mustard operation to correct **tetralogy of Fallot** (pulmonary stenosis, ventricular septal defect, dextroposition of the aorta, and right ventricular hypertrophy). In addition, the smallness of the patient contributes to the difficulty encountered in performing the surgery.

Cardiopulmonary Bypass. The purpose of the heart-lung bypass machine is to take over the patient's cardiac and pulmonary function while surgery is being performed on the heart. The machine includes a pumping mechanism to maintain blood pressure and circulation to vital organs. In addition, the machine functions as an oxygenator since the lungs are bypassed once the patient's heart is placed in cardiac arrest. Oxygen taken from the hospital's oxygen supply lines diffuses across a bubble oxygenator which comes in contact with the patient's blood as it passes through the cardiopulmonary bypass machine.

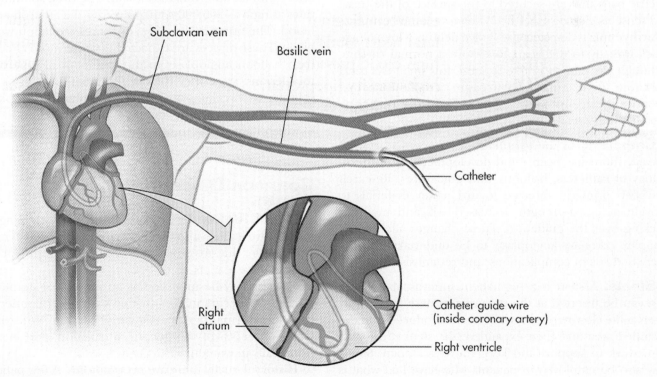

Subclavian vein

Basilic vein

Catheter

Right atrium

Catheter guide wire (inside coronary artery)

Right ventricle

Figure 8-4
Cardiac Catheterization

During this time the patient's red blood cells derive adequate oxygen from the machine even though the lungs are not functioning. Thus the surgeon can perform an intricate procedure on a nonbeating heart without jeopardizing the patient's vital organs.

Heart Transplant. Developments in the area of cardiac transplantation are currently centered on the production of new immunosuppressive drugs. The most common medical problem encountered in the treatment of cardiac transplant patients is rejection of the transplanted heart. Therefore, most investigative efforts are focused on development of newer classes of immunosuppressive agents that are specific for preventing rejection of the newly transplanted heart but do not suppress the patient's host defenses against life-threatening infections.

Pacemakers. New developments are occurring almost daily in the refinement of cardiac pacemakers. Pacemakers that can respond to the patient's metabolic work demands, as a normal heart would, are currently being evaluated. These ingenious devices are able to maintain variable heart rates depending on the body's demands in skeletal muscle activity, changes in core temperature, and changes in overall blood flow.

Defibrillators. Patients who have ventricular arrhythmias that do not respond to medical treatment are now given new hope with the development of automatic implantable cardiac defibrillators. These devices have electric pads that are secured to the surface of the heart and sense its electrical activity. When a sustained ventricular arrhythmia is detected, the device delivers a low-voltage shock directly to the heart to restore a normal rhythm. Although the patient is able to sense this small electrical discharge, this is a small price to pay in view of the fact that the odds are against surviving a cardiac arrest occurring outside the hospital.

Catheters. In the treatment of intracardiac arterial disease, there has been rapid development in the technology of catheters, balloons, and guidewires. Research has been primarily directed toward newer materials to provide increased strength, decreased bulk, and smoother tracking over the guidewire. These changes allow more complex coronary angioplasty to be undertaken with a decreased risk of complications and restenosis.

Stents. A stent is a permanent intravascular device that can be inserted at the time of coronary angioplasty when acute closure of a vessel occurs. Introduced into the occluded area and then expanded, the stent provides a framework to support and keep the vessel open. Stents may also be employed in patients who have had what is termed a chronic restenosis. These patients have undergone repeated angioplasty procedures for the same coronary artery lesion that continues to reappear despite multiple dilatations. The stent may be inserted immediately after balloon dilatation to form a supporting framework that will not allow the vessel to restenose.

Lasers. There is continuing research in the area of laser ablation (eradication and removal with a laser) of coronary artery lesions. Various kinds of laser systems are under development. These include laser catheters that have a metal cap tip in which laser energy is used to heat the cap to extremely high temperatures so that it can melt through atheromatous lesions.

Other catheter systems have what is termed direct laser energy emerging from the catheter tip to cut a channel through the atheromatous lesion. These catheters are currently able to reestablish only a small channel through an otherwise totally or subtotally occluded atheromatous lesion. After this procedure, a balloon catheter is advanced through the new channel, and balloon angioplasty is performed to make a larger channel for blood flow.

Another type of laser system is a laser balloon, which is essentially an angioplasty dilatation catheter with the capability of diffusing laser energy through the internal balloon surface outward to the endothelium of the coronary artery in contact with the balloon.

Other Devices. Mechanical ablation devices consist of either drill bits or coring tools that are placed into an artery with an atheromatous lesion. The drill, spinning at rates as high as 200,000 rpm, pulverizes the atheromatous lesion. The other device cores or shaves the lesion with a blade. These devices are expected to prove more effective than balloon angioplasty in the treatment of atheromatous lesions, since they remove the lesion instead of just splitting or breaking it apart as in balloon angioplasty. Cardiology is an exciting, rapidly expanding field, and one of which I am proud to be a part.

Common Diseases

Mitral Valve Prolapse. Abnormal bulging of mitral valve leaflets into the left atrium during left ventricular systole, due to structurally abnormal (floppy or billowing) valve leaflets.

Causes: May be inherited as an autosomal dominant trait. Often occurs in conjunction with other connective tissue abnormalities, particularly Marfan syndrome. Occurs in 1-5% of the general population, and is seen principally in women.

History: Usually there are no symptoms. A few patients experience nonspecific chest pain, palpitations with or without actual arrhythmia, dyspnea on exertion, fatigue, and syncope.

Physical Examination: Variable murmurs: usually midsystolic click and late systolic murmur. The patient may present other stigmata of connective tissue abnormality: thin body habitus, high palate, deformities of the chest wall (pectus excavatum, scoliosis).

Diagnostic Studies: Echocardiography confirms valve prolapse and indicates whether actual regurgitation occurs.

Course: Most patients have no symptoms and no complications. Rarely, regurgitation may have serious hemodynamic consequences. Endocarditis may develop on the mitral valve. Atrial fibrillation may occur. Sudden death may result from ectopic ventricular rhythms (**ventricular tachycardia**).

Treatment: Antibiotic prophylaxis of endocarditis before dental work and surgery. Beta-blockers usually control chest pain and arrhythmias. Rarely, surgical valve replacement.

Aortic Stenosis. Abnormal narrowing of the aortic valve opening, with reduction of left ventricular ejection volume during systole.

Causes: May be a consequence of acute rheumatic fever, but usually results from calcification of the valve with aging. Most patients are men over 50.

History: Weakness, dyspnea, chest pain, palpitations, syncope.

Physical Examination: Carotid pulsations are reduced. A precordial thrill may be noted. The second heart sound is reduced or absent. A harsh "diamond-shaped" (crescendo-decrescendo) murmur is heard at the base of the heart and transmitted to the carotids and cardiac apex.

Diagnostic Tests: Chest x-ray may show left ventricular dilatation and calcification of the aortic valve. Electrocardiogram, Doppler echocardiogram, and cardiac catheterization provide more precise and quantitative information.

Course: Left ventricular failure, arrhythmias, angina, syncope.

Treatment: Surgical replacement of the valve. Balloon dilatation of the valve may be successful.

Infective Endocarditis (Acute and Subacute Bacterial Endocarditis). Bacterial infection of one or more heart valves.

Cause: Usually, the combination of preexisting congenital or acquired valvular disease or abnormal communications (septal defects) and bacteremia (after dental or surgical procedures or in systemic infection or septicemia).

History: Fever, chills, dyspnea, cough, abdominal pain, muscle or joint pain.

Physical Examination: Fever, pallor. Audible cardiac murmur, or change in quality or loudness of a preexisting murmur. Signs of peripheral embolization of infective material (vegetations) from heart valves: petechiae of the palate and conjunctivae, splinter hemorrhages under fingernails, **Osler nodes** (tender purplish lumps in fingers, toes), **Janeway spots** (painless red spots of palms and soles), **Roth spots** (retinal exudates). Splenomegaly.

Diagnostic Tests: Anemia, leukocytosis, hematuria, proteinuria. Blood cultures may permit identification of the organism. Chest x-ray, electrocardiogram, echocardiogram supply diagnostic information.

Course: Valve leaflets may ulcerate and slough, with severe impairment of cardiac function. Fragments of infectious material (septic emboli) may be carried to brain, heart, kidney, and other tissues, or to the lung, causing local infective vascular lesions (mycotic aneurysms).

Treatment: Intravenous antibiotics for several weeks. Surgery may be undertaken in very severe cases.

Angina Pectoris. Paroxysmal chest pain due to myocardial ischemia, without permanent damage to heart muscle.

Cause: The primary cause is narrowing of one or more coronary arteries by arteriosclerosis. Arteritis, congenital vascular anomalies, emboli, severe anemia, cardiac hypertrophy, and cocaine intoxication can also lead to signs and symptoms of inadequate coronary blood flow. Risk factors for development of coronary arteriosclerosis include a family history of the disease, male gender, hypertension, cigarette smoking, diabetes mellitus, overweight, a sedentary lifestyle, and elevation of total cholesterol, LDL cholesterol, homocysteine, lipoprotein (a), or C-reactive protein.

History: Angina pectoris is a syndrome of anterior chest pain coming on abruptly and resolving spontaneously in less than 30 minutes. Pain is typically precipitated by physical exertion, strong emotion, exposure to cold, or eating a meal, and is relieved by rest or by taking nitroglycerin. The pain is described as a tightness, squeezing, or pressure; the patient often expresses this by holding a clenched fist in front of the chest. The pain may radiate into the neck, jaw, or arm, particularly the left. A variant, Prinzmetal angina, occurs at rest and is more common in women and younger patients than typical angina.

Physical Examination: There may be no abnormal findings, but the blood pressure is often elevated by pain and anxiety. Examination may disclose signs of underlying cardiovascular or systemic disease.

Diagnostic Tests: The electrocardiogram may be normal during an attack, but usually shows ST-segment depression and flattened or inverted T waves, indicating myocardial ischemia. There may also be evidence of conduction defects or ventricular hypertrophy. Holter monitoring allows recording of the ECG continuously for 24 hours. Stress testing records the electrocardiogram during standardized and closely supervised physical exertion. Angiography demonstrates narrowing of coronary vessels. Other studies (myocardial perfusion scintigraphy, radionuclide angiography, and echocardiography) can supply further information about the location and extent of coronary disease.

Course: Gradual progression to more severe disease (myocardial infarction, congestive heart failure) usually occurs, even with treatment. Unstable angina, which worsens with time despite treatment, has a less favorable prognosis.

Treatment: The standard treatment for an anginal attack is sublingual (under the tongue) nitroglycerin, which promptly abolishes pain of coronary ischemia by producing dilatation in the coronary arteries. Nitroglycerin can also be taken prophylactically before physical exertion. Longer-acting nitrate preparations, beta-blocking agents, and calcium-channel blockers taken regularly can prevent or mitigate attacks. Most patients are advised to take aspirin daily for its effect in inhibiting platelet aggregation and reducing the risk of myocardial infarction.

Coronary artery bypass graft (CABG) uses veins or other materials to conduct blood past narrowed places in coronary arteries. Percutaneous transluminal coronary angioplasty (PTCA, balloon angioplasty) dilates narrowed places with a balloon passed into the circulation through an arterial catheter. A metal stent implanted at the time of angioplasty may provide long-term freedom from restenosis.

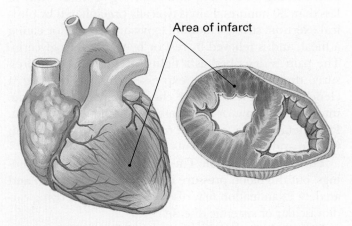

Area of infarct

Figure 8-5
Myocardial Infarction, Cross Section

Myocardial Infarction (Heart Attack, Coronary Thrombosis).

Damage to a segment of heart muscle by severe impairment of coronary blood flow (Figure 8-5).

Causes: The underlying causes are the same as for angina pectoris. Myocardial infarction (MI) is usually due to thrombosis in a coronary artery already narrowed by arteriosclerosis. Arteritis, vasospasm, embolism, sudden hypotension, or cocaine can also precipitate infarction.

History: Anterior chest pain, similar to angina but generally more severe and lasting more than 30 minutes. Pain often comes on at rest and is not relieved by nitroglycerin. Typically, men experience sweating, weakness, restlessness, shortness of breath, and nausea. Women may experience the same symptoms or may perceive jaw or shoulder discomfort and/or chest tightness or discomfort without actual crushing pain. Rarely, infarction occurs without pain (silent infarction).

Physical Examination: The pulse and blood pressure may be increased, normal, or decreased. Mild fever often develops after the first 12 hours. The heart sounds may be soft or distant. An **atrial gallop** (fourth heart sound) is often heard. A **seagull murmur** of mitral regurgitation indicates rupture of a papillary muscle. The cardiac rhythm may be abnormal. A pericardial friction rub is often heard. Jugular venous distention and rales of pulmonary edema are seen in heart failure.

Diagnostic Tests: The electrocardiogram shows ST-segment elevation (changing later to depression) and inversion of T waves in leads pertaining to the area of infarction. Q waves indicate severe myocardial damage and a graver prognosis. The white blood cell count may be slightly elevated. Serial determination of the serum levels of the cardiac enzymes LDH (lactic dehydrogenase), CK-MB (the MB isoenzyme of creatine kinase), myoglobin, and troponins (C, I, and T) show characteristic rises. Fluoroscopy or other imaging techniques may show segmental wall motion at the site of infarction. Scintigraphy with technetium 99m pyrophosphate shows a hot spot at the site. Doppler echocardiography may also confirm the extent and location of infarction.

Course: About 20% of persons who sustain myocardial infarction die before reaching a hospital. With intensive therapy, the prognosis for the other 80% is good. During the acute phase, arrhythmia, shock, and congestive heart failure are serious possibilities. Other dangerous complications include rupture of papillary muscle (one of the muscles in the ventricles that control movements of the mitral and tricuspid valves) with resulting serious valvular malfunction, cardiorrhexis (bursting of the ventricle), left **ventricular aneurysm** (extreme dilatation and thinning of the ventricle, with loss of contractile power), pericarditis, and formation of a **mural thrombus** (a localized clot adjacent to the infarcted area of ventricular wall).

Treatment: The standard treatment protocol includes hospitalization, administration of oxygen by inhalation and of narcotics for pain relief by injection, and continuous electrocardiographic monitoring. Thrombolytic agents (tPA [tissue plasminogen activator], streptokinase, or anistreplase) are administered intravenously to dissolve clots. Anticoagulants (aspirin, IV heparin) may also be administered. Beta-blocking agents are started early. In some centers, balloon angioplasty is performed during the acute phase of myocardial infarction.

Congestive Heart Failure (CHF). A syndrome of impaired hemodynamics due to inability of the heart to maintain normal circulation.

Causes: Any condition that impairs the contractile force of the heart (ischemia due to coronary artery disease; myocarditis) or that overtaxes a normal heart (systemic or pulmonary hypertension, congenital or acquired valvular disease, hyperthyroidism). Right ventricular failure may be due to pulmonary hypertension or cor pulmonale. A distinction is sometimes made between **forward failure** (inability of the heart to pump blood at a volume that is adequate for the needs of tissues) and **backward failure** (inability of the heart to distend adequately during diastole, with resulting increase of pressure in the venous system). Purely mechanical inadequacy of heart function is complicated by inappropriate hormonal and biochemical responses, including increase of peripheral vascular resistance due to sympathetic vasoconstriction and retention of sodium and water due to release of renin from kidneys whose blood flow is diminished.

History: Shortness of breath, particularly on exertion; orthopnea, paroxysmal nocturnal dyspnea, cough; fatigue, nocturia; anorexia and right upper quadrant fullness due to hepatic engorgement; ankle edema.

Physical Examination: Dyspnea, cyanosis, tachycardia, hypotension. Jugular venous distention. Left ventricular dilatation and hypertrophy. Diminished first heart sound. S3 gallop. Expiratory wheezes and rhonchi. Crepitant rales at bases; reduced breath sounds and dullness to percussion may indicate pleural effusion. Hepatomegaly, **hepatojugular reflux** (bulging of jugular veins when the liver is compressed because of increased pressure in the venous system). Pitting edema of the lower extremities, ascites.

Diagnostic Tests: The red blood cell count may be diminished. The electrocardiogram may indicate myocardial infarction, arrhythmia, or left ventricular hypertrophy. Echocardiography gives more precise information about ventricular size and function. Chest x-ray shows cardiomegaly, signs of pulmonary venous congestion (fine lines at the periphery of the lungs due to edema of pulmonary alveolar septa, called **Kerley B lines**), and sometimes pleural effusion. Radionuclide angiography shows that the **ventricular ejection fraction** (the fraction of the blood contained in the ventricle that is expelled during systole) is reduced.

Course: Congestive heart failure indicates a serious impairment of cardiovascular dynamics, and even with treatment the course is often steadily downhill. The prognosis for long-term survival is poor, and death often occurs suddenly.

Treatment: Rest, salt restriction, and early correction of identifiable precipitating factors. Diuretics (thiazides, loop diuretics, potassium-sparing diuretics), ACE inhibitors, and beta-blockers are used to reverse biochemical imbalances and hormonal effects that lead to sodium retention and circulatory volume overload. Digitalis glycosides increase the force of cardiac contraction.

Cardiomyopathy, Myocardiopathy. General terms for cardiac disorders that arise primarily from diseases of the heart muscle (myocardium) rather than from coronary artery disease, systemic or pulmonary hypertension, valvular disease, or congenital structural abnormality.

Cardiomyopathies vary widely in cause, pathophysiology, and clinical presentation and can accompany or complicate other cardiac disorders.

The heart muscle is vulnerable to damage by a broad range of harmful influences, including infection (viral, parasitic, rickettsial), drugs and toxins (cancer chemotherapy agents, alcohol, cocaine, arsenic), radiation, metabolic disorders (amyloidosis, hemochromatosis, glycogen storage diseases), connective tissue disorders (systemic lupus erythematosus, scleroderma), generalized diseases of muscle (muscular dystrophy), and deficiency states (beriberi, due to lack of dietary thiamine). Most cases of cardiomyopathy are, however, idiopathic. Some types of hypertrophic cardiomyopathy are familial and are associated with the risk of sudden death at an early age.

Depending on its cause, cardiomyopathy can present as a dilated, flabby heart with poor contractility and diminished **ejection fraction** (EF) or as a thick-walled, hypertrophic heart with inadequate diastolic relaxation and filling. Most patients develop some degree of congestive heart failure, with dyspnea, tachycardia, and pulmonary or peripheral edema, and the typical physical findings outlined in the preceding section. Other symptoms may include chest pain, palpitation, and syncope.

Diagnosis is by ECG, echocardiography, and cardiac catheterization. Apart from standard measures to combat cardiac failure, drug therapy of myocardiopathies is of marginal effectiveness.

Treatment consists of either a heart transplant or making appropriate lifestyle changes, providing general support, and eliminating underlying disorders when possible. The prognosis for long-term survival in most forms of cardiomyopathy is poor.

Acute Pulmonary Edema. An extreme form of left ventricular failure in which respiratory symptoms predominate. It can be precipitated by acute myocardial infarction or by any factors that increase the severity of existing cardiac failure. There are severe dyspnea, cough, and wheezing, with frothy pink sputum. The pulse is rapid and weak, the lips and nail beds cyanotic. Auscultation reveals rales and rhonchi in the lungs. The arterial oxygen is low. Chest x-ray shows cardiomegaly, increased vascular markings, Kerley B lines, pleural effusion. Treatment includes oxygen by inhalation, morphine, and intravenous diuretics.

Shock. A condition in which the systemic blood pressure is too low to maintain adequate tissue perfusion.

Causes: Hypovolemia (reduced blood volume due to hemorrhage, dehydration, severe burns, ascites); cardiogenic (impairment of cardiac function by arrhythmia, myocardial infarction, myocarditis, acute valvular failure); vascular obstruction (pericardial tamponade, pulmonary embolism); dilatation of the circulatory system (septic shock, anaphylactic shock, toxic shock syndrome, neurogenic shock, drugs).

History: Weakness, palpitations, thirst, sweating, anxiety, loss of consciousness.

Physical Examination: The blood pressure is low and the pulse rapid. Peripheral pulses are weak or absent. The **tilt test** is positive (rise in pulse and drop in blood pressure when patient is moved from recumbent to erect position). In hypovolemic shock the skin is pale, cold, and clammy. In septic shock there may be high fever and flushing. Agitation, confusion, and deteriorating level of consciousness.

Diagnostic Tests: Procedures used during early treatment to assess the degree of shock include blood tests (complete blood count, electrolytes, arterial blood gases), urine flow, cardiac monitoring, and central venous pressure or pulmonary wedge pressure with Swan-Ganz catheter.

Course: Without treatment shock may lead to irreversible damage: cerebral ischemia and infarction, myocardial infarction, renal failure.

Treatment: Vigorous treatment is required to maintain tissue perfusion and prevent irreversible consequences. The patient is placed in the **Trendelenburg position** (head lower than feet), and oxygen is administered. Morphine sulfate is given for pain (unless there is respiratory depression or head injury). Volume replacement with blood, plasma, or artificial plasma expanders in hypovolemic shock. Treatment of underlying conditions. Compression of the arms, legs, and abdomen by an inflatable MAST (military antishock trousers) garment can maintain cerebral, coronary, and renal blood flow until bleeding or other underlying condition is controlled and blood volume restored. Dopamine, adrenal steroids, and other drugs may be administered.

Hypertension. Sustained elevation of arterial blood pressure above 140 mmHg systolic or 90 mmHg diastolic.

Cause: Unknown in more than 90% of cases, which are thus called essential hypertension. Essential hypertension shows a genetic pattern, running in families and being much commoner in African Americans. Its development may depend on environmental factors, excessive dietary salt, sodium retention by the kidney, abnormalities of the renin-angiotensin system, obesity, alcohol abuse, and use of NSAIDs. Secondary hypertension is due to a demonstrable cause: renal parenchymal disease, renal ischemia, Cushing disease, primary aldosteronism, pheochromocytoma, or estrogen use in the form of oral contraceptives.

History: There may be no symptoms whatsoever until complications develop.

Physical Examination: Elevated blood pressure and accentuation of the second heart sound at the aortic valve area; otherwise there may be no findings. Retinopathy is indicated by detection of **Keith-Wagener-Barker changes** on ophthalmoscopic examination. Left ventricular hypertrophy may be indicated by precordial heave or by a systolic ejection murmur.

Diagnostic Tests: Laboratory studies may be normal. The search for a cause of secondary hypertension includes testing blood and urine for signs of renal disease.

Course: Some hypertensive patients experience a return of blood pressure to normal after a few weeks, months, or years. In most, however, elevation of blood pressure remains throughout life. Hypertension causes several forms of damage to the cardiovascular system (hypertensive cardiovascular disease), including left ventricular hypertrophy and dysfunction, arteriosclerosis, dilatation and dissecting aneurysm of the aorta, hypertensive encephalopathy, and hypertensive renal disease. In accelerated or malignant hypertension there is sustained high blood pressure responding poorly to treatment, and rapid progression of cardiovascular damage.

Treatment: Therapy of essential hypertension ideally includes lifestyle modification (reduction of alcohol intake, increased physical exercise), restriction of dietary salt, and control of overweight. Drug therapy is tailored to the severity of the disease, and typically starts with a single drug (a thiazide diuretic or a beta-blocker), others being added as needed: ACE inhibitors, angiotensin II receptor inhibitors, calcium channel blockers, methyldopa, alpha-

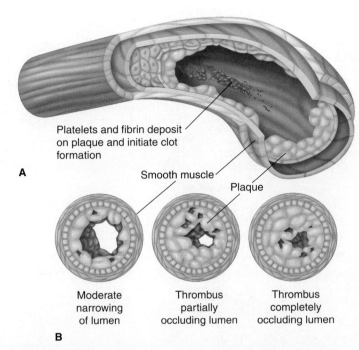

Platelets and fibrin deposit on plaque and initiate clot formation

Smooth muscle

Plaque

A

Moderate narrowing of lumen

Thrombus partially occluding lumen

Thrombus completely occluding lumen

B

Figure 8-6
Thrombus Formation in an Atherosclerotic Vessel:
(A) Initial Clot Formation, (B) Varying Degrees of Occlusion

receptor antagonists, guanethidine, and drugs of other classes.

Atherosclerosis. Hardening and even calcification of arterial walls, with narrowing of their lumens (see Figure 8-6).

Cause: Inflammation and degeneration of arterial walls, with diffuse or plaquelike deposition of cholesterol crystals in the tunica intima (inner lining) of systemic arteries. Various inborn metabolic abnormalities in lipoproteins may predispose to abnormal elevation of serum cholesterol level and abnormal deposition of cholesterol in arterial walls. (Involvement of coronary and cerebral arteries in the same process is a principal cause of coronary artery disease and cerebrovascular disease.)

History: Intermittent claudication: cramping muscle pain in calves, thighs, buttocks (depending on site of arterial obstruction) that is brought on by walking and relieved by rest. Erectile dysfunction.

Physical Examination: Weakness or absence of femoral, popliteal, or pedal pulses. Bruit over aorta, iliac or femoral arteries. Trophic changes (loss of hair, thinning of skin, pigmentation).

Diagnostic Tests: Evidence of reduced blood flow can be obtained by Doppler ultrasonography, transcutaneous oximetry, or other measures.

Treatment: Physical therapy and treatment with pentoxifylline or other agents may improve exercise tolerance slightly. Surgical treatment (endarterectomy or arterial

grafting) yields much better results. Percutaneous transluminal angioplasty (balloon dilatation) is effective in selected cases.

Deep Vein Thrombophlebitis. Inflammation in the wall of a tributary of one of the common iliac veins in the pelvis or lower limb, associated with clotting of blood within the vein.

Causes: Congestive heart failure, sudden immobilization because of recent surgery or injury, oral contraceptives, malignancy.

History: Pain or tightness in the calf or thigh, with edema distally. There may be no symptoms until pulmonary embolism occurs.

Physical Examination: Distal edema may be the only objective sign. There may be pain or tenderness on calf rocking, or a positive **Homans sign** (calf pain or tightness on passive dorsiflexion of the foot).

Diagnostic Tests: Doppler ultrasonography, impedance plethysmography, and venography confirm, localize, and quantify venous obstruction.

Course: There is considerable danger of pulmonary embolism. Healing may be followed by deep venous insufficiency, with chronic edema.

Treatment: Hospitalization. Intravenous or low-dose intramuscular heparin and oral anticoagulant.

Diagnostic and Surgical Procedures

aneurysm resection Surgical removal of a segment of vessel that has an abnormal ballooning and threatens to rupture.

arteriogram Injection of radiopaque dye directly into an artery to obtain x-rays of the vessel and its branches.

balloon angioplasty Stretching or breaking up atherosclerotic plaques in coronary arteries.

bypass See *coronary artery bypass graft.*

cardiac catheterization A procedure that involves passing a flexible catheter through the femoral artery and into the heart to measure pressures within the heart's chambers. Dye is then injected to show patency or obstruction of the coronary arteries.

carotid endarterectomy Removal of hardened plaque from an obstructed carotid artery.

commissurotomy Surgical enlargement of the aperture of a stenotic heart valve, particularly the mitral, by stretching or cutting.

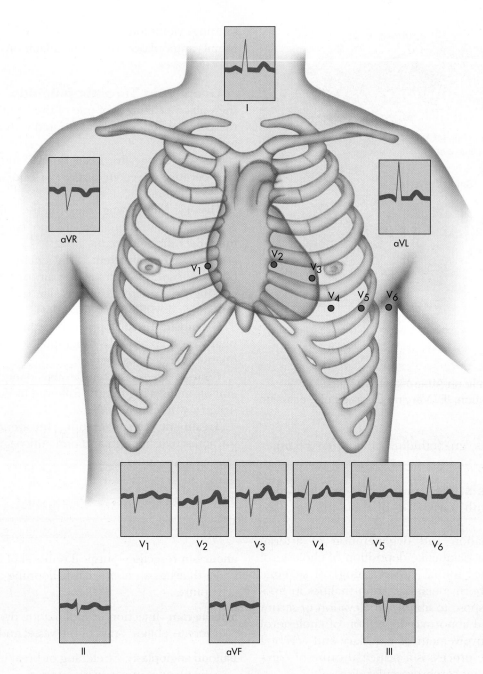

Figure 8-7
Electrocardiogram Tracing

coronary artery bypass graft (CABG) Surgical procedure done to bypass one or more occluded coronary arteries by using a vein graft (often from the leg).

CPR (cardiopulmonary resuscitation) The use of external compression of the heart coupled with breathing techniques to revive a victim whose heart and respirations have stopped.

ECG, EKG (electrocardiogram) A tracing of the electrical activity of the heart (Figure 8-7). An EKG traces

the conduction of the electrical impulse generated by the SA node as it travels through the atria (P wave on the EKG) and through the ventricles (QRS complex on the EKG). Then, during the recovery period as the heart prepares to contract again, the T wave is evident on the EKG. As this electrical impulse travels through the heart, it can be detected on the skin by EKG electrodes.

The basic EKG records 12 leads. Three peripheral electrodes are placed: on the right arm, left arm, and left leg. Six other electrodes are placed at precise locations on the chest around the heart area. The EKG technician can change from one lead to the next by using a dial on the EKG machine.

Leads I, II, and III (the so-called limb or bipolar leads) are obtained by simultaneously recording the electrical activity from the extremities. By combining the input from two of these three electrodes, the EKG machine generates a tracing for lead I (right arm and left arm,), lead II (right arm and left leg), and lead III (left arm and left leg).

The next three leads are called augmented leads because they increase or augment the amplitude or size of the tracing by 50%. The augmented leads are aVR (augmented voltage, right arm), aVL (augmented voltage, left arm), and aVF (augmented voltage, left foot).

The remaining six leads necessary to complete the 12-lead EKG are known as the precordial or chest leads. These electrodes are placed on the chest and are designated by a "V."

Lead V1 is positioned over the fourth intercostal space at the right sternal border and records the electrical activity of the right ventricle. Lead V2 is positioned over the fourth intercostal space at the left sternal border and records the electrical activity of the right ventricle. Lead V3 is positioned midway between V2 and V4 and records the electrical activity of the left ventricle. Lead V4 is positioned over the fifth intercostal space at the midclavicular line and records the electrical activity of the left ventricle. Lead V5 is positioned over the fifth intercostal space at the anterior axillary line and records the electrical activity of the left ventricle. Lead V6 is positioned over the fifth intercostal space at the midaxillary line and records the electrical activity of the left ventricle. Each of the 12 leads gives a different picture of the electrical condition of the heart.

echocardiography A noninvasive diagnostic procedure in which an ultrasonic beam is directed at the heart and the returning echoes are recorded and analyzed; valuable for the measurement of cardiac chambers (wall thickness and cavity volume), assessment of ventricular function, and identification of valvular malfunction.

exercise stress test Test during which the patient exercises on a treadmill to stress the heart and reproduce symptoms of angina and EKG changes.

femoral-popliteal bypass Implantation of a vessel graft (real or artificial) into the femoral and popliteal arteries to bypass one or more blockages.

Holter monitoring A continuously recorded EKG as monitored by a portable EKG machine worn by the patient. This procedure is done on an outpatient basis for 24 hours to detect arrhythmias.

"Nitro *Paste*"

Physicians often dictate "nitro paste" when the correct drug form is actually nitroglycerin ointment. The dosage of this coronary vasodilator is measured in inches of ointment (or fractions thereof) as it comes from the tube. The patient is supplied with disposable ruled applicators, with which the ointment is measured out and smeared over the skin in much the same way as one spreads mucilage or wallpaper paste—hence, probably, the popular misnomer "paste."

When "nitro paste" is dictated, "nitro" should be expanded to "nitroglycerin," and "paste" should be translated "ointment"—unless departmental rules forbid using the right words when the dictator uses the wrong ones. Note that the name of one brand of nitroglycerin, Nitrol, is easily mistaken for "nitro" in dictation.

Vera Pyle
Current Medical Terminology

MUGA scan Radiologic procedure in which a radioactive isotope is injected into the arteries with a subsequent scan showing uptake of the isotope by the heart. These radioactive emissions are electronically collected and analyzed by computer, resulting in a series of successive images all taken at the same point in the cardiac cycle. This test is used to assess heart size, shape, and function. MUGA stands for *multiple gated acquisition*.

pacemaker implantation Placement of pacemaker electrodes to the heart to correct heart block or control persistent irregular rhythms.

percutaneous transluminal angioplasty (PTA) Procedure used to dilate an occluded artery, usually a coronary artery, by passing a catheter (with a deflated balloon section) to the site of the occlusion and inflating the balloon to compress the obstruction and enlarge the lumen of the vessel.

treadmill stress test See *exercise stress test*.

valve replacement Excision and replacement of a valve of the heart because of stenosis or insufficiency.

vein stripping Surgical removal of (usually) the saphenous leg vein and its branches to treat varicose veins.

venipuncture Insertion of a needle into a vein for the purpose of removing blood for testing, or to inject fluids, medicines, or diagnostic materials.

Laboratory Procedures

cholesterol, serum A lipid (fatty) material formed in the liver and transported in the blood, which serves as a building block for various hormones and other substances. Elevation of serum cholesterol, which is usually due to an inherited disturbance of lipid metabolism, is associated with increased risk of atherosclerosis. See *HDL, LDL, VLDL.*

CPK (creatine phosphokinase) A serum enzyme that can be chemically distinguished into three isoenzymes or fractions: the BB isoenzyme is elevated in cerebral infarction, the MM in muscular dystrophy and muscle crush injury, and MB in myocardial infarction. When separated in the laboratory by electrophoresis, these isoenzymes appear as distinct bands in a visual display. Hence the expression *MB band* is roughly synonymous with *MB isoenzyme*. Do not confuse *creatine* with *creatinine.*

HDL (high-density lipoproteins) Lipid-carrying serum proteins associated with a relatively low risk of cholesterol deposition in arteries.

isoenzyme Any of a group of enzymes having similar chemical effects but differing in structure and often arising from different sources in the body. See *CPK, LDH.*

LDH Abbreviation for *lactic dehydrogenase,* an isoenzyme. LDH1 is found in heart muscle; levels are increased after myocardial infarction. LDH2 is normally found in higher amounts in the serum than is LDH1. When the level of LDH1 surpasses that of LDH2, this is called a "flipped LDH." *LDH* need not be translated in reports.

lipoproteins, serum Serum proteins that bind and transport lipid materials including cholesterol.

LDL (low-density lipoproteins) Lipid-carrying serum proteins associated with a relatively high risk of cholesterol deposition in arteries.

MB bands See *creatine phosphokinase.*

VLDL Abbreviation for *very low-density lipoproteins.*

Pharmacology

The drug treatment of cardiovascular disease is an exceedingly complex topic. Not only are diseases of the heart and circulation treated with many different kinds of drugs, but many of those drugs are effective in a variety of disorders, including ischemic coronary syndromes, congestive heart failure, hypertension, arrhythmia, and peripheral vascular disease. Nearly all patients with circulatory disorders receive balanced combinations of three or more drugs whose dosages, effects, and interactions must be tailored to individual needs.

Cardiac glycosides derived from the foxglove plant (*Digitalis lanata* and other species) were among the earliest drugs shown to have a favorable effect in heart disease, strengthening and steadying the beat of the failing heart. Digitalis (often abridged to *dig,* which rhymes with *bridge*) is a general term for drugs of this class. Because of unpredictable dosage requirements and a considerable risk of toxicity (including nausea and potentially dangerous cardiac arrhythmias), blood levels of these agents may need frequent checking. Though largely supplanted nowadays by safer and more specific drugs, cardiac glycosides still have a role in the management of congestive heart failure.

> digoxin (Lanoxin, Lanoxicaps)

Beta-blockers (beta-adrenergic blocking agents) reduce the stimulant effects of epinephrine and norepinephrine at various beta-adrenergic receptor sites in the circulatory system. They slow and stabilize the heart rate, diminish peripheral blood pressure, and reduce cardiac work and oxygen demand. They are widely used in the treatment of hypertension, angina pectoris, acute myocardial infarction, congestive heart failure, and some arrhythmias. The generic names of drugs in this class end in *-olol.*

> acebutolol (Sectral)
> atenolol (Tenormin)
> bisoprolol (Zebeta)
> esmolol (Brevibloc)
> metoprolol (Lopressor, Toprol-XL)
> nadolol (Corgard)
> pindolol (Visken)
> propranolol (Inderal)
> sotalol (Betapace)
> timolol (Blocadren)

Alpha-blockers (alpha-adrenergic blocking agents) are used principally in the treatment of hypertension.

> clonidine (Catapres, Duraclon)
> doxazosin mesylate (Cardura)
> guanabenz (Wytensin)
> guanadrel (Hylorel)
> guanethidine (Ismelin)
> guanfacine (Tenex)
> methyldopa (Aldomet)
> phenoxybenzamine (Dibenzyline)
> prazosin (Minipress)
> reserpine (Serpasil)
> terazosin (Hytrin)

A noncardioselective drug that blocks both alpha and beta adrenergic receptors is carvedilol (Coreg), used in the treatment of hypertension and congestive heart failure.

Calcium channel blockers. These drugs reduce heart rate and blood pressure and inhibit certain cardiac arrhythmias by blocking the passage of calcium ions across biologic membranes. They are used in the treatment of hypertension, angina pectoris, peripheral vascular disease, and some arrhythmias.

> amlodipine (Norvasc)
> diltiazem (Cardizem, Dilacor XR)
> felodipine (Plendil)
> nicardipine (Cardene)
> nifedipine (Adalat, Procardia)
> verapamil (Calan, Covera-HS, Isoptin, Verelan)

ACE (angiotensin-converting enzyme) inhibitors block the synthesis of angiotensin II, a hormone with vasoconstrictor and smooth muscle stimulant effects. Drugs in this class promote vasodilatation, decreasing pulmonary and peripheral vascular resistance and hence arterial pressure and cardiac work.

They are used in the treatment of hypertension and congestive heart failure. The generic names of drugs in this class end in -*pril*.

> benazepril (Lotensin)
> captopril (Capoten)
> enalapril (Vasotec)
> fosinopril (Monopril)
> lisinopril (Prinivil, Zestril)
> moexipril (Univasc)
> quinapril (Accupril)
> ramipril (Altace)
> trandolapril (Mavik)

Angiotensin II (two) **receptor antagonists** block the stimulant effect of angiotensin II on vascular smooth muscle. They are useful in the treatment of hypertension and left ventricular hypertrophy, particularly in patients intolerant to ACE inhibitors. The generic names of drugs in this class all end in -*sartan*.

> candesartan (Atacand)
> eprosartan (Teveten)
> irbesartan (Avapro)
> losartan (Cozaar)
> olmesartan (Benicar)
> valsartan (Diovan)

Nitrates are vasodilators, chiefly used to relieve the pain of angina pectoris by increasing coronary artery flow. All of the following are trade names for nitroglycerin. Their routes of administration are indicated.

> Nitro-Bid (sustained-release capsule)
> Nitrodisc (transdermal patch)
> Nitro-Dur (transdermal patch)
> Nitrogard (transmucosal tablet)
> Nitrol (topical ointment)
> Nitrolingual (sublingual spray)
> Transderm-Nitro (transdermal patch)
> Tridil (IV)

Other nitrates given orally include:

> isosorbide dinitrate (Isordil, Sorbitrate)
> isosorbide mononitrate (Imdur)

Diuretics promote an increase in the renal excretion of water, sodium, and other ions, thus reducing peripheral and pulmonary edema in congestive heart failure. They are also first-line agents in the treatment of essential hypertension. These drugs vary widely in their mechanisms of action and particularly in the circulating ions whose excretion they favor.

> amiloride (Midamor)
> bumetanide (Bumex)
> chlorothiazide (CTZ) Diuril
> chlorthalidone (Thalitone)
> eplerenone (Inspra)
> furosemide (Lasix)
> hydrochlorothiazide (HCTZ) (Esidrix,
>   HydroDIURIL, Microzide, Oretic)
> hydroflumethiazide (Diucardin)
> indapamide (Lozol)
> metolazone (Mykrox, Zaroxolyn)
> methyclothiazide (Enduron)
> spironolactone (Aldactone)
> torsemide (Demadex)
> triamterene (Dyrenium)

Each of the following antihypertensive drugs combines a diuretic with another antihypertensive agent. (Proprietary names are given first in this list.)

Aldactazide (spironolactone + HCTZ)
Aldoril (methyldopa + HCTZ)
Apresazide (hydralazine + HCTZ)
Combipres (clonidine + chlorthalidone)
Dyazide (triamterene + HCTZ)
Enduronyl (deserpidine + methyclothiazide)
Hydropres (reserpine + HCTZ)
Inderide (propranolol + HCTZ)
Moduretic (amiloride + HCTZ)
Renese-R (reserpine + polythiazide)
Salutensin (reserpine + hydroflumethiazide)
Tenoretic (atenolol + chlorthalidone)
Zestoretic (lisinopril + HCTZ)

Antiarrhythmic drugs. Cardiac arrhythmias can result from a variety of disturbances in the conduction system of the heart, and are treated with a correspondingly broad range of pharmacologic agents.

adenosine (Adenocard)
amiodarone (Cordarone)
bretylium (Bretylol)
disopyramide (Norpace)
flecainide (Tambocor)
ibutilide fumarate (Corvert)
lidocaine (Xylocaine)
mexiletine (Mexitil)
moricizine (Ethmozine)
procainamide (Procanbid, Pronestyl)
propafenone (Rythmol)
quinidine (Quinaglute Dura-Tabs, Quinidex)
tocainide (Tonocard)

Bile acid sequestrants promote the intestinal excretion of cholesterol and are used in the treatment of hypercholesterolemia.

cholestyramine (Prevalite, Questran)
colesevelam (Welchol)
colestipol (Colestid)

HMG CoA (3-hydroxy-3-methylglutaryl coenzyme A) reductase inhibitors block the synthesis of total cholesterol and LDL cholesterol. These drugs have been shown to delay progression of atherosclerosis and to decrease the risk of myocardial infarction and stroke in persons with hyperlipidemia. The generic names of drugs in this class end in *-statin*, and the drugs are collectively known as statins.

atorvastatin (Lipitor)
fluvastatin (Lescol)
lovastatin (Mevacor)
pravastatin (Pravachol)
simvastatin (Zocor)

Drugs that reduce serum triglyceride levels are used in selected hyperlipidemias.

clofibrate (Atromid-S)
fenofibrate (Tricor)
gemfibrozil (Lopid)

Vasopressors used in medicine are potent selective stimulants of arterial smooth muscle, increasing the heart rate, raising systemic blood pressure by boosting peripheral vascular resistance, but maintaining coronary and renal blood flow. Administered by continuous IV infusion, they are often valuable in the management of severe cardiovascular collapse

dobutamine (Dobutrex)
dopamine (Intropin)
isoproterenol (Isuprel)
norepinephrine (Levophed)

Anticoagulants are used to prevent thrombosis of coronary and cerebral arteries in persons at risk of myocardial infarction or stroke and to prevent or treat deep venous thrombosis (DVT).

anisindione (Miradon)
ardeparin (Normiflo)
dalteparin (Fragmin)
danaparoid (Organan)
dicumarol
enoxaparin (Lovenox)
heparin
warfarin (Coumadin)

Tissue plasminogen activators (tPA), synthesized by recombinant DNA technology, convert plasminogen in a blood clot to plasmin, which breaks down fibrin and so dissolves the clot. When administered within the first 2-3 hours after myocardial infarction, thrombotic stroke, and peripheral vascular occlusion, these drugs can restore blood flow. They are given intravenously.

alteplase (Activase)
reteplase (Retavase)

Thrombolytic enzymes are used for the same indications and also act by dissolving clots. They are given intravenously.

anistreplase (Eminase)
streptokinase (Kabikinase, Streptase)
urokinase (Abbokinase)

Transcribing Hematology Dictation

Hematology is the branch of medicine concerned with diagnosis and treatment of disorders of the formed elements of the blood (red blood cells, white blood cells, platelets) and of blood coagulation.

Red blood cells or erythrocytes are formed in bone marrow by repeated divisions of large cells called erythroblasts. Developing erythrocytes become gradually smaller, finally losing their nuclei just before being released into the circulation. The circulating erythrocyte is a round disc with both sides slightly hollowed, so that when seen on edge it has a dumbbell profile.

The function of the erythrocyte is to carry oxygen from the capillaries of the lungs to the capillaries of the rest of the body, and carbon dioxide from the tissues to the lungs for excretion. This chemical transport depends on hemoglobin, an iron-containing substance that is responsible for the red color of blood. An erythrocyte survives for about 120 days after entering the circulation. Then it disintegrates and is removed from the blood, principally by phagocytes in the spleen, which conserve and recycle its iron content.

White blood cells (leukocytes) are larger than erythrocytes and much less numerous in circulating blood, the ratio being about 600:1. Unlike erythrocytes, which perform their only function in circulating blood, leukocytes appear in the blood only when in transit from their point of production to their destination in tissues. All leukocytes have nuclei. They are divided into two major classes on the basis of the sites where they develop.

Although all leukocytes arise from precursor cells in the bone marrow, only myeloid leukocytes develop to maturity there. Leukocytes of myeloid origin are further divided into granulocytes, which show conspicuous granules in their cytoplasm, and monocytes, which do not. Granulocytes are also called polymorphonuclear leukocytes because their nuclei are typically divided by shallow clefts into two to five lobes. Granulocytes are subdivided according to the staining properties of their granules into neutrophils, eosinophils, and basophils.

Neutrophils, the most numerous of all white blood cells, have granules that show approximately equal affinity for acidic and basic stains. The function of neutrophils is to engulf and digest devitalized tissue, invading microorganisms, and other foreign material. Within minutes after injury, neutrophils begin to migrate from the blood into the affected tissue. The nuclei of immature neutrophils are elongated but not lobed. Such cells are called unsegmented neutrophils, stab cells, band cells, or simply bands.

Eosinophils, normally making up no more than 5% of circulating white blood cells, have coarse granules that attract eosin and other acid dyes. Their function is unknown but their numbers increase in parasitic infestation and allergic disorders, and decrease after administration of adrenocortical steroid drugs.

Basophils constitute 1% or less of circulating leukocytes. Their coarse granules stain with basic dyes. They produce histamine, serotonin, and other biochemically active substances. These three types of granulocytes (polymorphonuclear leukocytes) are formed in bone marrow by differentiation of precursor cells called myelocytes.

Monocytes are large cells that make up 5-8% of total circulating leukocytes. Their nuclei are large, kidney- or horseshoe-shaped, and eccentrically placed. Monocytes function as phagocytes in tissues and are perhaps identical with histiocytes.

Lymphocytes are white blood cells that develop from precursor cells in bone marrow but migrate to other tissues before maturing. They can be found in both lymphoid tissue (spleen, lymph nodes) and in the blood, where they normally make up about 25% of circulating white blood cells. Lymphocytes are slightly larger than erythrocytes and have relatively large, dark-staining nuclei. Their function is to produce antibodies, to modulate immune processes, and to perform other protective functions. Lymphocytes are divided into two major populations, designated B and T, whose activities are closely related.

B cells (B lymphocytes) migrate in an immature state from the marrow to lymphoid tissue. Here they undergo differentiation and maturation before moving to other lymphoid tissues via the bloodstream, where they constitute 5-15% of circulating lymphocytes. A mature B cell can synthesize antibodies in small amounts, but these remain attached to the cell surface. Under appropriate circumstances, however, B cells evolve into plasma cells, which produce antibodies in large amounts and release them into the circulation.

T cells (T lymphocytes) migrate from the marrow to the thymus for maturation before proceeding to other lymphoid organs and tissues. They make up 55-65% of circulating lymphocytes. On the basis of their surface proteins, T cells are subdivided into several types, each with its specific function.

Helper (or inducer) **T cells** stimulate or augment the production of antibody by B cells and plasma cells. Suppressor T cells modify or curb this production. **Cytotoxic** (killer) **T cells** destroy cells they recognize as antigenic.

A few large granular lymphocytes that are neither B nor T cells are known as **null cells**. Their functions are unknown, but some of them seem to operate as natural killer cells, attacking foreign cells directly without any true immune response.

Platelets are very small round or oval bodies found in circulating blood. They are formed in bone marrow as extrusions from the cytoplasm of giant cells with lobed nuclei called megakaryocytes. Platelets are not cells and do not have nuclei. They function in blood clotting.

Blood coagulates (clots) when the soluble plasma protein fibrinogen is converted to insoluble fibrin. Normally this occurs after another plasma protein, prothrombin, is converted to thrombin. Activation of prothrombin can come about through a number of alternative biochemical pathways, variously involving platelets, tissue factors, and plasma proteins other than prothrombin and fibrinogen. All known coagulation mechanisms require the presence of calcium. In addition, Factor V (labile factor), Factor VII (stable factor, proconvertin), Factor VIII (antihemophilic globulin, AHG), Factor IX (Christmas factor), Factor X (Stuart-Power factor), and Factor XI (plasma thromboplastin antecedent) are all necessary for normal coagulation.

Common Disorders of the Blood

Iron Deficiency Anemia. Anemia due to deficient iron stores; the most common type of anemia.

Cause: Depletion of iron stores usually results from chronic or recurring blood loss (gastrointestinal hemorrhage, menstruation, repeated blood donation). It can also occur in certain metabolic states (pregnancy, chronic infection) and, rarely, because of inadequate iron intake (vegetarians, dieters).

History: Fatigue, poor exercise tolerance, cardiac palpitation, shortness of breath. Dysphagia occurs in Plummer-Vinson syndrome (due to formation of esophageal webs). Pica (eating nonfood materials such as clay).

Physical Examination: Pallor, tachycardia, smooth tongue, brittle nails, cheilosis (chapping and fissuring of lips).

Diagnostic Tests: The red blood cell count is abnormally low. With advanced disease, cells become microcytic (smaller than normal; MCV reduced) and hypochromic (containing less hemoglobin than normal; MCH reduced). Abnormal cells, including target cells (cells so thin that the central portions of opposite sides touch, causing a bull's-eye appearance), may occur. The serum iron and serum ferritin are abnormally low. Administration of iron produces a prompt improvement in the red blood cell count, with elevated reticulocyte count. Diagnostic evaluation may include an aggressive search for a site of blood loss.

Treatment: Oral iron replacement continued for several months restores the red blood cell values and serum iron and ferritin to normal.

Pernicious Anemia. A chronic anemia due to deficiency of vitamin B_{12} absorption.

Cause: Pernicious anemia is an inherited autoimmune disorder that typically does not cause symptoms until after the age of 35. The biochemical cause is lack of secretion of intrinsic factor by glands in the gastric mucosa, with resultant failure to absorb vitamin B_{12}. All patients have gastric achlorhydria (lack of hydrochloric acid in gastric juice). Neurologic symptoms (ataxia, confusion, dementia) eventually occur.

History: Gradual onset of weakness, paresthesia in the fingers and toes, dysequilibrium, anorexia, sore tongue, and diarrhea.

Physical Examination: Pallor, icterus. The tongue appears red and smooth. Ataxic gait, diminished sense of vibration and position in extremities; later, loss of perception of light touch and pinprick.

Diagnostic Tests: The red blood cell count is low. Red blood cells are large (macrocytosis; increased MCV) and variable in size (anisocytosis). The reticulocyte count is low. Polymorphonuclear leukocytes have multilobulated nuclei. Bone marrow smear shows large precursors of red blood cells with abnormal morphology. The serum indirect bilirubin is elevated. The serum vitamin B_{12} is abnormally low. The Schilling test (administration of radioactively tagged B_{12} orally before and after administration of intrinsic factor) shows an increase in the urinary excretion of B_{12}. Endoscopy shows atrophic gastritis, and chemical studies indicate achlorhydria.

Course: This is an irreversible condition requiring lifelong treatment, without which neurologic damage may become irreversible. There is a heightened risk of gastric carcinoma in persons with achlorhydria.

Treatment: Administration of vitamin B_{12} regularly throughout life.

Aplastic Anemia. Failure of marrow production of red blood cells (also white blood cells and platelets).

Cause: Damage to bone marrow by chemicals (benzene), drugs (chloramphenicol), radiation, neoplastic infiltration, or autoantibodies.

History: Gradual onset of weakness, fatigue, dyspnea, headache.

Physical Examination: Pallor, purpura or petechiae, tachycardia, oral or pharyngeal infection or ulceration.

Diagnostic Tests: The red blood cell, white blood cell, and platelet counts are abnormally low. Marrow smear shows hypoplastic or acellular marrow.

Treatment: Blood transfusion to correct anemia. Oxygen and control of hemorrhage as needed. Antibiotics for infection. Corticosteroids, immunosuppressive agents, colony stimulating factors. Marrow transplantation if possible.

Erythroblastosis Fetalis (Hemolytic Disease of the Newborn).
Hemolytic anemia affecting a newborn, due to destruction of fetal red blood cells by antibodies formed by the mother's immune system.

Cause: The child's red blood cells contain some antigen not found in the mother's red blood cells. If fetal and maternal blood become mixed (as in antenatal trauma, amniocentesis, or chorionic villus biopsy), the maternal immune system may form antibody to this antigen, which then enters the fetal circulation and causes hemolysis. Mixing of blood during delivery stimulates maternal antibody that cannot affect the child just born, but will affect any future fetuses having the same red cell antigen.

The usual cause of severe erythroblastosis is presence of the D antigen of the Rh system in the red blood cells of a fetus borne by an Rh-negative mother. Milder degrees of hemolysis occur with other red blood cell incompatibilities, including those in the ABO system. The mother is unaffected in hemolytic disease of the newborn. The incidence of the disorder has been much reduced by the administration to Rh-negative mothers of high-titer Rh_o (D) immune globulin during each pregnancy and immediately after delivery.

History: Jaundice becoming evident within hours of birth. Pallor, generalized swelling, lethargy, poor feeding, spasms.

Physical Examination: Jaundice, pallor (often masked by jaundice), anasarca (generalized edema), pleural effusion, ascites (fluid in the abdominal cavity), enlargement of liver and spleen, cardiac murmurs, lethargy, spasticity, hyperactive reflexes, cardiac or pulmonary failure.

Diagnostic Tests: The red blood cell count is low and the unconjugated (indirect-reacting) bilirubin is high. Blood glucose may be depressed. Increased numbers of nucleated red blood cells and reticulocytes are found in the circulation. The direct Coombs test shows the red blood cells of the newborn to be coated with hemolytic antibody. The indirect Coombs test on the mother's blood confirms that she has formed antibody to fetal red cell antigen.

Course: Very mild cases may resolve spontaneously, but even with treatment a child showing profound jaundice and lethargy in the first 24 hours may die. Stillbirths are not uncommon. Anemia may correct itself over a few days once further exposure to maternal antibody ceases. However, severe anemia may lead to cardiac failure or death. A more severe threat is marked elevation of bilirubin, which is toxic in the newborn to the basal ganglia of the brain. Deposition of unconjugated bilirubin in the nerve tissue of the basal ganglia, called kernicterus, produces spasticity and unless quickly treated and reversed may lead to a parkinson-like movement disorder and often mental retardation and deafness.

Treatment: Exchange transfusion (replacement of fetal blood, a little at a time, with donor blood lacking harmful antigen) may be needed if anemia is profound or hyperbilirubinemia very high. Respiratory and cardiac function may require support.

Acute Lymphocytic Leukemia (Acute Lymphoblastic Leukemia, ALL).
A rapidly progressive hematologic malignancy of children (Figure 8-8).

Cause: Mutation of lymphocyte precursor cells, possibly due to drugs, radiation, or genetic predisposition or chromosomal aberration. Onset is in childhood, usually before age five.

History: Pallor, weakness, irritability, repeated infections, bleeding tendency, bone pain, headache, stiff neck, vomiting, cranial nerve palsies and other neurologic abnormalities.

Physical Examination: Pallor, lethargy, neurologic findings, evidence of opportunistic infections, hemorrhagic phenomena.

Diagnostic Tests: The white blood cell count may be low, elevated, or normal. Anemia and thrombocytopenia are often present. Serum levels of uric acid and creatinine may be elevated. Bone marrow examination shows replacement of normal elements by infiltrations of blast cells. Cerebrospinal fluid shows lymphoblasts (extremely immature lymphocytes) in central nervous system involvement. Imaging studies including radionuclide bone scans may show abnormalities due to infiltration of organs or tissues by malignant lymphoblastic cells.

Course: The disease is ordinarily fatal in less than six months. With vigorous treatment, many patients achieve long-term survival and apparent cure. Anemia, thrombocytopenia, susceptibility to infection, invasion of the central nervous system (50%), and infiltration and damage of the liver and other organs often prove lethal.

Treatment: Chemotherapy with vincristine, daunorubicin, or asparaginase, combined with corticosteroid. For central nervous system involvement, cranial irradiation and injection of methotrexate intrathecally (into the subarachnoid space). Control of anemia (transfusions if necessary), bleeding, and infection; personal and family counseling.

Chronic Myelogenous Leukemia (CML).
A malignancy of the marrow characterized by markedly elevated levels of circulating white blood cells formed there, with immature and abnormal cells.

Cause: The Philadelphia chromosome, the first oncogene to be associated with a specific malignancy; this is a reciprocal translocation of strands of genes between

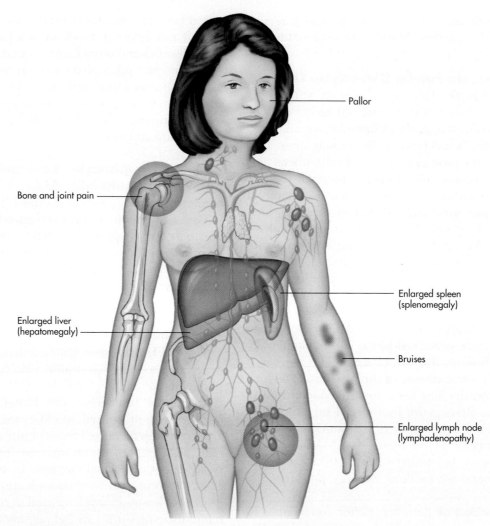

Pallor

Bone and joint pain

Enlarged spleen
(splenomegaly)

Enlarged liver
(hepatomegaly)

Bruises

Enlarged lymph node
(lymphadenopathy)

Figure 8-8
Signs and Symptoms of Leukemia

chromosomes 9 and 22. It results in malignant proliferation of myelogenous (marrow-produced) white blood cells (granulocytes and monocytes), which, however, retain their functions for years, until the disease reaches its terminal stage. Onset generally occurs in middle life (30s, 40s, and 50s).

History: Weakness, fatigue, fever, night sweats, bone pain.

Physical Examination: Low fever, enlargement of the spleen, tenderness over the sternum due to hyperactive marrow.

Laboratory Tests: Marked elevation of the white blood cell count, with modest increases in immature forms. Other cells in the circulation are generally normal in number and form. The uric acid may be elevated. Marrow smear shows increased cellularity and increased immature white blood cells. Chromosomal studies identify the Philadelphia chromosome.

Course: Usual survival is less than five years. However, long-term survival, and apparent cure, occur in half of patients who undergo successful bone marrow transplantation. The disease typically ends in a phase of greatly accelerated production of wholly immature and undifferentiated stem cells (blastic crisis), in which marrow dysfunction can lead to marked anemia, bleeding disorders, and toxemia.

Treatment: Largely supportive and palliative. Chemical suppressants of marrow activity (hydroxyurea, interferon alfa) lower white blood cell counts and mitigate symptoms. In the blast stage, chemotherapy protocols including vincristine, daunorubicin, and prednisone provide brief remission. Allogeneic bone marrow transplant (from a sibling or unrelated donor matched with respect to critical antigens, particularly HLA) is apparently curative in about one half of patients, and is more likely to be effective in younger patients.

Chronic Lymphocytic Leukemia. A malignancy of B lymphocytes.

Cause: Malignant change in a B-cell precursor, with formation of a clone of abnormal immunologically incompetent cells. This results in infiltration of bone marrow and other tissues with abnormal lymphocytes and failure of immune response. Most cases occur in the middle-aged and elderly.

History: Gradual onset of weakness and fatigue, often with enlarged lymph nodes. In some asymptomatic patients the condition is discovered incidentally on routine blood testing.

Physical Examination: Enlargement of lymph nodes, liver, spleen, or all of these. Pallor or jaundice may be present.

Diagnostic Tests: Relative and absolute **lymphocytosis** (increase in the percentage of lymphocytes among white blood cells, and in their total number). The lymphocytes are small but normal in appearance. Bone marrow may show infiltrations of lymphocytes. Red blood cell or platelet count may be reduced. There may be a deficiency of IgG in serum.

Course: Typically chronic, with mild or absent symptoms. Most patients survive 5-10 years after diagnosis. Possible complications include autoimmune hemolytic anemia, thrombocytopenia, and **lymphoma** (development of a malignant solid neoplasm of lymphoid tissue).

Treatment: Largely supportive and palliative. Chlorambucil, fludarabine, and adrenal corticosteroids may be used in severe or terminal disease. Splenectomy may be needed to control hemolytic anemia.

Hodgkin Disease

Cause: Unknown. Genetic influences and viral infection have been implicated, but without conclusive proof.

History: Painless enlargement of one or more lymph nodes, fever, sweats, pruritus, abdominal pain (aggravated by alcohol).

Physical Examination: Enlargement of lymph nodes, possibly spleen; fever. Infiltration of skin may occur (Figure 8-9).

Diagnostic Tests: Lymph node biopsy shows Reed-Sternberg cells (characteristic large cells with two nuclei).

Prognosis: The overall survival rate is about 50%; with early diagnosis and treatment, about 80%.

Treatment: Radiation, chemotherapy.

Non-Hodgkin Lymphoma. A variegated group of lymphocyte malignancies. Oncogenes have been identified for some types.

History: Painless enlargement of lymph nodes, fever, sweats, weight loss, abdominal pain.

Physical Examination: Enlargement of lymph nodes, spleen.

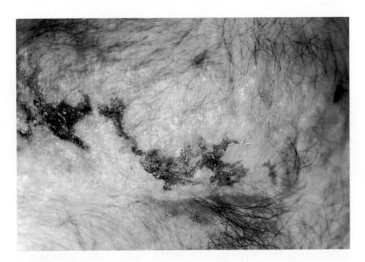

Figure 8-9
Cutaneous Hodgkin Disease

Diagnostic Tests: The peripheral blood may be normal. Lymph node biopsy shows characteristic malignant changes, and bone marrow biopsy shows infiltration of abnormal lymphoid aggregates. The serum LDH is elevated. Chest x-ray and CT scan of the abdomen and pelvis may show hilar and abdominal or pelvic lymphadenopathy.

Treatment: Radiation, chemotherapy, bone marrow transplantation.

Coagulation Disorders (Coagulopathies).

Deficiency or lack of any of the plasma clotting factors, including fibrinogen and prothrombin, can occur as an isolated genetic defect.

Classical hemophilia (hemophilia A), due to congenital deficiency of Factor VIII, is transmitted as a sex-linked recessive trait, carried by females but expressed only in males. Hemophilia B (Factor IX disease, Christmas disease) shows a similar pattern of inheritance. Acquired deficiency of prothrombin (hypoprothrombinemia) is more frequent than congenital deficiency. It can result from deficiency of vitamin K (an essential chemical building block for prothrombin), hepatic disease (particularly biliary obstruction, which blocks absorption of vitamin K by preventing passage of bile salts into the bowel), or treatment with coumarin anticoagulants. Acquired or congenital deficiency of plasma clotting factors causes a hemorrhagic tendency of variable severity characterized by prolonged bleeding from wounds, hematoma formation, hemarthrosis (bleeding into joints), and hematuria (blood in the urine).

Congenital or acquired deficiency of platelets (thrombocytopenia) is associated with petechiae (pinpoint hemorrhages in the skin) or purpura (larger skin hemorrhages). Frank or severe hemorrhage occurs less frequently. Idiopathic thrombocytopenic purpura (ITP) is an autoimmune disorder of children, usually benign and self-limited. In thrombotic thrombocytopenic purpura (TTP), deficiency of platelets may be accompanied by hemolytic anemia, renal impairment, and bizarre neurologic manifestations. The acute form may progress rapidly to a fatal termination. In Glanzmann disease (thrombasthenia), the platelet count is normal but platelet function is impaired.

Hemorrhagic manifestations, usually purpuric, also occur in certain diseases of blood vessels. In hereditary hemorrhagic telangiectasia (Osler-Weber-Rendu disease), recurrent bleeding occurs from telangiectases in the skin and mucous membranes. Von Willebrand disease is a hereditary hemorrhagic disorder, often mild, characterized by deficiency of Factor VIII, abnormal platelet function, and vascular abnormalities. Examples of acquired vascular disorders accompanied by purpuric bleeding include Henoch-Schoenlein purpura, Cushing syndrome, and scurvy.

Disseminated intravascular coagulation (DIC), which results from imbalance between the mechanisms of coagulation and of fibrinolysis, can be induced by infection (meningococcal meningitis, Rocky Mountain spotted fever, septicemia), trauma, shock, complications of pregnancy and parturition, and myelocytic leukemia. Clinical manifestations range from widespread bleeding to widespread intravascular thrombosis, and both of these may occur together.

Precise diagnosis of a hemorrhagic disorder depends on the results of several basic tests, which are often performed together as a coagulation panel: platelet count, bleeding time, clotting time, prothrombin time, partial thromboplastin time, and clot retraction. In addition, plasma assay for specific coagulation factors is possible.

Laboratory Procedures

band forms, bands Immature neutrophils whose nuclei appear as bands, in contrast to mature neutrophils whose nuclei are segmented or lobed.

basos An acceptable brief form for *basophils*.

blast forms, blasts Very immature cells, particularly leukocytes, not normally found in peripheral blood but present in acute leukemia.

bleeding time The number of minutes it takes for a small incision in the skin, made with a lancet, to stop bleeding. Either the Duke method (puncture of the earlobe) or the Ivy method (puncture of the forearm) may be used.

blood type A genetically determined and permanent characteristic of a person's red blood cells based on the presence of certain antigens. Two blood type systems of clinical importance are the ABO (comprising types A, B, AB, and O) and the Rh (comprising Rh-positive and Rh-negative). Blood for transfusion must be typed and then cross-matched (experimentally combined) with the prospective recipient's blood to avoid reactions due to incompatibility of bloods. Other red cell antigens not used for type and cross-matching include Duffy, Kell, Kidd, and Lewis. These are often used when blood typing is used as evidence of nonpaternity.

burr cell An abnormal red blood cell with a jagged contour.

CBC (complete blood count) A group of blood tests, including counts of red blood cells, white blood cells, and platelets; a differential count of the various types of white blood cells; and a determination of hemoglobin and hematocrit.

clotting factors See *factors, blood clotting*.

clotting time The time needed for a clot to form in a tube of freshly drawn blood under standard conditions. The Lee-White method is the one most often used.

coags Slang term for *coagulation studies*.

differential white blood cell count A determination of the relative numbers of the six types of white blood cells normally found in peripheral blood. When the count is performed visually, a technician observes 100 white blood cells in a stained smear of whole blood and reports the number of each cell type found as a percent. The differential count can also be done electronically. The six types of white blood cells are segmented neutrophils (PMNs or segs), band neutrophils (bands, representing the immature form), eosinophils (eos), basophils (basos), lymphocytes (lymphs), and monocytes (monos).

Duke bleeding time See *bleeding time*.

eos Brief form for *eosinophils*.

erythrocyte A mature red blood cell. Compare *reticulocyte*.

factors, blood clotting Substances present in the blood that participate in the clotting process.

Factor I fibrinogen
Factor II prothrombin
Factor III tissue thromboplastin
Factor IV calcium
Factor V labile factor (proaccelerin)
Factor VI (term not currently in use)
Factor VII stable factor (proconvertin)

Factor VIII antihemophilic globulin (AHG)
Factor IX Christmas factor
Factor X Stuart-Prower factor
Factor XI plasma thromboplastin antecedent
Factor XII Hageman factor
Factor XIII fibrin-stabilizing factor

granulocytes White blood cells with conspicuous cytoplasmic granules. According to the staining properties of these granules, the cells are classified as neutrophils, eosinophils, and basophils.

H&H Slang abbreviation for *hemoglobin and hematocrit.* The hemoglobin level is usually dictated first.

Hct, HCT Abbreviation for *hematocrit.*

hematocrit The percentage of a blood sample that consists of cells. The sample is spun in a centrifuge, which quickly drives all of the cells to the bottom of the tube. The length of the column of cells is expressed as a percent of the total length of the specimen. Red and white blood cells and platelets are all included, but red blood cells far outnumber the other formed elements.

hematocrit, central A hematocrit value determined by using a blood sample drawn from a central line catheter.

hemoglobin (Hgb, HGB) The oxygen-carrying complex of iron and protein in red blood cells. The hemoglobin level is reduced in anemia.

hemoglobin A1 Normal adult hemoglobin.

hemoglobin F Normal fetal hemoglobin, found also in adults with certain forms of anemia and leukemia.

hemoglobin S The abnormal hemoglobin found in the red blood cells of persons with sickle cell anemia.

left shift See *shift to the left.*

leukocytes White blood cells (WBCs), including neutrophils, eosinophils, basophils, lymphocytes, and monocytes.

MCH (mean corpuscular hemoglobin) The average weight of hemoglobin per red blood cell, calculated from the hemoglobin level and the red blood cell count.

MCHC (mean corpuscular hemoglobin concentration) The average concentration of hemoglobin in red blood cells, calculated from the hemoglobin level and the hematocrit.

mcL (microliters) Used in cell counts to avoid using such abbreviations as μL or mm³ or 10³ because special characters and superscript numerals do not transmit well electronically.

MCV (mean corpuscular volume) The average volume of a red blood cell, calculated from the hematocrit and the red blood cell count.

microhematocrit A hematocrit measurement performed on a small specimen of blood obtained by finger stick and centrifuged in a capillary tube.

monos Brief form for *monocytes.*

myelocytes White blood cells formed in bone marrow: neutrophils, basophils, eosinophils, and monocytes.

neutrophil, segmented A mature neutrophil with a segmented or lobulated nucleus. Also called *polymorphonuclear leukocytes* or *polys.*

ovalocytosis Abnormal oval shape of red blood cells, seen in various congenital disorders of red blood cell formation, including elliptocytosis.

platelets Noncellular formed elements in circulating blood, produced in bone marrow and active in blood coagulation. Also called *thrombocytes.*

PMNs Abbreviation for *polymorphonuclear leukocytes.*

poikilocytosis An abnormally wide variation in the shapes of red blood cells as seen in a stained smear.

polymorphonuclear leukocytes (PMNs, polys) White blood cells with segmented or lobulated nuclei. An acceptable brief form is *polys.* The term is often used synonymously with *neutrophils,* although eosinophils and basophils are also polymorphonuclear leukocytes.

polys Brief form for *polymorphonuclear leukocytes.*

PT, pro time (prothrombin time) The time required for a clot to form in blood treated with certain reagents. The result may be reported as both a time (in seconds) and a percent of normal prothrombin activity as detected by the same test in a control. The prothrombin time is prolonged in deficiency of certain coagulation factors and after treatment with heparin or coumarin anticoagulants.

PT/PTT Prothrombin time and partial thromboplastin time.

PTT (partial thromboplastin time) The time required for a clot to form in blood treated with certain reagents. Abnormal prolongation of this time occurs in deficiency of various coagulation factors and after treatment with heparin.

RBCs (red blood cells) The most numerous cells of the blood, which carry oxygen from the lungs to the tissues, and carbon dioxide from the tissues to the lungs.

red blood cell count The number of red blood cells per cubic millimeter of blood, as counted by a technician using a microscope or by an electronic cell counter. The count may be reported either as a simple numeral (e.g., 5,300,000/mcL [microliter]) or as the product of a number less than ten and 10^6 (e.g., 5.3×10^6). The count may be dictated simply as 5.3 and may be so transcribed or may be expanded to 5,300,000.

red blood cells, nucleated Immature red blood cells, released from the bone marrow before disappearance of their nuclei. Mature RBCs have no nuclei.

red blood cell indices Measures of the volume and hemoglobin content of red blood cells, derived by calculating from the hemoglobin, hematocrit, and red blood cell count. The red cell indices are the MCV, MCH, and MCHC.

reticulocyte An immature red blood cell whose cytoplasm contains an irregular network of degenerating nuclear material. An increase in the number of reticulocytes indicates increased red blood cell production in response to blood loss or hemolysis.

segs An acceptable brief form for *segmented neutrophils*.

shift to the left An increase in the relative number of immature neutrophils, as detected in a differential white blood count. The various types of cells were formerly recorded on forms arranged in columns, the more immature neutrophils being recorded at the extreme left of the form.

sickle cell An abnormal red blood cell found in persons with sickle cell anemia; the cell assumes a sickle or crescent shape at reduced oxygen levels (Figure 8-10).

sickling An abnormal sickle or crescent shape observed in red blood cells on a blood smear.

spherocytosis Abnormal spherical shape of red blood cells as noted in a stained smear of whole blood on microscopic examination.

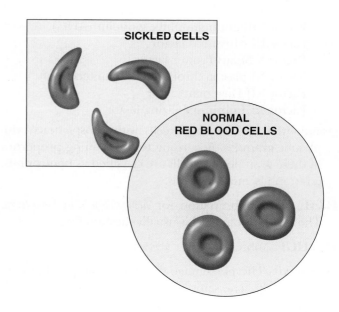

Figure 8-10
Sickle Cell Anemia

stabs Another name for *bands* (immature neutrophils). The German word *Stab* means *staff* or *rod*, referring to the unsegmented nucleus of an immature neutrophil.

target cell An abnormal red blood cell with a bull's-eye appearance due to flattening of the cell with a prominent spot of hemoglobin in the center.

thrombocytes See *platelets*.

triglycerides, serum The level of fat in the serum, usually measured in the fasting state.

WBCs (white blood cells) See *leukocytes*.

white blood cell count (white count, white cell count) The number of white blood cells per cubic millimeter of blood, as counted by a technician using a microscope or by an electronic cell counter. The count may be reported as either a simple numeral (e.g., $7,200/\text{mm}^3$ or mcL) or as the product of a small number and 10^3 (e.g., 7.2×10^3). In the latter case, the report may be dictated simply as 7.2 and may be so transcribed or may be expanded to 7,200.

TRANSCRIPTION**TIPS**

1. Unless you transcribe exclusively in a physician specialist's office, the majority of the reports you encounter will be from the three main specialties of cardiology, gastroenterology, and orthopedics. Diseases of the cardiovascular system are quite prevalent, and the medical terminology is extensive. Even patients with noncardiac chief complaints may have chronic secondary cardiovascular disorders such as arrhythmia, hypertension, or elevated cholesterol level. This is particularly true of elderly patients. Thus, you should be familiar with cardiovascular terminology.

2. There are several soundalike terms relating to the cardiovascular system. Memorize their meanings so that you can select the appropriate term for a correct transcript.

   hypertension (high blood pressure)
   hypotension (low blood pressure)

   palpitation (sensation caused by irregular heart beats)
   palpation (use of the hands to examine body surfaces)

   Buerger disease (a disease of the blood vessels)
   Berger disease (a kidney disorder)

3. These slang terms should be translated correctly when encountered in dictation.

"cabbage"	CABG (acronym for coronary artery bypass graft)
cardiac cath	cardiac catheterization
cath'd	catheterized
dig (dij)	digoxin
nitro	nitroglycerin
"romied"	ROMI (rule out myocardial infarction). Do not make a verb ("romied") of this abbreviation.
V fib	ventricular fibrillation
V tach ("tack")	ventricular tachycardia

4. Both combining forms *angio-* (Greek) and *vaso-* (Latin) mean *(blood) vessel.*

5. Heart sounds are transcribed with a capital letter followed by a subscript number or a numeral on the baseline. Special characters such as subscripts do not transmit well electronically; hence, the common use of numerals on the baseline.

   S1 or S_1 (first heart sound)
   S2 or S_2 (second heart sound)
   S3 or S_3 (third heart sound)
   S4 or S_4 (fourth heart sound)
   A2 or A_2 (aortic second sound, closure of the aortic valve)
   P2 or P_2 (pulmonic second sound, closure of the pulmonary valve)

6. Electrocardiogram leads ("leeds") may be transcribed with either regular or subscript numerals.

   V1 through V6 *or* V_1 through V_6

7. Both *EKG* and *ECG* are acceptable abbreviations for *electrocardiogram.* The *K* comes from the Greek word *kardia* (heart) and also from the German spelling, *Elektrokardiogramm.* Do not transcribe the abbreviated form unless it is dictated.

8. Note these difficult-to-spell cardiovascular drugs.

   Cardizem (*not* Cardiazem or Cardizyme)
   Catapres, Combipres (only one *s*)
   Inderal (*not* Inderol)
   Minipress and Lopressor (two *s*'s)
   Rythmol (an antiarrhythmic drug, the spelling of which differs from the word *rhythm*)

9. The abbreviation *AV* can mean either *arteriovenous* or *atrioventricular.* Be sure to translate the abbreviation correctly based on its meaning in the sentence.

AV fistula	arteriovenous fistula
AV node	atrioventricular node

10. In a cardiology context, the abbreviation *AAA* and the dictated form *triple A* stand for *abdominal aortic aneurysm.*

11. The abbreviation *ASHD* can mean either *arteriosclerotic heart disease* or *atherosclerotic heart disease.* Unless either term has been dictated in full elsewhere in the report, the abbreviation must be transcribed as dictated, even in a final diagnosis, because the transcriptionist has no way of knowing which of the disease processes is meant.

Spotlight on

Transcribing Cardiology Dictation

by Kathleen Mors Woods

In literature and in life, the heart is always depicted as the soul of a person and is described in vivid terms. One may be called a heartbreaker, a heart throb, a sweetheart. One may be heartless, heartsick, brokenhearted, fainthearted, good-hearted, lighthearted, lionhearted, or have a big heart, a cold heart, a hard heart, or a heart as good as gold. These glossy descriptions take on a more meaningful tone when placed in a medical context and discussion of cardiology emerges.

In the medical field, we are concerned with cardiology as the study of the heart, its functions, and its diseases, the identification of these diseases by diagnostic tests, and ultimately the correction of defects. When a newborn baby is diagnosed with a congenital heart defect, or a 16-year-old is stabbed in the chest, or a person's aorta is literally ripped out of the chest in an automobile accident (by hitting the steering wheel not wearing a seat belt), the cardiac surgeon is called upon to demonstrate a broad range of abilities in treating these patients. Transcribing reports on these procedures carries with it the excitement of a new technology, expanding every day through research and a commitment to life-saving techniques.

The various techniques cover pacemaker insertion for irregular rhythm, the automatic implantable defibrillator for sudden death, coronary artery bypass grafting for coronary (vessel) blockage, valve replacement and repair with either mechanical parts or real preserved harvested parts, to the ultimate procedure for end-stage disease—heart and heart-lung transplantation.

Cardiac Evaluation. Let's start by imagining the following scenario: Your neighbor has chest pain and goes to a cardiologist. The other factors for having this chest pain (for example, kidney stones or ulcers) have been ruled out. At the cardiologist's office, an electrocardiogram is performed. Twelve leads are attached, six at the wrists and ankles (leads I, II, III, aVF, aVL, aVR), and six on the chest (V_1 through V_6).

If the patient's pain is caused by the decrease in blood flow due to a narrowing or obstruction of an artery carrying oxygen to the heart, and if damage has been done or is occurring, this will show up on the EKG. The pain, then, is caused by an obstruction (clot) in the vessel. If this clot remains in the vessel, the vessel is occluded and the muscle of the heart (myocardium) is damaged, for the area the vessel feeds dies. If the patient is "evolving the infarction" (having a heart attack) and admitted to a hospital in a timely fashion, several other tests are performed, including a CPK (creatine phosphokinase) curve as a measure of the infarct. CPK-MB bands are located only in the heart muscle, and blood serum levels will rise if heart cells are damaged during an infarction (but not during angina). New drugs are used to either dissolve the clot within the vessel or work with the body's own clotting factors to dissolve it.

Another option is for the patient to have a treadmill exercise stress test and to be referred for a cardiac catheterization.

Catheterization. Cardiac catheterization was invented in 1929 by a physician named Werner Forssmann, who first tested the procedure by catheterizing his own circulatory system. Over the years it has progressed from a simple investigative technique to a powerful diagnostic procedure.

The patient is premedicated and taken to the catheterization laboratory. A puncture is made in the groin and a catheter is fed up into the heart. If the blood supply to the legs is poor, the catheter is inserted through a brachial cutdown in the arm, a small incision in the upper part of the arm which is later sutured closed. The catheter is properly positioned and radiopaque dye injected. While the dye is being injected and coursing through the vessels, it is recorded on running 35-mm film in black and white. This is later developed and shows where the blockages are in the coronary arteries, how the valves and heart muscle are functioning, and different pressures in these arteries. This film is called a *cineangiogram* (like cinema), or *cine* ("sin-ee") for short.

Although the catheterization is quite straightforward, the terminology is technical and specialized. Terms such as *aortic gradient, LVEDP, pigtail catheter, PCWP, assumed Fick method,* and *ejection fraction* might seem quite alien. Your reference sources should include a personal word list and equipment list.

Catheters are referred to by size and name. A *7-French JL4* catheter is translated *7-French Judkins left 4 cm curve* catheter. The word *French* refers to the French scale for sizing catheters and is often abbreviated *F;* thus, *7F* means *seven French*. The catheters are named for shape, size, inventor, or manufacturer, or have a trade name.

Angioplasty. When your neighbor's cardiac evaluation is completed, she may be told she has blockage of only one coronary artery. One of her options at this point is to have a PTCA (percutaneous transluminal coronary angioplasty). This procedure is often done immediately following the injection of a drug such as streptokinase or urokinase to lyse (break up) the clot. It can, however, be scheduled electively.

A catheter with a tiny balloon on the 4 or 5 mm tip is placed at the site of the narrowing of the artery, and the balloon is inflated by means of a hand pump, to compress or squeeze the plaque back against the artery wall and open the blood flow through the vessel.

The advantage of this procedure is that it does not involve open heart surgery. The disadvantage is that this narrowing can recur, especially in those carrying inherited (familial) diseases. An angioplasty must be done in a hospital setting that provides surgery. When an artery tears open (dissects), the patient is taken to surgery for repair of the artery.

Abbreviations. Although abbreviations are frequently dictated, the transcriptionist should exercise discretion when transcribing abbreviations in medical reports. When you are required to type abbreviations, use only those abbreviations that will not be misinterpreted; if you drop one letter of an abbreviation, you change the medical meaning and location. The posterior descending artery is abbreviated *PDA*, which also stands for the congenital heart defect of *patent ductus arteriosus*. When you translate abbreviations, be sure to transcribe the correct meaning as indicated by the context of the report.

A patient with multiple occlusions may opt for open heart surgery, or coronary artery bypass graft (CABG, pronounced "cabbage"). Open heart procedures occur in two ways—opening the chest down the middle (median sternotomy), or, less usual, spreading the ribs and entering through this area (thoracotomy). Bypasses are named for the number of vessels reconnected—single, double, triple, or whatever number.

In interpreting the dictation, the transcriptionist must become familiar with many abbreviations and eponyms. If a baby has a B-T shunt, it is the procedure named after the famous Blalock-Taussig blue baby operation first performed by those two physicians. Favaloro, Bovie, St. Jude, Carpentier-Edwards, and Björk-Shiley are all proper names (eponyms). If an eponym is the name of one person (Johns Hopkins, Austin Flint), it is not hyphenated. One must learn which compound terms are which electrical activity. For example, a DDD pacemaker serves the electrical activity of both the atrium and ventricle, paces (stimulates) both the atrium and ventricle to beat, and may cause (trigger) the atrium to contract while sending no signal (inhibited) to the ventricle, depending on what natural electrical activity is occurring in the heart at that time.

Of course, as soon as you have most of the common words down, you could be introduced to the exciting new field of the AICD (automatic implantable cardioverter defibrillator). In an AICD operation, a patch is placed on the heart and sewn on, with leads extending to a box (in the stomach area) which, like some types of pacemakers, can monitor the rhythm of the heart. When there is an arrhythmia (irregular rhythm), the generator box senses this, fires a jolt to the heart, and starts it back up again.

Pacemakers. Pacemakers are identified by a three-letter code system, such as *DDD* or *VVI*, which need not be translated. The first letter indicates the chamber that is paced; the second letter denotes the chamber that is sensed; the third letter indicates whether the pacemaker is inhibited or triggered by the heart's own electrical activity. For example, a DDD pacemaker serves the electrical activity of both the atrium and ventricle, paces (stimulates) both the atrium and ventricle to beat, and may cause (trigger) the atrium to contract while sending no signal (inhibited) to the ventricle, depending on what natural electrical activity is occurring in the heart at that time.

As a cardiology transcriptionist, you get to "know" a cardiology patient quite well through the medical history you transcribe, and you get a lot of satisfaction knowing that you are playing an essential role in a patient's return to good health.

Source: *The SUM Program Cardiology Transcription Unit*

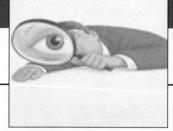

Proofreading Skills

Instructions: In the paragraphs below, circle the errors. Identify misspelled and missing medical and English words and punctuation errors, and write the correct words and punctuation in the numbered spaces opposite the text.

1 PRESENT ILLNESS
2 This 68-year-old caucasian male with a history of hyper-
3 tension and congestive heart failure was apparantly in
4 good health although he had failed to follow up on his
5 office appointments and ran out of refills on probably
6 his Lasix one week ago. The patient shortly thereafter
7 had some slight precordial chest pain which resolved.
8 The precordial chest pain returned again. The patient
9 obtained a good relief with nitroglycerin sublingual.
10 The patient has also been on Calan and Micro-K which
11 he has continued to take. He has had no chills or fever,
12 no nausea emesis or diarrhea, no unusual color change.
13 He did complain of being somewhat diaphoretic and
14 dizzy with the chest pain.
15
16 FAMILY HISTORY
17 No familial diseases known.
18
19 PHYSICAL EXAMINATION
20 General appearance: A slightly obese, well-developed
21 68-year-old Caucasian male.
22 HEENT: Head symetrical. Pupils equal, react to light
23 and accommodation, no scleral icterus. Ears, nose, and
24 throat cleer. Mouth moist.
25 Neck: Supple, no masses. Normal anterior carotid
26 pulsations bilaterally.
27 Chest: Clear to P&A.
28 Cardiovascular: Distant heart tones, no murmurs. Good
29 peripheral pulses, including dorsalis pedis.
30 Abdomen: Protuberant, no masses. Active bowel
31 sounds.
32
33 IMPRESSION
34 1. Probable angina pectorus.
35 2. Rule out MI.
36 3. CHF, compensated.
37 4. Hypertension.
38 5. ASHD.

1 _____
2 Caucasian _____
3 _____
4 _____
5 _____
6 _____
7 _____
8 _____
9 _____
10 _____
11 _____
12 _____
13 _____
14 _____
15 _____
16 _____
17 _____
18 _____
19 _____
20 _____
21 _____
22 _____
23 _____
24 _____
25 _____
26 _____
27 _____
28 _____
29 _____
30 _____
31 _____
32 _____
33 _____
34 _____
35 _____
36 _____
37 _____
38 _____

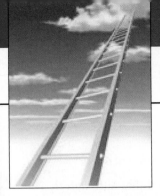

SkillsChallenge

Fill-in Exercise: Circulation of the Blood

Instructions: The following paragraphs describe the process by which blood is circulated throughout the body. The numbered blanks correspond to the numbers in the narrative. Fill in the blanks with the correct terms from the word list below.

Deoxygenated blood moves from the capillaries throughout the body to venules, to veins, and finally into the (1) before it enters the (2) of the heart.

Leaving this chamber, the blood is pumped through the (3) and into the right ventricle. From there, it goes through the pulmonary valve into the (4) that leads to the lungs. In the lungs, carbon dioxide is exchanged for (5), and the blood becomes oxygenated and bright red in color.

The oxygenated blood leaves the lungs via the (6) and enters the (7) of the heart. The valve between the left atrium and the left ventricle is known as the (8).

All heart valves have delicate (9) or leaflets that close tightly to prevent backflow of blood as the heart pumps. As the blood leaves the left ventricle, it passes through the (10) and into the (11), the largest artery in the body, to begin its journey again through the body.

aorta	aortic valve
cusps	left atrium
mitral valve	oxygen
pulmonary artery	pulmonary vein
right atrium	tricuspid valve
vena cava	

1. vena cava _____
2. _____
3. _____
4. _____
5. _____
6. _____
7. _____
8. _____
9. _____
10. _____
11. _____

Adjectives Exercise

Adjectives are formed from nouns by adding adjectival suffixes such as *-ac, -al, -ar, -ary, -eal, -ed, -ent, -iac, -ial, -ic, -ical, -ive, -lar, -oid, -ous, -tic,* and *-tous*. In addition, some adjectives have a different form entirely from the noun, which may be either Latin or Greek in origin.

Instructions: Test your knowledge of adjectives by writing the adjectival form of the following cardiology words. Consult a medical dictionary to select the correct adjectival ending as necessary.

1. heart _____
2. artery _____
3. vein _____
4. atrium _____
5. ventricle _____
6. aorta _____
7. systole _____
8. myocardium _____
9. cyanosis _____
10. hypertension _____
11. aneurysm _____
12. valve _____

Word Root and Suffix-Matching Exercise

Instructions: Combine the following word roots with suffixes to form words that match the definitions below. Fill in the blanks with the medical words that you construct.

Word Root	Suffix
cardio-	-plasty
endo-	-megaly
valvulo-	-ology
electro-	-gram
angio-	-ectomy
aneurysm-	-itis
phlebo-	

A. inflammation of a vein

_____

B. enlargement of the heart

_____

C. inflammation of the inner lining of the heart
(*Tip:* Use 2 word roots and 1 suffix.)

_____

D. the study of the heart

_____

E. surgical widening of a constricted valve

_____

F. record of the heart's electrical activity
(*Tip:* Use 2 word roots and 1 suffix.)

_____

G. surgical widening of narrowed blood vessels

_____

H. surgical removal of an aneurysm

_____

Soundalikes Exercise

Instructions: Circle the correct term from the soundalikes in parentheses in the following sentences.

1. (Cor, Core, Corps): The heart was not enlarged.

2. The cardiac catheterization showed that although there were obstructed major vessels, there was sufficient (recanalization, recannulation) that medical therapy rather than bypass could be tried.

3. After the first angioplasty, the patient's vessel restenosed, so a (recanalization, recannulation) was done.

4. The echocardiogram showed the patient's (ejection, injection) fraction to be acceptable.

5. The vessel (loops, loupes) were pulled up (taught, taut) and the aneurysm tied off.

6. (Canalization, Cannulation) was done via the femoral artery with a JL4 guiding catheter.

7. An (osteal, ostial) lesion was noted near the takeoff of the posterior descending artery from the right coronary artery.

8. The EKG showed irregular rhythm, and the patient complained of (palpations, palpitations, papillations).

9. The patient was having difficulty breathing and experienced (perfuse, profuse) diaphoresis.

10. The angiogram was nondiagnostic due to inadequate (perfusion, profusion) of dye into the aorta.

11. There was diffuse inflammation of the (pericardium, precordium) and severe congestive heart failure.

12. The patient complains of (pericardial, precordial) chest pain.

13. Prior to coronary artery bypass grafting, the patient was put on intra-aortic balloon (pump, sump).

14. A (pump, sump) drain was placed in the thorax and the chest closed.

15. The (chordae, chordee) tendineae of the atrioventricular valve cusp were severed.

Abbreviations Exercise

Common abbreviations may be transcribed as dictated in the body of a report. Uncommon abbreviations must be spelled out, with the abbreviation appearing in parentheses after the translation. All abbreviations (except laboratory test names) must be spelled out in the Diagnosis or Impression section of any report.

Instructions: Define the following cardiology abbreviations. Then memorize both abbreviations and definitions to increase your speed and accuracy in transcribing cardiology dictation.

AAA _____

ALL _____

ASHD _____

AV node _____

BP _____

CABG _____

CBC _____

CML _____

CPR _____

CVP _____

DIC _____

DVT _____

ECG, EKG _____

EF _____

H&H _____

Hct, HCT _____

HCTZ _____

ITP _____

JVD _____

LAD _____

LADD _____

LDH _____

LVF _____

MI _____

MUGA scan _____

PMI _____

PND _____

PT _____

PTT _____

PTCA _____

RBCs _____

RCA _____

tPA _____

TTP _____

Medical Terminology Matching Exercise

Instructions: Complete the following matching exercise to test your knowledge of word roots, anatomic structures, symptoms, and disease processes encountered in the medical specialty of cardiology by matching the definitions in Column A with their terms in Column B.

Column A	Column B
1. ___ blood vessel	**A.** sphygmomanometer
2. ___ irregular heartbeat	**B.** pericardium
3. ___ vein	**C.** angio-
4. ___ extremely rapid, ineffective heartbeat	**D.** arrhythmia
5. ___ leg pain on exercise due to blockage of arteries	**E.** coronary arteries
6. ___ supply heart muscle with oxygenated blood	**F.** -megaly
7. ___ membranous sac around the heart	**G.** heart-lung machine
8. ___ used to measure blood pressure	**H.** aneurysm
9. ___ fatty degeneration	**I.** athero-
10. ___ circulates blood during heart surgery	**J.** claudication
11. ___ ballooning of part of artery wall	**K.** phlebo-
	L. ventricular fibrillation

Dictation Exercises

Instructions: Prior to transcribing the dictations, complete these activities.

1. **Using the Style Guide**

    a. When, according to the Style Guide, do you expand brief forms?

    b. According to the Style Guide, how do you handle abbreviations in the body of the report?

    c. When, if ever, should abbreviations for laboratory and other diagnostic tests be expanded?

    d. Review style guidelines for EKG terms, both leads and findings. When do you hyphenate "T wave"?

    e. What is the appropriate way to transcribe murmurs? For example, the dictator says, "a grade three over six murmur"; how would you transcribe it?

    f. When is the use of ordinal numbers (1st, 2nd, 3rd, etc.) appropriate in medical transcripts?.

    g. Review the style recommendations for transcribing medication lists. (Look at Lists under Numbers.)

    h. What is the abbreviation for the unit of measure *milliequivalents*?

    g. What is the proper way to transcribe fractions used with English units of measure and fractions used with metric units of measure or percentages? Give examples.

    h. What is the difference between *post* and *status post*?

    i. The doctor dictates some drug dosages but fails to dictate the unit of measure to go with the numbers. What should you do?

    j. How do you transcribe metric fractions less than 1; for example, how would you transcribe the dictated "point five milliseconds"?

    k. Read the section in the Style Guide on editing. What does it say about correcting physicians' misspeaks?

    l. Review the Error-prone Abbreviations list under Abbreviations. What is the correct way to transcribe the dictated *q.h.s.* and *q.d.*? Is there a problem, according to the Error-prone Abbreviations list, with *q. day* as well?

    m. When do you use the article *a*, and when do you use the article *an* before a noun?

    n. Review the list of slang forms that need to be translated in medical reports. Which slang terms might be heard in cardiology and pulmonary reports and how would you transcribe them?

    o. The Style Guide recommends that the possessive form ('s) be dropped from eponyms (names) used as adjectives before a noun (for example, Alzheimer disease, not Alzheimer's disease), but what do you do if only the eponym is dictated without the noun?

    p. Sometimes abbreviations and acronyms are pronounced as words. To what is a dictator referring when he says "cabbage"?

2. **Problem Solving**
    This activity is to help you prepare ahead of time for some of the problems you'll encounter in the dictations. Some of these items may not have a definitive answer but are intended to simply get you thinking about how to handle a variety of situations that are common in transcription. If nothing else, they will help you recognize a problem when you encounter it in the dictations.

    a. A common problem for students is interpreting dictated abbreviations because so many of the letters of the English alphabet can sound like each other. For example, every vowel can sound like another vowel and the consonants *p, b, v, t,* and *d* can all, at times, sound like each other when not enunciated clearly. How would you handle an abbreviation you weren't quite sure of?

    b. You have an abbreviation that can be expanded in more than one way. How do you determine which expansion to use? What do you do if you can't determine which expansion to use?

    c. Sometimes physicians dictate punctuation; this can present problems, especially for students, on several levels. Speculate about the types of problems this may cause you as a student.

d. ESL physicians may dictate incorrect pronouns, verbs, and prepositions. How should you handle these types of dictation errors?

e. Laboratory test abbreviations are generally not expanded the way other abbreviations are. However, it's all too easy to mistake one letter for another—*b* for *v*, *t* for *p*, etc. What can you do to be sure that you are interpreting laboratory test abbreviations correctly?

f. Doctors sometimes coin words, that is, they make them up. For example, they may turn a noun like *Coumadin* into a verb, *coumadinize*. After a time, when these words have been used so much, they become acceptable, the words will appear first in word and phrase book references and ultimately in medical dictionaries. What do you do, however, if a doctor is dictating a word you cannot confirm in a word and phrase book or the dictionary, but you're pretty sure you're hearing it correctly?

g. Sometimes doctors misspeak and simply say one word for another. For example, one might say a patient's name is *Normal* when it's really *Norma* or that a patient has admitted to *martial* problems instead of *marital* problems. How would you handle such slips of tongue?

h. Sometimes dictators say "quote unquote." What types of information do physicians put in quotation marks, and how do you determine where to place the open and closing quotation marks?

3. **Preparatory Research**

Any information requested in these questions not readily available in your textbook (including the Appendix) or required references can easily be found using Internet search engines such as Google or on-line medical dictionaries.

a. Research pharmacologic (or chemical) cardiac stress test. What drugs are used to perform this test? For what reasons is it normally performed (as compared to a treadmill stress test)?

b. Look up the term *salvo*. Write its definition in your New Terms notebook.

c. Review laboratory reference values for total cholesterol, LDL, and HDL.

d. List three lipid-lowering drugs.

e. Look up the drug class *beta-blockers*. What are *beta-blockers* used for? List three.

f. Research an echocardiogram procedure. What are the indications for an echocardiogram? What diagnostic findings might one expect?

g. What is an *appendage*? How might this term apply to the heart?

h. Look up *foramen ovale*. Where is the foramen ovale found? Define this term.

i. What is another term for *cardiac ultrasound*? What are some of the indications for a cardiac ultrasound?

j. What is *SBE prophylaxis*? Why is it recommended for some patients?

k. Look up the word *interrogation*. What is the computer science definition? (That definition comes closest to its use in the context of checking pacemaker or ICD function.)

l. What does the term *regurgitation*, as applied to the heart, mean?

m. What does the term *ablation* mean? Research cardiac ablation in Google or some other search engine. Describe the procedure and its purpose.

n. The prefix *dys-* can be added to just about any medical word denoting a condition. How does it change the meaning of the word to which it is added?

o. Look up *lipid arcus* (in the eyes). What is the significance of lipid arcus if it's present?

p. What is a *Cardiolite stress test*? Why is it performed?

q. What is a *heart gallop*?

r. What does "oriented times three" mean?

s. What is an *ejection fraction*? On what kind of test would this be discussed? What is being measured with an ejection fraction?

Sample cardiology reports appear on the following pages, illustrating a variety of reports. Fictional names are provided for illustration of proper format, and no resemblance to actual persons is intended. Sample transcripts were prepared according to the *AAMT Book of Style*, where possible.

History and Physical Examination

OLSEN, NATALIE
Hospital #123456
Date of Admission: 11/17/XXXX
Attending Physician: Kathryn Pieper, MD

CHIEF COMPLAINT
Chest pain.

HISTORY OF PRESENT ILLNESS
This 65-year-old white female was admitted to the hospital with chest pain on the night of admission. This lasted off and on for some time, for probably several hours. It was not relieved by nitroglycerin, and because of this she presented herself to the emergency department. She also has type 1 diabetes mellitus, and her sugars are sporadically in the 300-400 range. She has been unable to lose weight and is grossly obese.

PAST MEDICAL HISTORY
Please see old records for past medical history.

SOCIAL AND FAMILY HISTORY
See old records.

SYSTEM REVIEW
System review is essentially unchanged from the last admission. She has occasional headaches. There is some decrease in her hearing. She has cough and congestion but no pneumonia or tuberculosis (TB). Appetite and digestion have been good, and she has not had any gastrointestinal (GI) bleeding. She has no urgency, frequency, or dysuria, but she has had urinary tract infections in the past. Neuromuscular is negative. Positive history for arthritis.

PHYSICAL EXAMINATION
VITAL SIGNS: Blood pressure is 140/80, pulse is 88 and regular, respirations 16 and regular.
GENERAL: This is a well-developed, obese female complaining of chest pain and shortness of breath.
HEENT: Head is normocephalic. She has bilateral arcus senilis and compensated edentulism.

(continued)

OLSEN, NATALIE
Hospital #123456
Page 2

NECK: Neck is supple. No bruits noted.
BREASTS: Breasts are without masses.
LUNGS: Lungs reveal scattered wheezes and basilar rales.
HEART: Heart reveals a regular sinus rhythm. She has a soft apical murmur.
ABDOMEN: Abdomen is 4+ protuberant. No masses are felt.
EXTREMITIES: Unremarkable with the exception of 1+ edema. Peripheral pulses are diminished but present.
NEUROLOGIC: Reflexes are equal and active. Neurologic is physiologic.

IMPRESSION
1. Arteriosclerotic heart disease with chest pain and congestive heart failure. Rule out myocardial infarction.
2. Diabetes mellitus.
3. Exogenous obesity.
4. Degenerative osteoarthritis.

KATHRYN PIEPER, MD

DH:hpi
D&T: 11/17/XXXX

BRYNER, CURTIS
#112538
DATE OF PROCEDURE: 5/25/XXXX

PREOPERATIVE DIAGNOSIS
Presyncope with intermittent junctional bradycardia.

POSTOPERATIVE DIAGNOSIS
Presyncope with intermittent junctional bradycardia.

OPERATION
Dual-chamber DDD transvenous pacemaker placement.

PACEMAKER GENERATOR
Pacesetter Model 2010T

SETTINGS
Bipolar leads: Atrial pulse width 0.6 msec. Sensitivity 1 mV. Pulse amplitude 4 volts. Refractory period 275 msec.
Ventricular bipolar lead: Pulse width 0.6 msec. Sensitivity 2 mV. Pulse amplitude 4 volts, and refractory period 250 msec.
Pacemaker mode: DDD. Rate: 70 pulses per minute. AV delay: 155 msec.
Lead threshold: Atrial lead model #P452PBV. Threshold 0.45 volts at 0.6 mA. Pulse width 0.6 msec. P-wave amplitude 3 mV. Lead impedance 490 ohms.
Ventricular lead: Bipolar lead model #10167. Threshold 0.7 volts with 0.8 mA at pulse width of 0.6 msec. R-wave amplitude 14.5 mV. Lead impedance 750 ohms.

OPERATION
The patient was prepped and draped in the usual manner. Using sedation and 1% Xylocaine anesthesia, an infraclavicular incision was made. The pocket was carried down to the fascia and placed subfascially. Then the subclavian vein was located with a needle and a guidewire placed into the vein. Two introducers were placed over this wire and the atrial and ventricular leads placed into the superior vena cava. Then the atrial lead was put into place and the leads screwed in. Then the ventricular lead was placed in the ventricular apex.

Thresholds were measured as obtained and were found to be quite adequate. The lead was checked for length on fluoroscopy and then attached into the pocket around a collar with a 2-0 silk suture. Then the leads and generator were connected together and the pacemaker placed into the pocket.

Hemostasis appeared to be good. The fascia was closed with interrupted 2-0 Vicryl and the subcutaneous tissue closed with running 3-0 Vicryl sutures. Skin was closed with a 4-0 Vicryl subcuticular stitch. The patient was taken to the recovery room in satisfactory condition.

JEFFREY REVENAUGH, MD

JR:hpi
d&t: 5/25/XXXX

Consultation Report

BLAUER, JAMES
#092796
Date of Consultation: 6/25/XXXX
Attending Physician: Brad Madsen, MD

The patient is seen in consultation because of chest pain and cardiac irregularity.

The patient tells me that about 10 years ago he had a severe episode of chest pain and was hospitalized for a heart attack.

About 3 days ago, he started having more shortness of breath. He also began having chest pains plus nausea and vomiting. His breathing was quite difficult, and he came to the emergency department, was found to be in congestive heart failure with cardiac irregularity, and was admitted to the hospital for further care.

The rest of his history can be obtained from his previous record.

On physical examination the patient does appear older than his stated age of 69 by at least 5 years. His blood pressure is 186/80, his pulse is 100 to 178, and he has runs of paroxysmal atrial tachycardia (PAT), frequent premature ventricular contractions, and he has had a couple of short runs of ventricular tachycardia. During one of his runs of PAT, I gave him 5 mg of verapamil intravenously, and this reduced the rate dramatically. His neck veins are distended. He has moist rales over both lungs. The heart is at the midclavicular line in the fifth interspace, and there is a systolic murmur at the apex. His abdomen is soft. No masses can be felt. He has 2+ edema in the lower extremities. Both of his knees have bruises from a previous fall. I did not do a rectal exam because of his respiratory difficulty.

It is my impression that he has a combination of arteriosclerotic and hypertensive cardiovascular disease with mild cardiomegaly, probable left ventricular hypertrophy, and congestive heart failure with functional classification of III. He also has pulmonary emphysema secondary to his smoking, with chronic obstructive pulmonary disease.

I have taken the liberty to discontinue the Theoclear L.A. for the present because I do not want to cause more cardiac irritability, and we will continue with the Calan, the diuretic, a low dose of Xylocaine, and we may have to go back to digoxin, but I would rather wait for a time in view of his ventricular ectopic beats.

Thank you for allowing me to see this patient, and I shall be glad to follow him with you.

GRANT CASTERELLA, MD

GC:hpi
d&t: 6/25/XXXX

Emergency Department Note

BOWMAN, CYNTHIA
#012465
Date of Visit: 4/13/XXXX
Attending: Lance Owens, MD

The patient is a 19-year-old white female who has a rather long and complicated medical history. Since 16 years of age, the patient has had chronic fatigue, extreme exercise intolerance, episodes of anorexia nervosa, and recurrent syncopal attacks. She is not able to walk up a flight of stairs or walk more than one block because of fatigue and dyspnea with exertion.

The patient was noted to have a sinus bradycardia with heart rates in the 40s at times. She had an echocardiogram which showed mitral valve prolapse. She had a treadmill exercise test, at which time she was able to go into stage 3 and achieved a maximum heart rate of 185 per minute. The test was remarkable for a rather flat blood pressure response with systolic blood pressure 114 at rest and into the exercise, with no appropriate increase during the exercise test. In addition, the patient developed a prolonged PR interval of 0.34, with some blocked atrial premature contractions (APCs) during the recovery phase of the exercise. She had evidence of both sinus node dysfunction and atrioventricular (AV) nodal disease.

IMPRESSION
1. Recurrent syncopal episode of unknown etiology. Patient does not have significant postural hypotension on examination. Patient has a history of sick sinus dysfunction. It is possible that the patient has a significant bradyarrhythmia precipitating syncopal episodes.
2. Possible sinus node dysfunction.

KATHERINE HORTON, MD

KH:hpi
d&t: 4/13/XXXX

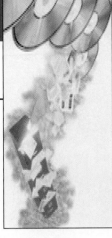

Transcription Practice

Key Words

The following terms appear in the cardiology/hematology dictations. Before beginning the medical transcription practice for Chapter 8, look up each term below in a medical or English dictionary and write out a short definition.

adenosine
angina
atrial fibrillation
cardiomyopathy
coronary stent
echocardiogram
Holter monitor
hypertension
LAD artery
lipids

pacemaker
PACs
PVCs
presyncope
renal artery stenosis
revascularization
status post CABG
stress test
stress echogram
tachycardia

After completing all the readings and exercises in Chapter 8, transcribe the cardiology/hematology dictation. Proofread your transcribed documents carefully, listening to the dictation while you read your transcripts.

Transcribe (*not* retype) the same reports again without referring to your previous transcription attempt. Initially, you may need to transcribe some reports more than twice before you can produce an error-free document. Your ultimate goal is to produce an error-free document the first time.

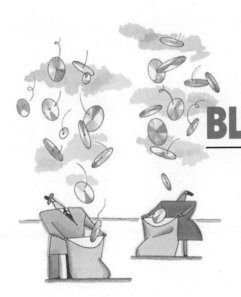

BLOOPERS

Incorrect	Correct
History of intermittent provocation.	History of intermittent claudication.
The EKG showed a wondering tape measure.	The EKG showed a wandering pacemaker.
Cardiospastic ratio.	Cardiothoracic ratio.
Patient with low bile hypertension.	Patient with labile hypertension.
Foraminal valley.	Foramen ovale.
The rhythm is sinus with primal eruptions by atrial interior beeps.	The rhythm is sinus with occasional atrial premature beats.
Memories, scallops, and rubs.	Murmurs, gallops, and rubs.

Gastroenterology

Chapter Outline

Learning Objectives

- Describe the structure and function of the gastrointestinal system.
- Spell and define common gastrointestinal terms.
- Identify types of questions a physician might ask about the digestive system during the review of systems.
- Describe common features a physician looks for on examination of the abdomen.
- Identify common diseases of the gastrointestinal system. Describe their typical cause, course, and treatment options.

- Identify and define diagnostic and surgical procedures of the gastrointestinal system.
- List common gastrointestinal laboratory tests and procedures.
- Identify and describe common gastrointestinal drugs and their uses.
- Demonstrate knowledge of anatomical, medical, pharmacological, adjectival, and soundalike terms by accurately completing the exercises in this chapter.

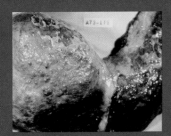
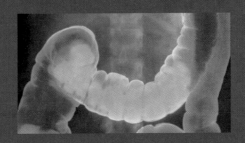
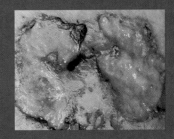

Transcribing Gastroenterology Dictation

The **gastrointestinal** (GI) **(digestive) system** (Figure 9-1) includes all those structures concerned with the ingestion of solids and liquids, their mechanical and chemical breakdown into usable nutrients, the absorption of these into the circulation, and the excretion of solid wastes.

Anatomy in Brief

The **alimentary canal** is a coiled but unbranched tube extending from the lips to the anus and divided into mouth, oropharynx, esophagus, stomach, small intestine (duodenum, jejunum, ileum), and large intestine (colon, rectum).

Numerous microscopic glandular structures occur in the walls of the digestive tract (gastric glands, intestinal glands), and in addition larger secretory organs (salivary glands, liver, pancreas) pour their products through ducts into parts of the tract. These secretions serve to liquefy and lubricate food and to break down fats, proteins, and carbohydrates to fatty acids, amino acids, and simple sugars, respectively.

The **peritoneum** is a delicate serous membrane that lines the abdominal and pelvic cavities (**parietal peritoneum**) and also covers the stomach, small intestine, and

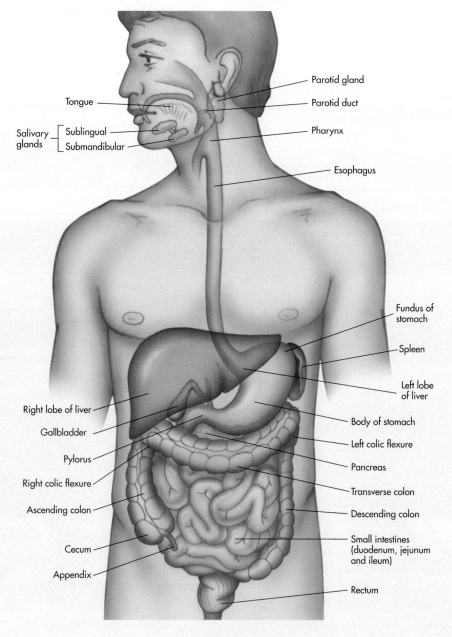

Figure 9-1
The Digestive System

colon (except for the distal part of the rectum), as well as the liver, spleen, uterus, ovaries, ureters, and dome of the bladder (**visceral peritoneum**). Structures such as the pancreas and kidneys that lie behind the peritoneal cavity are called retroperitoneal.

The **liver**, the largest gland in the body, lies in the right upper quadrant of the abdomen just below the **diaphragm** and is largely covered by peritoneum. The liver performs numerous vital functions and is intimately concerned with carbohydrate and nitrogen metabolism and with removal of certain waste products. **Bile**, the secretory product of the liver, passes through a duct into the duodenum. Bile contains **bile salts**, which help in the digestion of fats, and bilirubin, a breakdown product of hemoglobin. Bile does not flow steadily into the duodenum, but is stored in the **gallbladder**, a bulb or pouch connected by the cystic duct to the common bile duct. Ingestion of a fatty meal stimulates contraction of the gallbladder and increased flow of bile into the intestine.

The **pancreas** is a flat retroperitoneal organ lying behind and below the stomach, with its right end (head) embraced by the sweep of the duodenum. It is composed of two types of glandular tissue: groups of cells that secrete enzymes for the digestion of carbohydrate, protein, and fat, which are poured through a duct into the duodenum near the orifice of the common bile duct; and other groups of cells that secrete hormones (insulin, glucagon, somatostatin) and release them directly into the bloodstream.

Terminology Review

adenoma A benign tumor arising from glandular epithelium.

anaplastic Referring to tumor tissue containing primitive, undifferentiated cells, unlike the structurally differentiated cells of normal tissue.

anorexia Loss of appetite.

belching Burping.

bloating An overly full, distended feeling, usually from excessive intestinal gas.

borborygmi (singular, **borborygmus**) Audible rumbling and gurgling sounds in the digestive tract.

colic Sharp, crampy pains.

colon Term that can mean part or all of the large intestine.

constipation Firm, difficult stools.

diarrhea Abnormal frequency, urgency, and looseness of stools.

diverticulum An abnormal outpouching of a hollow organ such as the colon.

dysphagia Difficulty swallowing.

endorectal Inside the rectum; said of diagnostic or therapeutic instruments or procedures.

enterocolitis Inflammatory disease of both the small and large intestines.

eructation Belching; burping.

flatulence Excessive intestinal gas.

heartburn Burning pain in the epigastrium or chest due to digestive disorders.

hematemesis Vomiting blood.

hematochezia Passage of blood from the rectum.

hemorrhoids Anal varicose veins.

hepatic Referring to the liver.

hernia Protrusion of organ or tissue through an abnormal opening.

hyperplasia An increase in the number of cells in a tissue or organ.

ileus Intestinal obstruction.

intussusception Prolapse of one part of the intestine into another.

jaundice Discoloration of skin and sclerae by excessive bile pigment.

lientery Passage of undigested food in stools.

melena Black stools (often due to the presence of blood).

obstipation Total inability to pass stool.

odynophagia Pain on swallowing.

palliative Directed to the relief of symptoms rather than the elimination of their cause.

postprandial Following a meal.

rebound tenderness Additional stab of pain when pressure on abdomen is released, often indicating peritoneal irritation.

splenomegaly Enlargement of the spleen.

steatorrhea Excessive amounts of fat in the feces.

tenesmus Straining at stool, usually without result and often painful.

transrectal Said of a diagnostic or surgical procedure that is performed through the rectum.

volvulus Intestinal obstruction due to twisting of the bowel.

Lay and Medical Terms

belching	eructation
chewing	mastication
fart, pass gas	expel flatus
gallstones	cholelithiasis
gas in bowel	flatulence
heartburn	pyrosis
piles	hemorrhoids
vomiting	emesis

Medical Readings

History and Physical Examination

by John H. Dirckx, M.D.

Review of Systems. The gastrointestinal history is concerned mainly with two types of symptoms: abdominal pain of any type or degree (though abdominal pain often results from nondigestive causes); and any disturbances of digestive function, including **anorexia**, nausea, vomiting, and diarrhea. Symptoms due to disorders of the liver or biliary tract, the pancreas, or the rectum or anus are also included here.

In reviewing the past digestive tract history, the examiner inquires about previous diagnoses of hiatal hernia, ulcer, gallstones or gallbladder disease, pancreatitis, colitis; any tumors of the alimentary canal or associated structures; results of gastrointestinal x-rays or other diagnostic studies (esophagoscopy, gastroscopy, colonoscopy); operations on the digestive organs, including appendectomy and hemorrhoid surgery; and use of antacids, laxatives, enemas, or prescription medicines for digestive symptoms.

Abdominal pain may be described as burning, crampy, or dull. It may be constant, intermittent, or of varying intensity. It may remain in one place or radiate or migrate to another, perhaps in the back or chest. It may be brought on, aggravated, or relieved by eating, not eating, drinking, having a bowel movement, or assuming certain positions. It may be provoked by taking certain medicines or eating certain foods; a record of any food intolerances is an important part of the digestive history.

Symptoms besides abdominal pain that draw attention to the digestive system are anorexia, nausea, pain or difficulty in swallowing that seems to originate below the pharynx, vomiting, flatulence, constipation, diarrhea,

abnormal appearance of the stools, weight loss, jaundice, and anorectal pain, swelling, or bleeding. A history of vomiting prompts inquiries about its frequency and the volume and character of emesis. Blood that is mixed with gastric contents often has a characteristic coffee-grounds appearance. Jaundice (a yellow color of the skin, mucous membranes, and ocular sclerae) indicates an excessive quantity of bile pigment in blood and tissues. It can result from intrinsic liver disease (hepatitis, hepatic failure) or from obstruction of the biliary tract by a gallstone or a tumor.

Because constipation and diarrhea mean different things to different people, the interviewer must carefully determine the frequency and consistency of the patient's stools. Even with normal bowel habits, an abnormal stool color can indicate disease. Clay-colored stools occur in obstruction of the biliary tract because bile does not reach the intestine. Blood that has passed through much of the intestine before appearing in the stool may look tarry black (melena) because of chemical changes in blood pigment.

Inguinal hernia may also be considered with the gastrointestinal history because most hernias contain loops of bowel and eventually affect digestive or eliminative function. The patient is asked about swelling or bulging in the groin or scrotum that is accentuated by coughing or straining and diminishes or disappears in the recumbent position.

Physical Examination of the abdomen is performed to assess skin turgor and muscle tone, to determine the size, shape, and position of the abdominal and pelvic organs, and to detect any masses or tenderness. The physician starts with light palpation, which provides information about the abdominal wall and any zones of tenderness, and then progresses to deep palpation to study the internal organs and search for masses. An area of pain or tenderness known to the physician is examined last.

Throughout the examination, the physician closely observes the patient's face for signs of distress. Rebound tenderness, a transient stab of pain when the abdomen is pressed and then suddenly released, denotes local or generalized peritoneal irritation. The physician may look for tenderness in the liver or gallbladder by gentle fist percussion over the right lower ribs or by hooking the fingers of the examining hand under the right costal margin and asking the patient to inhale deeply. Costovertebral angle tenderness occurs in inflammation or infection of the kidney or ureter.

Most normal intra-abdominal structures cannot be distinctly felt through the abdominal wall. By vigorous palpation of a very thin patient, one can feel parts of the normal liver, spleen, and kidneys, but ordinarily these organs must be enlarged before they can be palpated. No part of the digestive tract can normally be felt, nor can the pancreas, gallbladder, or ureters. In an obese patient, even gross abnormalities can escape detection by palpation.

Percussion can be used to measure the **liver span** (the width of liver dullness between lung and bowel resonances) and to distinguish between a solid organ or tumor, which yields a dull or flat note, and bowel distended by gas, which yields a hollow or resonant note. It can also confirm the presence of **ascites** (free fluid in the peritoneal cavity) by detecting a change in the percussion note as the patient rolls from the supine position to the right or left side (shifting dullness).

A Doctor's View

A Surgeon's View of Gastroenterology and Practice

by Thomas L. Largen, M.D., FACS

As a board-certified general surgeon in private practice for 30 years, I have performed numerous surgical procedures. But one of my favorite subjects is gastroenterology, that branch of medical science concerned with the study of the stomach, intestines, and related structures, including the esophagus, liver, gallbladder, and pancreas.

The Gastroenterology Team. The advent of endoscopy and the specialization of gastroenterology have certainly made the field of GI surgery a more interesting one. At the hospital where I currently practice, we have several board-certified gastroenterologists—medical doctors trained in the treatment of diseases involving the gastrointestinal tract and trained in the use of flexible endoscopes to study the esophagus, stomach, pancreatic ducts, biliary ducts, the entire colon, and sometimes the distal small bowel.

Teamwork. A patient's presenting problem is first assessed by one of the gastroenterologists. If medical treatment methods are found to be unsuccessful—as in controlling hemorrhage, for example—then I am called upon to carry out definitive surgery. From a surgeon's viewpoint, it is a tremendous help to know exactly what I can expect to find when I begin the surgery, and the information from the gastroenterologist enables me to plan accordingly.

The Miracle of the Modern Endoscope. An endoscope is a long hollow tube with a light source that can be inserted into a hollow organ to view and assess the condition of the organ. In gastroenterology, there are three categories of endoscopes: the esophagogastroscope, the sigmoidoscope, and the colonoscope.

When I was a resident in the early 1950s, only rigid endoscopes existed. The rigid esophagoscope of that era was a very dangerous instrument. It could easily perforate the esophagus, which in essence is a flimsy, thin-walled tube. Additionally, it was of little value in examining the stomach because it could not negotiate the curves and corners of the organ.

The rigid sigmoidoscope of the 1950s was about 10 inches, or 25 cm, in length, and it too had its limitations. Because it was short, it didn't allow much exposure, and because it was rigid, there was the danger of perforating the lower colon.

Then in the early 1970s, Japan introduced the first **fiberoptic flexible endoscope**. That event alone drastically changed the direction and practice of gastroenterology. Up until 25 years ago, most gastroenterology work was performed by general surgeons. With the advent of flexible fiberoptics, medical doctors began to specialize in diagnosis, treatment, and procedures of the GI tract, and the field of gastroenterology became a specialty. Today, most endoscopes utilize state-of-the-art flexible fiberoptics.

Endoscopic Diagnosis and Treatment. This is an exciting time in gastroenterology practice. With the introduction of the flexible endoscope, new treatment modalities have evolved. People who present with gastrointestinal hemorrhage from either the upper GI tract (the esophagus, stomach, or duodenum) or the lower GI tract (the colon) are frequently diagnosed by means of upper and/or lower endoscopy.

Bleeding sites can be controlled by application of a heat probe through the endoscope or injection of a sclerosing (hardening) agent through a long needle passed through the endoscope. Bleeding esophageal varices are often controlled by sclerosing these dilated varicose veins through the esophagoscope.

Patients who have had strokes or other medical problems are sometimes unable to swallow or eat properly and require a temporary alternative means of securing nutrition. A feeding tube can be inserted into the stomach by way of an esophagogastroscope, eliminating the need to do open surgery for this purpose. Endoscopes are also useful in removing foreign bodies from the esophagus and occasionally from the stomach or duodenum.

Today, surgical procedures can actually be performed through endoscopes. For example, an experienced gastroenterologist can do a **sphincterotomy** through the scope (cutting the sphincter of Oddi, which is located in the second portion of the duodenum through which the pancreatic duct and the common bile duct enter the small intestine). Retained gallstones in the biliary ducts can be extracted using a wire basket-type catheter placed through the scope, eliminating the need for the patient to undergo an open operation.

There is a gastroenterologist in England who is so good at manipulating the **esophagogastroduodenoscope** (EGD) that he can actually go through the sphincter of Oddi, into the common bile duct, then into the cystic duct and into the gallbladder to remove stones! Unfortunately, this is more a feat of showmanship than practical application, because gallstones always come back if you do nothing but simply remove them.

Polypectomies (the surgical removal of outgrowths) are frequently performed to remove polyps in the stomach and colon. A wire snare is connected to an electrosurgical unit, placed through the endoscope, and the polyp is removed and the bleeding base coagulated. Polyps are a common occurrence and may or may not be malignant.

Endoscopes are leading the way to early diagnosis and treatment of malignancies. Directed laser beams can be used through the endoscope for palliative surgery such as burning a hole through a malignant tumor in the esophagus to allow a patient to swallow. Malignancies of the stomach and colon are diagnosed much earlier, thanks to endoscopes, and are increasing our chances for curing neoplasms of the entire GI tract.

Laparoscopy. Examination of structures in the abdomen by means of an endoscope inserted through a small incision in the abdominal wall has virtually replaced open procedures (exploratory laparotomy) undertaken for purely diagnostic reasons. In addition, many surgical procedures formerly requiring laparotomy, such as appendectomy, cholecystectomy, inguinal herniorrhaphy, and oophorectomy, are now routinely performed laparoscopically.

The patient undergoing laparoscopy is first given a general anesthetic. A Veress needle is then inserted through a skin puncture, usually just below the umbilicus, and carbon dioxide gas is introduced into the peritoneal cavity under pressure. This process is called **insufflation**, and the condition it creates—the presence of air or gas in the peritoneal cavity—is called **pneumoperitoneum**. The purpose of creating a pneumoperitoneum is to distend the abdominal cavity so as to permit manipulation of the laparoscope and visualization of abdominal and pelvic structures. An incision or port is then made through the abdominal wall at a location most suitable for the intended investigation, and the laparoscope is introduced. Further incisions may be made as needed. For surgical procedures, other instruments may be inserted through these incisions. Carbon dioxide gas is released from the abdomen at the end of the procedure.

Other Advances. Although the use of flexible fiberoptic endoscopes dominates modern gastroenterology practice, other diagnostic modes are also utilized. It may come as a surprise that the value of traditional **contrast media studies** (upper GI series, air-contrast barium enema) rests entirely with the radiologist. It takes a dedicated, interested radiologist to produce a diagnostic exam.

I have the good fortune to work with one of the finest radiologists in the country. He recently spent a great deal of time doing a Gastrografin enema on a patient of mine, massaging and filling the small bowel for a retrograde study. The radiologist was able to diagnose an **intussusception** of the distal small bowel, a feat which I have never seen before or since. His diagnosis was absolutely correct, as I proved that evening in surgery. Most radiologists would have missed this diagnosis.

Ultrasound (visualizing internal body structures by recording the reflections of ultrasonic waves) is useful in diagnosing biliary tract disease and pancreatic disease. **Nuclear studies** such as HIDA/DISIDA scans are helpful in identifying biliary tract involvement. There is also a nuclear scan that localizes gastrointestinal bleeding sites. **Computerized tomography** (CT) scans can help diagnose pancreatic and liver masses. **Magnetic resonance imaging** (MRI) studies are yet to be of much help in evaluating the gastrointestinal tract, although **arteriography** is of great help in localizing bleeding sites, and even therapeutically stopping a bleeding vessel by plugging (embolizing) the vessel with small debris, such as Gelfoam.

The use of mechanical bowel preparations and preoperative and perioperative antibiotics has markedly decreased postoperative wound infections and leaks. However, there is no substitute for good surgical technique. The gastrointestinal contents should never be allowed to spill into the wound or abdominal cavity. Gloves and instruments should be changed immediately upon completing a gastrointestinal **anastomosis** (sewing two ends together) and proceeding with closure of the surgical wound.

The advent of **surgical staplers**, originally introduced in Russia, has made gastrointestinal surgery safer, quicker, and more fun to do. Resections of various parts of the GI tract used to take two to three hours; now a resection can be accomplished in 30 to 45 minutes in most cases.

The world of gastroenterology is a fascinating one. I particularly enjoy being a gastrointestinal surgeon. It's like Christmas every day—I open a new package and I never know for sure what I am going to find!

Common Diseases

Gastroesophageal Reflux Disease (GERD).
Backflow of gastric juice into the esophagus.

Cause: Structural or functional incompetence of the lower esophageal sphincter (**LES**), associated with disordered gastric motility and prolonged gastric emptying time. In a few cases, reflux of gastric juice may be facilitated by **esophageal hiatus hernia** (weakness or dilatation of the opening in the diaphragm where the esophagus passes through, with herniation of part or all of the stomach into the thorax; often asymptomatic). Reflux of acid gastric juice into the esophagus causes inflammation because the esophageal mucosa is not adapted to resist acid and digestive enzymes.

History: Recurrent epigastric and retrosternal distress, usually described as heartburn; belching, nausea, gagging, cough, hoarseness in varying proportions. There is a strong association with asthma, obesity, and diabetes mellitus. Symptoms are triggered or aggravated by recumbency (especially after a meal), vigorous exercise, smoking, overeating, caffeine, chocolate, alcohol, and certain drugs.

Physical Examination: Unremarkable.

Diagnostic Tests: Imaging studies confirm reflux of swallowed barium from the stomach and may identify ulceration or stricture. The 24-hour monitoring of esophageal pH with a swallowed electrode proves a sustained abnormal acid state in the esophagus. Endoscopy gives direct visual proof of inflammation and may identify a zone of **Barrett esophagus** (cellular change due to chronic inflammation).

Course: The underlying disorder of the LES and of gastric motility is irreversible. Severe reflux disease can lead to peptic ulceration of the esophagus, with eventual stricture due to scarring. Another possible complication is Barrett esophagus, a metaplasia (transformation) of normal squamous esophageal epithelium into columnar epithelium; some cases of Barrett esophagus progress to adenocarcinoma.

Treatment: Avoidance of smoking, alcohol, caffeine, and large meals. Over-the-counter antacids may suffice to control symptoms. Otherwise, acid production may require suppression by H_2 antagonists (cimetidine, ranitidine, famotidine, nizatidine) or proton pump inhibitors (omeprazole, lansoprazole). Prokinetic drugs (bethanechol, metoclopramide, cisapride) may improve sphincter function and gastric motility.

Peptic Ulcer Disease (PUD) and Gastritis.
Inflammation and ulceration of the stomach, duodenum, or both by acid gastric juice (Figure 9-2).

Cause: Most commonly, infection of the gastric mucosa by *Helicobacter pylori*, a motile bacterium that survives in the

acid environment of the stomach by secreting urease, an enzyme that converts urea to ammonia and bicarbonate, thus providing a protective alkaline medium for itself. *H. pylori* infection, which is spread from person to person by the fecal-oral route, results ultimately in a marked increase of acid production.

Peptic ulceration can also result from regular use of prostaglandin-inhibiting drugs: adrenal corticosteroids and nonsteroidal anti-inflammatory agents such as ibuprofen and aspirin. In rare cases it is part of Zollinger-Ellison syndrome, in which a tumor of the pancreas produces

Barrett *Esophagus*

Barrett esophagus is a metaplastic change, first described by the British surgeon Norman Barrett in 1950, in which the normal stratified squamous epithelium of the lower esophagus is converted to columnar epithelium like that of the gastric and intestinal mucosa. The condition causes no symptoms and is diagnosed incidentally on endoscopy and confirmed by biopsy. A zone of columnar metaplasia has a velvety texture and an intense pink to red color, in contrast to the normal smooth, off-white surface of squamous epithelium.

About 10% of persons with GERD eventually develop this condition. Acid reflux is apparently instrumental in inducing cellular metaplasia. But since as many as one third of patients with Barrett esophagus do not have typical symptoms of GERD, it is suspected that some co-factor may heighten the risk that esophageal mucosa will undergo this change under the influence of refluxed gastric juice. According to one theory, bile salts in refluxed fluid constitute this co-factor. (In order for bile salts to appear in gastric juice, bile must first reflux from the duodenum through the pylorus and into the stomach.)

The chief significance of Barrett esophagus is that it is recognized as a premalignant change. Adenocarcinoma, a relatively uncommon type of esophageal cancer, is approximately 50 times as common in persons with Barrett esophagus as in the general population. Each year about 1% of patients with Barrett esophagus progress to carcinoma.

One recent study concluded that Barrett esophagus is also associated with a fivefold increase in the risk of cancer of the colon. In addition, persons with Barrett esophagus have a 30% risk of esophageal stricture, as opposed to a 10% risk in patients without columnar metaplasia.

For unknown reasons, the incidence of Barrett-related esophageal cancer is increasing rapidly. And although it has been thought of as typically a disorder of middle-aged white men, its incidence in women and African Americans appears to be rising.

John H. Dirckx, M.D.
Perspectives on the Medical Transcription Profession

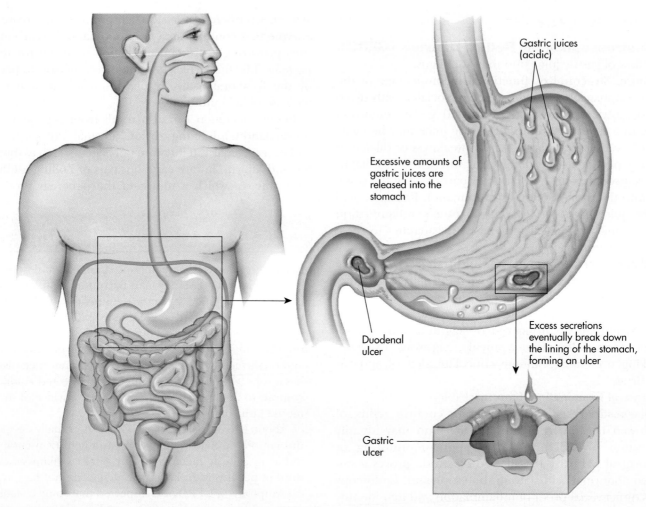

Figure 9-2
Peptic Ulcer Disease

excessive amounts of the hormone gastrin and thus causes hypersecretion of gastric acid. Severe stress, head injuries, and burns are sometimes complicated by peptic ulcer. Most peptic ulcers occur in the duodenum, but the stomach may be involved as well or instead.

History: Burning epigastric pain that comes on within an hour after meals and is relieved by taking antacids or food. Night pain is common. Tobacco, alcohol, caffeine, and certain foods aggravate symptoms, apparently by stimulating acid production. With complications: hematemesis, melena, **early satiety** (feeling that the stomach is full after only one or two mouthfuls of food), weight loss, severe abdominal pain, collapse.

Physical Examination: Unremarkable. Abdominal tenderness is variable and may be absent. With hemorrhage: pallor and tachycardia. With perforation: boardlike rigidity of the abdomen due to chemical peritonitis.

Diagnostic Tests: Upper GI studies with barium contrast medium can show ulceration, scarring, obstruction, or perforation. Endoscopy visualizes ulcers, bleeding sites, and scarring, and it is important to rule out carcinoma in

gastric lesions. Infection by *H. pylori* can be confirmed by culture, biopsy, serologic testing, or breath-testing for evidence of urease activity on orally administered isotopically tagged urea.

Course: Without treatment, peptic ulcer disease tends to persist, with remissions and exacerbations, for many years. The most serious complications are hemorrhage (the principal cause of ulcer mortality), obstruction due to scarring, perforation of the digestive tract with release of gastric juice into the peritoneal cavity, and penetration into the retroperitoneal space.

Treatment: Smoking cessation, avoidance of alcohol and caffeine. Acidity may be adequately controlled by over-the-counter antacids, H_2 antagonists (cimetidine, ranitidine, famotidine, nizatidine) in over-the-counter or prescription strength, or proton pump inhibitors (omeprazole, lansoprazole). Proven *H. pylori* infection is treated with a course of therapy including bismuth subsalicylate and two antibiotics, tetracycline or amoxicillin, and metronidazole or clarithromycin.

Gastroenteritis. Inflammation of the stomach and intestine, manifested by abdominal pain, vomiting, and diarrhea; usually acute, infectious, and self-limited.

Causes: Infection with viruses (adenovirus, echovirus, coxsackievirus, rotavirus), bacteria (*Escherichia coli* H157:O7 and other virulent strains, *Campylobacter, Yersinia, Salmonella, Shigella, Clostridium*), protozoa (*Entamoeba histolytica, Giardia lamblia*), fungi (*Candida albicans*). Most of these infections are acquired by the fecal-oral route. Some are much more likely to occur in immunocompromised persons. Outbreaks are usually due to contaminated food or water. "Food poisoning" is due to toxins produced by staphylococci, *Salmonella, Clostridium*, or other organisms. Gastroenteritis can also be a reaction to medicines, foods, poisonous plants, toxic chemicals.

History: Usually abrupt onset of abdominal distress or cramping, anorexia, nausea, vomiting, and diarrhea. Chills, fever, malaise. Hematemesis and bloody diarrhea are ominous signs. In severe or protracted disease, or in children or the elderly, dehydration and electrolyte depletion can lead to prostration, vascular collapse, and death.

Physical Examination: May be unremarkable. Abdominal tenderness, **tympanites** (hollow percussion note due to distention of bowel with gas), hyperactive bowel sounds. In severe disease, signs of dehydration and electrolyte depletion include dryness of mucous membranes, **decreased skin turgor** (loss of normal consistency and fullness), tachycardia, hypoactive deep tendon reflexes, and decreased urine output.

Diagnostic Tests: Stool examination for white blood cells and organisms, with culture for pathogenic bacteria. Blood studies may show hematologic abnormalities or fluid and electrolyte imbalance.

Course: Most cases of gastroenteritis, even those caused by bacteria such as *Salmonella, Campylobacter*, and *Yersinia*, resolve spontaneously without specific treatment. However, cholera (due to *Vibrio cholerae*, rare in the U.S.), bacillary dysentery (due to *Shigella* species), typhoid fever (due to *Salmonella typhi*), and **pseudomembranous enterocolitis** (due to toxin-producing *Clostridium difficile*, often following treatment with antibiotics that kill normal intestinal flora) are all severe and potentially fatal infections requiring prompt, aggressive antimicrobial treatment. Gastroenteritis in small children or in elderly or debilitated persons can lead to dangerous electrolyte and water depletion and vascular collapse.

Treatment: Largely symptomatic and supportive. Over-the-counter products may suffice to control nausea, cramping, and diarrhea. Water and electrolytes may be replaced orally or intravenously as indicated. Antibiotic treatment is indicated only in certain specific infections. Trimethoprim-sulfamethoxazole or ciprofloxacin are effective in bacillary dysentery (shigellosis), typhoid fever,

and cholera; pseudomembranous enterocolitis is treated with metronidazole or vancomycin.

Appendicitis. Acute inflammation of the appendix.

Cause: Obstruction of the appendiceal lumen by a **fecalith** (stonelike mass of hardened feces), seed, or parasite, or by swelling due to infection or neoplasm. Obstruction is followed by inflammation, impairment of blood supply, necrosis, and rupture.

History: Gradual onset of generalized abdominal distress gradually becoming more severe and steady and localizing in the right lower quadrant. Anorexia, nausea, vomiting, fever, chills, constipation. Sudden spontaneous relief of pain suggests perforation.

Physical Examination: Slight fever and tachycardia, tenderness and rebound tenderness over **McBurney point** (about one third of the distance from the right anterior superior iliac spine to the umbilicus), tenderness and rebound tenderness in the same area on rectal or pelvic examination. Diminished bowel sounds. After perforation, boardlike rigidity of the abdomen indicating peritonitis, signs of toxicity, vascular collapse. In infants, the elderly, and pregnant women, the findings may be atypical or deceptively mild.

Diagnostic Tests: Moderate elevation of the white blood cell count, with left shift (increase of band or immature forms). Focused CT may show a mass, ileus, or other signs of peritonitis, or an opacity in the appendiceal lumen; barium injected by rectum fails to fill the appendix.

Course: Without treatment the condition has a mortality rate over 90%. Most cases progress to perforation within 12-36 hours, followed by generalized peritonitis, septicemia, and collapse.

Treatment: Surgical removal of the appendix (by open procedure or laparoscopy) is the only effective treatment. Perforation requires surgical repair, intravenous fluids, and antibiotics.

Irritable Bowel Syndrome (IBS). Intermittent or chronic abdominal distress and bowel dysfunction without any demonstrable organic lesion.

Cause: Unknown. A derangement of the normal interaction between the brain and the bowel is postulated. IBS is more likely to occur with emotional stress, dietary irregularities, and heavy intake of caffeine. Lactose intolerance and abuse of antacids or laxatives may be partly responsible. The disorder is more common in women and in persons under 65. As many as 50% of patients report a history of verbal or sexual abuse.

History: Intermittent lower abdominal pain, often relieved by having a bowel movement; alternating diarrhea and constipation; a sense of inadequate evacuation after bowel movement; excessive mucus in stools; flatulence.

Physical Examination: Essentially negative.

Diagnostic Tests: Stool examinations, barium enema, colonoscopy, and blood studies are all negative.

Course: Symptoms tend to wax and wane for many years, with intervals of complete remission.

Treatment: Regular eating habits, avoidance of coffee and other triggering factors. Antispasmodics may be prescribed to reduce bowel motility and cramping. Alosetron and tegaserod usually provide control of severe symptoms, but only in women.

Crohn Disease (Regional Enteritis, Regional Ileitis).

A chronic inflammatory disease of the bowel that can lead to intestinal obstruction, abscess and fistula formation, and systemic complications.

Cause: Unknown. The disease shows a familial pattern of incidence.

History: Recurrent crampy or steady abdominal pain, nausea, diarrhea, **steatorrhea** (excessive fat in stool), hematochezia, weakness, weight loss, and fever.

Physical Examination: Abdominal tenderness, signs of complications.

Diagnostic Tests: The white blood count and erythrocyte sedimentation rate are elevated. There may be mild anemia and reduction of serum levels of potassium, calcium, magnesium, and other substances. Barium enema shows regional narrowing of the lumen ("**string sign**") alternating with areas of normal caliber. Sigmoidoscopy and colonoscopy show local inflammation with **skip areas** (intervening zones of normal mucosa). On biopsy, all layers of the bowel are seen to be involved, not just the mucosa as in ulcerative colitis.

Course: Complications include intestinal obstruction, formation of abscesses and fistulas, perforation of the bowel.

Treatment: Low-fiber diet, drugs to reduce intestinal motility, specific anti-inflammatory drugs (azathioprine, sulfasalazine, olsalazine). Surgery may be necessary to deal with perforation or fistula formation. In severe disease, segmental resection of the bowel, or colectomy with ileostomy, may be necessary.

Ulcerative Colitis.

A chronic inflammatory disease of the colon, chiefly the left colon, causing superficial ulceration.

Cause: Unknown.

History: Bloody diarrhea, abdominal cramps, tenesmus, anorexia, malaise, weakness, hemorrhoids or anal fissures. Bowel movements may occur more than 20 times a day and may awaken the patient at night.

Physical Examination: Fever, abdominal tenderness, signs of complications.

Diagnostic Tests: The white blood count and erythrocyte sedimentation rate are elevated. Anemia

may be present. Stool examination reveals mucus, blood, and pus, but no bacteria or parasites. Serum electrolytes and protein may be depleted. Sigmoidoscopy and colonoscopy show erythematous, friable mucosa with superficial ulceration, and sometimes polyp formation. Biopsy shows chronic inflammation and microabscesses of the crypts of Lieberkühn.

Course: The course is intermittent, with spontaneous remissions and exacerbations. Physical and emotional stress and dietary irregularities may increase symptoms. Possible complications include colonic hemorrhage, perforation, **toxic dilatation** (extreme dilatation of the colon, compounded by effect of bacterial toxins); polyp formation with progression to carcinoma; arthritis, spondylitis; iritis; oral ulcers.

Treatment: General supportive treatment and control of diet (high protein, low milk) are crucial to long-term control of the disease. Sulfasalazine, mesalamine, and corticosteroids suppress colonic inflammation and reduce symptoms. In severe disease, hospitalization with intravenous alimentation and fluid replacement and antibiotic treatment to combat sepsis may be necessary. In intractable disease, colectomy and ileostomy may be necessary.

Diverticulosis and Diverticulitis.

A **diverticulum** (plural, **diverticula**) is a blister- or bubble-like outpouching of a hollow or tubular organ. **Diverticulosis** of the colon (see Figure 9-3) is the formation of one or more such outpouchings of the colon. **Diverticulitis** means inflammation and infection of colonic diverticula.

Cause: Unknown; more common in middle-aged and elderly.

History: Most patients with diverticulosis have no symptoms. The diverticula may be discovered incidentally on routine examination (barium enema, colonoscopy). A few patients may experience irregular bowel habits or abdominal pain. Patients in whom diverticulitis develops experience acute abdominal pain, nausea, vomiting, constipation, and sometimes fever or blood in the stools.

Physical Examination: With the development of diverticulitis, there may be mild fever, abdominal tenderness, and even the sensation of a mass, most often in the region of the sigmoid colon (left lower quadrant of the abdomen).

Diagnostic Tests: The white blood count and sedimentation rate may be slightly elevated. The stool may be positive for occult blood. Barium enema, sigmoidoscopy, or colonoscopy may be performed to identify and localize the lesion, but are contraindicated in the presence of acute inflammation because of the danger of perforation of the bowel. X-ray studies may be used to identify free air in the peritoneal cavity due to perforation, and CT scan may be done to detect abscess formation.

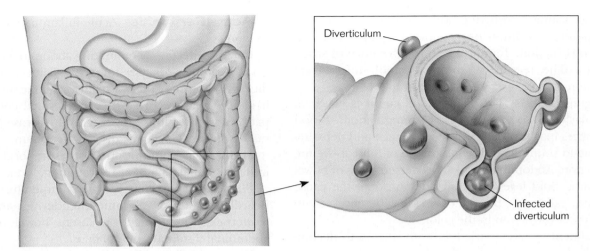

Figure 9-3
Colon with Diverticulitis

Diagnostic evaluation needs to be particularly thorough to rule out malignancy.

Course: Diverticulitis may lead to hemorrhage, perforation of the bowel, obstruction due to fibrous scarring, fistula formation, abscess formation.

Treatment: Patients with mild or no symptoms may require no treatment but are often advised to follow a high-fiber diet. During the acute phase of diverticulitis, patients are kept at bed rest, with nothing by mouth (n.p.o., NPO), intravenous fluids and nutrition, and, if necessary, a nasogastric tube. Usually antibiotic treatment is used because of the risk of peritonitis and abscess formation. Metronidazole, ciprofloxacin, and trimethoprim-sulfamethoxazole are the drugs usually used. As many as one third of patients with diverticulitis will need surgery to drain an abscess or to resect a segment of badly diseased colon.

Intestinal Obstruction. Blockage of the flow of digestive fluids through the small or large intestine.

Causes: Surgical adhesions, hernia, neoplasms, gallstones, **volvulus** (twisting of a loop of intestine) (see Figure 9-4), **intussusception** (passage of a segment of intestine into the segment distal to it), foreign body, fecal impaction. Obstruction due to causes outside the bowel (volvulus, hernia) are often complicated by **strangulation** (ischemia of the involved portion of bowel).

History: Crampy abdominal pain, nausea, vomiting, obstipation. Obstruction of the small intestine causes more severe and rapidly progressing symptoms than obstruction of the colon.

Physical Examination: Abdominal distention, **borborygmi** (gurgling sounds due to intestinal activity); increased bowel sounds, often high-pitched or in peristaltic **rushes** (urgent-sounding series of squeaking or

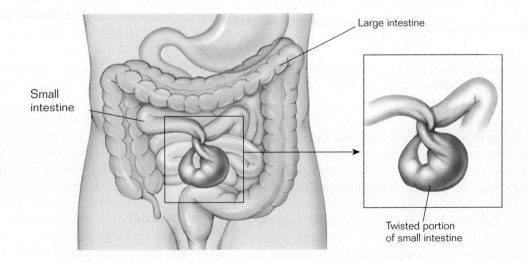

Figure 9-4
Volvulus

gurgling sounds occurring with overactive peristaltic movements). A fullness or mass may be palpated at the site of obstruction. Tenderness in the presence of strangulation. The rectum is empty of stool unless fecal impaction is the cause of obstruction.

Diagnostic Tests: The white blood count is elevated, particularly in the presence of strangulation. Blood chemistries may show electrolyte imbalance and dehydration due to vomiting and sequestration of fluid above the obstruction. Abdominal x-rays show dilated loops of bowel containing fluid levels, and may demonstrate the cause (volvulus, gallstone). Barium enema may be necessary to identify an obstruction in the colon.

Treatment: A nasogastric tube with suction to decompress the bowel proximal to the obstruction. Intravenous fluids to correct dehydration and electrolyte imbalance. Surgery is often necessary to relieve obstruction and to resect infarcted areas of bowel in cases of strangulation.

Adynamic Ileus. Failure of normal flow of materials through the digestive tract because of atony or paralysis of the bowel.

Causes: Recent abdominal surgery, peritonitis, mesenteric ischemia or infarction, medicines (opiates, anticholinergics).

History: Nausea, vomiting, obstipation, abdominal distention. Pain mild or absent.

Physical Examination: Abdominal distention, little or no tenderness, bowel sounds diminished or absent.

Diagnostic Tests: X-ray of the abdomen shows distended loops of small intestine with fluid levels.

Treatment: Nasogastric tube and suction, intravenous fluids, correction of the underlying cause if possible.

Hemorrhoids. Dilated veins just above or just below the anus.

Cause: Unknown. Constipation with straining at stool, prolonged sitting, and local infection have been implicated.

History: Anorectal discomfort or pain, swelling or protrusion, and bleeding.

Physical Examination: Dilated veins externally or internally, as seen by endoscopy. Sigmoidoscopy or colonoscopy and barium enema may be performed to rule out malignancy.

Course: Symptoms are typically mild and intermittent. Bleeding is occasionally significant. Thrombosis of stagnant blood within a hemorrhoid results in acute pain and swelling, but the problem resolves spontaneously in a few weeks.

Treatment: High-fiber diet, stool softeners, hot sitz baths, soothing applications, or suppositories. With severe pain or bleeding, surgery is indicated. Band ligation is used for internal hemorrhoids; external hemorrhoids are treated by excision or cryosurgery.

Acute Peritonitis. Acute inflammation of the peritoneum.

Causes: Infection (penetrating abdominal wounds, surgery, peritoneal dialysis for renal failure, spread from digestive or urinary tract or from a systemic site); chemical irritation (leakage of gastric or intestinal contents, bile, pancreatic secretions from injured, diseased, or perforated structure); systemic disease; neoplasm.

History: Fairly abrupt onset of severe local or generalized abdominal pain, nausea, vomiting, fever.

Physical Examination: Elevated temperature and pulse. Boardlike rigidity of abdomen, tenderness and rebound tenderness. Diminished or absent bowel sounds and abdominal distention due to ileus.

Diagnostic Tests: The white blood count is elevated. Blood studies may also show electrolyte imbalances due to peritoneal effusion, vomiting, and dehydration. Anemia may occur. Fluid obtained by abdominal paracentesis may show amylase or lipase (indicating leak of intestinal contents or pancreatic juice), significant cellular abnormalities, or infecting microorganisms. Various types of imaging may be of use in confirming and identifying intra-abdominal catastrophe.

Course: Without treatment the outlook is poor. Septicemia and vascular collapse often occur within a few hours of onset. In some patients, peritonitis becomes localized, with **abscess** formation, particularly **subphrenic** (just below diaphragm) or pelvic. Peritonitis often results in eventual formation of fibrous adhesions that may produce intestinal obstruction.

Treatment: Hospitalization, nothing by mouth (n.p.o., NPO), gastrointestinal suction to decompress the bowel and draw off secretions, intravenous fluids, narcotics for pain, antibiotics for infection, surgery to repair underlying abnormality.

Abdominal Hernia. A localized weakness in the musculoaponeurotic wall of the abdomen, with protrusion of abdominal contents. Abdominal hernias are classified according to position as:

umbilical (at the navel): often congenital, seldom requiring surgical repair because they resolve during infancy.

inguinal (in the groin) (Figure 9-5):

    direct inguinal: due to thinning and stretching of the lower abdominal wall, often with aging.

    indirect inguinal: (usually congenital) weakness and bulging in the inguinal canal, the passage through which, in the male fetus, the testicle descends from the abdominal cavity to the scrotum; a similar potential passage exists in women.

femoral: herniation into the femoral canal, through which the femoral artery and vein pass from the pelvis into the thigh.

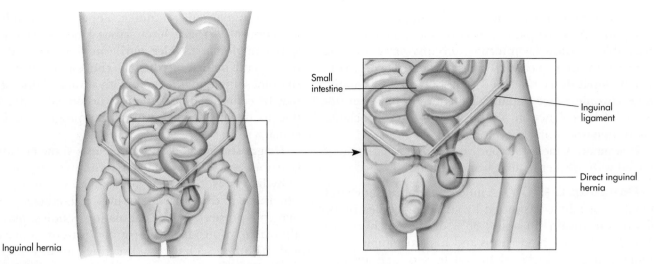

Small intestine

Inguinal ligament

Direct inguinal hernia

Inguinal hernia

Figure 9-5
Inguinal Hernia

Cause: Congenital weakness or malformation; thinning of the abdominal musculature by aging. Herniation may be precipitated or aggravated by vigorous or repeated straining of the abdominal wall (chronic constipation, urinary obstruction, heavy lifting, chronic cough).

History: A tender bulge in the abdominal wall that enlarges with straining. Intestinal obstruction may occur with severe abdominal pain, nausea, vomiting, weakness, shock, and collapse.

Physical Examination: A fluctuant bulge in the abdominal wall that enlarges with straining and can be reduced with manipulation or recumbency unless incarceration has occurred. A defect in the abdominal wall at the site of the hernia can be palpated. Visible or palpable mass, tenderness. Evidence of strangulation or bowel obstruction.

Diagnostic Tests: Barium enema and other studies may be done to rule out obstructive disease of the bowel or urinary tract.

Complications: **Strangulation** (compromise of blood supply), **incarceration** (inability to reduce hernia), bowel obstruction.

Treatment: Surgical repair of the defect, sometimes with implantation of reinforcing mesh.

Hepatitis A. **Hepatitis** is a general term referring to inflammation of the liver. Hepatitis can be caused by various drugs, toxic chemicals, and infections. Viral infections are the most important causes of hepatitis.

Cause: Hepatitis A virus. Transmission is by the fecal-oral route. Contaminated food and water are important means of infection.

History: Anorexia, nausea, vomiting, malaise, upper respiratory or flulike symptoms, fever, joint pain, aversion to tobacco, abdominal discomfort, diarrhea or constipation. Infection may be asymptomatic in children.

Physical Examination: Fever, jaundice, enlargement and tenderness of the liver, splenomegaly, cervical lymphadenopathy.

Diagnostic Tests: The serum bilirubin is elevated, and liver function tests are abnormal. Atypical lymphocytes may appear in the blood. Anti-HAV (IgM) antibody appears early in the course of the disease and disappears after recovery. IgG antibody develops later and persists indefinitely, indicating past history of, and immunity to, the disease.

Course: Symptoms characteristically resolve within 2-3 weeks. The mortality is very low.

Treatment: Supportive and symptomatic.

Hepatitis B

Cause: Hepatitis B virus. Transmission is by blood (shared needles, needle stick injury in healthcare workers) or sexual contact. Maternal transmission to neonates occurs also.

History: Fever, anorexia, nausea, vomiting, malaise, joint pain and swelling, rash, aversion to tobacco, abdominal pain, bowel irregularities.

Physical Examination: Fever, jaundice, enlargement and tenderness of liver. Splenomegaly, cervical lymphadenopathy.

Diagnostic Tests: The serum bilirubin is elevated, and liver function tests are abnormal. Atypical lymphocytes may appear in the blood. Hepatitis B surface antigen (HB_SAg) appears early in the disease and indicates presence of infection and infectivity of the patient. Antibody to surface antigen ($AntiHB_S$) indicates recovery, immunity to future infection, and lack of infectivity. Presence of HB_SAg after the acute phase suggests chronic infection.

Course: The incubation period may be 6-12 weeks or longer, and acute illness may persist for as long as 16 weeks. The mortality rate is somewhat higher than that of hepatitis A. Some patients become carriers of the disease, able to transmit infection months or years after recovery. In some, a chronic phase occurs. **Chronic persistent hepatitis** is mild and generally asymptomatic, while **chronic active hepatitis** leads to gradual deterioration of liver function, cirrhosis, and an appreciable risk of hepatocellular carcinoma.

Treatment: Chiefly supportive. Chronic hepatitis is treated with interferon alfa-2b and lamivudine.

Hepatitis C (HCV).

A mild or asymptomatic viral hepatitis usually transmitted by sharing needles or by blood transfusion. In about 85% of cases it becomes chronic, with risk of cirrhosis and hepatocellular carcinoma. Carriers can be identified by serologic testing. Treatment is with interferon alfa or ribavirin. Liver transplantation.

Cirrhosis (Portal Cirrhosis, Cirrhosis, Laënnec Cirrhosis).

A chronic disorder of the liver characterized by inflammation of secretory cells followed by nodular regeneration and fibrosis (Figure 9-6).

Causes: The principal cause is chronic alcohol abuse. About 20% of persons with hepatitis C eventually develop cirrhosis. Other toxic, metabolic, nutritional, and infectious factors may play a part in the genesis of cirrhosis. The cirrhotic liver contains various combinations of fatty change and fibrosis forming small and large nodules.

History: Usually gradual onset of anorexia, nausea, weakness, weight loss, abdominal swelling due to **ascites** (accumulation of fluid in the abdominal cavity), and often jaundice. Disturbance of sex steroid hormone metabolism causes impotence in men and amenorrhea in women.

Physical Examination: Fever, muscle wasting, pleural effusion, **ascites**, peripheral edema. The liver is usually enlarged and may be firm or even hard. The spleen may also be enlarged. Jaundice appears relatively late. Elevation of estrogen level causes gynecomastia in men, spider angiomas (**spider nevi**) on the face and upper trunk, and palmar erythema. The tongue may appear smooth, shiny, and inflamed. With advanced disease there may be coarse, flapping tremors (**asterixis**) and delirium due to hepatic failure, which may progress to hepatic coma.

Diagnostic Tests: Laboratory tests show elevation of bilirubin and enzymes such as aminotransferases, lactic dehydrogenase (LDH), and alkaline phosphatase, which rise in the presence of liver cell damage. Anemia may be present, and coagulation studies may yield abnormal results. Liver biopsy confirms presence of typical histologic changes. Imaging studies including radioactive liver scans provide further information. Esophagoscopy may show esophageal varices.

Course: Symptoms may wax and wane over a period of years, often in response to varying levels of alcohol consumption. Progressive hepatic failure often occurs. Fibrosis within the liver typically shuts off branches of the portal circulation and increases the pressure in the portal vein (**portal hypertension**). In consequence, other vessels (particularly the lower esophageal venous plexus) dilate and become varicose (bulging) or tortuous (coiled, twisted). Hemorrhage from bleeding esophageal varices is often life-threatening, particularly when hepatic disease causes a coagulation disorder. There is an increased incidence of hepatocellular carcinoma in persons with cirrhosis.

Treatment: Abstinence from alcohol, attention to nutrition, particularly carbohydrate, protein, vitamins. Rest, sodium restriction, and diuretics for edema and ascites. Severe ascites may require abdominal **paracentesis** (removal of peritoneal fluid with a needle passed through the abdominal wall). Patients with portal hypertension and bleeding esophageal varices may need a **portacaval shunt** (surgical procedure allowing portal vein blood to bypass the liver and empty directly into the inferior vena cava).

Cholelithiasis (Gallstones).

The formation of gallstones is a common disorder, generally due to some disturbance in the flow of bile from the gallbladder or in the composition of bile. Gallstones are more common in women and in elderly persons. Risk factors include pregnancy, diabetes mellitus, high serum cholesterol, Crohn disease, and sickle cell anemia. In the latter condition, stones consist primarily of bilirubin from hemolyzed red blood cells. In the other conditions, gallstones are composed primarily of cholesterol.

Gallstones are often asymptomatic (**"silent"**), but about 90% of persons with **cholecystitis** (inflammation of the gallbladder) have pre-existing **cholelithiasis** (Figure 9-7).

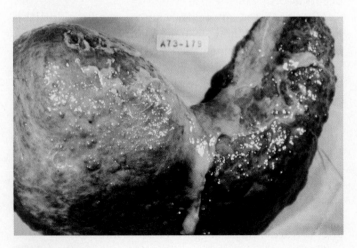

Figure 9-6
Cirrhosis

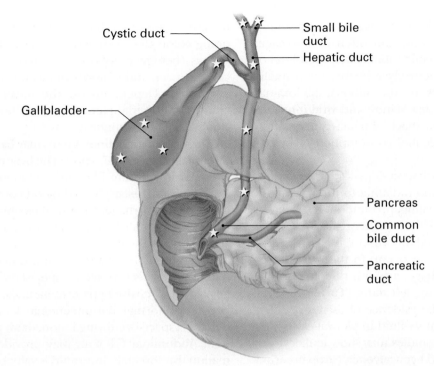

Figure 9-7
Common Sites for Cholelithiasis

Stones may be demonstrated on plain abdominal films, but ultrasound and imaging after injection of opaque medium are more sensitive and specific. Potential serious complications are blockage of the **common bile duct** by a stone with ensuing obstructive jaundice, blockage of the **cystic duct** with ensuing cholecystitis, and passage of a stone into the intestine with the potential for causing bowel obstruction (**gallstone ileus**).

Treatment of symptomatic gallstones is surgical removal (along with the gallbladder), usually through a **laparoscope**. Stones can also be crushed and flushed out with instruments passed through an endoscope inserted through the mouth and threaded into the common bile duct. Oral bile salts (chenodeoxycholic acid, ursodeoxycholic acid) and extracorporeal shock wave lithotripsy (ESWL) sometimes dissolve stones.

Acute Cholecystitis. Acute inflammation of the gallbladder.

Causes: Most patients with cholecystitis have preexisting cholelithiasis. Impaction of a stone in the cystic duct leads to obstruction of the flow of bile from the gallbladder, with ischemia, acute inflammation, and sometimes abscess formation or perforation.

History: Fairly acute onset of severe epigastric and right upper quadrant pain, nausea, and vomiting.

Physical Examination: Fever and jaundice may be present. In the right upper quadrant of the abdomen there are tenderness, rebound tenderness, and **involuntary guarding** (spasm of abdominal muscles on palpation). Bowel sounds are reduced or absent. Occasionally a mass can be felt below the liver edge, representing a distended gallbladder.

Diagnostic Tests: The white blood cell count, bilirubin, and levels of serum enzymes reflecting hepatic damage may all be elevated. Imaging studies (plain abdominal x-ray, ultrasound, scans with radiotagged media) may precisely identify the problem.

Course: Acute cholecystitis may resolve spontaneously. Often relapses occur with gradual development of chronic cholecystitis. Inflammation may culminate in **gangrene** (tissue death due to compromise of blood supply) or perforation of the gallbladder, or may ascend into the liver via the biliary tract (ascending cholangitis).

Treatment: Chiefly supportive, with narcotics for pain, intravenous fluids, and close observation. Impending or actual perforation is treated by surgical (laparoscopic) decompression (drainage) of the gallbladder or, preferably, by removal of the gallbladder (cholecystectomy).

Acute Pancreatitis. Acute inflammation of the pancreas.

Causes: Most cases occur in alcoholics or in persons with chronic biliary tract disease (cholelithiasis, cholecystitis). In these instances, obstruction of the pancreatic duct by edema, or backflow of bile from the duodenum into the pancreatic duct, causes release of pancreatic enzymes into the substance of the gland, with resulting intense inflammation, necrosis, and often hemorrhage. Other causes are **hypercalcemia** (abnormally high level of calcium in the blood), **hypertriglyceridemia** (abnormally high level of triglycerides in the blood), abdominal trauma or surgery, certain medicines, and viral infection including mumps. An acute attack of pancreatitis is often precipitated by excessive alcohol consumption or by eating a large meal.

History: Abrupt onset of severe, persisting epigastric pain, worse on lying flat, and radiating to the flanks and back. Nausea, vomiting, sweating, prostration, restlessness.

Physical Examination: Pallor, tachycardia, fever, epigastric tenderness, reduced or absent bowel sounds. Jaundice or hypotension may occur. In the presence of severe pancreatic hemorrhage, a bluish discoloration of the skin may appear over the left flank (**Turner** or **Grey Turner sign**). There may be evidence of ascites or a left **pleural effusion** (inflammatory fluid in pleural cavity).

Diagnostic Tests: Blood studies may show leukocytosis, hyperglycemia, anemia, and **hypocalcemia** (drop in serum calcium). Blood levels of pancreatic enzymes (amylase, lipase) are typically elevated. Imaging studies may show gallstones, a mass representing the swollen pancreas, left **atelectasis** (collapse of part of left lung caused by shallow breathing at site of pain), or left pleural effusion (inflammatory fluid in pleural cavity).

Course: Acute pancreatitis has a high mortality rate and, among survivors, a high recurrence rate. Possible outcomes include abscess formation, splenic vein thrombosis, ileus, shock, renal failure, adult respiratory distress syndrome, severe hypocalcemia with tetany, formation of **pseudocysts** (pockets of inflammatory fluid and debris between the pancreas and surrounding tissues), and progression to chronic disease.

Treatment: Hospitalization, narcotics for pain relief, nasogastric suction, intravenous fluids with attention to water balance, nutritional needs, and replacement of calcium. Surgery may be required to control hemorrhage, correct underlying disease, or drain pseudocysts.

Adenocarcinoma of the Colon and Rectum.
A malignant neoplasm arising from glandular epithelium in the large intestine. In both men and women, colon cancer ranks second as a cause of cancer deaths in the U.S. One half of all colon cancers are situated in the sigmoid colon or rectum. These tumors tend to grow slowly but may eventually become bulky; they may encircle and constrict the bowel.

Causes: Most colon cancers arise by malignant transformation of benign polyps (adenomas). Several oncogenes are associated with heightened risk of developing primary cancer in the colon; some of these predispose to formation of multiple malignant tumors, which may involve organs other than the bowel. Risk factors for developing colon cancer include age over 40, a history of adenomas (benign polyps) of the colon, a family history of colon cancer, and a history of ulcerative colitis.

History: Depending on the location of the tumor, crampy abdominal pain, change of bowel habits, bloody stools, weakness, fatigue.

Physical Examination: A mass may be felt on abdominal or digital rectal examination. The liver may be enlarged or irregular in contour if hepatic metastases are present.

Diagnostic Tests: The red blood count may be low as a result of hemorrhage. Chemical examination of the stool may detect occult blood. The carcinoembryonic antigen (CEA) titer in the serum may be elevated. This is not a reliable diagnostic indicator of colon cancer but is useful in watching for recurrence or metastatic disease after surgery. With extensive hepatic metastases, liver function tests become abnormal. Barium enema demonstrates mucosal defects, a space-occupying lesion, or an encircling obstruction. Abdominal CT scan may provide additional information. Endorectal ultrasound is valuable in distal lesions. Chest x-ray may show pulmonary metastases. Colonoscopy with biopsy provides definitive diagnosis.

Course: The overall survival rate in treated colon cancer is about 35%. If complete resection of primary tumor can be carried out, the survival rate is about 55%.

Treatment: The procedure of choice is surgical resection. **Rectal carcinoma** may require **abdominoperineal resection** (removal of the entire lower bowel, including the anus) with sigmoid colostomy. Tumors higher in the colon may be able to be resected with simple anastomosis of normal bowel above and below the surgical site. Chemotherapy and radiation therapy are valuable adjuncts to surgery in colon carcinoma.

Abdominal Injury.
Blunt injury to the abdomen can cause bruising, laceration, or severe hemorrhage of internal organs (liver, spleen, kidney, digestive tract, urinary bladder). In penetrating abdominal injuries, the risk of damage and particularly of hemorrhage is much increased. Puncture of the stomach or intestine releases digestive fluids into the peritoneal cavity and causes chemical peritonitis. Hemorrhage into the abdominal cavity is called hemoperitoneum.

The diagnosis of abdominal injury depends on careful physical examination, x-ray studies and scans, and **peritoneal lavage** (injection of fluid through a needle passed through the abdominal wall, followed by its withdrawal and laboratory examination). This procedure can detect blood, digestive fluids, urine, or other substances not normally present.

Management includes supportive care and prompt surgical intervention to repair leaking blood vessels or punctured organs.

Diagnostic and Surgical Procedures

anastomosis Surgical joining of two organs or vessels.

appendectomy Surgical excision of the vermiform appendix.

barium enema (BE) An x-ray that uses barium given rectally to outline the colon and rectum (Figure 9-8).

cholecystectomy Surgical removal of the gallbladder. It can be done either through an open incision or through minimally invasive laparoscopy.

colectomy Surgical excision of part or all of the colon.

colonoscopy Endoscopic procedure to view the colon using a flexible (fiberoptic) endoscope (Figure 9-9).

colostomy A surgically created opening from the colon to the abdominal wall, through which feces are passed rather than by the rectum; may be temporary or permanent.

endoscopy Insertion of a tube with a light source into a body cavity to view and often to biopsy the structures. Common types of endoscopies are esophagoscopy, gastroscopy, gastroduodenoscopy, anoscopy, sigmoidoscopy, and colonoscopy.

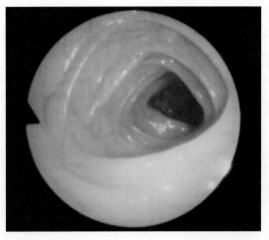

Figure 9-9
Colonoscopy Examination of the Transverse Colon

esophagogastroduodenoscopy (EGD) Endoscopic procedure to view the esophagus, stomach, and duodenum.

exploratory laparotomy Inspection of the abdominal and pelvic cavities through an incision in the abdominal wall.

gastrectomy Excision of a portion or all of the stomach.

gastroscopy Endoscopic procedure to view the stomach.

hemicolectomy Surgical excision of approximately half the colon.

hemorrhoidectomy Surgical excision of hemorrhoids (anal varicose veins).

herniorrhaphy Surgical repair of a hernia (protrusion of organ or tissue through an abnormal opening).

imaging studies Flat, upright, and (usually left) lateral decubitus films of the abdomen; fluoroscopic studies with swallowed or injected barium or other contrast medium (barium swallow, upper GI series, small bowel series, barium enema); CT or MRI for specific indications (for example, to assess gallbladder, masses); and ultrasound studies.

KUB x-ray Plain x-ray to image the kidneys, ureters, and bladder (hence KUB).

laparoscopy Inspection of abdominal cavity through an endoscope inserted through an incision in the abdominal wall.

portacaval shunt Surgical procedure allowing portal vein blood to bypass the liver and empty directly into the inferior vena cava.

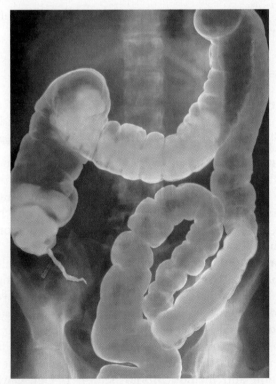

Figure 9-8
Normal Barium Enema with Enhanced Color

pyloroplasty Incision of the pylorus and reconstruction of the pyloric channel to relieve pyloric obstruction.

resection Surgical removal.

splenectomy Surgical removal of the spleen, usually precipitated by splenic injury.

upper GI series (UGI) with small bowel follow through An x-ray series that uses barium taken orally to outline the esophagus, stomach, and small intestine.

Laboratory Procedures

absorption tests Based on determination of blood or stool levels of substances that have been ingested in measured amounts.

alkaline phosphatase An enzyme whose level in the serum is often increased in bone disease and obstructive liver disease.

ALT (alanine aminotransferase) Formerly called *SGPT*. An enzyme whose level in the serum is elevated in hepatitis, cirrhosis, and other liver diseases.

ammonia, serum A breakdown product of protein metabolism, increased in hepatic failure.

amylase, serum An enzyme whose level is increased in pancreatitis and mumps.

AST (aspartate aminotransferase) Formerly called *SGOT*. An enzyme whose level in the serum is elevated in myocardial infarction, liver disease, and other conditions.

bilirubin, conjugated Bilirubin that has been conjugated (combined with glucuronic acid) by the liver so that it is water-soluble.

bilirubin, direct Bilirubin that reacts directly with testing chemicals because it has been rendered water-soluble (combined with glucuronic acid) in the liver. Its level is increased in biliary obstruction.

bilirubin, indirect Bilirubin in the serum that does not react directly with testing chemicals because it has not yet been conjugated (combined with glucuronic acid) in the liver. Its level is increased in disorders that impair the function of liver cells.

bilirubin, unconjugated Fat-soluble bilirubin that has not been conjugated (combined with glucuronic acid) by the liver.

bilirubin, urinary Bilirubin in the urine; it can be measured with a dipstick. Any amount is considered abnormal; usually it indicates obstructive liver disease or hepatitis.

Campylobacter pylori Former name for the organism now called *Helicobacter pylori*.

carcinoembryonic antigen (CEA) Not a reliable diagnostic indicator of colon cancer, but useful in watching for recurrence or metastatic disease after surgery.

CLO (Campylobacter-like organism) test To detect *H. pylori* in acid peptic disease.

examination of stool For occult blood, fat, pathogens (bacteria, fungi, parasites), abnormal constituents.

5'-nucleotidase (pronounced "five prime nucleotidase") A serum enzyme whose level increases in biliary obstruction. Testing for this enzyme helps to distinguish liver disease from bone disease as possible causes of elevated serum alkaline phosphatase.

Helicobacter pylori (*H. pylori*) A gram-negative organism formerly known as *Campylobacter pylori*, which is the cause of many peptic ulcers.

Hemoccult test For occult blood in the stool.

LFTs (liver function tests).

occult blood Blood present in quantities too small to be detected by naked-eye observation but detected by microscopic or chemical examination.

SGOT (serum glutamic-oxaloacetic transaminase) Former name for *AST*.

SGPT (serum glutamic-pyruvic transaminase) Former name for *ALT*.

stool for ova and parasites (O&P) Examination of stool for parasites or their ova (eggs).

Pharmacology

Drugs for peptic ulcers. Several types of drugs are used to treat peptic ulcers, including antacids, H_2 blockers, antispasmodics, and others.

Antacids. Antacids were the original, and for many years the only, treatment for peptic ulcers. They are weak bases that exert a therapeutic effect by neutralizing hydrochloric acid. This raises the pH of the stomach contents, which decreases mucous membrane irritation and also inhibits the action of pepsin.

Antacids contain aluminum, magnesium, calcium, sodium, or a combination of these as the active ingredients. Some antacids contain simethicone to relieve flatulence and gas; simethicone acts by changing the surface tension of air bubbles trapped in the GI tract to allow them to be expelled. Others contain aspirin or acetaminophen for pain relief. Antacids are available without a prescription and include Bromo Seltzer, Di-Gel, Gaviscon, Maalox, Mylanta, Phillips' Milk of Magnesia, Riopan, Rolaids, and Tums.

H$_2$ blockers. The release of gastric acid is triggered by histamine, which acts on special histamine receptors (known as H$_2$ receptors) in the gastric parietal cells lining the stomach. Drugs that block these receptors and prevent release of acid are known as H$_2$ blockers and are used to treat ulcers and gastroesophageal reflux disease (GERD). Examples include cimetidine (Tagamet), famotidine (Pepcid), nizatidine (Axid AR), and ranitidine (Zantac).

Proton pump inhibitors for peptic ulcer disease and GERD (gastroesophageal reflux disease). Unrelated to H$_2$ blockers, proton pump inhibitors decrease gastric acid by blocking the final step of acid production within the gastric parietal cell. This final step involves an enzyme system known as the proton pump, hence the name of this drug category.

> esomeprazole (Nexium)
> lansoprazole (Prevacid)
> omeprazole (Prilosec)
> pantoprazole (Protonix, Protonix IV)
> rabeprazole (AcipHex)

Drugs used to treat *H. pylori* infections. Successful eradication of *H. pylori* requires the use of two antimicrobial agents combined with bismuth (such as Pepto-Bismol) and either an H$_2$ blocker or a proton pump inhibitor such as lansoprazole (Prevacid) or omeprazole (Prilosec). Antimicrobials and bismuth disrupt the cell walls surrounding bacteria, causing cell death. Antimicrobials for *H. pylori* infections include:

> amoxicillin (Amoxil, Trimox, Wymox)
> clarithromycin (Biaxin)
> metronidazole (Flagyl, Protostat)
> tetracycline (Achromycin V, Panmycin, Sumycin)

GI stimulants for GERD. GI stimulants increase the rate of gastric emptying in order to keep excess acid from accumulating in the stomach. An example is metoclopramide (Maxolon, Reglan).

GI spasm. Spasm of the smooth muscle layer of the GI tract is responsible for much of the pain caused by a wide variety of digestive disorders. GI spasms can be relieved by antispasmodic drugs, which are also known as **anticholinergic drugs**. Anticholinergic drugs exert their therapeutic action in the following way. Muscle contraction and peristalsis in the GI tract are controlled by the parasympathetic nervous system through the release of the neurotransmitter acetylcholine. Acetylcholine acts on cholinergic receptors to stimulate muscular contractions and begin peristalsis to move food through the GI tract. If peristalsis is too strong and causes spasms, anticholinergic drugs can be given to block the effects of acetylcholine to stop the spasms and slow peristalsis.

> dicyclomine (Bentyl, Di-Spaz)
> L-hyoscyamine (Anaspaz, Levbid, Levsin,
>   Levsin Drops, Levsin/SL, Levsinex Timecaps)
> methantheline (Banthine)
> propantheline (Pro-Banthine)

These drugs combine an antispasmodic drug with the central nervous system sedative phenobarbital or the antianxiety drug Librium.

> Bellergal-S (belladonna, phenobarbital)
> Donnatal, Donnatal Extentabs (L-hyoscyamine,
>   scopolamine, phenobarbital)
> Librax (clidinium, Librium)

Antidiarrheal drugs produce a therapeutic effect by slowing peristalsis in the intestinal tract or by absorbing extra water in diarrheal stools. Some antidiarrheal drugs exert their effect because they contain opium or related narcotic drugs. Although these drugs have pain-relieving properties, a common side effect is constipation. This side effect then becomes the therapeutic effect in treating diarrhea.

Drugs for diarrhea which contain opium or related substances are classified as narcotics and may be controlled substances, depending on the actual addictive properties of the particular drug. Examples include difenoxin (Motofen), diphenoxylate (Lomotil), and paregoric (Pantopon). Non-narcotics include loperamide (Imodium).

Nonprescription drugs for diarrhea contain nonopiate substances such as kaolin and pectin which absorb water. Examples include Donnagel, Kaolin, and Kaopectate. Drugs used to treat bacterial or protozoal diarrhea or traveler's diarrhea include ciprofloxacin (Cipro) and doxycycline (Doryx, Vibramycin, Vibra-Tabs).

Laxatives are used for short-term treatment of constipation, with attention also given to adequate water intake, dietary fiber/bulk, and other measures to promote regularity. OTC laxatives are frequently overused and even abused. There are several classifications of laxatives: magnesium laxatives, irritants, bulk-producing laxatives, stool softeners, mechanical laxatives, and others.

Magnesium laxatives include the active ingredient of magnesium, which attracts water from the bloodstream into the intestines to soften the stool. These drugs include Epsom salt, MOM (milk of magnesia), and Phillips' Milk of Magnesia.

Irritant laxatives act directly on the intestinal mucosa to stimulate peristalsis. Examples include bisacodyl (Correctol, Dulcolax, Fleet Laxative), cascara, and sennosides (Ex-Lax, Ex-Lax chocolated, Fletcher's Castoria, Senokot).

Bulk-producing laxatives use fiber and other substances to hold water in the intestines that is normally absorbed into the bloodstream. Their action is the most natural and safest of all the laxatives. Examples include Citrucel, Fiberall, Metamucil, and Perdiem. Laxatives that act as stool softeners are emulsifiers that allow water and fat in the stool to mix; they include docusate (Colace, Dialose, Surfak).

Mechanical laxatives include glycerin suppositories (Colace, Fleet Babylax) that directly stimulate the urge to defecate by their presence in the lower colon. Bowel preps and enemas may be prescribed to evacuate the colon prior to surgical or endoscopic procedures. These include CoLyte, Fleet enema, GoLYTELY, HalfLytely, Evac-Q-Kit, and X-Prep.

Drugs used to treat irritable bowel syndrome. The traditional treatment of IBS includes modification of diet and lifestyle and the use of antispasmodics, antidiarrheals, and laxatives as appropriate. More specific agents that alter the response of the bowel to hormones of the serotonin family are effective in women but not in men. In patients whose predominant symptom is diarrhea, the 5-HT$_3$ receptor antagonist alosetron (Lotronex) reduces stool frequency and cramping. In patients with constipation, the 5-HT$_4$ partial agonist tegaserod (Zelnorm) increases stool frequency and reduces bloating and discomfort.

Ulcerative colitis drugs. Ulcerative colitis is a chronic disease characterized by abdominal pain, diarrhea, rectal bleeding, and abscesses. The cause is unknown. Antispasmodic and anti-inflammatory drugs used to treat ulcerative colitis include 4-ASA (Pamisyl, Rezipas), mesalazine (Dipentum), sulfasalazine (Azulfidine), and topical corticosteroids such as hydrocortisone (Cortenema, Cortifoam).

Antiemetics are used to control nausea and vomiting arising from illnesses of the GI tract, as a side effect of drugs, surgery, radiation or chemotherapy, or from vertigo or motion sickness. Vomiting patients may be given medication in rectal suppository form because they are unable to keep oral medications down.

For severe nausea and vomiting, chlorpromazine (Thorazine) and prochlorperazine (Compazine) are prescribed. Medications such as promethazine (Phenergan), thiethylperazine (Torecan), and trimethobenzamide (Tigan) are prescribed for moderate nausea and vomiting.

Vertigo is caused by irritation to the inner ear which upsets balance and stimulates the vomiting center. Motion sickness arises from repeated motion, such as in a car, which also overstimulates the inner ear. Drugs to treat these problems seem to act by either reducing the sensitivity of the inner ear to motion or inhibiting the increased inner ear stimuli from reaching the chemoreceptor trigger zone and the vomiting center in the brain.

> dimenhydrinate (Dramamine)
> diphenhydramine (Benadryl)
> meclizine (Antivert, Bonine)
> promethazine (Phenergan)
> scopolamine (Transderm-Scop)

Note: All of these drugs are given orally, with the exception of scopolamine (Transderm-Scop), which is manufactured as a small transdermal patch worn behind the ear.

Antiemetics for patients undergoing chemotherapy. Chemotherapy drugs directly stimulate the vomiting center in the brain. In addition, some cause release of serotonin in the small intestine; this stimulates the vomiting reflex. Because the nausea and vomiting in response to chemotherapy can be severe and prolonged, antiemetic drugs are often given prophylactically prior to beginning chemotherapy.

> chlorpromazine (Thorazine)
> dronabinol (Marinol)
> granisetron (Kytril)
> metoclopramide (Reglan)
> ondansetron (Zofran)
> prochlorperazine (Compazine)
> promethazine (Phenergan)
> trimethobenzamide (Tigan)

Immunosuppressants. The following are immunosuppressant drugs given to liver transplant patients to prevent rejection of donor organs.

> cyclosporine (Neoral, Sandimmune)
> muromonab-CD3 (Orthoclone OKT3)
>   (monoclonal antibody)
> tacrolimus (Prograf)
> Xomazyme-H65

TRANSCRIPTION**TIPS**

1. Common soundalikes:

   peritoneal (the serous membrane lining the abdominopelvic walls)
   perineal (the area between the genitalia and anus)

2. The following slang terms should be translated when dictated:

appy	appendectomy
bili	bilirubin
procto	proctoscopy
sig	sigmoidoscopy
tic	diverticulum

3. These abbreviations should be translated for clarity when encountered in dictation:

BE	barium enema
RUQ	right upper quadrant
RLQ	right lower quadrant
LUQ	left upper quadrant
LLQ	left lower quadrant

4. Spelling tips:

inflamed	*but*	inflammation
spleen	*but*	splenectomy

   diverticulum (singular)
   diverticula (plural), *not* diverticuli

5. The spelling *distention* is preferred; *distension* is an acceptable alternative.

6. Memorize the spelling of these difficult gastrointestinal terms:

borborygmus	cirrhosis
hemorrhoid	intussusception

7. Note the challenging spellings of these common gastrointestinal drugs:

   AlternaGEL
   CoLyte
   Dulcolax (the first *l* is often not pronounced by the dictator)
   Fleet enema (often dictated incorrectly as Fleet's)
   GoLYTELY
   Maalox (double *a*)
   Mylanta (*y*, not *i*)
   Mylicon (*y*, not *i*)
   Phillips' Milk of Magnesia (note placement of the apostrophe)
   Zantac (not to be confused with Xanax, an antianxiety drug)

8. Although *antacids* have an anti-acid effect, the *i* is omitted from *anti-* in the correct spelling. In contrast, *antiemetic* is correct even though the first *i* is often not clearly pronounced.

9. Physicians often dictate *melanotic* when what they really mean is *melenic* (the passage of dark bloody stools). *Melanotic* refers to melanosis, the presence of excessive melanin (pigment), usually in the skin, and is not related to the stool.

10. Although you will often hear "coffee-ground emesis" dictated, common sense demands the plural, "coffee-grounds," in this phrase.

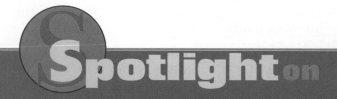

Spotlight on

Transcribing Gastroenterology Dictation

by Bron Taylor

Transcription of gastrointestinal system dictation is relatively straightforward, which isn't to say it can be mastered overnight. We can work for years in this area and still be challenged by hearing strange and wonderful new things from the doctors.

Patients with GI complaints are in considerable distress, not only from the painful and sometimes life-threatening conditions themselves, but also from the embarrassment many of them can cause. Physicians working with these problems have learned to put the patients at ease and acquire, if they didn't start out with it, a good sense of humor.

The relief that many patients obtain from correct diagnosis and treatment of GI problems is considerable, too, and all of this, plus the many organ systems involved with these problems and the interfaces with other specialties, make this a very dynamic and ever-changing field, with new drugs and new treatments being constantly introduced.

GI transcription problems. The problems we face in transcribing GI dictation are those all transcriptionists face, and the same solutions apply—acquiring good reference material; establishing links with other transcriptionists, with physicians, with nurses in the Endoscopy Room and staff who work in Central Supply; keeping an accurate personal notebook; reading medical journals—all help one to master and stay on top of this material.

There are several specific GI questions that baffle most beginners, such as the *perineal/peritoneal/peroneal* soundalikes. Careful listening will often distinguish *peritoneal* from *perineal*, and in an operation such as an abdominoperineal resection (in which both terms appear), one has to be alert to this. The word *peroneal*, referring to an area of the outer side of the leg, is much less likely to appear in GI dictation.

Another problem is *ileum/ilium*, and I'm indebted to Vera Pyle for a mnemonic device for distinguishing these. The "e" in *ileum*

is a letter made with a loop, like the loops of bowel of the ileum.

Another frequent source of confusion is the word *ascitic*, from *ascites*. It sounds like *acidic*, and the only way to resolve this one is by context. An *ascitic wave* is the fluid wave seen on palpation of the abdomen in patients with ascites. I have seen students transcribe "acidic wave" and insist "that's what the doctor said." Similarly, in the early stages of doing this work, one can confuse *cirrhosis* with *serositis*, and, again, context saves the day.

Here as with all transcription, the more one learns about the anatomy and what's going on, the more interesting and enjoyable the work is and the less likely one is to make such errors.

As with transcription of any type, dictators can sometimes lead us astray. One of the typical dictation errors is the plural of *diverticulum*, which is *diverticula*, not *diverticulae*, *diverticuli*, *diverticulee*, or *diverticulas*.

Another source of confusion from the physicians is when they "helpfully" (and sometimes it is) dictate punctuation, without any warning that they've deviated from the body of their reports to talk to us directly. One dictator where I work baffled many of us for months in talking about the retroflexion maneuver used in endoscopy, also called the *J-turn maneuver*. He'd say, very fast, "with the J, that's-J-as-in-the-letter-J turn maneuver." (When we finally deciphered this, we immediately wrote the term on our bulletin board, which is a good practice to follow so that others won't have to reinvent the wheel.) Also, the dictated punctuation mark *colon* can cause a problem in gastrointestinal dictation, much of which concerns the colon itself.

Editing and speed. Beginners can be intimidated by listening to experts transcribe at high speed and can be overwhelmed by real-world expectations of productivity. It can all seem hopeless when first listening to dictations, many of which seem to be dictated in a foreign language. How can one be expected to do meticulous, accurate work—as *fast* as it has to be done?

It's one thing to say NEVER GUESS, look up everything if you have any doubt, and ask everyone questions—and another to produce work *fast*. And if that's not confusing enough, medical transcriptionists are expected to edit errors in the dictation as they become capable and experienced.

Editing requires great delicacy, sensitivity, and knowledge. The official policy in some medical records departments is that the transcriptionists must never edit what the doctors say; they must type exactly what the doctors say. When confronted directly about editing, many doctors will tell you NOT to edit their dictation, yet when they meet you in the hall they'll thank you for making their work read so beautifully. And when a beginner asks an experienced transcriptionist or supervisor how to handle an obvious error in dictation or inappropriate language, they will often tell the beginner to type what the dictator *means* rather than *says* in that particular instance. It can all be incredibly confusing.

Gaining speed in spite of all these pressures and areas of potential conflict is not hopeless. It's *knowledge of medicine* that increases speed and accuracy, not learning to move one's fingers faster on the keyboard. By understanding what's going on in dictated procedures, by knowing the anatomy well, by being familiar with the most frequently used medications, you eventually will arrive at the point where you almost know what's going to be dictated before the doctor says it, and that's the point where speed comes almost before you know it. Suffering through the learning process, not being tempted to take shortcuts—this is the real road to speed. You'll get to the point where you don't have to look up words so often because you understand how the dictator is thinking.

The foreign accent problem, which is formidable for beginners, solves itself by the same method. You will get to the point where you KNOW what the dictator wants to say, no matter how odd the words sound, and people will tell you that you have a wonderful ear. This really *will* happen, although it has to be taken on faith in the beginning.

One of the satisfactions of this work is the degree to which you can teach yourself about medicine. You don't have to major in anatomy or become a pharmacy student, if you keep your ears and eyes open and soak up all the medical information you can, all the time. The amount of anatomy to be learned is finite—there are a certain number of muscles and bones and nerves to learn,

and no more, and anatomy can be learned so well that using it becomes automatic. New drugs and procedures are being constantly introduced, but once one knows the bulk of them, most of the work is done.

We don't want to give the impression that there is so much new information to be learned with every report that the transcriptionist must spend every day in a time-consuming search for new information. There are patterns that underlie what the dictators are saying, and it all makes good sense, and it's a great satisfaction to learn these—by any means. The reports themselves will teach you a great deal.

It's especially important in the beginning stages to resist pressure to *guess* and thus avoid leaving blanks in reports. Unfortunately, there *are* supervisors who encourage guessing and who will not allow blanks in reports, who think that pages without gaps are "good enough." You have to *resist this pressure* because it is just not safe to guess when you're working on a patient's permanent medical record.

Too many words sound alike. One of the best tools you can develop is a little bell of doubt that rings for you when you're really not sure what you're transcribing. When this little bell goes off, trust it—if you have a hunch it might be wrong, it probably IS wrong. Look it up, ask someone, and, if you have to leave a blank, do that—and attach a note to the dictator.

With study and experience, one acquires a picture of what's happening behind the dictation, and everything starts to make sense. Mumbles become clear, your questions to the doctors become more astute and generate more interesting answers, you catch more mistakes, and you begin to see the bigger picture and realize how it all fits together. Some days you'll have the satisfaction of having a new procedure or drug already in mind before it's dictated, which is a nice "a-ha" feeling and brightens your day.

Not every day will be fascinating, for much of the dictation will be repetitive, but there are many rewards hidden in the dictation.

Source: *The SUM Program Gastrointestinal Transcription Unit.*

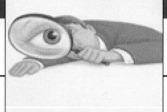

Proofreading Skills

Instructions: In the paragraphs below, circle the errors. Identify misspelled and missing medical and English words and punctuation errors, and write the correct words and punctuation in the numbered spaces opposite the text.

1	PREOPERATIVE DIAGNOSIS	1	_____
2	Anal stricture.	2	_____
3		3	_____
4	PROCEDURE	4	_____
5	Resection of perianal skin tags, posterior midline, partial	5	_____
6	sphincterotomy anal dilatation, and Y-V anoplasty.	6	_sphincterotomy, anal_ (add comma)
7		7	_____
8	The perineum and perianal areas were prepped with	8	_____
9	Betadine and suitably drapped. Anterior midline and	9	_____
10	left posterolateral skin tags was resected, bleeding	10	_____
11	controled by electrocoagulation. A half-shell retractor	11	_____
12	was placed, and a partial posterior midline sphincter-	12	_____
13	otomy was carried out. Then, gently, anal dilatation was	13	_____
14	carried out with one finger, two fingers, and finally	14	_____
15	three fingers. A Y-shaped incision had been made	15	_____
16	begining up just above the upper border of the anal	16	_____
17	sphincter, coming down partway linearly, and then	17	_____
18	going in the Y shape on each side. Some scar tissue was	18	_____
19	ressected. The perianal skin posteriorly was dissected	19	_____
20	away from underlying scar tissue and sphincter, and	20	_____
21	bleeding was controlled by electrocoagulation. The tip	21	_____
22	of this skin was then sutured to the end of the Y and	22	_____
23	mucosa-to-skin was approximated with interupted 3-0	23	_____
24	chronic sutures, turning the Y into a V and effectively	24	_____
25	widening the anal canal. Surgicel gauze was placed in	25	_____
26	the cannal and the procedure terminated.	26	_____

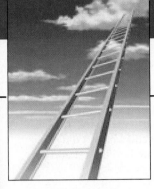

SkillsChallenge

Fill-in Exercise

Instructions: The numbered blanks correspond to the numbers in the narrative paragraphs. Fill in the blanks with the correct entry from the word list following.

Digestion begins in the (1), where food is chewed thoroughly, a process known as (2). There it is mixed with saliva. Saliva contains the digestive enzyme (3), which begins the digestion of starch. The food then passes through the (4), or throat, where it is swallowed, a process known as (5). From the throat, food passes through a long tube known as the (6), through the (7) sphincter, and finally into the stomach.

The body of the stomach is called the (8). Folds in the stomach wall are known as (9). Within the stomach, gastric glands secrete (10) acid and pepsin, which digest proteins. The partially digested food is then moved by wavelike contractions known as (11) through the pyloric sphincter into the small intestine.

The first part of the small intestine is the (12). The digestion of fats begins when bile, which is produced by the (13), passes from its storage site, the (14), through the common bile duct into the duodenum and combines with food. The pancreatic enzyme (15) completes the digestive process for fats. The food then moves into the second and third parts of the small intestine, the (16) and (17). The walls of the small intestine contain microscopic projections of mucous membrane called (18) that allow digested food to pass through the intestinal wall and into capillaries for distribution throughout the body.

Waste products from food digestion continue to pass through the digestive tract, passing from the ileum through the (19) valve and into the first part of the large intestine, the (20). A long, wormlike structure known as the vermiform (21) is found here; its purpose is unknown, but if it becomes inflamed, it must be surgically removed.

Food waste then moves progressively through the large intestine as more water is absorbed and the waste becomes firmer. The section of large intestine that follows the cecum is the (22). It has three segments that are named according to their orientation within the abdomen. The (23) colon ascends upward from the cecum toward the liver. Under the liver it bends, forming the (24) flexure. It then continues across the abdomen; this section is the (25) colon. When it reaches the spleen, the (26) colon turns downward and forms the splenic flexure.

The next segment of the large intestine is the (27) colon, named for the S-shape resembling the Greek letter *sigma*. The last segment of the large intestine is the (28). Waste passes through a final sphincter at the base of the rectum called the (29), or (30) sphincter. The final solid waste product excreted from the body is known as (31) or (32).

The process of excretion is called (33). The entire digestive tract is also known as the (34) canal or (35) tract, and the small and large intestines are known by the general term (36).

alimentary	hepatic
amylase	hydrochloric
anal	ileocecal
anus	ileum
appendix	jejunum
ascending	lipase
bowel	liver
cardiac	mastication
cecum	oral cavity
colon	peristalsis
defecation	pharynx
deglutition	pyloric
descending	rectum
duodenum	rugae
esophagus	sigmoid
feces	stool
fundus	transverse
gallbladder	villi
gastrointestinal	

1. _____   19. _____
2. _____   20. _____
3. _____   21. _____
4. _____   22. _____
5. _____   23. _____
6. _____   24. _____
7. _____   25. _____
8. _____   26. _____
9. _____   27. _____
10. _____   28. _____
11. _____   29. _____
12. _____   30. _____
13. _____   31. _____
14. _____   32. _____
15. _____   33. _____
16. _____   34. _____
17. _____   35. _____
18. _____   36. _____

Medical Terminology Matching Exercise

Complete the following matching exercise to test your knowledge of the word roots, anatomic structures, symptoms, and disease processes encountered in gastroenterology.

Instructions: Match each definition in Column A with its term in Column B.

Column A

1. ___ stones in the gallbladder
2. ___ twisting of segment
3. ___ word root meaning *anus* and *rectum*
4. ___ varicose vein in anal area
5. ___ inflammation of ileum, causing diarrhea and fever
6. ___ loss of appetite
7. ___ inflammation of liver, caused by a virus
8. ___ jaundice
9. ___ word root meaning *stomach*
10. ___ difficulty swallowing
11. ___ fluid in the abdomen
12. ___ pouch in intestinal wall that can become inflamed
13. ___ lack of peristalsis due to intestinal obstruction
14. ___ occurring after eating
15. ___ severe constipation
16. ___ suffix for *hernia*
17. ___ degeneration of liver cells, usually caused by alcoholism
18. ___ growth in colon, often on a stalk
19. ___ bright red blood in stool
20. ___ word root for *small intestine*
19. ___ word root for *common bile duct*
20. ___ word root for *abdomen*

Column B

A. hemorrhoid
B. diverticulum
C. -cele
D. cholelithiasis
E. polyp
F. paralytic ileus
G. entero-
H. hematochezia
I. choledocho-
J. volvulus
K. cirrhosis
L. procto-
M. postprandial
N. gastro-
O. anorexia
P. icterus
Q. ascites
R. obstipation
S. dysphagia
T. Crohn disease
U. laparo-
V. hepatitis

Adjectives Exercise

Adjectives are formed from nouns by adding adjectival suffixes such as *-ac, -al, -ar, -ary, -eal, -ed, -ent, -iac, -ial, -ic, -ical, -ive, -lar, -oid, -ous, -tic,* and *-tous.* In addition, some adjectives have a different form entirely from the noun, which may be either Latin or Greek in origin.

Instructions: Test your knowledge of adjectives by writing the adjectival form of the following gastroenterology words. Consult a medical dictionary to select the correct adjectival ending as necessary.

1. liver _____
2. esophagus _____
3. stomach _____
4. intestine _____
5. pylorus _____
6. ileum _____
7. colon _____
8. appendix _____
9. feces _____
10. nausea _____
11. jaundice _____
12. constipation _____
13. anorexia _____

Abbreviations Exercise

Instructions: Define the following common GI abbreviations. Then memorize both abbreviations and definitions to increase your speed and accuracy in transcribing GI dictation.

BE _____
CEA _____
EGD _____
GERD _____
GI _____
IBS _____
LES _____
LFTs _____
LLQ _____
NG (tube) _____
n.p.o. _____
p.o. _____
RLQ _____
RUQ _____
UGI series _____

GI Questions

1. Distinguish between the following GI words: diverticulum, diverticula, diverticulitis, diverticulosis.

   _____

   _____

   _____

   _____

   _____

2. Where is a peptic ulcer located?

   _____

3. Distinguish between cholelithiasis and choledocholithiasis.

   _____

   _____

Word Root and Suffix-Matching Exercises

Instructions: Combine the following root words with suffixes to words that match the definitions below. Fill in the blanks with the medical words you construct.

Word Root	Suffix
appendic(o)-	-ectomy
cholecyst-	-itis
colo-, colon(o)-	-logy
entero-	-scopy
gastro-	-stomy
laparo-	-tomy

A. inflammation of the stomach and intestines

   _____

B. surgical removal of the gallbladder

   _____

C. using a scope to visualize the colon

   _____

D. a surgical incision into the abdomen

   _____

E. using a scope to visualize the stomach

   _____

F. a new opening for the colon

   _____

G. a surgical incision into the stomach

   _____

H. inflammation of the appendix

   _____

I. a study of the stomach and intestines

   _____

J. surgical removal of the appendix

   _____

Soundalikes Exercise

Instructions: Circle the correct term from the soundalikes in parentheses in the following sentences.

1. There was an (acidic, ascetic, ascitic) fluid wave in the abdomen on examination.

2. The patient insisted he did not drink to excess, but he had advanced (cirrhosis, psoriasis) of the liver.

3. On palpation of the abdomen over the rectus muscles, it was clear that the patient had a (diaphysis, diastasis, diathesis).

4. The patient complained of constant burning chest pain and on gastroscopy was shown to have severe gastroesophageal (efflux, reflex, reflux).

5. On anal examination the patient was noted to have a small tear or (fissure, fistula).

6. On bimanual exam the patient was suspected of having a rectovaginal (fissure, fistula).

7. The colostomy procedure was considered a success, but the patient developed a colovesical (fissure, fistula).

8. The lesion was seen just beyond the hepatic (flexor, flexure).

9. The colonoscope was (passed, past) beyond the hepatic (flexor, flexure) but could not be advanced (passed, past) the splenic (flexor, flexure).

10. The patient experienced significant pain from (fundal, fungal) pressure on the stomach.

11. The colonoscopy was performed all the way to the terminal (ilium, ileum) and the entire colon examined.

12. The (perianal, perineal) tissues were irritated, probably from the cleansing enemas prior to the procedure.

13. The baby was placed on (gavage, lavage) after it was discovered that he could not swallow.

14. The (perineum, peritoneum) was entered and the bowel pushed back with a wet lap.

15. (Aural, Oral) mucosa was pink and moist.

16. A brownish (mucous, mucus) discharge was oozing from the (mucous, mucus) fistula.

17. (Palpation, Palpitation, Papillation) of the abdomen revealed no masses.

18. The patient was placed on (parental, parenteral) feedings after the gastrectomy.

19. After the abdominal hysterectomy, (perineal, perennial, peritoneal, peroneal) closure was accomplished with 0 silk.

20. The patient was placed on a (regimen, regime, regiment) of laxatives and tap-water enemas in preparation for the colonoscopy.

Dictation Exercises

Instructions: Prior to transcribing the GI dictations, complete these activities.

1. **Using Chapter 3, Style Guide**

   a. When, according to the Style Guide, do you expand brief forms and abbreviations?

   b. Review the list of acceptable and unacceptable brief forms and slang. What should you do if *preop* and *postop* are dictated in a heading or in the body of a report? What if *H&H* is dictated?

   c. Review the Style Guide for the correct way to transcribe abbreviations for Latin terms used with drug dosages.

   d. Review the style guidelines for handling numbers. When do you spell out numbers? What do you do if a sentence starts with a number?

   e. Read what the Style Guide says about clipped sentences. What distinguishes a clipped sentence from a sentence fragment?

   f. What does the Style Guide say about adjectives following the noun? How do you punctuate a phrase like "diabetes mellitus insulin-dependent poorly controlled"?

   g. What does the Style Guide say to do when a department or specialty name is used to refer to an entity (person)?

   h. Review the error-prone abbreviations list. What should you transcribe if *cc* is dictated?

   i. What does the Style Guide say to do when two consecutive numbers are dictated?

   j. What does the Style Guide say about possessive eponyms?

   k. Read the General Information and the Editing and Style sections in the Style Guide. Ask your instructor whether you are allowed to edit for clarity or should transcribe verbatim.

   l. Review *post* and *status post* in the Style Guide. What is the difference between the two?

   m. Sometimes physicians will dictate items in a series with conjunctions between the items instead of the usual commas. Would it be appropriate to edit out the conjunctions and insert commas?

   n. Review the Style Guide for transcribing suture sizes. How do you transcribe "three oh" suture? How do you transcribe "number 2" suture?

   o. Read the paragraph about combined anatomical and directional terms (such as *anterior-posterior* versus *anteroposterior*) in the Spelling section of the Style Guide. When should you hyphenate the terms and when should you combine them?

2. **Problem Solving**
   This activity is to help you prepare ahead of time for some of the problems you'll encounter in the dictations. Some of these items may not have a definitive answer but are intended to simply get you thinking about how to handle a variety of situations that are common in transcription. If nothing else, they will help you recognize a problem when you encounter it in the dictations.

   a. Acronyms (abbreviations pronounced as though they are words) are common in medical documentation. Knowing that, consider this situation. The patient has just had an operation and the dictator says the patient was taken to what sounds like the "pack-yoo" in stable condition. How would you initially spell this term? How would you research it?

   b. Doctors, especially radiologists and pathologists, often like to be descriptive in their dictation. Students may think some of the words they dictate are medical words when they're actually just descriptive English terms used in a medical context. What are some ways you might research descriptive phrases used in radiology reports, when these phrases may not appear in your references?

   c. Occasionally, physicians just misspeak. It's probably happened to you in conversation as well. You're thinking one way, but by the time it comes out of your mouth, it's been changed, and sometimes the original thought gets garbled in the process. Find out from your instructor how much leeway you have to edit physician misspeaks. For example, if a physician dictates an incorrect verb tense, does the instructor allow you to edit it?

   d. In a dictation on a postop patient, the physician dictates an abbreviation that you're not quite sure of. There's no context to help you figure out what the abbreviation is or stands for except that it "put out 70 cc and it was removed." What might this object be? What might be left in after surgery and removed later? Once you determine what the object was, how would you determine what the abbreviation might be?

   e. In laboratory values, the addition of a "point zero" to the numeric value is considered an indication of a precise measurement. What do you think would be an appropriate action to take if a dictator dictated the word approximately before such a measurement? Can a value be both precise and approximate?

f. Sometimes it's difficult to verify the exact term dictated in a medical report, and you have to use your knowledge of spelling rules to determine the spelling based on a related word. Adjectives frequently fall into the category of hard-to-verify terms, but sometimes verbs do as well. If a physician dictates what you recognize to be an adjective (remember your adjective suffixes from medical terminology?) or perhaps a verb (there are suffixes that identify a word as a verb as well), how would you define and spell such a term if you can't find it in the dictionary?

g. There are many ways that experienced transcriptionists use to decipher terms they can't quite hear or that may be garbled. Frequently, they may use context clues or their knowledge of word components (prefixes, combining forms, and suffixes) and how words are put together. Another technique is to continue transcribing and see if the word in question is repeated, perhaps more clearly later or in a context where the term is more obvious. Suppose that there is a term you keep hearing but you can't quite get every syllable, and the term is followed almost every time by the same phrase "with air." Can you think of some ways you might be able to decipher the term that precedes the phrase?

3. **Preparatory Research**
Any information requested in these questions not readily available in your textbook (including the appendix) or required references can easily be found using Internet search engines such as Google or online medical dictionaries.

a. What is an older abbreviation/acronym for CT scan that may be pronounced as a word?

b. Find a list of generic and brand medications that are used to treat diabetes mellitus. Are any used in combination? What is the benefit of a combination of drugs to treat a condition like diabetes or hypertension? (*Hint*: It's not just that two drugs are stronger or more effective than one drug.)

c. Perform a Google (or other search engine) search for "CT scan" + fat + appendicitis. Make a note of descriptive terms that are associated with the word *fat* on CT scan findings. (*Tip*: Once you click on a link, use your Ctrl-F search function to find the

word *fat* on the page and note the words around it. Keep searching for fat until you've found all the instances where it is present.)

d. Define *purulent*.

e. Research *patient-controlled anesthesia*. Under what circumstances is it provided? What type(s) of drugs are used in patient-controlled anesthesia? What is the abbreviation for this phrase?

f. What is a *Roux-en-Y procedure*? Why is it performed?

g. Research signs and physical findings that point to a diagnosis of appendicitis.

h. What medical and surgical treatments are used for ulcerative colitis?

i. What is the plural of *diagnosis*? If the dictator gives more than one diagnosis in a list, what should the heading be?

j. The prefix *pan-* can be added to many medical terms, and you may not be able to verify them in a dictionary. What does the prefix *pan-* mean? List 3-4 words that begin with the prefix *pan-* and define them. (*Note*: Not all *pan* words begin with the prefix *pan-*.)

k. Define the anatomic landmark, *Z line*.

l. Review the anatomy and anatomic landmarks of the upper and lower gastrointestinal tract.

m. Sometimes medical terms sound like inflated versions of simpler English words. *Insufflate* is one such term. What does it mean?

n. What does *titrated* mean?

o. What is the adjectival form of *appendix*?

p. What is the plural of *ostium*? What is a synonym for *ostium*?

q. When one hears the term *emphysema*, one generally thinks of pulmonary emphysema. What does *emphysema* mean? How does it apply to organs other than the lungs? What is the adjective form of *emphysema*?

r. What does *edema* mean? How does *edema* differ from *emphysema*?

s. What is the difference in meaning between *emergency* and *emergent*? (*Note*: Look in an English rather than a medical dictionary.)

t. What is the correct spelling for the noun and adjective form of *inflame*?

u. What is the difference in meaning between attained and obtained?

v. What does *ligate* mean? What is a *ligature*?

w. What does *tenesmus* mean?

Sample Reports

Sample gastroenterology reports appear on the following pages, illustrating a variety of reports. Fictional names are provided for illustration of proper format, and no resemblance to actual persons is intended. Sample transcripts were prepared according to the *AAMT Book of Style*, where possible.

Letter

July 3, XXXX

Kevin Walsh, MD
3567 Union Avenue
Laborville, CA 93025

Re: Kent Whisenant

Dear Dr. Walsh:

I was embarrassed to find out that through a clerical slip-up, this consultation note was not dictated promptly as it should have been. Please accept my apology.

I personally reviewed the air-contrast barium enema. The radiologist's impression was that there was a soft tissue mass in the terminal ileum. My impression was that this could possibly be a Meckel's, although this would be very unusual. This is probably lymphoid hyperplasia and is unimpressive.

My impression is irritable bowel syndrome and possibly a Meckel diverticulum. Therapeutically, I suggested he go on a high-fiber diet, and our nursing staff talked to him extensively about the use of bran. He was given three Hemoccult test cards and these were returned, and all three were negative.

Unless symptoms recur, I do not believe a further investigative workup is necessary at this time.

Thank you very much for referring me this patient, and again I apologize for the delay in sending you this note.

Sincerely,

Richard Callihan, MD

RC:hpi

Gastroenterology Consultation

ANDING, SCOTT
#82741
July 4, XXXX
Medical 502B

The patient received multiple transfusions for his multiple vascular surgeries. There was no history of any jaundice following any of these transfusions, although he relates some jaundice many, many years ago, with the etiology at that time being unclear. He has manifested no symptoms referable to liver disease and generally remains asymptomatic in this regard. There is no history of significant alcohol intake or recent travel, and the only drug one could implicate in his hepatitis is Aldomet, which he has been on for only 1 year.

His physical examination revealed that his liver extended 3-4 fingerbreadths below his right costal margin and was firm; however, no other signs of liver disease, namely, spider angiomata or palmar erythema, were present. We have found that his AST was elevated at least as far back as February. Several repeat blood tests have shown varying degrees of elevation of the bilirubin and transaminases. Additionally, his globulins have been elevated, and his prothrombin time has been mildly prolonged to approximately 50% of control.

It seems likely that the patient has chronic liver disease from his transfusions in the 1990s, the etiology being hepatitis C. It is unlikely that Aldomet is contributing to his elevated transaminases, as the elevations have been documented prior to the Aldomet usage. The possible chronic liver diseases include chronic persistent hepatitis, chronic active hepatitis, and the possible development of cirrhosis. I am concerned about the development of cirrhosis in view of the prolonged pro time and the elevated globulin level, although one cannot be sure regarding this diagnosis without a liver biopsy.

In view of his mild enzyme elevations and his asymptomatic state in regard to his liver disease, despite a liver biopsy showing chronic active hepatitis, I could not imagine treating him with immunosuppressive therapy in view of his age and general medical condition. Additionally, it is still unknown at this time what the natural history of this disease is, as well as whether there is any significant response to steroid therapy in terms of prognosis. As well, with his mildly prolonged prothrombin time, this would pose a slightly increased risk for the liver biopsy that at this time I do not feel is warranted in view of the unlikelihood of any treatment based on the liver biopsy findings.

We will simply watch him and have repeat liver tests in approximately 3 months. Should the disease progress in any way or he become symptomatic or new data become available on the use of steroids in the treatment of hepatitis C liver disease, then we may reassess the need for liver biopsy at that time.

DENISE LOEWEN, MD

DL:hpi
d: 7/4/XXXX
t: 7/5/XXXX

CHICHESTER, MARK
#90438
Admitted: 6/1/XXXX
Medical 302C

ADMISSION DIAGNOSIS
Metastatic colon cancer.

HISTORY OF PRESENT ILLNESS
A 61-year-old white male who is status post sigmoid resection and segmentectomy of the liver for colon cancer, who presents because of liver metastasis on CT scan despite one year of 5-FU therapy. He is without complaint of loss of appetite, weight loss, nausea, vomiting, jaundice, melena, or hematochezia. He denies change in bowel habits since the operation but does chronically have bulky stools.

PAST MEDICAL HISTORY
Resection of the sigmoid with segmentectomy of the left lobe of the liver, secondary to metastases, and a primary colocolostomy. Metastases were also noted to the regional and retroperitoneal lymph nodes, which were also resected. Therapy with 5-FU was given as above.

MEDICATIONS ON ADMISSION
None.

ALLERGIES
None.

FAMILY HISTORY
There is no family history of cancer.

SOCIAL HISTORY
The patient does not smoke or drink.

PHYSICAL EXAMINATION
VITAL SIGNS: Blood pressure 110/70, pulse of 60, respiratory rate 18, temperature 36.
GENERAL: This is a well-developed, well-nourished white male in no acute distress.
HEAD & NECK: HEENT unremarkable. Neck is supple without jugular venous distention (JVD), adenopathy, or bruit.
CHEST: Lungs are clear.
HEART: Regular rate and rhythm.
ABDOMEN: Soft, nondistended, and nontender. Liver is approximately 8-10 cm in span and does not descend below the right costal margin. There is no splenomegaly or masses.
LYMPH NODES: There is no palpable adenopathy throughout.
RECTAL: Normal anal sphincter tone. No masses. Stool was Hemoccult-negative.
NEUROLOGIC: Neurologically the patient is intact.

(continued)

CHICHESTER, MARK
#90438
Admitted: 6/1/XXXX
Medical 302C
Page 2

ADMISSION LABORATORY
Hemoglobin 14.4. White blood cells 6.9 with 66 segs, 19 lymphs, 5 monos, 9 eos, and 1 baso. Platelets 295,000. Astra was within normal limits. The profile showed an alkaline phosphatase of 141, AST of 29, total bilirubin of 0.5, total protein 7.5, albumin 3.9. PT is 11.5 and PTT is 28.1. Chest x-ray showed a small, approximately 1-cm nodule in the right lower lung and was otherwise normal.

PRINCIPAL DIAGNOSIS
Metastatic colon cancer.

KAREN ZEMPOLICH, MD

KZ:hpi
d: 6/1/XXXX
t: 6/1/XXXX

LACOURSIERE, SUZANNE
February 5, XXXX

The patient has primary biliary cirrhosis. I refilled the patient's colchicine. Articles were sent to the patient on primary biliary cirrhosis. The patient should have LFTs and a serum cholesterol drawn every 8 months, and I ordered a chem-25, CBC, iron, and TIBC. The results of these tests were within normal limits with the following important exceptions: serum iron was 45, which is low; TIBC was 433, which is high; and percent iron saturation was 10, which is low. Her ferritin was 10, which is also low. These results taken together indicate that the patient was iron deficient, and so I started her on Feosol 1 p.o. b.i.d. Her GGT was 105, which is elevated, and alkaline phosphatase was 209, which is also elevated. A CT scan of the abdomen has been done and was negative.

She continued to have abdominal pain. I gave her a trial of Reglan 10 mg p.o. q.i.d. and also scheduled an upper GI with small bowel follow through. The upper GI showed hesitancy in opening of the duodenal bulb, but the bulb was intrinsically normal and the duodenum was normal as well. The remainder of the upper GI series and small bowel series was normal. I don't believe the hesitancy in the opening of the duodenal bulb to be significant.

I saw the patient again with continued complaints of abdominal pain. At that time her friend had just died of colon cancer. She complained of fatigue and malaise, as well as new symptoms of reflux and heartburn.

My impression is that she has irritable bowel syndrome as well as esophageal reflux. I gave her a prescription for Sinequan 25 mg q.d. and a sample supply of Tagamet 400 mg b.i.d. The Tagamet improved her symptoms, as she called in for a refill.

KZ:hpi
d: 2/25/XXXX
t: 2/26/XXXX

Operative Report

JONES, PARKER
#802741

DATE OF SURGERY
October 1, XXXX

PREOPERATIVE DIAGNOSIS
Recurrent right inguinal hernia.

POSTOPERATIVE DIAGNOSIS
Recurrent right inguinal hernia.

OPERATION
Right inguinal hernia repair.

PROCEDURE
After the patient was placed supine on the operating table and a proper level of anesthesia was attained, the abdomen was prepped and draped in the usual sterile fashion.

A right groin incision was made and carried through the subcutaneous tissue, through Scarpa's fascia, and to the external oblique fascia. The external oblique fascia was opened from the internal inguinal ring to the external inguinal ring. The ilioinguinal nerve was identified and preserved. The cord was mobilized and a defect was found medially. This was a direct inguinal hernia recurrence. The floor was entirely opened up, and a hernia repair was carried out by reapproximating the conjoined tendon down to Cooper's ligament with a running 0 Prolene stitch. This was carried out until a transition suture was placed, and then the conjoined tendon was reapproximated to the shelving edge until the internal inguinal ring was snug. The external oblique was closed over the cord with a running 3-0 Vicryl suture, the subcutaneous tissue with 3-0 plain, and the skin with a running 4-0 subcuticular Dexon stitch. The patient's wound was dressed, and he was sent to the recovery room in satisfactory condition.

PAUL VAN HORN, MD

PVH:hpi
d: 10/2/XXXX
t: 10/3/XXXX

Operative Report

MELLO, MARSHA
PATIENT #010152

DATE OF SURGERY
December 2, XXXX

PREOPERATIVE DIAGNOSIS
Acute appendicitis.

POSTOPERATIVE DIAGNOSIS
Contained perforated acute appendicitis.

PROCEDURE PERFORMED
Laparoscopic appendectomy.

ANESTHESIA
General endotracheal.

ESTIMATED BLOOD LOSS
100 cc.

FLUIDS
Approximately 900 cc of Ringer's lactate.

CLINICAL NOTE
This 58-year-old female gives a greater than 48-hour history of vague abdominal pain with anorexia that has localized in the last several hours into the right lower quadrant. She has peritonitis by her physical exam. Her temperature was 101°F. The CT scan was consistent with acute appendicitis. The patient gave informed consent and was given ciprofloxacin and Flagyl in the ED in preparation for this surgery. The patient has an allergy to cephalosporin.

PROCEDURE NOTE
The patient was brought into the operating room, placed in a supine position, general anesthesia induced, and intubated by the anesthesia staff. A Foley catheter was placed under sterile conditions into the bladder. The abdomen was shaved and then prepped and draped in a sterile fashion.

An approximately 4-cm incision was made vertically above the umbilicus and taken down sharply to the linea alba. The peritoneum was incised sharply, and a Hasson trocar was placed in the abdomen after securing the linea alba with 2-0 Vicryl on each side. The abdomen was insufflated to more than 15 cm of water pressure with carbon dioxide and maintained there throughout the case. Two other trocars were introduced, a 5-mm trocar in the midline suprapubic area and a second 12-mm trocar in the midclavicular line, halfway between the umbilicus and the suprapubic trocar. Using these trocars, and with blunt dissection and gravity, the small bowel was taken out of the pelvis and demonstrated a contained perforation in the distal third of the appendix. The small bowel and part of the peritoneum had sealed this area off. Despite this, the small bowel with its thickened mesentery was fairly easily removed superiorly to allow good exposure to the appendix.

(continued)

284

MELLO, MARSHA
PATIENT #010152

DATE OF SURGERY
December 2, XXXX
Page 2

The base of the appendix was easily dissected, and a staple was fired across its base. A second staple was fired across the mesoappendix, and there was no bleeding noted. The appendix was removed and placed into a specimen bag through the midline Hasson trocar site. The abdomen was then irrigated with approximately 1.5 L of saline with bacitracin. The pelvis in particular and the right lower quadrant were irrigated, and some irrigant was removed from the right gutter near the liver.

At the conclusion of this, the 12-mm trocar was removed and the site noted to be bleeding. A figure-of-8 suture was placed through the fascia, which demonstrated good control of the bleeding. The 5-mm trocar was removed under direct vision without any bleeding. The Hasson trocar was removed without any problems. There were noted to be adhesions just to the left of the Hasson trocar site; however, these adhesions remained out of our way for the course of the procedure. The Hasson trocar site was closed with three sutures of 0 Vicryl, the middle suture being a figure-of-8, with good reapproximation of that fascia.

All three wounds were irrigated with saline and closed with interrupted 4-0 Vicryl in a subcuticular fashion. Steri-Strips were applied to all these wounds, as well as a dry sterile dressing. The patient was extubated without difficulty, no complications were noted, and she was sent to the PACU in stable condition.

REX EASLEY, MD

RE:hpi
D: 12/02/XXXX
T: 12/03/XXXX

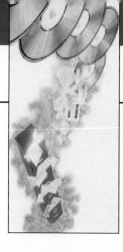

Transcription Practice

Key Words

The following terms appear in the gastroenterology dictations. Before beginning the medical transcription practice for Chapter 9, look up each term below in a medical or English dictionary and write out a short definition.

appendicitis
cholecystectomy
cholecystitis
bowel obstruction
colonoscopy
esophagectomy
EGD (esophagogastro-
   duodenoscopy)

hemorrhoidectomy
intussusception
laparoscopic cholecys-
   tectomy
open cholecystectomy
pancreatic carcinoma
ulcerative colitis

After completing all the readings and exercises in Chapter 9, transcribe the gastroenterology dictation. Proofread your transcribed documents carefully, listening to the dictation while you read your transcripts.

Transcribe (*not* retype) the same reports again without referring to your previous transcription attempt. Initially, you may need to transcribe some reports more than twice before you can produce an error-free document. Your ultimate goal is to produce an error-free document the first time.

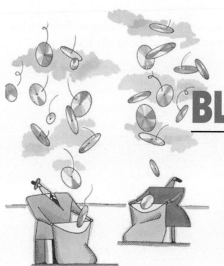

BLOOPERS

Incorrect	Correct
No history of tardy stools.	No history of tarry stools.
The abdomen became somewhat permanent.	The abdomen became somewhat prominent.
Bronchoscopic exam revealed hemorrhoids.	Proctoscopic exam revealed hemorrhoids.
Rectal examination defurred.	Rectal examination deferred.
The abdomen had shifting pelvis.	The abdomen had shifting dullness.
The patient had exclusive bowel movements.	The patient had extrusive bowel movements.
No stool packagings were discovered.	No stool pathogens were discovered.
We just had time for a kosher exam.	We just had time for a cursory exam.
Soft balls equal in traction.	Soft, small fecal impaction.
An SS cinema was prescribed.	An SS (soapsuds) enema was prescribed.

Endocrinology

Learning Objectives

- Describe the structure and function of the endocrine system.
- Spell and define common endocrine terms.
- Identify types of questions a physician might ask about endocrine symptoms during the review of systems.
- Describe common signs of endocrine disorders a physician looks for on examination of the eyes, face, and neck.
- Identify common diseases of the endocrine system. Describe their typical cause, course, and treatment options.

- Identify and define diagnostic and surgical procedures of the endocrine system.
- List common endocrine laboratory tests and procedures.
- Identify and describe common endocrine drugs and their uses.
- Demonstrate knowledge of anatomical, medical, pharmacological, adjectival, and soundalike terms by accurately completing the exercises in this chapter.

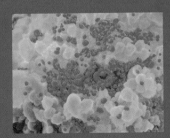
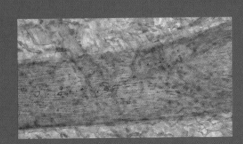
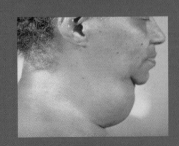

Transcribing Endocrinology Dictation

Endocrinology is the study of the glands that make up the endocrine system (Figure 10-1). These glands are located in different areas of the body, and many important hormones are produced by endocrine glands (also called ductless glands because their secretions pass directly into the circulation).

Endocrine literally means "internal secretion." The endocrine glands are described below. Some of these endocrine glands (for example, the pancreas and the gonads) perform nonhormonal functions as well.

Anatomy in Brief

The **pituitary gland**, or **hypophysis**, situated on the undersurface of the brain, consists of two distinct masses of endocrine tissue. The anterior pituitary (**adenohypophysis**) produces hormones that regulate the development and function of other endocrine glands: **thyroid-stimulating hormone (TSH)**, **adrenocorticotropic hormone (ACTH)**, which stimulates the adrenal cortex, and the gonadotropins: **follicle-stimulating hormone (FSH)** and **luteinizing hormone (LH)**, which stimulate gonadal functions. The anterior pituitary is also the source of **growth hormone (somatotropin)**, which regulates the natural growth process, and **prolactin** (required for lactation after pregnancy).

The posterior pituitary (**neurohypophysis**) is in direct continuity with the part of the brain called the **hypothalamus**. It produces two hormones: **oxytocin**, which stimulates uterine contractions in labor, and **vasopressin (antidiuretic hormone, ADH)**, which helps to control water balance by promoting reabsorption of water by the kidneys.

The **thyroid gland**, whose name means "shield-shaped," is situated in the front of the neck overlying the junction of the **larynx** and **trachea**. The thyroid gland produces two iodine-containing hormones, **thyroxine (T_4)** and **triiodothyronine (T_3)**, which circulate in the blood bound to a plasma protein (**thyroid binding globulin, TBG**). These hormones influence general metabolism, chiefly by regulating gene transcription of body proteins (including growth hormone).

The four **parathyroid glands** are so-called because they lie on or in the capsule of the thyroid gland. These glands produce **parathyroid hormone (PTH)**, which regulates the serum calcium level within narrow limits. Calcium control is important for proper maintenance of bones and teeth; more critically, the level of calcium in the serum and in tissue fluids exerts a potent influence on nerve and muscle function. Parathyroid hormone maintains the level of calcium in serum by moving calcium ions out of the bones, reducing the renal clearance of calcium, and increasing the rate of intestinal absorption of calcium. **Calcitonin**, a hormone produced by the thyroid gland, is also involved in regulation of serum calcium.

The **adrenal glands** are two crescent-shaped caps of endocrine tissue, one situated on top of each kidney. Each adrenal gland consists of two essentially different bodies of endocrine tissue: the outer **cortex** and the inner **medulla**.

The adrenal cortex produces three classes of hormones, two of which play crucial roles in the control of sugar, protein, and mineral metabolism. The **glucocorticoids** (principally **cortisol**) increase glucose production by the liver, affect protein and fat metabolism, help to regulate blood pressure, mediate many of the responses of the body to stress, and tend to suppress immune and inflammatory responses.

The **mineralocorticoids** (principally **aldosterone**) regulate electrolyte and water balance by promoting renal retention of sodium ions of potassium, hydrogen, and ammonium ions. **Adrenal androgens** play a minor role in reproductive physiology in both men and women. They are chiefly of interest as a cause of hirsutism and virilization in certain adrenal diseases.

The **adrenal medulla** is part of the **sympathetic nervous system**. Cells of the adrenal medulla are stimulated directly by sympathetic nerve endings to produce **epinephrine**, **norepinephrine**, and **dopamine**, which although not essential to life play a critical part in the body's response to severe stress. These hormones affect many tissues, increasing the rate and force of cardiac contractions, relaxing the smooth muscle of the bronchi, constricting some blood vessels and dilating others, stimulating liver and muscle tissue to produce and release glucose, and controlling fat breakdown and insulin production.

The **pancreas** (see Figure 10-2) is an **endocrine** gland as well as an **exocrine** one (one that produces a secretion released through a duct). The endocrine function of the pancreas is performed by the **islets of Langerhans**, tiny aggregations of endocrine cells interspersed among the exocrine secretory elements.

The **B** or **beta cells** of the islets of Langerhans produce insulin, which increases glucose utilization and exerts other complex influences on the metabolism of carbohydrates, proteins, and fats. The **A** or **alpha cells** produce **glucagon**, an inhibitor of glucose activity, and the **D** or **delta cells** produce somatostatin, which inhibits secretion of growth hormone by the anterior pituitary.

Terminology Review

acromegaly Abnormal growth of the body, especially facial features and extremities due to excess of pituitary growth hormone.

alopecia Hair loss.

amino acid A relatively simple nitrogen-containing organic compound. Of the 20 amino acids that are essential to human metabolism, half can be manufactured in the body and the others must be obtained in the diet.

body mass index (BMI) A measure of the proportion of fat to lean body mass.

bruit A vascular hum synchronous with heartbeat, heard with a stethoscope.

calorie A measurement of the energy released by food.

carbohydrate One of three basic food types, it is the source of energy in the diet which is consumed in the form of starches and sugars.

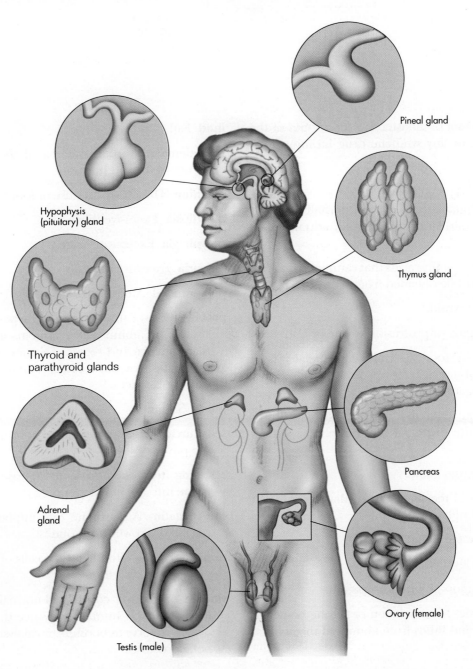

Pineal gland

Hypophysis (pituitary) gland

Thymus gland

Thyroid and parathyroid glands

Adrenal gland

Pancreas

Testis (male)

Ovary (female)

Figure 10-1
The Endocrine Glands

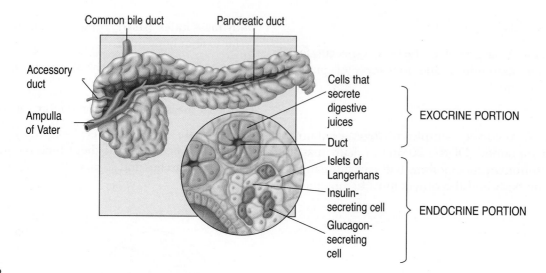

Common bile duct
Pancreatic duct
Accessory duct
Ampulla of Vater
Cells that secrete digestive juices
Duct
EXOCRINE PORTION
Islets of Langerhans
Insulin-secreting cell
Glucagon-secreting cell
ENDOCRINE PORTION

Figure 10-2
The Pancreas

corticosteroid Cortisol or aldosterone (hormones of the adrenal cortex), or any synthetic drug having similar effects.

diaphoresis Sweating.

endocrine gland A gland that secretes internally (directly into the circulation): pituitary, thyroid, adrenal, pancreas, gonads.

essential amino acids Amino acids that cannot be made in the body and must be obtained from diet.

euthyroid Normal thyroid.

exophthalmos Bulging or protrusion of one or both eyes.

fat One of three basic food types, also called *lipid*. It is an oily or greasy substance built up of fatty acids (long, straight-chain organic acids).

glucose A 6-carbon sugar that is the most plentiful in the blood and the principal fuel of cellular energy metabolism.

goiter Enlarged thyroid gland.

hormone A chemical messenger or mediator produced by a cell, tissue, or gland.

hyperglycemia Elevated blood glucose.

hypoglycemia Low level of blood glucose.

hyperkalemia Elevation of serum potassium.

ketoacidosis, diabetic Accumulation of ketone bodies in the body tissues and fluids from abnormal metabolization of fat.

lid lag Slowness of upper eyelids to move with eye movements.

lipid Fat.

myxedema Abnormal swelling of the skin due to deficiency of thyroid hormone.

nutrition The intake and use of foods by the body.

polydipsia Excessive thirst.

polyphagia Excessive hunger.

polyuria Excessive urination.

postprandial After meals.

protein One of three basic food types, made up of long strands of amino acids, proteins are responsible for maintenance and repair of tissues and organs, and for production of intracellular enzymes, hormones, and other substances.

ptosis Sagging.

sella turcica The saddle-shaped bony depression in which the pituitary rests.

releasing hormone Promotes release of a specific hormone into the circulation.

somatostatin A hormone that inhibits production and release of growth hormone.

tropic hormone Stimulates the cells of a remote gland to produce its secretion.

vitamin An organic compound normally present in many foods that the human body needs in trace amounts, usually to serve as boosters or catalysts in essential metabolic processes.

Lay and Medical Terms

losing hair	alopecia
sex drive	libido
sugar diabetes	diabetes mellitus
sweating	diaphoresis

Medical Readings

History and Physical Examination

by John H. Dirckx, M.D.

Review of Systems. The physician asks if there are problems with the patient's vision (bulging eyes may be a sign of thyroid disease; loss of vision could indicate retinopathy secondary to diabetes mellitus). Difficulty swallowing or swelling in the neck could be due to thyroid disease. Excessive thirst or urination might indicate diabetes mellitus. Heat or cold intolerance and hair changes might be symptomatic of thyroid disease.

Physical Examination. The amount, distribution, texture, and color of the scalp hair are observed, as well as the pattern of any hair loss. The patient's face not only registers current emotional state but often reflects systemic disease as well. Myxedema, acromegaly, and Cushing syndrome each produce characteristic changes in facial features.

Any swellings or masses in the neck are palpated for size, shape, consistency, mobility, pulsatility, and tenderness. The thyroid gland is felt and its size and consistency assessed. For this examination the physician may stand behind the patient and have the patient swallow in order to move the gland up and down under the palpating fingers.

Normally the patient sits upright for the eye examination. The orbital margins are inspected for swelling. The lids are observed for evidence of deformity and swelling. Bulging or protrusion of one or both eyes (exophthalmos) can result from the type of hyperthyroidism called Graves disease.

A Doctor's View

Metabolism and Nutrition

by John H. Dirckx, M.D.

Metabolism. Metabolism is a general term for the sum of all the chemical and electrical processes that occur in the living body. A principal part of metabolism is the **oxidation** of foods so as to release energy in tiny amounts that are usable at the cellular level. Most metabolic processes are at least partially under the control of hormones.

A **hormone** is a chemical messenger or mediator produced by a cell, tissue, or gland. Hormones are released into the circulation and perform their functions at sites remote from their origins. Some hormones stimulate cellular functions, while others inhibit them. A **tropic hormone** stimulates the cells of a remote gland to produce its secretion, and a **releasing hormone (relin)** promotes release of a specific hormone into the circulation.

Nutrition. Nutrition refers to the intake and use of foods by the body. Each of the three main types of food (**protein, fat, carbohydrate**) has its own function in human nutrition.

A normal adult requires one gram of **protein** per kilogram of body weight per day to supply sufficient materials for maintenance and repair of tissues and organs, and for production of intracellular enzymes, hormones, and other substances. Proteins are built up of long strands of **amino acids**, which are relatively simple nitrogen-containing organic compounds that serve as building blocks for all the complex proteins of the human organism. About half of these can be synthesized in the body; the rest, called **essential amino acids**, must be obtained from the diet.

Carbohydrate (consumed in the form of **starches** and **sweets**) is the most important source of energy in most diets. Carbohydrate foods are chemically degraded in the digestive system to simple sugars, especially **glucose**, a 6-carbon sugar that is the most plentiful in the blood and the principal fuel of cellular energy metabolism.

Fats (lipids) are oily or greasy substances built up of **fatty acids** (long, straight-chain organic acids). Fats in the diet come mainly from animal foods, but the term *fat* is often extended to include oils of plant origin.

All three basic types of food can be and are burned in the body as fuel. The amount of energy that a foodstuff can supply can be determined by burning the food outside the body in a **calorimeter** (a small furnace equipped with a sensitive means of measuring heat production). The energy released by food is measured in calories per gram (cal/g). The large calorie or kilocalorie (kcal, 1000 calories) is a more convenient unit of measure in nutrition; in modern parlance, **kilocalories** are usually called simply **calories**.

Whereas proteins and carbohydrates both supply about 4 calories (kcal) per gram, fats supply about 9. The active adult requires 2500-4000 kcal/day: 1200-1800 kcal to meet the energy demands of basic life processes, plus those needed for physical exertion. In the average middle-class American diet, 50% of calories come from carbohydrates, 35% from fat, and 15% from protein.

Water, Minerals, and Vitamins. By convention, the subject of nutrition also includes materials usually not thought of as foods: water, minerals, and vitamins. **Water** is the most abundant substance in the body and the principal constituent of blood. **Intracellular fluid** accounts for about 40% of total body weight, **interstitial fluid** (in tissue spaces, outside of cells) another 15%, and **plasma** (the fluid part of blood) about 5%. The water content of plasma, and indirectly that of the intracellular and interstitial compartments, is regulated within narrow limits by a complex system of checks and balances involving the sensation of thirst, perspiration, gastrointestinal fluid loss, renal excretion and reabsorption of water and electrolytes, and other chemical processes.

Essential dietary **minerals** include iron (needed for the production of red blood cells and as a catalyst in many metabolic processes), calcium (a principal constituent of bones and teeth), sodium, potassium, zinc, magnesium, and many more.

Vitamins are organic compounds, normally present in many foods, that the human body needs in trace amounts, usually to serve as boosters or catalysts in essential metabolic processes.

Disorders of nutrition are relatively common and have many causes, among them overeating, alcoholism,

Hazards *of Obesity*

What's so bad about being overweight? Obesity is known to be an independent risk factor for many life-threatening and life-shortening conditions (hypertension, hypercholesterolemia, type 2 diabetes mellitus, myocardial infarction, obstructive sleep apnea, and hypoventilation syndrome) as well as for others capable of causing severe distress or disability (osteoarthritis and other orthopedic disorders, infertility, lower extremity venous stasis disease, gastroesophageal reflux disease, and urinary stress incontinence). Certain common malignancies (cancer of the colon, rectum, and prostate in men, and of the breast, cervix, endometrium, and ovary in women) occur more commonly in obese persons than in those of normal weight.

Lesser degrees of obesity can constitute a significant health hazard in the presence of diabetes mellitus, hypertension, heart disease, or other risk factors. Distribution of excess body fat in central depots (abdominal or male pattern, with an increased waist-to-hip ratio) rather than in peripheral ones (gluteal or female pattern) is associated with higher risks of many of these disorders.

Obese persons are more liable to injury than persons of normal weight. Because they move more slowly, they are more likely to be hit while crossing a street. A larger body is more unwieldy: obese persons are more likely to fall on stairs or in the shower.

An overweight person is more difficult for a physician to examine. Palpation of masses in the abdomen, breasts, or subcutaneous tissues may be virtually impossible. Excess fat also disperses x-rays and renders other imaging techniques less useful. Overweight persons are notoriously poor candidates for thoracic and abdominal surgery, and have a much higher incidence of unsuccessful outcomes, complications, and intraoperative and postoperative mortality.

Not least among the adverse consequences of obesity are social stigmatization, poor self-image, low self-esteem, and the anxiety and depression resulting from them. Overweight persons face occupational discrimination, social rejection, and derision from persons of normal weight, including friends and relations, who are apt to attribute their obesity to a lack of self-discipline or even to moral degeneracy. The obese tend to have higher rates of unemployment and a lower socioeconomic status, and this is only partly related to their inability to qualify for certain jobs because of size or weight restrictions.

In public they are often the target of rude and disparaging remarks and other tokens of hostility from ignorant and ill-disposed strangers. They can't travel comfortably in compact cars, be accommodated comfortably in restaurants, or fit comfortably into seats in theaters, sports arenas, buses, or airplanes (all of which are designed to cram the maximum number of paying customers into the available space).

Excessive size of trunk and limbs makes for clumsiness in performing many of the activities of daily living. Bathing and personal hygiene may be awkward or impossible for the overweight, particularly in public facilities. Physical exercise, part of any rational program for the treatment of obesity, is often far more difficult for the obese than for persons of normal weight. Their choice in clothing is sharply limited. Euphemisms used by manufacturers and vendors of clothing who cater to overweight persons (*stout, portly, stocky, corpulent, full-figured, large framed*) can seem almost as offensive as intentionally derogatory street terms.

Surely it must be evident to even the slenderest intelligence that obesity, besides being a very prevalent condition, poses harrowing health risks and generates devastating psychological trauma.

John H. Dirckx, M.D.
Perspectives on the Medical Transcription Profession

stringent dieting, anorexia nervosa, malabsorption due to inherited abnormalities or to gastrointestinal disease or surgery, and any severe chronic disease including metastatic carcinoma. Specific vitamin deficiencies occur but are rare in our culture. Most nutritional deficiencies are complex and occur as part of a more general pattern of illness.

The most common nutritional disorder, except among the extremely poor, is not undernutrition but **obesity**, an excess of subcutaneous fat in proportion to lean body mass.

Body Mass Index (BMI).

Body mass index (BMI), the weight in kilograms divided by the body surface in square meters, is a useful measure of the proportion of fat to lean body mass. The National Institutes of Health (NIH) has defined obesity as a BMI of 30 or more, and overweight as a BMI between 25 and 30. By these criteria, about two thirds of adults in the United States are either overweight or obese, and the prevalence of obesity is increasing in both children and adults. The cause of obesity is unknown, but in most cases it appears to be genetically determined. Most obese persons do not have faulty eating habits or endocrine disease.

Obesity is an independent risk factor for hypertension, hypercholesterolemia, type 2 diabetes mellitus, myocardial infarction, some cancers, osteoarthritis, gastroesophageal reflux disease, and a number of other conditions.

Weight reduction leads to reduction in many of these risks, but cannot repair damaged arteries or joints. Most safe and effective weight-reduction programs include a diet low in fat and in total calories and 30 minutes of strenuous physical exercise on most or all days of the week. Other methods include the use of behavior modification therapy, hypnosis, or drugs to suppress appetite, and gastrointestinal surgery to reduce the size of the stomach or diminish intestinal absorption of food.

Common Diseases

Acromegaly, Gigantism. Overgrowth of body structures in adulthood (acromegaly) or in childhood (gigantism) due to excessive somatotropin (growth hormone).

Cause: Benign pituitary adenoma producing abnormal amounts of somatotropin. May occur as part of multiple endocrine adenomatosis.

History: Excessive long-bone growth (when onset is before puberty); excessive growth of hands, feet, jaw. Weakness, amenorrhea, headache, hoarseness, obstructive sleep apnea, sweating.

Physical Examination: Coarse facial features, hypertension, visual field defects, cardiomegaly.

Diagnostic Tests: Serum level of growth hormone is elevated and is not suppressed by administration of oral glucose. The blood sugar is elevated. X-ray of the skull may show an enlarged **sella turcica** (the saddle-shaped bony depression in which the pituitary rests). MRI may show a pituitary tumor.

Course: Premature cardiovascular disease. Other complications include pituitary failure, hypertension, diabetes mellitus, cardiac enlargement and failure, carpal tunnel syndrome, and visual field defects.

Treatment: Surgical excision of the tumor is usually successful. Radiation may also be used. Bromocriptine is administered to reduce the level of growth hormone. Octreotide, a synthetic analog of somatostatin (a hormone that inhibits production and release of growth hormone) is also effective.

Hypothyroidism. A syndrome resulting from deficiency of circulating thyroid hormone. When the disorder appears at birth or in early infancy, it is called **cretinism**; hypothyroidism occurring after early childhood is called **myxedema**.

Causes: Congenital absence or hypoplasia of the thyroid gland (Figure 10-3); intrinsic thyroid disease (Hashimoto thyroiditis); deficiency of dietary iodine, goitrogenic foods, or medicines; deficiency of pituitary thyroid-stimulating hormone.

History: Weakness, lethargy, myalgia, constipation, depression, intolerance to cold, polymenorrhea, weight gain, hoarseness.

Physical Examination: Dry, sallow skin, brittle hair and nails, thinning of scalp hair and outer thirds of eyebrows, puffy face, sluggish speech, bradycardia, nonpitting edema. A goiter may be present when disease is due to iodine deficiency, antithyroid agents, or thyroiditis.

Diagnostic Tests: The T_4 and other measures of thyroid hormone are depressed, the TSH level elevated (except when disease is due to pituitary TSH deficiency). There may be reduction of red blood cells, blood sugar, and sodium, and elevation of cholesterol. Antibody to thyroid may be found in Hashimoto thyroiditis.

Course: With treatment the prognosis is excellent. Complications of untreated disease include coronary artery disease, congestive heart failure, heightened susceptibility to infection, psychosis, and coma.

Treatment: Deficiency of thyroid hormone can be corrected by administration of levothyroxine. Maintenance treatment must be continued indefinitely unless a treatable cause of hypothyroidism can be found and eliminated.

Hyperthyroidism (Thyrotoxicosis). A syndrome resulting from excessive thyroid hormone in the circulation.

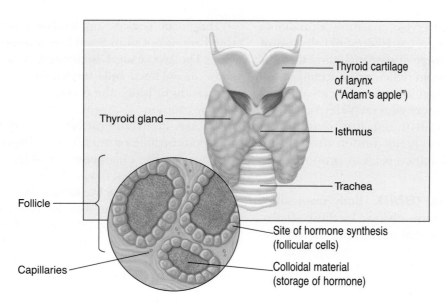

Figure 10-3
The Thyroid Gland

Causes: The principal cause is autoimmune disease of the thyroid gland, with production of thyroid-stimulating immunoglobulin by the immune system. This condition (**Graves disease**) is eight times commoner in women and usually comes on between ages 20 and 40. Graves disease may be accompanied by other autoimmune disorders (pernicious anemia, myasthenia gravis, diabetes mellitus). Less common causes of hyperthyroidism are acute thyroiditis and inappropriate administration of thyroid hormone.

History: Restlessness, nervousness, fatigue, intolerance to heat, sweating, cardiac palpitations, weight loss, frequent bowel movements, menstrual irregularities, enlargement of thyroid gland (goiter). In Graves disease, bulging of eyes, conjunctival drying or irritation.

Physical Examination: Tachycardia, warmth and moistness of skin, resting tremor of hands, hyperactive deep tendon reflexes, loosening of nails. In Graves disease, diffuse or nodular enlargement of thyroid, sometimes with arterial **bruit** (a vascular hum synchronous with heartbeat, heard with a stethoscope); **exophthalmos** (undue prominence of eyes due to edema of orbital contents), staring gaze, **lid lag** (slowness of upper eyelids to move with eye movements).

Diagnostic Tests: The levels of T_3 and T_4 are elevated, and TSH is depressed. The radioactive iodine uptake is increased. Thyroid-stimulating immunoglobulin is present in the serum. Antinuclear antibody may also be present. There may be mild anemia and hypercalcemia.

Course: Complications include atrial fibrillation, paralysis, and hypercalcemia.

Treatment: End-organ effects of thyroid hormone (tachycardia, tremor, restlessness) can be reduced by beta-blocker treatment. Glandular hyperactivity can be reduced by antithyroid medicines (propylthiouracil, methimazole), radioactive iodine, or thyroidectomy.

Hypoparathyroidism

Causes: The most common cause is accidental removal of the parathyroid glands during thyroidectomy. Rarely the parathyroid glands may be damaged by trauma, infection, neoplasm, or chemical poisons, or by autoantibodies, which may be formed in the polyglandular autoimmune syndrome.

History: With acute onset, tetany, tingling of face, hands, and feet, muscle cramps, **carpopedal spasm** (painful cramps of wrists and ankles), laryngospasm with respiratory obstruction, seizures. With more chronic onset, mental retardation, abnormalities of bones and teeth, cataract, parkinson-like disorder due to calcification of basal ganglia.

Physical Examination: The skin may be dry and coarse. Deep tendon reflexes are hyperactive, and the **Chvostek sign** (twitching of face after percussion over facial nerve in front of ear) and **Trousseau sign** (spastic contraction of the hand after application of a constricting cuff to the arm) are present.

Diagnostic Tests: The serum calcium is low and the serum phosphorus is high. Excretion of phosphorus in the urine is reduced. The level of parathyroid hormone in the serum is low.

Treatment: Calcium replacement, intravenously in acute tetany, and vitamin D. Treatment must be continued indefinitely.

Adrenal Insufficiency (Addison Disease). An acute or chronic deficiency of cortisol and related hormones from the adrenal cortex.

Causes: Degeneration of the adrenal cortices, usually as an autoimmune phenomenon sometimes involving other endocrine glands as well. Other diseases (infection, malignant tumors) may account for destruction of the adrenal glands in rare cases. Deficiency of pituitary ACTH also causes some adrenal insufficiency, but not the full-blown clinical picture of Addison disease. Adrenal crisis may be precipitated by severe physical stress (surgery), systemic disease (meningococcemia), or by sudden withdrawal of steroid therapy.

History: Weakness, easy fatigability, anorexia, nausea, vomiting, diarrhea, abdominal pain, amenorrhea, emotional lability. In addisonian crisis, fever, confusion, collapse, coma.

Physical Examination: Weight loss, wasting, hypotension, sparseness of axillary hair; increased pigmentation of skin, especially over pressure points, skin creases, and nipples. In crisis, severe hypotension and evidence of dehydration.

Diagnostic Tests: The eosinophil count is elevated. The serum sodium is low, the potassium and BUN (blood urea nitrogen) elevated. Serum cortisol is abnormally low and does not rise in response to administration of ACTH. Chest x-ray shows a small vertical heart.

Course: Without treatment, steady progression is likely. Addisonian crisis can be rapidly fatal. Fluid and electrolyte depletion, wasting, cardiovascular collapse.

Treatment: The basic treatment is replacement of missing corticosteroids. Supportive treatment and elimination of any identifiable underlying or precipitating cause are important. In crisis, intravenous fluid and electrolyte replacement may be lifesaving.

Cushing Syndrome (Hyperadrenocorticism). A syndrome due to prolonged elevation of adrenal cortical hormones in the circulation.

Causes: The most frequent cause of Cushing syndrome today is medicinal administration of adrenocortical hormones. The condition can also result from production of excessive adrenocortical hormones by a neoplasm of the adrenal cortex, from medicinal administration of ACTH, or from production of ACTH-like substances by other neoplasms (such as bronchogenic carcinoma). When excessive adrenal cortical activity results from an elevated level of ACTH from a tumor (basophil adenoma) of the pituitary, the condition is called Cushing disease.

History: Increasing obesity, stretch marks (especially on trunk and thighs), acne, easy bruising, impaired wound healing, weakness, thirst, headache, amenorrhea or impotence, increased body hair, personality change.

Physical Examination: Truncal obesity, moon face, **buffalo hump** (soft tissue prominence over upper back), protuberant abdomen with purple striae (stretch marks), hirsutism, acne, hypertension.

Diagnostic Tests: Blood glucose is elevated and potassium is low. The serum level of cortisol is high and does not fall after administration of dexamethasone, a synthetic corticosteroid. Urinary excretion of cortisol is also increased. In Cushing disease and other disorders due to excessive ACTH, the blood level of ACTH is elevated. Otherwise the ACTH level is subnormal, its production by the pituitary having been suppressed by high circulating levels of corticosteroid. An adrenal tumor may be shown by abdominal CT scan. Tumor of the pituitary is identified by cranial MRI.

Course: Depends on the origin of the problem. Untreated Cushing syndrome can be complicated by osteoporosis, nephrolithiasis, psychosis, heightened susceptibility to infection, and consequences of hypertension and diabetes mellitus; it is generally fatal within a few years.

Treatment: Discontinuance of corticosteroid treatment, or reduction of dose. Surgical removal of a causative pituitary or adrenal neoplasm. Ketoconazole or metyrapone can be used to suppress cortisol levels when surgery is not feasible.

Type 1 Diabetes Mellitus

Cause: A lack of insulin in the circulation due to failure of pancreatic B cells to respond to normal stimuli to insulin production. Failure of insulin production may be due to toxic, infectious, or autoimmune damage to B cells in genetically predisposed persons.

History: Polyuria (increased output of urine), **polydipsia** (excessive thirst), **polyphagia** (excessive appetite), weakness, and weight loss, coming on gradually or suddenly, usually in a person under 40 years of age. With fulminant onset, type 1 diabetes mellitus may present as **ketoacidosis** with dyspnea, drowsiness, collapse, and coma.

Physical Examination: Unremarkable in uncomplicated diabetes. In ketoacidosis: tachypnea, tachycardia, hypotension, flushing, fruity breath, and stupor or coma. Symptoms of cardiovascular, neurologic, or ocular complications may be evident in long-established or neglected disease.

Diagnostic Tests: Fasting blood sugar is over 140 mg/dL, and 2-hour postprandial blood sugar is over 200 mg/dL. Sugar is present in the urine. Serum cholesterol is often elevated. In ketoacidosis, ketones are found in the serum and the urine, and there is chemical evidence of metabolic acidosis (low blood pH, low blood HCO_3^-). Glycosylated hemoglobin (HbA_{1c})

reflects blood sugar levels over the preceding few weeks and is used to monitor control. Laboratory studies may also show evidence of systemic complications (infection, renal disease).

Course: Type 1 diabetes mellitus is a lifelong derangement of carbohydrate metabolism. In most patients, careful attention to diet and general health and proper use of insulin permit good control of blood sugar and fair protection against complications. Diabetes predisposes to numerous other conditions, including hypercholesterolemia, atherosclerosis, ocular cataracts and retinopathy, renal disease, infections of the urinary tract, skin, and other tissues, neuropathy, and microvascular disease in the extremities.

Treatment: Type 1 diabetes mellitus is by definition a disease that must be treated with insulin as a condition of the patient's survival. The mainstay of treatment, however, is diet, with limitation of total calories and restriction of carbohydrate and cholesterol. Increased fiber helps to stabilize carbohydrate metabolism, and artificial sweeteners are substituted for sugar. Injections of insulin are given 1-4 times a day. The patient monitors plasma glucose level by self-testing of fingerstick blood with a portable electronic meter. A variety of insulin products are available with different patterns of absorption and peak activity. The proper management of diabetes requires scrupulous attention to general health, care of the skin and the feet, and vigorous treatment of complications. Regular eye examinations and periodic testing for microalbuminuria provide early detection of retinopathy and nephropathy respectively. Diabetic ketoacidosis is treated with intravenous fluids, insulin, and general supportive measures.

Type 2 Diabetes Mellitus

Cause: A relative deficiency of circulating insulin accompanied by insensitivity or resistance of tissues, particularly liver and muscle, to insulin effect. There is a genetic predisposition to this form of diabetes, but the mechanism of transmission is unknown. Type 2 diabetes mellitus accounts for 90% of all cases of diabetes mellitus. Most patients are over 40 and obese.

History: The condition may remain asymptomatic for months or years. Polyuria, polydipsia, and sometimes weakness or fatigue occur as in insulin-dependent disease, but weight loss and ketoacidosis do not occur.

Physical Examination: Unremarkable except for obesity, unless complications have developed. Hypertension is often present.

Diagnostic Tests: Fasting blood sugar over 140 mg/dL; 2-hour postprandial blood sugars over 180 mg/dL. There is often sugar in the urine. Ketones are not found in serum. The cholesterol is often elevated. With advanced disease there may be chemical or electrocardiographic evidence of complications.

Course: Mild type 2 diabetes mellitus may cause few symptoms, particularly with treatment. Complications are the same as those for type 1 diabetes mellitus, with the exception of ketoacidosis. Complications typically do not develop as rapidly or become as severe as type 1 diabetes.

Treatment: Dietary restriction of carbohydrate alone may suffice to control blood sugar levels and abolish symptoms of polyuria and fatigue. Cholesterol restriction is also advised. Drugs such as pioglitazone and rosiglitazone help to overcome insulin resistance. Alpha-glucosidase inhibitors (acarbose, miglitol) impede absorption of dietary carbohydrate. To achieve optimal control, the use of insulin may be required. Care of general health and avoidance of skin injury and infection are important in the management of all forms of diabetes.

Carcinoma of the Pancreas

Causes: Carcinoma of the pancreas ranks fourth among malignant tumors as a cause of death in the U.S. It is more common in men, and most cases occur after age 60. Other risk factors are obesity, cigarette smoking, and type 2 diabetes mellitus. Most tumors are ductal cell adenocarcinomas arising in the head of the gland.

History: Symptoms are insidious in onset and include anorexia, indigestion, weight loss, weakness, and fatigue.

Diagnostic Tests: Imaging studies (CT, MRI, ultrasound), laparoscopy, and pancreatic biopsy can provide a specific diagnosis but are often not performed early enough. Serum markers such as pancreatic oncofetal antigen (POA), alpha fetoprotein (AFP), carcinoembryonic antigen (CEA), CA 19-9, and CA 125 are often useful in following the progress of the disease once it is recognized but are too nonspecific to establish a diagnosis.

Course: By the time clear-cut indications of trouble such as abdominal pain, jaundice, ascites, and sudden onset of diabetes mellitus appear, most patients have invasion of the portal vein or the superior mesenteric artery, metastases to regional nodes, liver, adrenals, lungs, bone, and elsewhere, or tumors too large for resection.

Treatment: Such patients are candidates only for palliative treatment (radiation, chemotherapy, surgery to relieve biliary obstruction). Resectable tumors are treated with the Whipple procedure (pancreaticoduodenectomy). The overall five-year survival rate for pancreatic carcinoma is less than 3%.

Metabolic Syndrome.
A combination of metabolic disorders (obesity, hypertension, insulin resistance, hyperlipidemias, and others) associated with a high incidence of cardiovascular disease and premature death.

Cause: Genetic predisposition to insulin resistance, compounded by overeating and a sedentary lifestyle.

History: Overweight, often from childhood. Inactive lifestyle. Hypertension, hyperglycemia often noted early in life. Premature symptoms of cardiovascular disease.

Physical Examination: Obesity (waist circumference over 40 inches [102 cm] in men and over 35 inches [88 cm] in women). Systolic blood pressure over 130, diastolic pressure over 85. Signs of premature cardiovascular disease may be evident on examination of ocular fundi, heart, peripheral vessels.

Diagnostic Tests: Fasting plasma glucose of 100 mg/dL (5.55 mmol/L) or higher. High-density lipoprotein (HDL) cholesterol less than 40 mg/dL (1.04 mmol/L) in men and less than 50 mg/dL (1.30 mmol/L) in women. Triglyceride 150 mg/dL (1.70 mmol/L) or more. Elevated low-density lipoprotein (LDL) cholesterol, plasma insulin, and uric acid.

Course: Characterized by early and rapid development of the usual complications of obesity, hypertension, hyperglycemia, and dyslipidemia. Progression to type 2 diabetes mellitus is expected.

Treatment: Weight control, regular aerobic exercise. Drug treatment of hypertension, hyperglycemia, and lipid abnormalities as appropriate.

Phenylketonuria (PKU). An inborn error of metabolism causing mental retardation unless diagnosed and treated in early life.

Cause: Decreased activity of phenylalanine hydroxylase, an enzyme that normally converts phenylalanine to tyrosine. Phenylalanine is an essential amino acid whose principal dietary source is milk. In phenylketonuria, abnormally high levels of phenylalanine accumulate and cause irreversible damage to the central nervous system. Transmitted as an autosomal recessive trait, it occurs in one of 10,000 Caucasian births. Several clinical patterns are recognized.

History: The child appears normal at birth, but within a few months may display **psychomotor retardation** (delayed development in muscle strength and coordination and impairment in the ability to understand and learn), **hyperactivity** (increased mobility, restlessness, inability to sit or lie still), seizures, movement disorders, paralysis, and abnormally fair skin with a tendency to eczema.

Physical Examination: Fair skin, mental retardation, muscle weakness or paralysis, **myoclonus** (involuntary jerking or twitching of certain muscles or muscle groups), **eczema** (an acute or chronic inflammation of the skin with itching, redness, blistering, weeping, crusting, and scaling). The urine has a mousy odor.

Diagnostic Tests: The serum level of phenylalanine is abnormally elevated, the level of tyrosine reduced. The urine contains phenylketones (phenylpyruvic acid and 2-hydroxyphenylacetic acid), hence the mousy odor and the name of the disease. Early detection of phenylketonuria is mandatory if treatment is to be successful.

Note: Testing of newborn blood for phenylalanine is standard pediatric practice. Testing is required by law in many states before hospital discharge of the newborn. With hospital stays for uncomplicated delivery restricted to 24 hours, many infants are tested before phenylalanine levels have begun to rise. Repeat testing must therefore be done a few days later in an outpatient setting.

Course: With dietary restriction of phenylalanine begun early, most patients lead normal lives. Sensitivity to phenylalanine may be outgrown in some cases.

Treatment: Restriction of dietary phenylalanine by feeding low-phenylalanine substitutes for milk. Avoidance of the artificial sweetener **aspartame**. Treatment should be begun before one month of age and continued as long as blood tests show a rise in phenylalanine after consumption of milk.

Diagnostic and Surgical Procedures

Chvostek test, sign Twitching of the face after percussion over the facial nerve in front of the ear, a sign of latent tetany due to hypocalcemia.

fine-needle biopsy of the thyroid gland Sampling of the thyroid gland tissue via insertion of a fine-bore needle into the thyroid.

Glucometer A small portable device from Bayer used to measure blood sugar.

lobectomy Surgical removal of a lobe of the thyroid gland.

parathyroidectomy Surgical removal of one more more of the parathyroid glands.

Trousseau test, sign Spastic contraction of the hand after application of a constricting cuff to the arm, a sign of latent tetany.

thyroidectomy Surgical removal of the thyroid gland.

Laboratory Procedures

acetone, urinary Acetone in the urine can be measured with a dipstick. Small amounts are found in starvation and other abnormal metabolic states, larger amounts in uncontrolled diabetes mellitus.

blood sugar The level of glucose in the blood.

calcitonin, serum A hormone produced by the thyroid gland and affecting the metabolism of calcium. It is markedly elevated in certain malignancies of the thyroid and lung.

fasting blood sugar (FBS) Determination of serum glucose in a specimen drawn from a patient who has been fasting for several hours, usually overnight.

glucose tolerance test (GTT) Measurements of blood sugar made at various intervals after ingestion of a standard carbohydrate meal.

glucose, urinary Should be negative. Glucose (sugar) in the urine usually indicates diabetes mellitus or other endocrine dysfunction.

glycosylated hemoglobin (hemoglobin A1$_c$) Measurement of the amount of glucose bound to the hemoglobin of red blood cells. Useful in monitoring long-term control of diabetes mellitus.

GTT (glucose tolerance test).

ketones, serum A group of waste products resulting from abnormal metabolism of fat in uncontrolled diabetes mellitus. Ketones may be called ketone bodies or simply "acetone."

17-ketosteroids Urinary breakdown products of adrenal cortical hormones, increased in certain disorders of the adrenal gland.

T3, T$_3$ (triiodothyronine) Thyroid hormone.

T4, T$_4$ (thyroxine) Thyroid hormone.

thyroid-stimulating hormone (TSH) Hormone secreted by the anterior pituitary gland that stimulates the thyroid gland and promotes is normal function.

thyroxine Principal hormone of the thyroid gland. Also called T$_4$.

Pharmacology

Thyroid supplements are used to treat hypothyroidism. They are obtained from natural sources such as desiccated (dried) ground beef or pork thyroid glands, or they are synthetically manufactured. These drugs contain both T$_3$ and T$_4$.

desiccated thyroid (Armour Thyroid)
liotrix (Thyrolar)

The drug **liothyronine (Cytomel, Triostat)** contains only T$_3$, whereas levothyroxine (Levo-T, Levothroid, Synthroid, Unithroid) contains only T$_4$.

Antithyroid drugs are used to treat hyperthyroidism. They act by inhibiting the production of T$_3$ and T$_4$ in the thyroid gland.

methimazole (Tapazole)
propylthiouracil
radioactive sodium iodide 131 (Iodotope)

Corticosteroids prescribed to systemically inhibit inflammatory reactions throughout the body are given orally.

betamethasone (Celestone)
cortisone (Cortone)
dexamethasone (Decadron, Dexameth, Dexamethasone Intensol, Dexone, Hexadrol)
hydrocortisone (A-Hydrocort, Cortef, Hydrocortone, Solu-Cortef)
methylprednisolone (A-Methapred, Medrol, Solu-Medrol)
prednisolone (Hydeltrasol, Orapred, Pediapred, Predalone 50, Prelone)
prednisone (Deltasone, Meticorten, Orasone)
triamcinolone (Aristocort, Kenacort, Kenalog-40, Tac-40, Trilog, Trilone)

Cortisone replacement. Adrenal gland malfunction and resultant low levels of cortisone cause Addison disease. The drug fludrocortisone (Florinef) is used for cortisone replacement.

Anabolic (androgenic) steroids. These synthetic substances, which resemble male sex hormones chemically, change the natural balance of the body between anabolism (tissue building) and catabolism (tissue breakdown). They have been used for years by athletes to increase muscle mass, strength, and endurance. Although the use of these drugs is illegal in professional sports, the practice continues.

In AIDS patients, anabolic steroids have been legitimately prescribed to counteract the wasting syndrome. Oxandrin (oxandrolone) is an example.

Insulin. Insulin is secreted by beta cells in the islets of Langerhans in the pancreas. This hormone plays an essential role in sugar metabolism. Traditionally, insulin has been derived from beef or pork pancreas. Human insulin is synthetically produced by means of recombinant DNA techniques; this avoids the potential for allergic reactions. The trade name for all such human insulin is Humulin. Regardless of the original source, all insulins are classified according to how quickly they act in the body to lower the blood glucose level (which depends on the size of the insulin crystal) and how many hours their therapeutic action continues (which is lengthened by the addition of protamine and zinc).

Rapid-acting insulins include:
regular (Regular Iletin I, Regular Iletin II, Humulin R, Novolin R, Velosulin BR)

Intermediate-acting insulins include:
NPH (NPH Iletin, Humulin N, Novolin N, NPH-N)
Lente (Iletin II Pork Lente, Lente Iletin II, Novolin ge Lente)

Long-acting insulins (Ultralente) include:

Novolin ge Ultralente

Mixtures of NPH and regular insulin include:

Humulin 50/50
Humulin 70/30; Novolin 70/30 PenFill

Human insulin analogs are created by making small changes in the sequence of amino acids in the insulin molecule during synthesis by recombinant DNA technology. Insulin analogs preserve the metabolic activity of the naturally occurring hormone but have a more rapid onset (usually in 15 minutes or less) and, in some cases, a smoother, more prolonged rise and fall in serum level. For many patients the use of one or more insulin analogs improves control of diabetes while reducing the number of injections needed each day.

insulin aspart (NovoLog)
insulin detemir (Levemir)
insulin glargine (Lantus)
insullin glulisine (Apidra)
insulin lispro (Humalog)

An **insulin pump** is a portable or implantable electronic device that delivers insulin from a reservoir through an indwelling subcutaneous catheter. A small basal dose of rapidly acting insulin is infused continuously. In addition, bolus doses are administered manually by the patient before meals or as needed to deal with marked elevations of plasma glucose, as determined by routine fingerstick testing.

Oral antidiabetic drugs. The pancreas of a patient with type 2 diabetes mellitus is still producing limited amounts of insulin. With diet control and weight loss, this amount of insulin may be sufficient. If not, an oral antidiabetic drug will be prescribed. Some oral agents used in type 2 diabetes mellitus stimulate the pancreas to produce more insulin. Contrary to popular belief, these drugs are not "oral insulin" and are ineffective in type 1 diabetes.

chlorpropamide (Diabinese)
glimepiride (Amaryl)
glipizide (Glucotrol)
glyburide (DiaBeta, Glynase PresTabs, Micronase)
metformin (Fortamet, Glucophage)
repaglinide (Prandin)

The following drugs help to control type 2 diabetes by increasing the sensitivity of muscle and fat cells to the patient's own insulin. They do not stimulate the pancreas to produce more insulin.

pioglitazone (Actos)
rosiglitazone (Avandia)

Another class of antidiabetic drugs inhibit an enzyme in the intestine that digests carbohydrate. This delays the absorption of glucose and thus keeps the blood sugar lower after meals.

acarbose (Precose)
miglitol (Glyset)

Drugs used to treat diabetic neuropathy. Diabetic neuropathy is a chronic complication of diabetes mellitus that is characterized by degenerative changes in the nerves of the lower extremities, pain, and altered sensation (paresthesia).

Most of the drugs used to treat this disease are antidepressants. Although antidepressants do not have a direct analgesic effect, they are effective in treating various types of pain syndromes.

amitriptyline (Elavil)
amoxapine
desipramine (Norpramin)
doxepin (Sinequan, Sinequan Concentrate)
imipramine (Tofranil, Tofranil-PM)
lamotrigine (Lamictal)
nortriptyline (Aventyl, Pamelor)
protriptyline (Vivactil)

A drug used to treat both diabetic neuropathy and diabetic retinopathy is tolrestat (Alredase).

TRANSCRIPTION**TIPS**

1. Use of Arabic numerals is preferred by the American Diabetes Association. Type 1 and type 2 diabetes mellitus have replaced the use of Roman numerals.

2. The oral antidiabetic drug *Diabinese* is often pronounced *DiabinASE* in dictation, and the transcriptionist must be alert to its correct spelling.

3. Note the lack of capitalization:

Choice dm   Novolin ge

4. Memorize the correct spelling:

euthyroid: Patients who do not have either hypothyroidism or hyperthyroidism are said to be *euthyroid*.

Synthroid: Although thyroid has a *y*, the *y* has been deleted in the spelling of the medication *Synthroid*.

5. Note the unusual internal capitalization:

BetaRx
DiaBeta
NovoLog

Spotlight on

Fat Chance

by Judith Marshall

It really all started the night my husband put his arm around me and told me I was as cute as a baby Clydesdale. Then he reminisced about his youth and romantic adventures, recalling fondly that he loved going out with big women because "fat women are so grateful." I had another male saboteur on my hands. The myth had caught up with me. I had been brought up to believe that men would take care of me. First my father, then husband, and always and forever, the doctor.

My health was in my doctor's hands through pregnancy ("Now you can eat for two!"); minor health complaints ("If you are tired and can't sleep, have some Valium, take up bridge, do volunteer work; dye your hair, buy a new dress, stop dwelling on yourself"); and menopause ("Menopause is a consideration but don't worry. In a few years you'll dry up and that will be that!").

It must have been a neurotic need for punishment which drew me back to him for help with weight control. He listened to me intently and solicitously patted my hand. His voice sounded like dry leaves scraping against a sidewalk. "Diet and exercise, my dear. What is it you, ah, do for a living?" I reminded him that I work full time as a medical transcriptionist. He gave me that constipated smile of his and nodded sagely. "Yes, I have a young girl who does my work for me at home. A mother, you know. Has the child in the playpen beside her. It's wonderful. She's managed to learn all my words."

As I sat there, I knew I made him uncomfortable. To him I represented failure. There was nothing he could bandage, splint, or remove surgically (never mind suction lipectomy). Worse, I was a medical transcriptionist who knew the lingo and wanted answers. There were no pills, no ointments to be dispensed. He had nothing to offer except his contempt.

The last I heard they had already built the great railroads out West so I couldn't join a labor gang. I had a career anyway, one which burned about 250 calories a day if I counted picking up *Gray's Anatomy*, several brisk hikes to the copy machine, and riffling through the *PDR*. I was no longer just an endomorph. I WAS Jabba the Hutt. My fat cells were indestructible, like cockroaches constantly evolving to meet any chemical challenge to their extinction, and surviving, always surviving.

Why couldn't I lose weight on 1000 calories a day? Why was I so ravenously hungry? Why, after 40, was it so hard to lose even a pound and why were my hips pulling downward to my ankles? I lost time, I lost money, I lost my temper, I lost my nerve, I lost face, and I even lost teeth. Why couldn't I lose weight?

I had so many risk factors I should have been dead at 35. Time was running out. I had just sustained an eight-pound gain on a weekend in Cleveland (Slovenian-style pork roast and Rudy's fresh kielbasa with homemade dumplings). My porcine proportions yearned for a glimpse of the physiology of anorexia nervosa and bulimia. I would no longer be called the Sow City Wrangler at the square dances on Thursday night. I would take the fat out of *femme fatale*.

If the medicine man had failed me, I would hotfoot it to the best qualified female internist in Boston. This physician would understand my problems. She would be a nutritional Whiz Kid, a Phi Beta Kappa of calories. With great trepidation and after pinning my clothes together (the buttons had popped), I visited the doctor. Her tiny frame was sheathed in a size six designer dress in a bold brown check, and she wore a heavy, expensive gold chunky bracelet around her neck. She was about 30 years old. After a thorough review, examination, and blood work, she peered at me across the desk and said, "You simply follow this 1200-calorie diet and stop noshing between meals. See you in six months and you should be 10 pounds lighter by then." She looked pointedly at her watch.

Lordy, lordy, nothing had changed. The lard continued to expand. I began to transcribe frenetically. I never could eat and type at the same time. Besides, we are not allowed food in the work area, so I worked a lot of overtime. The diet the doctor had given me was preprinted and not realistic unless you had someone to do the food shopping, then prepare all the meals three times a day plus snacks, then lock it all up in the garage for the night. The doctors' battle to fight obesity is so monumentally time-consuming and frustrating, no wonder they just hand out a form diet.

Obesity, of course, is a uniquely female problem in a world that took centuries to recognize premenstrual syndrome. (Now it's trendy. We have a PMS clinic in the neighborhood, for heaven's sake.) I insinuated myself into a cluster of doctors at a cocktail party and whispered, "Female, fat, and forty," just to see them recoil in horror.

I had been told by doctors that I had no will power, that I was secretly bingeing. My one experience with diet pills led me to try to fly by jumping off the Mass General Hospital. Reading diet books took no fat off me but padded the wallets of the authors. Watching Jane Fonda's exercise tape sank me into a deep depression.

The language of food, cookbooks, and restaurant critic columns holds more prurient interest for me than pornography. I could even salivate over a well-written history, the doctor recounting the patient's daily dietary habits. My transcription, however, was suffering. I typed that the patient with pneumonia had "congested lunches" and that an asthmatic patient was to be "weighed off from steroids on a tapering basis."

Desperate and disgusted, seeking supernatural cures, I waddled into a weight loss clinic. They listened to me as if the most important thing in the world was my weight problem. Without pills, shots, packaged foods, or gimmicks, I am on a 500-calorie diet. I am walking three miles a day and dancing six hours a week. Richard Simmons, eat your heart out. A program of behavior modification and fat restriction gave me a lipid profile and a blood pressure reminiscent of my salad days.

It's not perfect. I hate going there five days a week. The nurses are all gorgeous, tall and willowy. The closest any of them ever came to cholesterol was walking through a field of buttercups. They keep meticulous records. "Going fishing again? Watch yourself. You always tend to drink beer when you go fishing." Some of them don't have to say anything to make me feel guilty. They just stand there, looking like my mother. But this time I am paying for feeling guilty. Mother did it for nothing.

My doctor thinks the clinic is owned and run by charlatans, that the program is unhealthy, that the weight loss is too fast. My doctor warned me that when I finish this ridiculous and dangerous program, I will put every single pound back on and then some.

Fat chance, doc.

Whining and Dining

by Judith Marshall

About five years ago, I wrote a column entitled "Fat Chance" in which I was truly obnoxious, hooting about a spectacular weight loss achievement. I was convinced I would never gain any of it back. Pass the humble pie. As soon as I quit starving and square dancing, it was do-si-do into old bad habits.

All of my recipes were marked, "Serves six, or two if they are Marshalls." If my professional organization charged people like me by the pound, there would be no dues increase. They could add a wing onto their building. But how could someone as smart as me evidently not know how to eat?

LOW-FAT DIET AND EXERCISE is the answer to permanent weight control. Why are we spending millions of collars in the diet industry? I have paid people to starve me, brainwash me, exercise me, puncture me, humiliate me, and weigh and measure me like a piece of pork (they probably thought so, too). And that was just the diet merchants, not the gyms and salons. I bought an

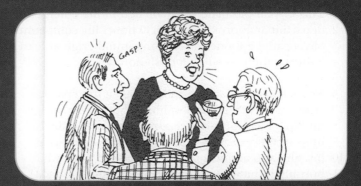

I insinuated myself into a cluster of doctors at a cocktail party and whispered, "Female, fat, and forty," just to see them recoil in horror. **Source**: Judith Marshall, *Medicate Me*, illustrated by Cindy Stevens.

exercise bike that tells me my pulse, blood pressure, rate of speed, and even croaks encouragement in a hoarse staccato computer voice—*you can do it, you can do it, you can do it.*

I have done it. I keep doing it. Veterans of fat wars have chomped through it all. Lose 70, put back 50, lose 50, put back 90. If the equation is fat equals stupid, take me to the head of the class. How easy to rationalize that large sizes are okay, but my tired frame with small bones was never meant to carry more than 120 pounds. Once again, I searched for thinness. . . .

Folks, I don't know what the answer is. I only know what it isn't. For me. For now. I thought a women's group experience would help us to deal with anger, depression, and self-hatred. I thought we could transcend talk about junk food. I thought we would discuss sexuality and life changes and not just regurgitate what some smart ad executive wrote up in the manual.

I agree with something Barbara Edelstein, M.D., wrote many years ago in *The Woman Doctor's Diet for Women*. "My feeling is that the overweight female responds best to a one-to-one relationship where you can challenge her, refute her without embarrassing her, and compel her to come to grips with herself, her own tricks and evasions."

So what am I eating and what's really eating me? I am nibbling back to the basics. Low-fat, low-calorie diet, and moderate exercise, for which I will pay no one. Many women volunteered to talk to me about their successes. I rejoice with them while mourning my own perceived failure. Perhaps I will find a therapist who does not take my problem lightly. As for my dollars perpetuating the bloated diet industry, well, I am just fed up.

Source: Judith Marshall, *Medicate Me*, illustrated by Cindy Stevens; and *Medicate Me Again*.

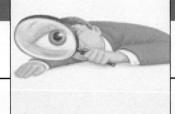

Proofreading Skills

Instructions: In the paragraphs below, circle the errors. Identify misspelled and missing medical and English words and punctuation errors, and write the correct words and punctuation in the numbered spaces opposite the text.

#	Text	#	Correction
1	This 67-year-old male was evaluated in the emergency	1	
2	departmt at approximately 0630 hours for complaints	2	department
3	of repeated episodes of vomiting, numberign at least	3	
4	5 during the preceding 8 or so hours.	4	
5		5	
6	She is a known diabetic and has taken fingerstick	6	
7	readings of 423 and 241 at home. She is on	7	
8	multiple medications including Regular Insulin 10	8	
9	units in the a.m., along with Ultralente 16 units at	9	
10	h.s. She also admits to some chest pane, somewhat	10	
11	burning in nature, without radiation into her face	11	
12	neck or arms. There is no history of diarrhea. She	12	
13	has a previous history of coranary artery bypass	13	
14	sugrery some 4 years earlier.	14	
15		15	
16	Physical assessment reveals her temp to be 98.2,	16	
17	pulse 60, respirations 20, and blood pressure 102/50.	17	
18	Initialy her color was pale. Her mucous membranes	18	
19	did appear dry. Her hart rate was regular without	19	
20	murmurs. There was a well-healed cicatrix to the	20	
21	anterior midsternal region. Lungs were clear to	21	
22	auscultation. The abdomen was soft with generalizd	22	
23	tenderness. No unusual pulsating masses. Lower	23	
24	extremties are free of any pretibial edema.	24	
25		25	
26	IMPRESSION	26	
27	1. Diabetes melitus, out of control.	27	
28	2. Dehydration.	28	
29	3. Electrolyte imbalance.	29	

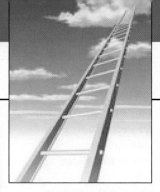

SkillsChallenge

Medical Terminology Matching Exercise

Instructions: Match the definitions in Column A with their terms in Column B.

Column A

1. ___ oral antidiabetic drug
2. ___ secreted by the adrenal cortex
3. ___ female hormone
4. ___ insulin-dependent
5. ___ a thyroid hormone
6. ___ non-insulin-dependent
7. ___ male hormone
8. ___ enlarged thyroid
9. ___ thyroid supplement
10. ___ regulates serum calcium levels
11. ___ hyperthyroidism
12. ___ antidiabetic injection
13. ___ produce insulin

Column B

A. thyroxine
B. parathyroid gland
C. glipizide
D. islets of Langerhans
E. Graves disease
F. estrogen
G. Humulin
H. corticosteroids
I. diabetes mellitus type 1
J. androgen
K. goiter
L. diabetes mellitus type 2
M. Synthroid

Abbreviations Exercise

Common abbreviations dictated in the body of a medical report may be transcribed as dictated. Uncommon abbreviations must be spelled out, with the abbreviations appearing in parentheses after the translation. All abbreviations (except laboratory test names) must be spelled out in the Diagnosis or Impression section of any report.

Instructions: Define the following endocrine abbreviations. Then memorize both abbreviations and definitions to increase your speed and accuracy in transcribing endocrinology dictation.

ACTH _____

ADA diet _____

ADH _____

BMI _____

FBS _____

FSH _____

GTT _____

LH _____

PKU _____

PTH _____

TBG _____

TFT _____

TSH _____

Dictation Exercises

Prior to transcribing the dictations, complete these activities.

1. **Using Chapter 3, Style Guide**
   a. The Style Guide states, "The use of a hyphen to separate two identical vowels or consonants when joining prefixes and combining forms is changing." List examples from the Style Guide of words beginning with the prefixes *re-* and *pre-* that no longer contain hyphens.
   b. When, according to the Style Guide, do you expand brief forms?
   c. What does the Style Guide recommend you do when a sentence begins with a number?
   d. Review the Brief Forms and Medical Slang list in the Style Guide. What should you do if you encounter "alk phos" or "satting" in dictation?
   e. According to the error-prone abbreviations list, how should you transcribe the term *units* when part of a medication dose? What is the appropriate translation for *h.s.* and *q.d.*?
   f. What symbol is used for the word *over* in the expression "grade four over five"?
   g. What is the recommended style for a department name referred to as an entity (person)?
   h. Read the first paragraph under General Information and the section on Editing in the Style Guide. Ask your instructor what to do if a dictator fails to dictate pronouns and conjunctions or subjects and helping verbs.
   i. According to the Style Guide, what is the difference between the terms *post* and *status post*?
   j. According to the error-prone abbreviations list, what is the acceptable abbreviation for *microgram*?
   k. Read the section in the Style Guide on suture sizes. How do you transcribe "three-oh" suture? How do you transcribe "number oh" suture?

2. **Problem Solving**
   a. The dictator says that the pulse rate is in the "one teens." How would you handle this?
   b. The dictator drops syllables when dictating a couple of medication names. What are some of the auditory and research techniques you could use to help you decipher the words?

3. **Preparatory Research**
   a. Where is the pituitary located? What is a pituitary adenoma?
   b. What does *prudent* mean? (*Note. Prudent* is an English word, not a medical term.)
   c. Define *Propionibacterium acnes.*
   d. Define *arthralgia* and *myalgia.*
   e. What is the difference between *discreet* and *discrete*? Which one is more likely to be used in a medical context?

   f. Perform an Internet search for TSH + "reference values" (keep the quotation marks around *reference values*). What is the reference range? What is the abbreviation for the units of measure used?
   g. Perform a similar search for the reference range and units of measure used for vitamin B_{12}.
   h. What does the hemoglobin A_{1c} value tell the physician about a patient's diabetic control?
   i. What does *proliferative* mean?
   j. When transcribing laboratory test results, it is customary to include the values for related tests in a single sentence, usually separated by commas unless the sentence is complicated by extraneous information. For example, all of the individual tests and values included on a CBC would be included in one sentence. The results of a chemistry panel (which can be anywhere from 3 to over 20 individual tests) would be included in a single sentence. Other common test groupings including thyroid profile, liver function tests, and electrolytes. Which individual tests or values would be included in CBC results? Which tests might be included in a chemistry panel?
   k. What contrast agents are used in angiography procedures? What are the side effects of these agents?
   l. What is the correct expansion for the imaging study, *MRCP*? (*Hint.* The *MR* stands for magnetic resonance).
   m. When people see or hear the word *manifest*, they usually think of it as a verb or a noun, but it can also be an adjective (and that's the way it's often used in dictation). What is the definition of *manifest* as an adjective? (*Hint.* You'll need to look it up in an English dictionary.)
   n. Define *anorexia, ascites, mesentery, debilitated.*
   o. In what anatomical area of the brain would a vertebrobasilar stroke occur?
   p. What does *FNA* stand for? (*Hint.* It's a procedure for obtaining a biological sample for pathological analysis.)
   q. Perform an Internet search for thyroid anatomy and read the discussion at **www.eMedicine.com**, paying particular attention to the muscles and nerves that are mentioned. Make a list of the nerves and muscles that are mentioned.
   r. What are the *strap muscles*? Why do you think they're called *straps*?
   s. Many of the organs in the body have sections or compartments called *lobes.* This is true of the thyroid gland. What is/are the names of the lobes of the thyroid gland that are mentioned in the thyroid anatomy discussion at **www.eMedicine.com**? (*Note.* You can search an individual browser page using the key combination control-F.)
   t. Define *platysma.*

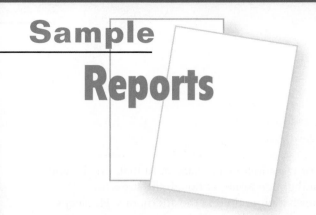

Sample Reports

Sample endocrinology reports appear on the following pages, illustrating a variety of reports. Fictional names are provided for illustration of proper format, and no resemblance to actual persons is intended. Sample transcripts were prepared according to the *AAMT Book of Style*, where possible.

Chart Note

BEARNSON, SARA
Age: 42
12/14/XXXX

CHIEF COMPLAINT
Increasing fatigue, nocturia, and vaginal pruritus.

HISTORY OF PRESENT ILLNESS
Brief exam for this obese 42-year-old female with a 2-year history of mild hypertension and type 2 diabetes mellitus, controlled by diet. Medications include Ortho-Novum 10/11. The patient was started on hydrochlorothiazide 50 mg 2 weeks ago because of elevated diastolic pressures.

Blood sugar by glucose meter is 417. Urine negative for ketones. Apical pulse of 90. Blood pressures are 144/94 and 140/98. Height 5 feet 2 inches, weight 186.

PHYSICAL EXAMINATION
Unremarkable.

RECOMMENDATIONS
1. Instruction to patient to push fluids for the next several days.
2. Discontinue hydrochlorothiazide and birth control pills to end possible drug-induced hyperglycemia.
3. Start Micronase 2.5 mg every other day and Capoten 25 mg b.i.d.
4. Set up appointment on Friday for fasting blood sugar.
5. Patient to see the nurse practitioner for fitting of a diaphragm and nutritional counseling on a 1200-calorie ADA diet.

AF:hpi

BRADLEY, MITCH
#090438
DATE OF OFFICE VISIT: 7/25/XXXX

This 36-year-old man was doing well until 3 years ago, when he developed progressively severe fatigue. At that time he had been in a stressful job situation. However, these symptoms have persisted and gotten worse, although the stress has improved. There is no relation to meals or time of day, although he is somewhat more tired in the afternoons. He sleeps 7-8 hours during the week and 12 hours on weekends. Chem-2, CBC, Epstein-Barr studies, and thyroid function tests have been normal. He was tried on Thyrolar 1/2 grain because of low normal T4, but there was no benefit. He has received Prozac, imipramine, and other antidepressants, including vitamin B12 injections, without any benefit. He has a 3-year history of constant burning in the eyes. An ophthalmologist did not find anything wrong.

REVIEW OF SYSTEMS
He has periodic dizziness, particularly when standing up rapidly, occasional tinnitus, frequent constipation and occasional diarrhea, nocturia x2-3, cold extremities, and dry skin of relatively recent onset. He has some anxiety and insomnia and is depressed, apparently in relation to his condition.

FAMILY HISTORY
The father has heart disease. The brother has retinitis pigmentosa.

HABITS
He drinks coffee. His diet is balanced and low in sugar.

EXAMINATION
Height 6 feet 1 inch, 190 pounds. Blood pressure 130/72, pulse is 68. HEENT, neck, heart, lungs, abdomen, pulses, extremities, gross neurologic, and skin are normal. Rectal not done.

ASSESSMENT
1. Chronic fatigue.
2. Burning eyes.
3. Depression.
4. Signs of possible hypothyroidism.
5. Constipation and diarrhea.

PLAN
Will check basal temperatures and begin thyroid prescription if low. Gave therapeutic trial of 6 mL vitamin C, 4 mL calcium/magnesium, 1 mL of B6, B12, B5, and B complex intravenously. Will repeat if helpful. Other recommendations as noted. Return in 4 weeks.

SANDRA BEECH, MD

SB:hpi
d: 7/25/XXXX
t: 7/26/XXXX

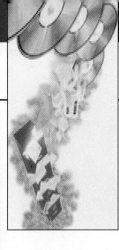

Transcription Practice

Key Words

The following terms appear in the endocrinology dictations. Before beginning the medical transcription practice for Chapter 10, look up each term below in a medical or English dictionary and write out a short definition.

diabetic ketoacidosis
multiple sclerosis
pancreatic carcinoma
pituitary adenoma

thyroidectomy
type 1 diabetes
type 2 diabetes
ulceration

After completing all the readings and exercises in Chapter 10, transcribe the endocrinology dictation. Proofread your transcribed documents carefully, listening to the dictation while you read your transcripts.

Transcribe (*not* retype) the same reports again without referring to your previous transcription attempt. Initially, you may need to transcribe some reports more than twice before you can produce an error-free document. Your ultimate goal is to produce an error-free document the first time.

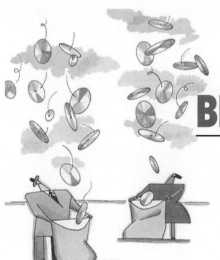

BLOOPERS

This child will probably be shorter than he wants to be, but he should have picked different parents.

Physical examination revealed a garrulous, obese woman who was short of breath on motion but not on talking.

The patient had waffles for breakfast and anorexia for lunch.

At 2 a.m. the patient was found dead in bed after otherwise having had a good day.

Mr. Blank is a giant of a man who appears to be roughly 24 months' pregnant.

The doctor's basic suggestions were that treatment remain conservative, and that procrastination be the procedure of choice for the time being.

It should be noted that this history was obtained in the patient's broken English and my broken Spanish.

In the morning the patient refused further examination, diagnostic procedures, or treatment and demanded release from the hospital. She said that she was too sick to be in the hospital and would return when she felt better.

The patient celebrated her wedding anniversary last evening with a ham dinner and a tiff with her husband.

Review of her past history showed that she had had a very uneventful life.

Chapter 11

Urology and Nephrology

Chapter Outline

Transcribing Urology and Nephrology Dictation

Anatomy in Brief

Terminology Review

Lay and Medical Terms

Medical Readings

History and Physical Examination

Common Diseases

Diagnostic and Surgical Procedures

Laboratory Procedures

Pharmacology

Spotlight

Transcription Tips

Proofreading Skills

Skills Challenge

Sample Reports

Transcription Practice

Bloopers

Learning Objectives

- Describe the structure and function of the urinary tract and male reproductive system.
- Spell and define common genitourinary terms.
- Identify types of questions a physician might ask about the genitourinary system in the review of systems.
- Describe common signs of abnormality a physician looks for on examination of the external genitalia and male reproductive organs.
- Identify common diseases of the excretory and male reproductive system. Describe their typical cause, course, and treatment options.

- Identify and define diagnostic and surgical procedures of the genitourinary system.
- List common genitourinary laboratory tests and procedures.
- Identify and describe common genitourinary drugs and their uses.
- Demonstrate knowledge of anatomical, medical, pharmacological, adjectival, and soundalike terms by accurately completing the exercises in this chapter.

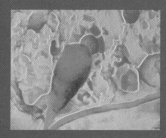
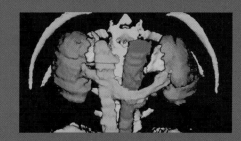
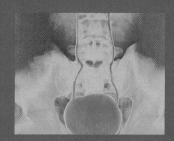

Transcribing Urology and Nephrology Dictation

The genitourinary (GU) system traditionally includes the urinary excretory organs as well as the male reproductive organs. Because of its complexity, the female reproductive system is given its own chapter of study. It is often categorized as obstetrics and gynecology (Ob/Gyn) or gynecology and fertility.

Anatomy in Brief

The **excretory system** includes the **kidneys**, the **ureters**, the **bladder**, and the **urethra** (see Figure 11-1). The function of this system is to regulate the composition of the blood by disposing of wastes and excessive amounts of water, electrolytes, and other substances.

The **kidneys** lie in the upper abdomen behind the peritoneal cavity, protected by cushions of fatty tissue. Each has a pronounced **hilum** at which an artery, a vein, and a ureter are attached.

The **male reproductive system** (see Figure 11-2) consists of the paired **testes (testicles)**, each with its collecting system (the **epididymis**, a coiled tubular structure attached to the testicle; and the **spermatic duct** or **vas deferens**, a tube that conducts sperm to the prostate), the **penis**, the **scrotum** (a cutaneous sac containing the testicles), the **prostate** (a gland surrounding the urethra just below the bladder), and the **seminal vesicles** (small pouchlike glands adjacent to the vas deferens).

The **testicle** produces **spermatozoa** (singular, spermatozoon), each one of which is capable of fertilizing a female ovum and carries the paternal contribution to the genetic makeup of the offspring. In addition, the testicles produce male hormones that are responsible for the development and maintenance of secondary sexual characteristics (facial and body hair, male body build, deep voice). The prostate contains secretory cells that produce the fluid component of semen. It also contains smooth muscle, and under sexual stimulation it closes off the bladder from the urethra and brings about ejaculation of semen (prostatic fluid + spermatozoa) through the urethra.

Terminology Review

albuminuria Proteinuria.

anuria Total cessation of urinary output.

azotemia See *uremia.*

bacteriuria The presence of bacteria in the urine.

casts Plugs of material formed in renal tubules, detected on urinalysis.

condyloma Genital wart.

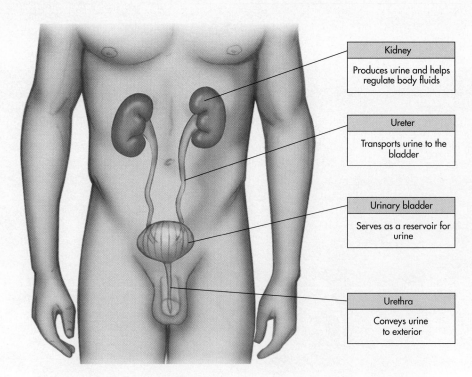

Figure 11-1
The Urinary Organs

Kidney
Produces urine and helps regulate body fluids

Ureter
Transports urine to the bladder

Urinary bladder
Serves as a reservoir for urine

Urethra
Conveys urine to exterior

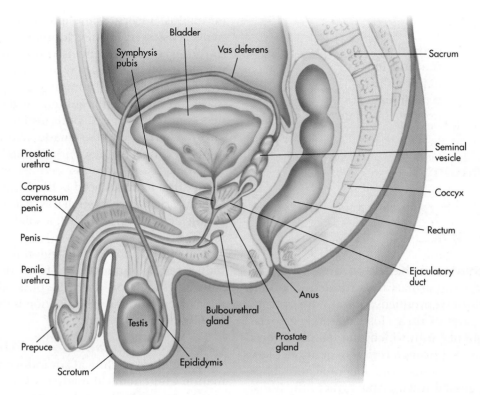

Figure 11-2
Male Reproductive Organs

crystals Detected on urinalysis.

diuresis An increase in the production of urine by the kidneys as a result of renal or systemic disease, toxic substances, or drugs administered to reduce body water, sodium, or both.

dribbling Uncontrollable passage of drops of urine, particularly just after voiding.

dysuria Pain with urination.

glycosuria The abnormal presence of glucose in the urine.

hematuria Blood in the urine.

hesitancy Difficulty initiating the urinary flow.

incontinence Involuntary passage of urine.

ketonuria The abnormal presence of ketones in the urine.

KUB Kidneys, ureters, and urinary bladder.

lues Syphilis.

micturition Voiding; urination.

nephritis Inflammation of the kidney.

occult blood Blood in the urine in such small amounts as to be undetected by the naked eye.

oliguria Marked reduction in the volume of urine excreted in 24 hours.

pH A measure of alkalinity or acidity of the urine.

pollakiuria Increased frequency of urination without increase in total volume excreted in 24 hours.

polyuria Increase in the 24-hour excretion of urine.

proteinuria The abnormal presence of protein in the urine.

pyuria Pus in the urine.

reflux The backward flow of urine within any part of the urinary tract.

UPJ Ureteropelvic junction.

uremia Refers to increased levels of urea, creatinine, and other nitrogen-containing waste products because of impairment of kidney function.

UVJ Ureterovesical junction.

Lay and Medical Terms

clap	gonorrhea
kidney stone	renal calculus
	nephrolithiasis
	renal lithiasis
pass water, pee	urinate, micturate, void

Medical Readings

History and Physical Examination

by John H. Dirckx, M.D.

Review of Systems: Kidneys and Urinary Tract. The kidneys and urinary tract (ureters, bladder, and urethra) and the reproductive system are considered together because of their close anatomic association and the frequency with which one disease affects both organ systems. A thorough review of genitourinary history includes past diagnoses of congenital anomalies of the urinary or genital tract; urinary tract infections; stone in a kidney, ureter, or bladder; sexually transmitted (venereal) diseases; genitourinary surgery; and menstrual and reproductive history.

Symptoms suggesting renal or urinary tract disease are pain in one or both flanks, increase in frequency of urination (as opposed to increase in urine volume), **nocturia** (being awakened at night by the urge to void), burning or pain on voiding, difficulty voiding, diminution in the urinary stream, incontinence of urine, bed-wetting in an older child or adult, blood in the urine, and any other marked change in the appearance of the urine.

Men are questioned about urethral discharge or burning; itching, rash, ulcers, or other lesions of the genitals; pain or swelling in the testicles; scrotal masses; and infertility.

Most persons are reticent about sexual matters, and not much is gained by determined probing unless the chief complaint involves the reproductive system in some way. When necessary, the interviewer may ask about the subject's sexual preference, frequency of sexual activity, number of different partners, participation in oral or anal sex, masturbation, and satisfaction with sexual activity. In addition, men are asked about difficulty in achieving or maintaining erections and premature or delayed ejaculation, women about pain during intercourse and any difficulty in attaining orgasm.

Physical Examination. With the patient standing, the physician inspects the **penis** and **scrotum** for dermatitis, ulcers, scars, and other skin lesions. The penis is assessed for developmental abnormalities, and the foreskin, if present, is retracted for inspection of the **glans**. The **urethra** may be milked to express any discharge. The scrotal contents are palpated, and any masses, testicular enlargement or deformity, or tenderness is noted. If one or both testicles are not felt in the scrotum, an attempt is made to locate them in the inguinal canals (undescended testis).

Scrotal masses are assessed by transillumination. A bright focal light is placed behind and in contact with the scrotum, and the room lights extinguished. A cyst or hydrocele will transmit light; a solid tumor or hernia will not.

The examination of this region in the male concludes with a rectal examination. This is described under the gastrointestinal portion of the physical examination. The female genitourinary examination is discussed in Chapter 12, Obstetrics and Gynecology.

Laboratory Examination of Urine

In the modern clinical laboratory, microscopic examination and chemical analysis of urine can yield information not only about the urinary tract but also about other body systems, water and acid-base balance, nutrition, and the presence of toxic substances. A major advantage of urine examinations is that, under ordinary circumstances, specimens are readily available, without the need for invasive procedures or elaborate equipment.

For most of the tests done in the urinology laboratory, the preferred specimen is 60-90 mL of freshly voided urine. Although a random specimen is usually suitable, a **first-voided specimen** (the first urine passed after arising in the morning) may be more satisfactory in testing for trace substances because it is usually more concentrated.

A **clean-voided specimen** (clean catch) is one obtained after cleansing of the area around the urethral meatus (usually with liquid soap and cotton balls) to prevent contamination of the specimen with material from outside the urinary tract.

A **midstream specimen** is one that contains neither the first nor the last portion of urine passed. It is obtained by introducing a specimen container into the urine stream after voiding has begun and removing it before voiding ceases. The purpose of this procedure is to obtain as pure as possible a sample of bladder urine, with minimal admixture of cells or other material from the urethra.

A **catheterized specimen** is obtained by urethral catheter (less often by suprapubic needle puncture of the bladder), either because the patient cannot void or to prevent contamination of the specimen. A **24-hour**

urine specimen consists of all the urine passed by the patient during a 24-hour period.

A urine specimen is usually collected in a clean, dry bottle or cup of glass, plastic, or waxed or plasticized paper. The container need not be sterile except for bacteriologic work. Examination of urine is carried out as soon as possible after the specimen is obtained because blood cells in urine rupture early and bacterial growth in a standing specimen may alter its chemical composition. When a delay is expected, the specimen is refrigerated. A 1- or 2-gallon jug is used to collect a 24-hour urine specimen. The jug may be kept on ice during the collection period, and one of several preservatives may be placed in the jug before collection begins to inhibit the growth of bacteria in the specimen.

The principal diagnostic procedure in urinology is the urinalysis, a set of routine physical and chemical examinations. In most laboratories, the urinalysis includes direct observation of the specimen for color, turbidity, and other obvious characteristics; determination of specific gravity; microscopic examination of sediment for cells, crystals, and other formed elements; determination of pH; and chemical testing for glucose, protein, occult blood, and perhaps bilirubin and acetone.

Variations in color and clarity of urine usually reflect variations in concentration of solutes, including pigment. Because the daily solute load is fairly constant, changes in concentration are nearly always due to changes in volume of water excreted. Turbidity (cloudiness) may be due to the presence of phosphates, which are insoluble in alkaline urine. A smoky brown color ("**Coca-Cola urine**") often indicates the presence of hemolyzed blood. Color changes may be due to abnormal waste products (bilirubin, porphyrins), drugs (methylene blue, phenazopyridine), or pigments from foods (beets, blackberries). Mucus shreds, fragments of tissue, or calcareous material may be grossly evident in the specimen.

Microscopic examination of the urine is usually preceded by centrifugation of the specimen to concentrate any cells or other formed elements present. A polychrome stain such as the Sternheimer-Malbin stain (crystal violet and safranin in ethanol) may be added to the sediment to enhance the distinctive features of various cells, but is not essential. Microscopic examination is carried out on a small volume of fluid urine placed on a slide and covered with a cover slip. Dried smears of urine are not ordinarily suitable for examination.

Formed elements frequently found in urine are red blood cells, white blood cells, casts, crystals, bacteria, epithelial cells, and amorphous sediment. Cell counts are recorded as cells per high-power field, obtained as an average after examination and counting of several fields. A small number of red and white blood cells are present in normal urine.

A finding of more than 1 or 2 **red blood cells per high-power field (RBC/hpf),** called **microscopic hematuria,** indicates either bleeding in some part of the excretory system or contamination of the specimen with blood, possibly menstrual. Hematuria occurs in acute glomerulonephritis, urolithiasis, hemorrhagic diseases, infarction of the kidney, tuberculosis of the kidney, benign or malignant tumors of any part of the urinary tract, and many cases of simple cystitis. The presence of more than 1 or 2 **white blood cells per high-power field (WBC/hpf),** known as **pyuria**, usually indicates infection in some part of the urinary tract.

Casts are microscopic cylindrical bodies that have been formed by concretion of cells or insoluble material within renal tubules and subsequently excreted in the urine. Casts are always abnormal. They are reported as the number counted per low-power field. Hyaline and waxy casts are homogeneous casts varying in refractivity. They consist of coagulated protein and are found in conditions associated with leakage of protein through glomeruli: nephritis, nephrotic syndrome (including lupus nephrosis, and Kimmelstiel-Wilson disease), toxemia, and congestive heart failure. Granular casts are formed by aggregation of red or white blood cells or both in renal tubules and occur in many of the same conditions as hyaline and waxy casts.

A variety of **crystals** may be found on microscopic examination of the urine. Their chemical composition can usually be deduced from their shape. Crystals of uric acid, cystine, calcium oxalate, and triple phosphate may appear in the urine of persons who excrete abnormal quantities of these materials and are subject to stone formation. **Bacteria** in significant numbers in a freshly voided specimen (bacteriuria, bacilluria) suggest urinary tract infection. Some squamous **epithelial cells** (squames) are often found in urine and have little significance. **Amorphous sediment** is a general term for ill-defined solid material seen on microscopic examination of urine. It consists of chemical and cellular debris and is of no diagnostic importance.

Routine chemical testing of urine is usually performed with a dipstick, a commercially produced strip of plastic or paper bearing a series of dots or squares of reagent, each designed to assess a specific chemical property of urine. The **dipstick** is immersed briefly in the urine, and the test squares are observed for color changes. These tests are semiquantitative and are read by comparing the degree of color change in each square with an appropriate color chart. Results of dipstick tests other than pH and specific gravity are reported as either positive on a scale of 1 to 4 (1+, 2+, 3+, 4+) or negative.

Kidneys, *More than a Filter*

The kidneys are usually thought of as organs that merely filter water and wastes from the circulation. They actually perform many highly selective excretory functions, conserving essential substances, preserving water and electrolyte balance, and supplying chemical mediators necessary for the maintenance of normal blood pressure, red blood cell production, and bone mineralization.

The kidneys (Figures 11-3, 11-4) are paired structures whose shape is so familiar that expressions like *kidney beans* and *kidney-shaped swimming pool* are readily understood by all. They lie on either side of the midline just below the posterior attachments of the diaphragm, at the level of the twelfth rib and the first three lumbar vertebrae—much higher than lay persons usually seem to think.

The right kidney is slightly lower than the left, probably because of the presence of the liver above it. Each kidney is surrounded by a cushioning envelope of fat and lies deeply imbedded in the posterior abdominal wall. The kidneys are retroperitoneal, that is, they lie behind and outside the peritoneal cavity, which encloses most of the abdominal organs (stomach, small intestine, liver, spleen, and most of the large intestine).

The hilum or notch of each kidney is the point of entry of the renal artery and the point of exit of the renal vein and the ureter. Nerves and lymph vessels also enter and leave at the hilum. The paired renal arteries are the last major branches given off by the abdominal aorta before it bifurcates into the common iliac arteries to supply the pelvic organs and lower limbs. The renal veins have an analogous relation to the inferior vena cava, being the first major tributaries received by it after it is formed by the union of the common iliac veins.

Each kidney is about 12 cm in height, 6 cm in breadth, 3 cm in thickness, and weighs about 150 g. That's very close to the proportions, size, and weight of a standard computer mouse. The kidney is enclosed by a smooth connective tissue capsule, somewhat like the skin of a sausage. The capsule can easily be peeled away from a normal kidney (although this does tear through a meshwork of fine blood vessels), but not from one that has been scarred by chronic inflammation or infarction.

The renal arteries not only deliver blood to the kidneys to be purged of wastes, but also provide oxygen and nutrients to the tissues of the kidney and carry away carbon dioxide to be excreted by the lungs. The blood flow through the kidneys constitutes about one fourth of the total cardiac output at rest. As blood passes through the capillaries making up the glomerulus, water and dissolved substances diffuse from it into the space between the two layers of the Bowman capsule.

John H. Dirckx, M.D.
Perspectives on the Medical Transcription Profession

The **pH** of urine (sometimes called simply the "reaction") is normally about 5.5. The urine may be alkaline (pH 8) in vegetarians and in persons with urinary tract infection due to urease-producing organisms such as *Proteus*, which split urinary urea to ammonia in the bladder.

The **specific gravity** of urine varies in direct proportion to the concentration of dissolved materials. It is ordinarily measured by means of a color change in the relevant square on a dipstick. A more precise measurement can be made by noting the depth to which a hydrometer, a precisely weighted float, sinks in the specimen. The normal specific gravity is 1.001 to 1.030 (which a dictator may pronounce "ten oh one" and "ten thirty"). The specific gravity is increased in dehydration (with normal renal function), toxemia, congestive heart failure, acute glomerulonephritis, and diabetes mellitus with glycosuria. The specific gravity is decreased (hyposthenuria) after ingestion or infusion of fluid (with normal renal function), in diabetes insipidus, and in renal failure with loss of concentrating ability.

The presence of **protein in the urine (proteinuria)** is usually due to leakage of albumin from the glomeruli. Hence it is often termed **albuminuria**, even though routine tests for protein in urine do not distinguish which proteins are present. Protein loss from the kidney occurs in glomerulonephritis, nephrotic syndrome, renal infarction, fever, and toxemia. In addition, most chemical tests for protein are positive in the presence of hematuria or pyuria.

Normally all of the plasma glucose that appears in glomerular filtrate is reabsorbed in the renal tubules. The detection of **glucose in the urine** (glycosuria) generally indicates an abnormal elevation of plasma glucose. The renal threshold for glucose is about 180 mg/dL. That means that at plasma levels above 180 mg/dL, more glucose appears in glomerular filtrate than can be reabsorbed by the tubules. Glycosuria is a cardinal finding in diabetes mellitus. It also occurs after rapid absorption of dietary glucose (alimentary glycosuria) and in some persons with abnormally low renal thresholds for glucose (renal glycosuria).

Occult blood refers to blood present in insufficient quantity to alter the color of the urine. A positive test for occult blood has generally the same significance as the finding of red blood cells in urine. **Acetone and other ketones** appear in the urine in diabetes mellitus with acidosis, in starvation, thyrotoxicosis, and high fever. Only bilirubin that has been conjugated with glucuronic acid is soluble in water. Hence the appearance of **bilirubin in the urine (bilirubinuria, choluria)** is noted in obstructive jaundice, in which conjugated bilirubin enters the blood stream from bile, but not in

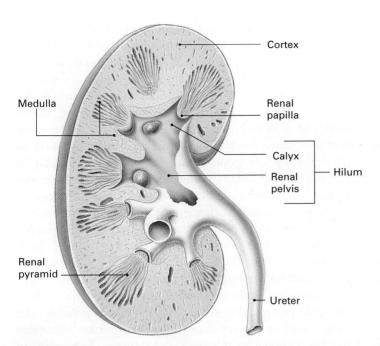

Figure 11-3
Sectioned Kidney

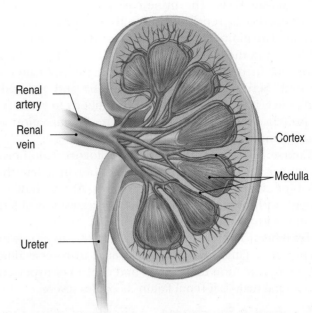

Figure 11-4
Renal Artery and Vein

jaundice due to hemolysis or liver disease, in which only unconjugated bilirubin is elevated in the plasma.

Common Diseases

Acute Renal Failure. An abrupt, severe decline in kidney function, with retention of nitrogenous waste products of protein metabolism (**azotemia**, **uremia**).

Cause: The abnormality may be **prerenal** (impaired blood supply to kidney), **renal** (also called parenchymal or intrinsic; disease of the kidney proper), or **postrenal** (obstruction of the outflow of urine from the kidney). Prerenal azotemia can result from renal artery stenosis, hypotension, or the effects of certain drugs (NSAIDs, ACE inhibitors) on renal blood flow. Renal azotemia can result from any severe disease of kidney tissue, including **acute glomerulonephritis**, **vasculitis** affecting the intrinsic renal circulation, and **acute tubular necrosis**.

History: Malaise, weakness, anorexia, nausea, reduced urine volume (**oliguria**). In advanced disease, vomiting, hematemesis, diarrhea, drowsiness, seizures, pruritus, cardiac arrhythmias, peripheral edema, dyspnea.

Physical Examination: Essentially negative. A pericardial friction rub may be heard in uremic pericarditis. In advanced disease, pallor, peripheral edema, pulmonary edema, congestive heart failure, coma.

Diagnostic Tests: The levels of BUN and creatinine are markedly increased in the blood. The serum pH is low (**metabolic acidosis**). Serum potassium and phosphorus levels are elevated and calcium is depressed. Anemia may be severe.

Course: The case mortality rate is 20-50% depending on the cause and underlying diseases. If the inciting cause is reversible, the renal failure itself may completely resolve. Most patients with reversible disease recover completely within six weeks. Typically there is an oliguric acute phase, followed by copious diuresis as renal function improves, and at length a return to normal urine volume. Infection is a common complication.

Treatment: Largely supportive. Restriction of water, protein, and potassium intake, with high carbohydrate diet and vitamin supplementation. Close monitoring of water and electrolyte balance. Renal dialysis or intravenous administration of glucose, insulin, and sodium bicarbonate, and oral sodium polystyrene sulfonate, to reduce serum potassium.

Acute Glomerulonephritis. Acute inflammation of renal glomeruli, with failure to excrete nitrogenous wastes.

Causes: Poststreptococcal glomerulonephritis is an autoimmune disease that follows infection (usually pharyngitis) with group A beta-hemolytic streptococci, type 12. In **Berger disease** (IgA nephropathy), immune complexes form in the glomerulus, often after a respiratory or gastrointestinal infection or a flulike illness.

History: Sudden appearance of tea-colored or Coca-Cola-colored urine, with reduction in urine volume and possibly peripheral edema.

Physical Examination: Blood pressure elevation (in poststreptococcal glomerulonephritis); peripheral edema.

Diagnostic Tests: The urine contains red blood cells, white blood cells, renal tubular epithelial cells, casts, and protein. Creatinine clearance and urinary sodium are reduced, and the 24-hour urinary excretion of protein is increased. In poststreptococcal disease, the ASO titer is elevated. Serum protein electrophoresis and antibody studies may indicate the presence of antibody to glomerular protein. Renal biopsy allows precise identification of tissue changes.

Course: Most patients with poststreptococcal glomerulonephritis recover without sequelae, but in a few the renal damage is rapidly progressive. About half of patients with Berger disease suffer progressive loss of kidney function.

Treatment: Largely supportive. Antibiotic to eradicate streptococci. Fluid restriction. Diuretics to reverse fluid retention. Attention to nutrition and control of hypertension. Renal dialysis if renal failure becomes severe.

Nephrotic Syndrome.
A disorder of kidney function in which a large amount of protein is lost in the urine from damaged glomeruli.

Causes: Various abnormalities of glomeruli due to systemic disease (diabetes, systemic lupus erythematosus, amyloidosis); other forms: minimal change disease (lipoid nephrosis), focal glomerular sclerosis, membranous nephropathy, membranoproliferative glomerulonephritis.

History: Gradual onset of peripheral edema, with weight gain, dyspnea.

Physical Examination: Edema, ascites (excess fluid in abdominal cavity), anasarca (generalized edema); pulmonary edema, pleural effusion.

Diagnostic Tests: Marked increase in 24-hour urinary excretion of protein. Reduction of total protein and albumin in the serum. Increase in serum cholesterol level. There may be no cellular elements in the urine and no evidence of nitrogen retention. Renal biopsy provides histologic identification of the underlying disease process.

Treatment: Limitation of protein and salt intake; diuretics, cholesterol-lowering agents.

Diabetic Nephropathy.
Progressive renal insufficiency with albuminuria and hypertension, occurring in persons with diabetes mellitus.

Cause: Thickening and degeneration of glomerular basement membrane and other pathologic changes that eventually occur in most patients with type 1 diabetes mellitus and in some patients with type 2. The incidence is higher in males, African Americans, Hispanics, and Native Americans. Most patients also have hypertension, which hastens the advance of renal damage.

History: Symptoms, which do not occur until damage is far advanced, are those of nephrotic syndrome (see above), chronic renal failure, or both.

Physical Examination: Edema, ascites. Hypertension.

Diagnostic Tests: Periodic determination of 24-hour urinary protein excretion (part of the routine surveillance of patients with diabetes mellitus) can detect microalbuminuria, a reliable marker of renal damage, early in the course of disease. With further progression, larger amounts of albumin are excreted, and measures of renal function show decline in glomerular filtration and in clearance of nitrogenous wastes. Serum levels of BUN, creatinine, and potassium are elevated. Metabolic acidosis may occur as a result of renal tubular dysfunction.

Course: Continual deterioration of renal function is usual. Use of certain drugs and injection of radiographic contrast media can precipitate acute renal failure. Diabetic nephropathy is currently the chief cause of end-stage renal failure requiring renal dialysis.

Treatment: Rigorous control of diabetes, with maintenance of plasma glucose as near normal as possible, can delay onset or progression of disease, but no treatment has been shown to reverse renal damage. Limitation of dietary protein and aggressive treatment of hypertension with ACE inhibitors or angiotensin II receptor blockers can delay progression of nephropathy. Urinary tract infections are promptly treated, and radiographic contrast media and drugs known to be toxic to the kidney are avoided. End-stage renal failure is treated with kidney transplantation, hemodialysis, or peritoneal dialysis.

Urolithiasis (Kidney Stones).
Formation of stonelike concretions (calculi) (Figure 11-5) in the urinary tract, which may obstruct a ureter at a site of natural narrowing such as the **ureteropelvic junction** (UPJ) or **ureterovesical junction** (UVJ).

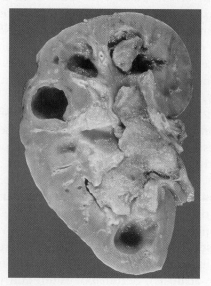

Figure 11-5
Kidney with Calculi

Causes: Changes in the concentration of dissolved minerals or other substances in the urine: uric acid in gout; cystine in cystinuria; calcium in disorders of calcium metabolism. Local infection may play a part. Men are affected four times more often than women, and the disorder tends to run in families.

History: Passage of a stone into a ureter causes severe flank pain or abdominal pain radiating to the groin (ureteral colic), nausea, vomiting, restlessness, and often hematuria.

Physical Examination: There may be tenderness over the involved kidney in the flank or abdomen. Fever suggests infection resulting from urinary obstruction.

Diagnostic Tests: The urine shows microscopic or gross blood. X-ray or ultrasound examination identifies and localizes most stones, but about 15% are not radiopaque. Intravenous pyelography can be done to demonstrate obstruction of the tract. Examination of stones shows them to be aggregates of crystalline and organic materials. Chemical analysis of stones indicates which of five common types is present: calcium oxalate, calcium phosphate, ammoniomagnesium phosphate (struvite), uric acid, or cystine.

Course: Most stones pass spontaneously without treatment. Recurrences are common. Obstruction of a ureter can result in **renal failure** (obstructive uropathy), infection, or both.

Treatment: Strong analgesics are prescribed, and all urine is collected and strained to identify stones or fragments. If infection is present or renal function is compromised, obstruction may be relieved by passing a ureteral catheter endoscopically from the bladder, or by **percutaneous nephrostomy** (inserting a drain through the skin into the renal pelvis). Stones lying low in a ureter may be extracted from below. **Extracorporeal shock wave lithotripsy (ESWL)** can be used to break stones into fragments, which then pass with the urine. A stone lodged in the renal pelvis or proximal ureter may be removed by percutaneous nephrolithotomy.

Acute Pyelonephritis. Acute inflammation of kidney tissue and the renal pelvis due to infection.

Cause: Bacterial infection with *Escherichia coli, Proteus, Pseudomonas, Klebsiella, Enterobacter,* or *Staphylococcus aureus.* Infection usually ascends from the lower urinary tract (bladder and urethra), but may be spread through the circulation from a remote focus. Obstruction to urine flow caused by prostatic enlargement, a ureteral stone, or pregnancy may be the underlying cause. **Vesicoureteral reflux** of urine or anomalies of the urinary tract (tortuous or duplicated ureter) are also risk factors.

History: Fever, chills, nausea, vomiting, flank pain, urinary urgency, pollakiuria, dysuria.

Physical Examination: The temperature and pulse are elevated. Tenderness at one or both costovertebral angles is usually noted on palpation.

Diagnostic Tests: The white blood cell count is elevated. Examination of the urine shows white blood cells, red blood cells, and bacteria. Urine culture identifies the infecting organism.

Course: Pyelonephritis resolves promptly with antibiotic treatment unless an underlying problem of septicemia or urinary obstruction remains unresolved.

Treatment: Antibiotics (trimethoprim-sulfamethoxazole, ciprofloxacin) are administered orally or intravenously. Urinary obstruction must be relieved by catheterization, **nephrostomy** (draining urine from the renal pelvis), or other procedure.

Acute Cystitis. Acute inflammation of the bladder, usually due to bacterial infection.

Cause: Usually infection due to *Escherichia coli* or other organisms ascending from the urethra. Cystitis is much commoner in women, in whom the urethra is short and straight, with its orifice in the vaginal vestibule where it is exposed to fecal contamination and trauma from sexual intercourse. Less commonly, cystitis may be due to urethral obstruction (principally in males), viral infection, bladder trauma, or spread of infection from adjacent pelvic organs. Pregnancy, diabetes mellitus, presence of an indwelling catheter, and advanced age are risk factors.

History: Fairly sudden onset of pollakiuria, urgency, urinary burning, and bladder spasms after voiding. Hematuria may occur. Often there is suprapubic or low back discomfort.

Physical Examination: Essentially unremarkable. Fever is absent. There may be suprapubic tenderness.

Diagnostic Examination: Laboratory studies of urine show white blood cells (sometimes clumped), red blood cells or occult blood, and bacteria. Tests for leukocyte esterase (an enzyme released by white blood cells in urine) and nitrites (formed by reduction of urinary nitrates by certain bacteria) are often positive. Urine culture identifies the causative organism, and sensitivity studies show which antibiotics are effective against it. However, culturing is not routinely performed except in atypical or recurrent disease. Cystitis is so uncommon in men that aggressive evaluation is usually undertaken in the male to identify any serious underlying cause such as obstruction or malignancy.

Course: The response to treatment is rapid, but many sexually active women experience frequent recurrences.

Treatment: Antibiotics (trimethoprim-sulfamethoxazole, cephalexin, ciprofloxacin) are often effective in courses of just two or three days. Urinary symptoms may be relieved by phenazopyridine (a bladder anesthetic taken orally) or antispasmodics. The frequency of recurrences in women can be reduced by regularly voiding just after intercourse. Long-term low-dose antibiotic prophylaxis also helps to prevent recurrences.

Urinary Incontinence. Four distinct types of involuntary leakage of urine from the bladder are recognized. **Urge incontinence**, which occurs after a sudden, intense, irresistible urge to void, is the commonest type of incontinence in elderly persons. It is due to overactivity of the detrusor muscle of the bladder and often responds to treatment with the antispasmodic oxybutynin or the muscarinic antagonist tolterodine.

Stress incontinence, which is seen almost exclusively in women, occurs when mechanical stress is placed on the bladder, as by coughing, laughing, or changing position. It may result from structural damage to the bladder as in childbirth. Treatment with pelvic muscle exercises (**Kegel exercises**) or estrogens may help. Surgical correction of anatomic abnormalities is often necessary and is highly successful.

Overflow incontinence is leakage of urine from an overdistended bladder, occurring almost exclusively in men with urinary obstruction due to prostatic disease. Treatment is correction of the obstruction.

Total incontinence is complete lack of control over voiding, usually due to neurologic disease, spinal cord injury, or radical prostatectomy. Continuous or intermittent catheterization may be the only effective means of controlling this type of incontinence. Incontinence is primarily a disorder of the elderly; besides the causes mentioned above, it may be due to dementia, urinary tract infection, diuresis, drugs, diminished mobility, and, in women, atrophic vaginitis.

Prostatitis. Inflammation of the prostate (Figure 11-6), typically due to bacterial infection, which may be acute or chronic. In acute prostatitis the presenting complaints are fever, urinary frequency and burning, occasionally urinary retention, and pain in the perineum or back. On digital rectal examination the prostate is found to be enlarged, warm, and exquisitely tender. The white blood count is elevated, and the urine contains white blood cells, red blood cells, and bacteria. Treatment is with oral or intravenous antibiotics.

In chronic prostatitis, symptoms are milder but of longer duration. Fever is absent and prostatic tenderness not so marked. Urinalysis yields normal results. Treatment is with antibiotics and must often be continued for a long time.

Benign Prostatic Hyperplasia (BPH). Enlargement of the prostate accompanying aging, with varying degrees of urinary obstruction.

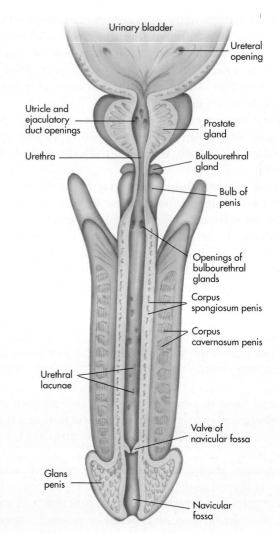

Figure 11-6
Bladder, Prostate, and Penis

Cause: Some prostatic enlargement due to overgrowth of androgen-sensitive glandular elements occurs naturally with aging. Causes of severely symptomatic enlargement are unknown.

History: Gradual onset of urinary symptoms, which may be **obstructive** (decreased force and caliber of urinary stream, hesitancy, intermittency) or irritative (frequency, urgency, nocturia).

Physical Examination: The prostate is symmetrically enlarged on digital rectal examination, firm but not hard. Abdominal examination may indicate distention of the bladder. Catheterization after voiding may indicate residual urine.

Diagnostic Tests: Urinalysis may indicate evidence of infection (white blood cells) or of bladder irritation (red blood cells). The blood urea nitrogen may be elevated if obstruction is advanced (**obstructive uropathy**). Intravenous pyelography may show bladder distention and bilateral ureteral dilatation. Urinary flowmetry gives an objective measure of the rate of flow from the bladder. Cystoscopy and urethroscopy may be of value in confirming the benign nature of the disorder.

Course: Symptoms may remain relatively mild for years, even decades. Obstruction may lead to infection and even to kidney failure. Benign prostatic hyperplasia does not evolve into carcinoma.

Treatment: Medical treatment with finasteride (an alpha-reductase inhibitor) or terazosin or doxazosin (alpha-adrenergic blocking agents) can reduce obstructive symptoms. In more severe cases, surgical excision of prostate tissue is indicated. **Transurethral resection** (TUR) is the usual procedure, but in some cases suprapubic (open) resection is preferred. Balloon dilatation of the prostate and transurethral laser excision are alternative procedures.

Adenocarcinoma of the Prostate. A malignant tumor arising from glandular epithelium of the prostate gland.

Cause: Adenocarcinoma of the prostate is the most common cancer in men (31% of all cancers diagnosed). The incidence of prostatic cancer found at autopsy in men over 50 is about 40%. However, prostate cancer causes only 11% of all cancer deaths in men. The risk of developing prostatic carcinoma is higher in men with a family history of it and in those who have undergone vasectomy. The tumor is testosterone-dependent (that is, it does not occur in men who have undergone orchidectomy). Adenocarcinoma of the prostate does not arise from benign prostatic hyperplasia.

History: There may be no symptoms. Diminished urine flow, urinary frequency, nocturia, and dribbling of urine may occur as in benign prostatic hyperplasia. The first symptom may be bone pain due to metastasis.

Physical Examination: The prostate, as palpated on digital rectal examination, may be unusually firm, nodular, or asymmetric.

Diagnostic Tests. The level of prostate-specific antigen (PSA), or acid phosphatase, or both in the serum is elevated in many cases of prostate carcinoma, particularly when metastasis has occurred. Transrectal ultrasound may detect abnormally dense areas within the prostate gland, representing tumor. Transrectal biopsy discloses zones of malignant tissue. The **Gleason grading system** gives a histopathologic estimate of malignancy and likely future behavior. X-ray studies and radionuclide bone scans may show metastases to bones of the spine or pelvis.

Course. Progression of disease is typically slow, and most patients die of other causes before the prostatic cancer has reached a lethal stage. Metastasis to lymph nodes and to the spine or pelvis eventually occurs.

Urinary obstruction may lead to urinary tract infection and even renal failure.

Treatment. Surgical excision (usually radical prostatectomy), radiation by external beam or implanted radioactive needles; in advanced (metastatic) disease, castration or administration of estrogen (or an antiandrogen such as flutamide) to suppress tumor growth.

Gonorrhea. Infection of the genital tract by the gonococcus.

Cause: *Neisseria gonorrhoeae* (gonococcus), a gram-negative diplococcus that is transmitted almost exclusively by sexual contact. It attacks genitourinary mucous membranes, producing a purulent inflammation that may spread to adjacent organs or the peritoneum, and may progress to scarring. Infection of the pharynx or rectum can be acquired through oral or anal sex.

History: Men: After an incubation period of three to five days, severe pain on urination and a thick green urethral discharge. Women: Similar symptoms sometimes occur, along with vaginal or vulvar inflammation. Often, however, there are no symptoms unless **pelvic inflammatory disease (PID)** (spread of infection to the uterus and uterine tubes) occurs. PID causes pelvic pain and fever, with variable other symptoms.

Physical Examination: In men, evident purulent urethral discharge, with inflammation of the meatus. In women, acute disease may be manifested by urethritis, cervicitis, vaginitis, inflammation of **Bartholin glands** (secretory glands lateral to the vaginal vestibule), or proctitis. If PID ensues, fever, abdominal tenderness, extreme tenderness on manipulation of cervix.

Diagnostic Tests: DNA amplification tests performed on material obtained by cervical or urethral smear and on urine are valuable for diagnosis as well as for screening asymptomatic persons of either sex. Stained smear of pus or secretions shows gram-negative diplococci inside WBCs. Culture on appropriate medium grows gonococci. Oral and anal specimens are positive when infection is in those areas.

Course: Acute urethral infection may resolve spontaneously, but in men it often spreads to the epididymis or prostate, or progresses to a stage of scarring, with resultant infertility. In women, spread to the vagina, cervix, uterus, tubes, and rectum often occurs. Tubal infection (**salpingitis**, PID) with scarring causes infertility and a heightened risk of ectopic pregnancy. In either sex, infection occasionally involves the skin, conjunctivae, joints, tendon sheaths, cardiac valves, or meninges. Spread of infection from mother to newborn can cause conjunctivitis with ensuing blindness.

Treatment: Antibiotic treatment with a single dose of intramuscular ceftriaxone or oral ciprofloxacin is usually

Sexually Transmitted Diseases

Sexually transmitted diseases (STDs) are statistically more likely to occur in persons under 25 years of age, in members of ethnic minorities, in persons of low socio-economic status, in persons with many sexual partners (especially prostitutes), and in sexually active gay men (but not in sexually active lesbians). Their incidence is also higher in urban areas. The only absolute protection against acquiring an infection through sexual contact is lifelong celibacy or maintenance of a permanently and mutually monogamous sexual relationship.

The overall incidence of sexually transmitted infections has increased substantially during the past two decades, and some diseases have shown a marked increase. Several factors have contributed to these changing statistics. The discovery in the 1940s that penicillin could cure syphilis and gonorrhea and the development during the 1950s of safe and effective oral contraceptives paved the way for the sexual revolution of the 1960s. Against a background of civil unrest and widespread drug abuse, this revolution led to social acceptance of sexual promiscuity.

The diagnosis and treatment of STDs are rendered more difficult by the reluctance of most people to discuss their sexual behavior with health professionals and by the refusal of many patients to believe that a sexual partner has become infected by some third person. Diagnosis often demands alertness and a high degree of suspicion on the part of the healthcare worker. History-taking must be searching but nonthreatening and nonjudgmental.

John H. Dirckx, M.D.
Perspectives on the Medical Transcription Profession

curative. It is standard practice to administer treatment for **chlamydial infection** at the same time since the infections so often occur together.

Chlamydial Infection. Urogenital infection with *Chlamydia trachomatis*.

Cause: Sexually transmitted infection of genital mucous membranes and related tissues with *Chlamydia trachomatis*, an intracellular gram-negative bacterium. Genital chlamydial infection (urethritis and cervicitis) is the commonest bacterial STD. Screening tests are positive in 10% of asymptomatic sexually active women.

History: Men: Urethral itching or burning, dysuria, thin serous discharge, one to four weeks after exposure. Anorectal pain and bleeding with rectal infection, common in gay men. Women: Dysuria and pollakiuria due to **acute urethral syndrome; dyspareunia** (pain with intercourse), vaginal bleeding, and vaginal discharge due to cervicitis; abdominal pain and fever due to

pelvic inflammatory disease. Most women with chlamydial infection are asymptomatic.

Physical Examination: May be unremarkable. Thin, watery urethral discharge may be noted in males. In women, cervical erythema with mucopurulent discharge indicates cervicitis. With development of PID, fever, abdominal pain, and cervical tenderness become evident.

Diagnostic Tests: DNA amplification testing of urine is used for both diagnosis and for screening of asymptomatic persons. A urethral or cervical smear may show organisms with direct fluorescence antibody examination, enzyme-linked immunosorbent assay, or DNA probe.

Course: Spontaneous resolution often occurs, but in many patients chlamydial infection has long-term consequences. In men, infection can spread to the epididymis, produce urethral stricture with resulting urinary obstruction or infertility, or trigger an autoimmune disorder called **Reiter syndrome** (arthritis, conjunctivitis, mucocutaneous lesions). In about one fifth of infected women, infection spreads to the uterus and tubes (salpingitis, PID). Complications of PID include **tubo-ovarian abscess, Fitz-Hugh–Curtis syndrome** (localized peritonitis in the region of the liver), and **tubal scarring** with infertility or sterility and heightened risk of **ectopic pregnancy**. A child born to an infected mother is at risk of chlamydial conjunctivitis, with the danger of blindness.

Treatment: Oral antibiotic therapy with tetracycline, erythromycin, or a single dose of azithromycin is ordinarily curative. Treatment is often instituted on suspicion (urethritis or cervicitis with negative cultures of urine and discharge) because of the high probability of chlamydial infection in such cases. Persons treated for gonorrhea are also routinely treated for chlamydial infection as well.

Erectile Dysfunction (Impotence). Failure of the penis to become erect after sexual stimulation, or to maintain sufficient rigidity for intercourse. Among many possible causes are atherosclerosis, neurologic disease or spinal cord injury, hormonal deficiency, side effects of medicines, anxiety, and depression. Diabetes mellitus, obesity, and cigarette smoking are risk factors. Most patients respond to oral phosphodiesterase inhibitors (sildenafil, tadalafil, vardenafil). Other methods of treatment include local injection of a vasodilator, induction of erection by means of a vacuum device, and implantation of a penile prosthesis.

Diagnostic and Surgical Procedures

intravenous pyelogram (IVP) X-ray examination of the urinary tract after intravenous injection of contrast material that is quickly excreted in the urine.

percutaneous nephrolithotomy Procedure in which a lodged stone in the renal pelvis or proximal ureter is surgically removed through the skin.

transurethral resection of the prostate (TURP) Surgical procedure to remove hyperplastic prostatic tissue obstructing the urethra.

vasectomy Surgical division of the vas deferens in the male to effect sterility.

voiding cystourethrogram (VCUG) X-ray film of the act of voiding with contrast medium in the urine.

Laboratory Procedures

acid phosphatase Enzyme whose level in the serum is often increased in prostatic carcinoma.

amorphous sediment Unformed and generally insignificant debris seen in a urine specimen under microscopic examination.

blood urea nitrogen (BUN) The serum level of urea nitrogen, a waste product of protein metabolism. Elevation indicates an impairment of kidney function.

catheterized urine specimen Specimen of urine obtained by passing a sterile catheter into the bladder.

clean-voided specimen (clean catch) Obtained after cleansing of the area around the urethral meatus to prevent contamination of the specimen with material from outside the urinary tract.

creatinine clearance A measure of kidney function, calculated from the serum creatinine level and the amount of creatinine excreted in the urine in 24 hours.

E. (Escherichia) coli Gram-negative bacterium normally found in the intestine and responsible for many urinary tract infections.

electrolytes, urinary Sodium, potassium, and chloride ions in the urine. Abnormal concentrations could indicate kidney disease.

first-voided specimen The first urine passed after arising in the morning.

midstream specimen One that contains neither the first nor the last portion of urine passed.

FTA-ABS Fluorescent treponemal antibody absorption test, to detect syphilis.

prostate-specific antigen (PSA) Blood test to screen for prostatic carcinoma.

RPR (rapid plasma reagin) Test for syphilis.

specific gravity The weight of a substance per unit of volume compared to pure water, which by definition has a specific gravity of 1.000. The specific gravity of urine (normally 1.001 to 1.030) is a rough measure of the amount of material dissolved in it.

24-hour urine specimen Consists of all the urine passed by the patient in a 24-hour period.

urinalysis (UA) A group of standard laboratory examinations of the urine, including determination of pH and specific gravity, chemical testing for sugar, albumin, occult blood, leukocyte esterase, nitrite, acetone, bilirubin, red and white blood cells, crystals, casts, and other materials.

urine culture Usually with colony count and sensitivity studies, to identify urinary pathogens.

VDRL Venereal Disease Research Laboratory test for syphilis. Abbreviation does not need to be expanded.

Pharmacology

Urinary tract drugs include antibiotics and other anti-infection agents, urinary tract analgesics, and urinary antispasmodics.

Antibiotics. The choice of an antibiotic for a urinary tract infection (UTI) depends not only on the causative organism but on the physiology of the excretory system. Because most UTIs are due to *E. coli* or other gram-negative pathogens, the drug selected must have proven effectiveness against such organisms. In addition, the drug chosen must be able to establish an effective tissue level despite the tendency of the kidneys to flush foreign chemicals out of the body as rapidly as possible.

cinoxacin (Cinobac)
ciprofloxacin (Cipro)
fosfomycin (Monurol)
nitrofurantoin (Furadantin, Macrobid, Macrodantin)
norfloxacin (Noroxin)
ofloxacin (Floxin)

Sulfonamides. Urinary tract infections can also be treated with sulfonamides (often called **sulfa drugs**). These drugs are not true antibiotics because they only inhibit the growth of bacteria, rather than killing bacteria as antibiotics do.

sulfadiazine
sulfamethoxazole (Gantanol, SMX)
sulfisoxazole (Gantrisin Pediatric)

The combination of sulfamethoxazole with the folic acid inhibitor trimethoprim (Bactrim, Septra) is widely used in the treatment of upper and lower urinary tract infections, although strains of *E. coli* resistant to it are increasingly isolated.

Urinary tract analgesics. Urinary tract infections and other diseases have associated symptoms of burning with frequent and painful urination. Urinary tract analgesics exert a topical pain-relieving effect on the mucosa of the urinary tract, even though the drugs are taken orally.

> Dolsed (L-hyoscyamine, methenamine)
> Pyridium (phenazopyridine)
> Urised (L-hyoscyamine, methenamine, methylene blue)
> Urogesic Blue

Antispasmodics. Irritation in any part of the urinary tract from infection, catheterization, urinary retention, or kidney stones can result in painful spasm. Overactive bladder and urge incontinence result from irritability and spasticity of the detrusor muscle. Antispasmodic drugs (anticholinergics and others) relieve symptoms by relaxing smooth muscle.

> flavoxate (Urispas)
> L-hyoscyamine (Anaspaz, Cystospaz)
> oxybutynin (Ditropan)
> solifenacin (VESIcare)
> tolterodine (Detrol LA)
> trospium (Sanctura)

Drugs for treatment of benign prostatic hyperplasia (BPH).

> alfuzosin (Uroxatral)
> dutasteride (Avodart)
> finasteride (Proscar)
> tamsulosin (Flomax)
> terazosin (Hytrin)

Drugs used to treat male erectile dysfunction (ED).

> alprostadil (Caverject, Muse)
> sildenafil (Viagra)
> tadalafil (Cialis)
> vardenafil (Levitra)

TRANSCRIPTION**TIPS**

1. Both the Romans and the Greeks studied the body and disease processes extensively. Different medical terms may describe the same anatomic structure because a relevant word can be found in both Latin and Greek.

2. Both the Latin stem *ren- (renal)* and the Greek *nephr- (nephric)* refer to the *kidney*.

3. Both the Latin stem *vesic- (vesical neck)* and the Greek *cyst- (cystoscopy)* refer to the urinary bladder.

4. The Latin stem *test- (testosterone)* and the Greek *orchi- (orchiectomy)* both refer to the *testicle*.

5. Do not confuse the term *prostate* (a gland of the male reproductive system through which the urethra passes) and the word *prostrate* (which describes a posture of submission or a state of exhaustion or extreme grief).

6. The abbreviation *UA (urinalysis)* is acceptable and clearly understood; it may be transcribed if dictated. The combined form *urinalysis* should be used, rather than *urine analysis.*

7. Learn to distinguish between *ureter/ureteral* and *urethra/urethral,* which refer to two totally different anatomical structures. (*Hint:* From head to toe and in alphabetical order, the ureter is found above the urethra.)

8. Some words have more than one acceptable spelling. For example, *calix/calices* is preferred; *calyx/calyces* is an acceptable alternative. Preferred spellings may vary among English and medical references. Examples:

anulus	annulus
calix, calices	calyx, calyces
curet	curette
distention	distension
tocolysis	tokolysis
transected	transsected

9. *Cath* is a slang term for *catheterization, cysto* for *cystoscopy.* Slang terms should be translated to their complete forms in medical reports. An exception would be the term *prepped (prepared),* which has become acceptable in its brief form through usage.

The patient was prepped and draped.
The skin was prepped prior to injection.

10. Note that the accent falls on different syllables in *CYS-to-scope* and *cys-TOS-copy.*

11. Urine specific gravity is always written as the number *1* followed by a decimal point and three other numbers. Normal values range from 1.001 to 1.030. If the dictator says "ten ten," the value should be transcribed as 1.010.

12. The presence of *K* in every trade name for potassium supplements refers to the chemical symbol for potassium (K^+).

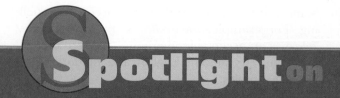

It's All Right to Laugh

by Judith Marshall

It never was a marriage made in heaven. I would tell people he was having a birthday . . . if I let him live. Or that I never thought of divorce. Murder yes, divorce never. All those old vaudeville jokes. Recently I told a friend that my husband and I were like two prehistoric monsters, throttling each other while plunging into an abyss. "What a pretty picture," he said dryly.

Many medical transcriptionists go to great lengths to stay out of the medical mill. Maybe we know too much, we hear too much, we understand too much. But I dragged the old goat down to Boston Union Hospital because I wanted to go dancing and he needed a total knee replacement. The internist agreed and ran a routine blood panel, including the relatively new PSA. When the results came back elevated, we paid little attention. When the test was repeated, both of us were sucked into the whirling vortex of healthcare and the business of cancer treatment. We forgot about the dancing.

In Surgery's chilly preop room, I stopped arguing with him long enough to promise I would not let him get chewed up and spit out by that business, sick with chemotherapy, radiation therapy, and radical surgery, only to face a certain demise.

The operative report and the pathology report revealed status post transurethral resection of the prostate, Stage D, with metastases to right pubic ramus.

We met with the surgeon, that technically perfect smarmy son-of-a-gun, who alternately pressured and patronized us. He said we should make up our minds in a week. Orchiectomy and Lupron injections were what he could offer us. Leuprolide, the wonder drug of the mid-80s, was expensive, he said, patting his knees thoughtfully. About $600 for each monthly injection. And he would administer it.

"What about diethylstilbestrol?" I piped up. The surgeon-god frowned and asked, "Are you a nurse?" "No," I countered, "I just read a great deal." Here was a man about to sell us the Cadillac of therapy and I had just mentioned a Volkswagen. He admitted he had one or two patients on DES, but the side effects were considerable and it was not his best recommendation.

We began the trek for another opinion, but not before I was hyperventilating into a paper bag, screaming about the cost of what I called the $600 erection. That is what Lupron does. It allows for an erection. So the Blue Cross folks get the Lupron and the Medicare-without-supplement group gets DES. And everyone gets an orchiectomy.

We saw a kind oncologist. At least he asked about our marriage and our hobbies, which at this point were dwindling rapidly. We asked for better odds and got none. But it was worth the time to speak with someone who had no vested interest in our decision. My stoic husband sat impassively through these interviews, like a sleepy toad on a rock. I thought he was not even paying attention. But he was. He reminded me that only 30% of patients receiving orchiectomy are alive at the end of three years. That meant 70% were dead.

The Veterans Administration told my husband (captain in the U.S. Army for five years, overseas, during World War II) he was not eligible for Lupron there because our income is more than $23,000. "Don't worry," I said to Stu. "Take the DES and we'll go through hot flashes together, and I can lend you the underwear for the gynecomastia. We can both feel like a blast furnace and save on the heating bill."

He developed other symptoms. His medication was changed in the hospital, and he developed shortness of breath and swollen ankles. I urged him to call his internist and tell him. " "I am out of shape," he said, "just a bit winded." "You need Lasix," I said. He demurred and he suffered. Heartless and cruel that I am, off I went to bingo. "Call 911 if you get worse. I am going out." He did call his doctor, who told him to relax and called in a prescription to our pharmacy. Xanax. The doctor prescribed an antianxiety agent. More screaming from me, but I took my husband's Xanax and I was fine. He again visited his internist and came out with Lasix, of course.

Truly, I have no magical bag of tricks as a medical language specialist. Not even Wonder Woman can ward off all these bullets with her bracelets. But I will see to it he does not become like my Uncle Ralph, a devastated man after castration, who put on his bathrobe and never left his house again. Women really do handle some things much better. We literally hand over a breast or a uterus, have our surgery, get cured or not, put on our suits or our aprons, and go back to work.

Well, the Bickersons called a truce and decided to have as much fun as possible. Maybe April in Paris, or limping around the dance floor, movies, candlelit dinners, friends, family, golden retrievers, pinochle, fishing, books, whatever we can do each day to feel good. The great American move to national healthcare came a little late for us. We will take one day at a time, enjoy life as much as possible, and he will die with his orchids on.

Source: Judith Marshall, *Medicate Me Again*

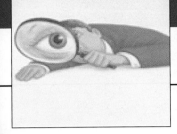

Proofreading Skills

Instructions: In the paragraphs below, circle the errors. Identify misspelled and missing medical and English words and punctuation errors, and write the correct words and punctuation in the numbered spaces opposite the text.

1 HISTORY AND PHYSICAL EXAMINATION

2

3 HISTORY

4 This 38-year-old mail was admitted threw the emergency

5 department with a hsitory of less than one day of a cute

6 ureteral colic on the left side. The patinet had an IVP in

7 the emergency department earlier today which shows

8 partial to complete obstruction of the left ureter at the

9 ureteravesical junction with a large stone approxi-

10 mately 8 x 5 mm lodged at the UV junction. The

11 patient has no other clacifications visible. The patient

12 denies any previous history of urinary tract stones or

13 other GU problems except for prostratitis a couple of

14 years ago. The patient has no other significant medical

15 problems.

16

17 FAMILY HISTORY

18 No familial history of kidney stones or other signifcant

19 hereditary disease.

20

21 PHYSICAL EXAM

22 A well-nourished, well-developed male in no acute

23 distress. Pupils equal, round, react to light. Ears, nose,

24 and throat clear. Neck supple, no JV distention or bruit.

25 Lungs clear to P&A. Heart: Regular rhythm,, no

26 murmur. Abdomen soft, slight left CVA tenderness,

27 slight left lower quadrant tenderness, no rebound.

28 Genitalia are within normal limits. Penis: Normal male.

29 Extremities: No cyanosis clubbing or edema.

30 Neurologic: Oriented x 3 with no gross deficits.

31

32 IMPRESSION

33 Left lower ureteral stone with obstruction.

1 _____

2 _____

3 _____

4 _male_____

5 _____

6 _____

7 _____

8 _____

9 _____

10 _____

11 _____

12 _____

13 _____

14 _____

15 _____

16 _____

17 _____

18 _____

19 _____

20 _____

21 _____

22 _____

23 _____

24 _____

25 _____

26 _____

27 _____

28 _____

29 _____

30 _____

31 _____

32 _____

33 _____

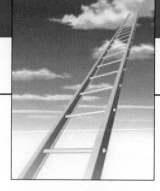

SkillsChallenge

Anatomy Fill-in Exercise

Instructions: The following paragraphs describe the process by which urine is formed. The numbered blanks correspond to the numbers in the narrative paragraphs. Fill in the blanks with the correct term from the word list following.

During the process of metabolism, proteins taken into the body are broken down into (1). This nitrogenous waste must be removed continuously by the kidneys. Other nitrogenous waste products removed by the kidney include creatinine and uric acid. In addition, the kidneys regulate blood electrolytes by excreting or retaining sodium and potassium. Circulating blood (carrying urea, creatinine, uric acid, sodium, and potassium) flows through the (2), which enters the kidney through a small depression on the medial aspect of the kidney called the (3). The renal artery divides into arterioles and then into capillaries within the cortex of the kidney.

Special capillary tufts called (4) are where the process of urine production actually begins. These capillary tufts are surrounded by a cuplike structure called (5) that collects filtrate taken from the capillary blood. This filtrate contains water, waste products, and electrolytes. The combination of the capillary tuft and the cuplike collecting tube is known as a (6), which is considered the functional unit of the kidney.

As the filtrate passes through the proximal convoluted tubule, the (7), and the distal convoluted tubule, water and electrolytes needed to maintain body functions are absorbed back into the blood. At this point, the filtrate is urine. The many renal tubules containing urine empty into cuplike collecting areas in the renal pelvis known as the (8). The collected urine then flows through the hollow tubes known as (9) into the urinary bladder.

The bladder has three orifices within it: one opening from each of the two ureters and one opening leading to the urethra. The triangular area within these three openings is called the (10). The urethra ends at the (11), where the urine is expelled from the body.

The process of urination is also known as (12) and (13). In the male, the urethra passes through a gland at the base of the bladder, called the (14) gland. This gland often enlarges in elderly men and can block the flow of urine.

1. urea _____
2. _____
3. _____
4. _____
5. _____
6. _____
7. _____
8. _____
9. _____
10. _____
11. _____
12. _____
13. _____
14. _____

Bowman capsule
calices or calyces
glomeruli
hilum
loop of Henle
micturition
nephron
prostate
renal artery
trigone
urea
ureters
urinary meatus
voiding

Adjectives Exercise

Adjectives are formed from nouns by adding adjectival suffixes such as *-ac, -al, -ar, -ary, -eal, -ed, -ent, -iac, -ic, -ical, -lar, -oid, -ous, -tic,* and *-tous.* In addition, some adjectives have a different form entirely from the noun, which may be either Latin or Greek in origin.

Instructions: Test your knowledge of adjectives by writing the adjectival form of the following urology words. Consult a medical dictionary to select the correct adjectival ending as necessary.

1. urine _____
2. kidney _____
3. bladder _____
4. ureter _____
5. urethra _____
6. hilum _____
7. calix, calyx _____
8. glomerulus _____
9. incontinence _____
10. uremia _____

Word Root and Suffix-Matching Exercises

Instructions: Combine the following root words with suffixes to create words that match the definitions below. Fill in the blanks with the medical words you construct.

Word Root	Suffix
oligo-	-oscopy
cyst–	-itis
noct–	-iasis
nephro-	-uria
litho-	-ectomy
glycos-	-ology
pyo-	
uro-	

A. the study of the urine

_____

B. inflammation of the bladder

_____

C. the urge to void at night

_____

D. scanty production of urine

_____

E. using a scope to see the bladder

_____

F. surgical removal of kidney

_____

G. pus (white cells) in urine

_____

H. sugar in the urine

_____

I. condition of kidney stones

_____

   (*Tip*: Use 2 word roots and 1 suffix)

Combined Forms Exercise

Instructions: Make combined words out of the following compounds.

costal-vertebral	_____
genital-urinary	_____
posterior-lateral	_____
rectal-vaginal	_____
superior-lateral	_____
ureteral-pelvic	_____
ureteral-vesical	_____
urethral-vesical	_____
vesical-ureteral	_____

Medical Terminology Matching Exercise

Complete the following matching exercise to test your knowledge of the word roots, anatomic structures, symptoms, and disease processes encountered in urology/nephrology.

Instructions: Match each definition in Column A with its term in Column B.

Column A	Column B
1. ___ blood in the urine	**A.** retroperitoneal
2. ___ cuplike structure that surrounds the glomerulus	**B.** trigone
	C. micturition
3. ___ urge to urinate during the night	**D.** hilum
4. ___ inflammation of the glomerulus	**E.** pole
	F. glomerulus
5. ___ kidney stones	**G.** Bowman capsule
6. ___ decreased production of urine	**H.** nephrolithiasis
7. ___ painful urination	**I.** meatus
8. ___ no urine production	**J.** glomerulonephritis
9. ___ collection of capillaries shaped like a ball in the kidney	**K.** calix *or* calyx
	L. pyelo-
10. ___ upper or lower end of kidney	**M.** nocturia
11. ___ area where blood vessels and nerves enter the kidney	**N.** oliguria
	O. anuria
12. ___ triangle in the bladder formed by end of ureters	**P.** pyuria
13. ___ opening of urethra to outside of body	**Q.** incontinence
14. ___ region where urine collects within the renal pelvis	**R.** dysuria
15. ___ position of kidneys in body	**S.** hematuria
16. ___ pus in the urine	
17. ___ voiding	
18. ___ inability to hold urine in the bladder	
19. ___ word root meaning *renal pelvis*	

Abbreviations Exercise

Common abbreviations may be transcribed as dictated in the body of a report. Uncommon abbreviations should be spelled out, with the abbreviation appearing in parentheses after the translation. All abbreviations (except laboratory test names like *VDRL* and *ALT*) should be spelled out in the Diagnosis or Impression section of a medical report.

Instructions: Define the following common urologic abbreviations. Then memorize both abbreviations and definitions to increase your speed and accuracy in transcribing dictation from urology.

BPH _____

BUN _____

ESWL _____

GU _____

IVP _____

KUB _____

TNTC _____

TURP _____

UA _____

UTI _____

VCUG _____

Spelling Exercise

Instructions: Look up each of the following words in a medical dictionary and circle the preferred spelling.

aneurism	aneurysm
calices	calyces
caesarean	cesarean
dysfunction	disfunction
fetal	foetal
fontanel	fontanelle
hydroma	hygroma
leucocyte	leukocyte
liter	litre
trepanation	trephination
venipuncture	venopuncture

Soundalikes Exercise

Instructions: Circle the correct term from the soundalikes in parentheses in the following sentences.

1. Genitalia: The patient has hypospadias and (chordae, chordee).

2. The mother brings her 10-year-old son in today because of frequent nighttime (anuresis, enuresis).

3. Intravenous pyelogram revealed bilateral poorly functioning (atopic, atrophic, ectopic) kidneys.

4. Clear (efflux, reflex, reflux) of urine was seen coming from both ureteral orifices.

5. It was felt the (anuresis, enuresis) was caused by severe prostatic hypertrophy, completely obstructing the prostatic urethra.

6. Due to benign hyperplasia of the (prostate, prostrate), a decision was made to do a prostatectomy.

7. A (ureteral, urethral) discharge was present, and gonococcus was diagnosed.

8. Both (urethras, ureters) were patent on intravenous pyelogram.

9. The (vesical, vesicle) neck of the bladder was obstructed by prostatic hypertrophy.

10. Vesicoureteral (efflux, reflex, reflux) was felt to be the cause of the patient's recurrent urinary (track, tract) infections.

Dictation Exercises

Prior to transcribing the dictations, complete these activities.

1. Using Chapter 3, Style Guide

a. Read the section in the Style Guide on obstetrical terms. What does gravida 5, para 5 mean? What is the TPAL system of recording a patient's obstetrical history?

b. When should you expand an abbreviation in the body of a report?

c. When, according to the Style Guide, do you expand brief forms?

d. According to the error-prone abbreviations list, what is the appropriate way to transcribe *q.h.s.*?

e. Read the section on Adding Headings Not Dictated in the Format section of the Style Guide.

f. Read the section on adjectival number compounds in the Style Guide under Hyphens. How would you transcribe "eighty pound child"?

g. What does the Style Guide say about starting a sentence with a numeral?

h. According to the Brief Forms and Medical Slang list, is *prepped* (for *prepared*) an acceptable form?

2. Problem Solving

This activity is to help you prepare ahead of time for some of the problems you'll encounter in the dictations. Some of these items may not have a definitive answer but are intended to simply get you thinking about how to handle a variety of situations that are common in transcription. If nothing else, they will help you recognize a problem when you encounter it in the dictations.

a. The physician clearly dictates the term *urethrolysis*, but you cannot confirm it in a medical dictionary. How do you verify the spelling and definition? What do you think *urethrolysis* means?

b. A physician spells a medication for you. Do you accept the spelling and keep transcribing or confirm the spelling? Why?

3. Preparatory Research

Any information requested in these questions not readily available in your textbook (including the Appendix) or required references can easily be found using Internet search engines such as Google or online medical dictionaries.

a. Perform a Google search for grammar + "has got" and make a note of when it is appropriate to use this expression.

b. What does *urolithiasis* mean?

c. What are the reference ranges for PSA? What is the significance of an elevated PSA?

d. What is *lithotripsy*? What are the different methods for performing lithotripsy?

e. Define *hydronephrosis*.

f. What does *end-stage* mean?

g. Why would a patient require *hemodialysis*?

h. What is the difference between *creatine* and *creatinine*?

i. What causes Lyme disease?

j. Where is the epididymis? What is the medical term for inflammation of the epididymis? What is the adjective form of *epididymis*?

k. Perform a Google search for stages + grades + "prostate cancer" and also for "Gleason score" and make a note of the way the values are transcribed.

l. What is the difference in meaning between *discreet* and *discrete*? Which is more likely to be found in a medical report?

m. What does *trabeculation of the bladder* mean? If found, what is its significance?

n. What is the trigone of the bladder?

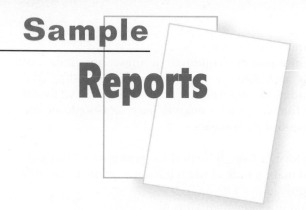

Sample Reports

Sample urology/nephrology reports appear on the following pages, illustrating a variety of reports. Fictional names are provided for illustration of proper format, and no resemblance to actual persons is intended. Sample transcripts were prepared according to the *AAMT Book of Style*, where possible.

Chart Note

MORGAN, EMILY
June 20, XXXX

SUBJECTIVE
This is a 24-year-old white married female who complains of urinary burning and frequency beginning approximately 5 days ago. She denies any prior urinary problems. She has had no chills, fever, flank pain, or hematuria. She has noted nocturia x3 since the onset of her symptoms. She has had no nausea or abdominal pain. She denies vaginal discharge or itching. Last menstrual period began 17 days ago. She is on Demulen 1/35-28 for birth control but has taken no other medicines. She is sexually active in a stable and apparently exclusive marital relationship. Her general health is good, and she denies recent upper respiratory infection (URI). She has never been pregnant.

OBJECTIVE
Temperature 98.6, pulse 72 and regular, blood pressure 116/80. The patient is alert and in no distress. Her skin is pale, warm, and dry. There is no costovertebral angle tenderness, and palpation of the abdomen indicates no masses or organomegaly. The bladder is not palpable or tender. On pelvic exam there is no evidence of vulvar edema or erythema and no discharge. The cervix is clean, and only scant mucoid material is seen in the vault. She had a negative (class 1) Pap smear about 8 months ago. Bimanual exam reveals a normal-sized uterus which is slightly retroflexed. The adnexal areas are normal. There are no masses or abdominal tenderness, and the rectal examination is negative.

A clean-voided urine shows 15-20 wbc/hpf, 8-10 red cells, 4+ occult blood, 1+ protein, negative for sugar, pH 5.5.

ASSESSMENT
Acute cystitis.

PLAN
1. Cipro 250 mg q.12 h. x3 days.
2. Pyridium 200 mg q.4-6 h. p.r.n. burning.
3. Increase oral fluids.
4. I discussed the probable origin of her condition with the patient and advised her to make a practice of voiding immediately after intercourse in the future.
5. The patient is to call in the day after tomorrow if she has any persisting symptoms.

JF:hpi

ROTH, JAMES
#987123456
Admitted 6/1/XXXX
Jeffrey Lyons, MD
Page 2

HISTORY
This 43-year-old male was admitted through the emergency department with a history of less than 1 day of acute ureteral colic on the left side. The patient had an intravenous pyelogram (IVP) in the emergency department earlier today which shows partial to complete obstruction of the left ureter at the ureterovesical (UV) junction, with a large stone approximately 8 x 5 mm lodged at the UV junction. The patient has no other calcifications visible. The patient denies any previous history of urinary tract stones or other genitourinary (GU) problems except for prostatitis a couple of years ago. The patient has no other significant medical problems.

PAST MEDICAL HISTORY
Otherwise negative.

ALLERGIES
None.

MEDICATIONS
None. Follows usual diet.

FAMILY HISTORY
No familial history of kidney stones or other significant hereditary disease.

PHYSICAL EXAMINATION
GENERAL: A well-nourished, well-developed male in no acute distress.
HEAD AND NECK: Eyes: Pupils equal, round, react to light. Ears, nose, and throat clear. Neck supple; no jugular venous (JV) distention or bruit.
CHEST: Lungs clear to percussion and auscultation (P&A).
HEART: Regular rhythm, no murmur.
ABDOMEN: Soft. Slight left costovertebral angle (CVA) tenderness; slight left lower quadrant tenderness. No rebound.
GENITALIA: Within normal limits. Penis: Normal male.
EXTREMITIES: No cyanosis, clubbing, or edema.
NEUROLOGIC: Oriented x3 with no gross deficits.

IMPRESSION
Left lower ureteral stone with obstruction.

RECOMMENDATION
Hydration, analgesia, observation, and if the stone does not pass within 72 hours or less, will probably recommend patient for ureteroscopy and stone basketing, and if needed, ultrasonic lithotripsy. If the stone cannot be mobilized downward, push back and extracorporal shock wave lithotripsy (ESWL) might be considered.

JEFFREY LYONS, MD

JL:hpi
D: 6/1/XX
T: 6/2/XX

Urology Consultation

ROTH, JAMES
#987123456
June 1, XXXX
Medical 701B

HISTORY

Apparently this patient presented to the emergency department last night about midnight with excruciating left flank pain radiating down into the left groin and testicle, chills, nausea, vomiting, and slight urinary burning, all of about 2 hours' duration, and a stat urine showed 60-80 red cells. Apparently he was given Stadol 2 mg IM for analgesia and some IV fluids, and he had an emergency intravenous pyelogram (IVP) run which showed a radiopaque stone measuring about 0.5 cm partially blocking the left ureter at a point about 2 cm above the ureterovesical (UV) junction. There was moderate hydronephrosis without appreciable dilatation of the caliceal system, and some dye was getting past the block. I have reviewed these films, and they show normal urinary tract anatomy on the right and on the left, except as noted.

When I examined him about 10 a.m., he was still in considerable distress although noticeably obtunded by a dose of Demerol given about one-half hour prior to my visit. He was sufficiently alert, however, to give a good clear history. Apparently this man has had two previous episodes of left-sided ureteral colic followed by spontaneous passage of stones, once while on military service in Turkey and once since then, but on neither occasion were the stones preserved for analysis.

His general health is good, and he takes no medicine. He has never had a urinary tract infection. There is no known family history of renal lithiasis, gout, or bone or joint disease; however, he is adopted. He is 41 years of age, married, with two daughters, and is employed as a manager of a bowling alley.

EXAMINATION

Temperature is 99.2, pulse 100, blood pressure 150/80. Physical exam is quite benign except that he is pale, sweating, restless, and in considerable distress and tender at the left costovertebral angle (CVA) and in the left upper quadrant over the kidney and ureter. External genital exam is unremarkable. I did not attempt to do a rectal exam. He has an IV running, even though he is now taking oral fluids and he is not nauseated. He is voiding painlessly, and his urine is being strained. I did not see his urine, but according to the patient and the attendant, it is not grossly bloody.

DIAGNOSIS

Left ureterolithiasis with partial ureteral obstruction and hydronephrosis.

RECOMMENDATIONS

1. Continue analgesia and hydration.
2. Continue straining urine and preserve any solid material passed for chemical analysis.
3. Clean-voided midstream urine for culture and sensitivity.
4. After this has been obtained, start Cipro 500 mg q.12 h. orally.

(continued)

ROTH, JAMES
#987123456
Page 2

5. He is now about 12 hours post onset of symptoms, but there is still a good statistical chance that he will pass his stone spontaneously. We are going to get another IVP at 4 p.m., and if he is still obstructed, I think we had better attempt to bring this stone down with a snare before he gets enough local edema to obstruct completely or gets into trouble with a red-hot ascending pyelonephritis.
6. In any event, he needs a biochemical analysis of his problem, and depending on that, he may need dietary or drug prophylaxis against further calculus disease.

Thank you for the privilege of collaborating in the care of this patient.

MICHAEL GIOVANNIELLO, MD

MG:hpi
D: 6/1/XX
T: 6/2/XX

Operative Report

PRICE, RICHARD
#082741
SURGERY 400-C

DATE OF SURGERY
June 4, XXXX

PREOPERATIVE DIAGNOSIS
Recurrent bladder neck obstruction.

POSTOPERATIVE DIAGNOSIS
Recurrent bladder neck obstruction.

TITLE OF OPERATION
Cystoscopy and transurethral resection of the prostate.

TECHNIQUE
Upon administration of satisfactory spinal anesthesia, the patient was placed on the cystoscopy table in the lithotomy position. The external genitalia were prepped and draped in the usual manner for endoscopy. The #24 Wappler instrument was passed under direct vision, revealing a normal distal urethra. There is no evidence of stricture or other localized lesion. As one enters into the prostatic urethra, he has a normal-appearing verumontanum. There is a small apical growth on the patient's left side, but this is not impressive. He has a very large obstructing-appearing lobe coming in from the right side, mainly superiorly, with only a relatively small amount near the floor. As one enters the prostatic urethra, there is a slightly scarred bladder neck contracture apparent; however, it is of wide caliber and would not be considered significant. The instrument was then irrigated, and cystoscopy was done with both right-angle and Foroblique lens systems. The main thing one sees here is a heavily trabeculated bladder, multiple bands and ridges, no true diverticulum. No stones are identified. There is no evidence of inflammation or tumor.

At this point, the McCarthy-Storz Foroblique resectoscope sheath was introduced, size 28 in character, after accepting comfortably 28 and 30 van Buren sounds. A standard transurethral resection of the prostate was done. The ureteral orifices sat nicely back from the bladder neck, and I instilled indigo carmine just for security. Once the bladder neck was cut down on the bladder side, I then started at 11 o'clock and subsequently 1 o'clock cutting lateral lobe tissue out bilaterally and then cut the tissue as it fell in. Because of his decompensating bladder, I did a fairly radical and deep transurethral resection of the capsule throughout. I did stay within the verumontanum but took out apical lobes as safely as I could. At the end of the resection, there was some venous bleeding but no evidence of arterial bleeding. The prostatic urethra was wide open. All chips were then irrigated from the bladder and a #26 three-way Foley inserted. It was inflated to 55 mL. We observed him for venous bleeding; this stopped almost immediately and remained clear. At that point he was transferred to the recovery room with vital signs stable, in good general condition.

ROY TRAWICK, MD

RT:hpi
d: 6/4/XXXX
t: 6/5/XXXX

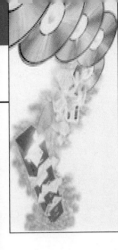

Transcription Practice

Key Words

The following terms appear in the urology/nephrology dictations. Before beginning the medical transcription practice for Chapter 11, look up each term below in a medical or English dictionary and write out a short definition.

bladder outlet obstruction
bladder tumor
cystoscopy
end-stage renal disease
epididymitis
hematuria

left flank pain
papillary tumor
prostatic carcinoma
testicular pain
urolithiasis

After completing all the readings and exercises in Chapter 11, transcribe the urology/nephrology dictations. Proofread your transcribed documents carefully, listening to the dictation while you read your transcripts.

Transcribe (*not* retype) the same reports again without referring to your previous transcription attempt. Initially, you may need to transcribe some reports more than twice before you can produce an error-free document. Your ultimate goal is to produce an error-free document the first time.

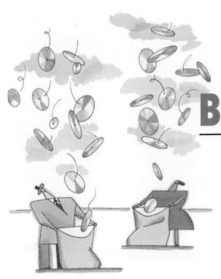

BLOOPERS

Incorrect	Correct
An undefended testicle.	An undescended testicle.
The patient is sexually impudent.	The patient is sexually impotent.
Exophthalmos of prostate, normal.	Examination of prostate was normal.
The bladder is never fully pacified.	The bladder is never fully opacified.
The patient was prepped and draped in a civil manner.	The patient was prepped and draped in the usual manner.
The patient had a temperature with blaze.	The patient had a temperature with malaise.

Chapter 12

Obstetrics and Gynecology

Learning Objectives

- Describe the structure and function of the female reproductive system.
- Spell and define common Ob/Gyn terms.
- Identify types of questions a physician might ask about the female reproductive system in the review of systems.
- Describe common abnormalities a physician looks for on examination of the external genital and internal pelvic examination.
- Identify common diseases of the female reproductive system. Describe their typical cause, course, and treatment options.

- Identify and define diagnostic and surgical procedures of the female reproduction system.
- List common Ob/Gyn laboratory tests and procedures.
- Identify and describe common Ob/Gyn drugs and their uses.
- Demonstrate knowledge of anatomical, medical, pharmacological, adjectival, and soundalike terms by accurately completing the exercises in this chapter.

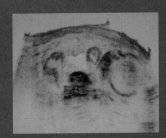
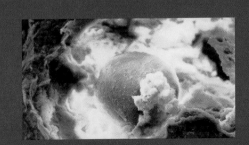
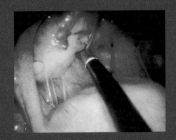

Transcribing Obstetrics and Gynecology Dictation

The **female reproductive system** is concerned exclusively with **procreation**; unlike that of the male, it does not share structures with the urinary tract to any significant extent.

Anatomy in Brief

The **female reproductive system** consists of the **internal genitalia** and **external genitalia** (see Figure 12-1 and Figure 12-2). The internal genitalia are the **ovaries, uterus, and vagina**. The external genitalia consist of the **vulva**, which contains the labia majora, labia minora, clitoris, and vaginal vestibule.

The **uterus** is divided into the **cervix** (the lowermost portion, protruding into the vaginal vault) and the **body** or **corpus** (the remainder of the uterus, which lies in the pelvic cavity between bladder and rectum). The system also includes the **breasts**, which provide nourishment to the newborn child.

Fertilization usually occurs in a uterine tube, and considerable embryonic development has already occurred before implantation in the uterine lining takes place.

Terminology Review

adnexa (singular **adnexum**, seldom used) Organs adjacent to the uterus—ovaries and tubes.

amenorrhea Absence of menstruation.

anovulation Failure of ovulation to occur at the expected times.

Bethesda system A uniform system for reporting findings on Pap (Papanicolaou) smear of the uterine cervix.

BUS Bartholin glands, urethra, and Skene glands.

dysfunctional uterine bleeding Irregular, unpredictable menstrual flow (too frequent or too infrequent, too heavy or too light), or amenorrhea, occurring in the absence of pregnancy, infection, or neoplasm.

dysmenorrhea Pain occurring with menstruation, typically felt low in the pelvis and in the low back, and often severe. The lay term for dysmenorrhea is "(menstrual) cramps."

dyspareunia Pain in the vulva, vagina, or pelvis with sexual intercourse.

dysplasia Cell abnormalities heralding eventual development of malignancy.

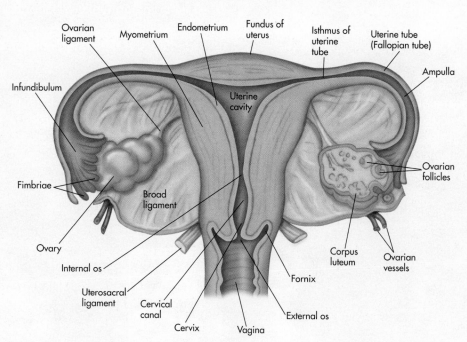

Figure 12-1
Female Reproductive Organs

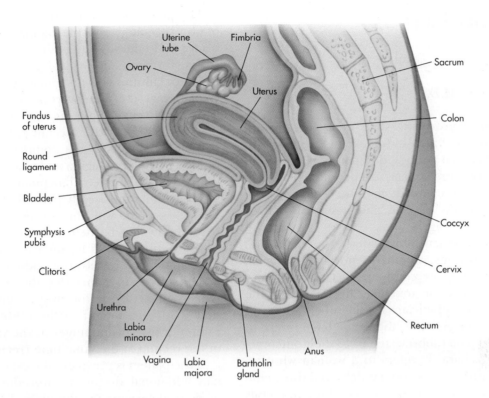

Figure 12-2
Female Reproductive Organs, Sagittal Section

dysuria Pain in the urethra or vulva with urination.

gravida Pregnant.

hypermenorrhea Abnormally high volume of menstrual discharge.

hypomenorrhea Abnormally low volume of menstrual discharge.

introitus Entrance to the vaginal vault.

IUD Intrauterine device. Most intrauterine devices have been removed from the market.

lactation Producing milk from the breasts.

meconium Stool formed in the fetal intestine before birth.

menarche The onset of the first menstrual period.

menometrorrhagia Excessive menstrual bleeding occurring both during menses and at irregular intervals.

menopause The cessation of regular menstrual periods.

menorrhagia Regularly occurring menstrual flow that is excessive in volume and lasts longer than a normal menstrual period.

metrorrhagia Menstrual bleeding occurring at irregular but frequent intervals.

mittelschmerz Intermenstrual pain due to peritoneal irritation by a small volume of blood escaping from the ovary at the time of ovulation.

oligomenorrhea Infrequent or scanty menstrual bleeding.

para Live birth.

polymenorrhea Menstrual bleeding that occurs with abnormal frequency.

primary amenorrhea Failure of menses to start at puberty (by age 14-16).

secondary amenorrhea Cessation of menses that have been normal in the past.

STD Sexually transmitted disease.

Lay and Medical Terms

afterbirth	placenta
bag of waters	amniotic membranes and fluid
birth control	contraception
change of life	menopause
cramps	dysmenorrhea
periods	menses
tubal pregnancy	ectopic pregnancy
womb	uterus

Medical Readings

History and Physical Examination

by John H. Dirckx, M.D.

Review of Systems. The **menstrual history** includes age at onset of menses (menarche), regularity of cycles, interval between periods, duration of periods, and the date of the last normal menstrual period. In addition, the interviewer inquires about menstrual cramps (dysmenorrhea), heaviness of flow, and intermenstrual or postmenopausal bleeding.

The **female reproductive history** covers pregnancies, miscarriages, abortions, stillbirths, normal deliveries, and cesarean births; any complications of pregnancy such as hemorrhage or toxemia. In recording the reproductive history, physicians use a kind of shorthand in which the term *gravida* (abbreviated G) refers to pregnancies and *para* (abbreviated P) to their outcome. Thus "gravida 3, para 3" refers to a woman who has been pregnant three times and has delivered three children. A more elaborate notation uses four numerals after "para," denoting, respectively, full-term deliveries, preterm deliveries, miscarriages or abortions, and living children. This recording system sometimes proves ambiguous with respect to multiple pregnancies (twins, triplets) and their outcome.

Women are also questioned about the use of condoms, diaphragms, oral contraceptives, or other contraceptive methods; pelvic pain, vaginal discharge, vulvar itching, sores, or rash; and any breast complaints (pain, swelling, masses, bleeding or discharge from the nipple.

Physical Examination. In women the examination of the external and internal genitourinary organs and the rectum and anus is normally performed with the patient in the lithotomy position. The patient lies on her back on a specially equipped examining table with her feet in stirrups, her thighs flexed sharply on her abdomen, and her knees spread wide apart. If she cannot assume the lithotomy position, the left lateral (Sims) position may be used instead.

The physician inspects the pubes and vulva for hair distribution, developmental anomalies, cutaneous lesions, swellings, and signs of inflammation. The urethral meatus and Bartholin and Skene glands are inspected and palpated. The integrity of the pelvic floor is assessed by having the patient bear down while the examiner observes for **cystocele** (bulging of the urinary bladder through the anterior vaginal wall), **rectocele** (bulging of the rectum through the posterior vaginal wall), or uterine prolapse. Any vaginal discharge is also observed, and the perineum and anus are examined.

The physician then inserts a warmed and lubricated bivalve speculum into the vagina and by spreading its blades and adjusting its position obtains a view of the cervix, fornices, and vaginal walls. Specimens may be taken for cultures or cytologic study at this point. A gynecologist may use a colposcope, which provides bright light and strong magnification, to inspect the cervix.

After removing the speculum, the examiner inserts one or two fingers of the dominant hand, gloved and lubricated, into the vagina and places the other hand on the patient's abdomen (bimanual pelvic examination). In this manner the size, shape, and position of the uterus can be assessed, and any masses or tenderness in the pelvic cavity can be detected. Normal uterine adnexa (ovaries, tubes, broad ligaments, round ligaments, and associated blood vessels) can seldom be felt.

The physician concludes the examination of the female subject by performing a digital rectal examination. With the patient in the lithotomy position, the examiner inserts one finger in the vagina and another in the rectum at the same time (**rectovaginal exam**).

If the patient is pregnant, the examiner performs certain additional diagnostic procedures. An attempt is made to determine the duration of the pregnancy by a consideration of uterine size. The size and shape of the pelvic outlet are assessed to determine whether it will accommodate the fetus during labor. If the pregnancy is sufficiently advanced, the examiner will attempt to learn by palpation (**Leopold maneuvers**) the position in which the fetus lies within the uterus. Finally, again if the pregnancy is sufficiently advanced, an attempt is made to hear fetal heart tones by auscultation through the mother's abdomen. A special stethoscope (fetoscope) may be used for this purpose.

A standard **breast examination** consists of the following elements:

Inspection of the breasts with the subject in the upright position, first with arms at sides, then with arms raised, and finally with hands pressed against hips to render underlying muscles taut.

Palpation of each breast in both the upright and supine positions, with attention to the axillae.

Assessment of nipples for inflammation, bleeding, or discharge.

A Doctor's View

A Brief Look at STDs in Women

by John H. Dirckx, M.D.

A **sexually transmitted disease (STD)** is any infectious disease that is transmitted from one person to another through sexual contact. The only thing all STDs have in common is their mode of transmission. In other respects they vary widely among themselves. Changes in national sexual mores have led to the emergence of sexually transmitted infections that were not previously known or recognized, such as **chlamydia** and **AIDS**, and to marked increases in the incidence of some formerly rare infections such as **genital herpes** and **genital warts**. Some of the viruses that cause genital warts induce cervical cancer.

All of the classically recognized STDs can be transmitted through vaginal intercourse. Most of them can also be transmitted through oral-genital contact and anal intercourse with resulting oropharyngeal, anorectal, or systemic infection. STDs affecting the skin (genital warts, pubic lice) or transmitted through the skin (syphilis, AIDS) can be acquired during intimate contact even though genital exposure is avoided or a condom is used.

The only absolute protection against acquiring an infection through sexual contact is lifelong celibacy or maintenance of a permanently and mutually monogamous sexual relationship. Some degree of protection against STDs is afforded by practicing "safe (or safer) sex"—which basically means using condoms and avoiding high-risk behaviors such as anal intercourse—and by limiting the number of sex partners.

The diagnosis and treatment of STDs are rendered more difficult by the reluctance of most people to discuss their sexual behavior with health professionals and by the refusal of many patients to believe that a sexual partner has become infected by some third person. Diagnosis often demands alertness and a high degree of suspicion on the part of the healthcare worker. History-taking must be searching but nonthreatening and nonjudgmental. Often the most suggestive point in the history is exposure to a new sexual partner within two months before the appearance of symptoms.

In treating any patient with an STD, the physician must reckon with two epidemiologic realities: the fact that at least one of the patient's sexual partners (and possibly all of them) is also infected, and the statistical probability that a person with one STD has other STDs. Failure to treat sexual partners prophylactically will lead to eventual reinfection of most patients. Moreover, unless both partners in a relationship are treated at the same time, they may keep reinfecting each other, a phenomenon known as "ping-ponging." STD screening tests are a standard part of prenatal care as well.

Common Diseases

Dysfunctional Uterine Bleeding. Unusually heavy or light bleeding from the uterus, typically unpredictable, or amenorrhea, in the absence of pregnancy or any demonstrable abnormality (neoplasm, infection) of the uterus.

Causes: Most cases are due to **anovulation** (failure to ovulate). This is a common occurrence and can result from physical or emotional stress, marked weight loss (as in anorexia nervosa or stringent dieting), strenuous exercise (running, gymnastics), excess or deficiency of thyroid hormone, polycystic ovary disease, recent discontinuance of oral contraceptives, lactation, and other causes. About one third of patients with amenorrhea have elevated levels of **prolactin**; in rare cases, this is due to overproduction of prolactin by a pituitary tumor.

History: Unusually heavy or light bleeding, typically irregular; often amenorrhea lasting for three or more cycles. Symptoms of underlying disease may also be present.

Physical Examination: Generally unremarkable. May show obesity or emaciation, stigmata of thyroid or ovarian disease (goiter, exophthalmos, hirsutism), or other evidence of an underlying disorder. Cysts may be palpable in the ovaries. Presence of normal breast development and axillary and pubic hair confirms normal estrogen effect. A palpable, nontender uterus of normal size and shape rules out congenital absence of the uterus (in primary amenorrhea) and helps to exclude uterine tumors or infection.

Diagnostic Tests: A pregnancy test is always done to rule out normal or **ectopic pregnancy** or recent miscarriage or abortion. Determination of blood levels of estrogen, LH, FSH, T_4, TSH, and prolactin is standard. In amenorrhea in which pregnancy has been ruled out, oral administration of a progesterone (medroxyprogesterone acetate) for five days is normally followed within 10 days by a discharge of blood from the uterus if the endometrium is healthy and the estrogen level adequate. Absence of a response suggests a severe uterine disorder (endometrial scarring) or estrogen deficiency due to pituitary or ovarian disease.

Pelvic ultrasound may help to confirm the presence or absence of uterine or ovarian disease. Laparoscopy may be needed for definitive diagnosis. CT or MRI of the head may be performed if a pituitary tumor is suspected.

Course: Depends on the underlying condition. Extremely heavy bleeding can lead to shock or anemia.

Treatment: Depends on the underlying condition. For many patients, a course of oral contraceptive provides cyclical hormone levels sufficient to induce what seem like normal menstrual cycles and flow. Clomiphene may be given to an anovulatory woman who wants to conceive. **Hyperprolactinemia** (abnormal elevation of prolactin) in the absence of a pituitary neoplasm is treated with bromocriptine. Thyroid, ovarian, or pituitary disease, or abnormalities of pelvic anatomy and physiology, may require other specific treatment.

Premenstrual Syndrome (PMS), Premenstrual Tension, Late Luteal Phase Dysphoria. A group of distressing physical and psychologic symptoms experienced in varying degrees and proportions by many women during the week preceding onset of menstruation: swelling of breasts, waist, and ankles, breast soreness, weight gain, irritability, drowsiness, depression, changes in appetite and libido (see Figure 12-3).

The cause is unknown, but hormonal and possibly psychological or psychosocial factors are thought to play a part. Cyclical treatment with fluoxetine is often effective. Other measures that may help are counseling, a regular program of exercise, and restriction of sodium, caffeine, alcohol, and sugar.

Dysmenorrhea. Pelvic pain occurring with menstruation.

Causes: *Primary*: "Normal" menstrual cramps, occurring in 50-75% of all women, and due to uterine vasoconstriction and spasm resulting from withdrawal of progesterone effect. *Secondary*: Endometriosis, pelvic inflammatory disease (PID), use of an **IUD (intrauterine device)**, tumor of the uterus, cervical stenosis (due, for example, to scarring after induced abortion).

History: Cramping pain felt low in the pelvis, often radiating to the back or inner thighs, often accompanied by nausea, diarrhea, headache, or prostration. Pain begins usually on the first day of the menstrual period and lasts 1-2 days. In secondary dysmenorrhea, symptoms are more variable.

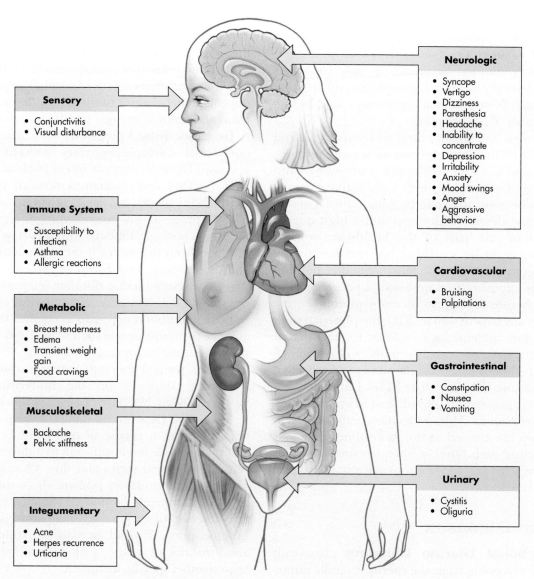

Sensory
- Conjunctivitis
- Visual disturbance

Immune System
- Susceptibility to infection
- Asthma
- Allergic reactions

Metabolic
- Breast tenderness
- Edema
- Transient weight gain
- Food cravings

Musculoskeletal
- Backache
- Pelvic stiffness

Integumentary
- Acne
- Herpes recurrence
- Urticaria

Neurologic
- Syncope
- Vertigo
- Dizziness
- Paresthesia
- Headache
- Inability to concentrate
- Depression
- Irritability
- Anxiety
- Mood swings
- Anger
- Aggressive behavior

Cardiovascular
- Bruising
- Palpitations

Gastrointestinal
- Constipation
- Nausea
- Vomiting

Urinary
- Cystitis
- Oliguria

Figure 12-3
Multisystem Effects of Premenstrual Syndrome

Physical Examination: Generally unremarkable in primary dysmenorrhea. Endometriosis, salpingitis, or uterine neoplasm may be detected as a cause of secondary dysmenorrhea.

Diagnostic Tests: In secondary dysmenorrhea, pelvic ultrasound or MRI may identify the underlying cause. Diagnostic D&C may disclose a cause within the uterine cavity. Laparoscopy identifies endometriosis or PID.

Course: Primary dysmenorrhea tends to diminish in severity after age 25, and particularly after childbirth. Without treatment, secondary dysmenorrhea may continue throughout the reproductive years.

Treatment: Nonsteroidal anti-inflammatory drugs (ibuprofen, naproxen, mefenamic acid) usually provide good symptomatic relief. Oral contraceptives may be prescribed for more sustained control. Endometriosis is treated with drugs or surgery.

Endometriosis. Growth of endometrial tissue outside of the uterus, particularly in the ovaries and on the pelvic walls.

Cause: Unknown. The problem affects about 2% of American women. Implants of endometrial tissue can occur in a wide variety of locations, including any peritoneal surface, the rectal mucosa, and the ovaries (causing **endometrial** or **"chocolate" cysts**, so-called because of their color).

History: Onset is usually during the middle to late 20s. Severe dysmenorrhea, often beginning days before the onset of menstruation and continuing for a week or more. Pain is constant and may be diffuse, with rectal pain and dyspareunia. Many patients are infertile (unable to conceive). Rectal bleeding may occur from implants in the rectum.

Physical Examination: Tender nodules of endometrial tissue may be palpated in the pelvis, particularly the **cul-de-sac** (lowermost part of pelvic cavity, between uterus and rectum), the ovaries, or the rectum.

Diagnostic Tests: Ultrasound, MRI, or barium enema may identify endometrial implants. Often laparoscopy is required to arrive at a definitive diagnosis. At laparoscopy, endometrial implants often appear as hemorrhagic cysts or **"powder burn" lesions** on peritoneal surfaces.

Course: Pain (including dyspareunia) and infertility tend to persist throughout the reproductive years. Medical or surgical treatment may diminish pain, but most treatment methods may further impair fertility.

Treatment: Analgesics and various hormone analogues (leuprolide, nafarelin, oral contraceptives) or hormone inhibitors (danazol) may help. Focal endometriosis may be ablated laparoscopically with a laser. For severe or generalized disease, **hysterectomy** (removal of uterus), **oophorectomy** (removal of ovaries), or both may be indicated.

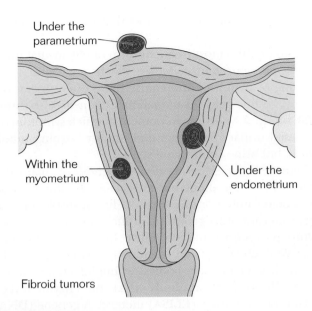

Figure 12-4
Uterine Fibroid Tumors

Uterine Myoma (Fibromyoma, Fibroid). A benign neoplasm of uterine muscle (Figure 12-4).

Cause: Unknown.

History: There may be no symptoms. Abdominal or pelvic pain or pressure, heavy vaginal bleeding, dysmenorrhea, urinary frequency, infertility.

Physical Examination: Pelvic examination shows one or more discrete, firm masses in the uterine wall. With heavy bleeding there may be tachycardia, pallor, or even shock.

Diagnostic Tests: With heavy bleeding the hemoglobin level may be low. Ultrasound or MRI studies can clearly delineate the nature of the problem.

Course: Uterine myomas tend to grow larger and more numerous with time. With significant bleeding there is a risk of chronic anemia or sudden onset of shock. Myomas in the pregnant uterus can lead to fetal loss, premature or difficult labor, or severe postpartum hemorrhage.

Treatment: Small or solitary myomas can be removed surgically (**myomectomy**). If tumors are large or numerous, **hysterectomy** (removal of the uterus) may be indicated. Before surgery, leuprolide or nafarelin is administered to reduce the size and vascularity of tumors.

Urethritis and Pelvic Inflammatory Disease. Genital infections due to **chlamydia** are currently the most common of all bacterial STDs. Although, strictly speaking, chlamydia is the name of the causative organism, in clinical parlance genital infections due to this organism are often called simply "chlamydia." *Chlamydia trachomatis* is highly contagious; at least 50% of sexual partners of persons with chlamydia are also infected. Moreover, 20% of men and 80% of women with the disease have no symptoms and do not know that they are infected (and infectious).

In women the most frequent form of chlamydial infection is mucopurulent cervicitis, which may cause slight bleeding or pain with intercourse but is often discovered only on routine pelvic examination. Chlamydia also causes acute urethral syndrome in women, in which symptoms of increased urinary frequency and urinary burning mimic cystitis, but urine cultures are sterile.

Because facilities for laboratory diagnosis of chlamydial infection are not altogether satisfactory, treatment must often be instituted on the basis of clinical suspicion. The organism cannot be grown on artificial media, and tissue culture is expensive and insensitive. In practice, a urethral or cervical smear is usually examined for chlamydial inclusion bodies (elementary bodies) within infected cells by a direct **fluorescent antibody (FA)** or enzyme-linked immunosorbent assay (**ELISA**) method. A genetic (**DNA**) **probe** procedure can also be used, and serologic tests are available.

As many as 20% of women with untreated chlamydia will eventually develop **acute salpingitis**, also called **pelvic inflammatory disease (PID)**, due to spread of infection to one or both uterine tubes. PID is more likely to occur in a woman with an **intrauterine device (IUD)**, and acute attacks are more common during menstruation. The symptoms of pelvic pain and fever are fairly nonspecific, but severe tenderness on manipulation of the cervix and on palpation of the uterine adnexa during pelvic examination is highly suggestive of the diagnosis. This is known as the **chandelier sign**; the term fancifully implies that the pain causes the patient to leap into the air and cling to the chandelier.

PID may progress to **tubo-ovarian** abscess or to perihepatitis (**Fitz-Hugh–Curtis syndrome**). A more common consequence of PID is scarring of the uterine tubes with resulting infertility or sterility and heightened risk of ectopic pregnancy.

Chlamydia responds to treatment with various antibiotics. Currently recommended drugs are doxycycline (Doryx, Vibramycin, Vibra-Tabs), tetracycline (Panmycin, Sumycin, Tetracyn, Tetralan), or azithromycin (Zithromax). All of the patient's sexual partners must be treated prophylactically, regardless of symptoms or laboratory test results. Tubo-ovarian abscess and salpingitis that do not respond to antibiotics may require surgical treatment.

Gonorrhea is infection of the genital tract of either sex by *Neisseria gonorrhoeae*, a gram-negative diplococcus. This disease has been known for centuries and goes by the colloquial name of "clap." Physicians often refer to the causative organism as the **gonococcus, GC** for short, and this abbreviation frequently stands for the disease itself in medical slang. Like chlamydia, gonorrhea is an infection of the genital mucous membranes, causing urethritis in men but frequently asymptomatic in women; it too is capable of progressing to PID with its complications of tubo-ovarian abscess and Fitz-Hugh–Curtis syndrome and its aftermath of tubal scarring with resultant infertility or sterility and increased risk of tubal pregnancy. Also like chlamydia, gonorrhea can cause severe eye infection, resulting in blindness, in an infant born to an infected mother.

The diagnosis of gonorrhea can be made by examination of a gram-stained smear of urethral discharge for the typical intracellular diplococci or by culture of urethral, cervical, or other material on special media such as Thayer-Martin agar, which is designed to favor the growth of gonococci. Highly sensitive rapid tests based on antigen detection or nucleic acid probe have largely supplanted cultures. Increasing problems of resistance to penicillin have led to the abandonment of this drug for the treatment of gonorrhea. A single intramuscular injection of ceftriaxone is highly effective in eradicating gonococcal infection. In addition, several cephalosporins (cefixime, cefuroxime, cefpodoxime) and quinolones (ciprofloxacin, ofloxacin) are effective in a single oral dose.

All patients treated for gonorrhea are also treated prophylactically for chlamydia because of the high frequency with which these diseases occur together. In addition, all sexual contacts of patients with gonorrhea are treated prophylactically against both diseases, regardless of symptoms or results of tests.

Genital Herpes. Herpes simplex is a local infection of skin or mucous membranes caused by a virus (Figure 12-5). Type 1 herpes simplex virus (HSV-1) typically causes lesions of the lips and face (orofacial herpes, herpes labialis, cold sore, fever blister), while type 2 causes lesions of the genitals (**genital herpes, herpes progenitalis**). Although the types are distinguishable in the laboratory, there is no difference in their clinical effects, and a 10-20% overlap of their preferred infection sites occurs.

Transmission is by direct contact with an infected person. The incubation period may be as short as one week, but sometimes the virus remains dormant for months or years before causing symptoms. Apparently persons with latent infection (no active lesions) can spread the disease to others, at least in certain circumstances. Genital herpes is always spread through sexual contact.

Regardless of its location, herpes simplex appears as a small cluster of vesicles surrounded by a reddened zone of skin or mucous membrane. Itching or burning is often intense and may precede the appearance of lesions. Within a day or two the vesicles slough and become shallow, painful ulcers. A first attack of herpes simplex may be accompanied by swelling and inflammation of regional

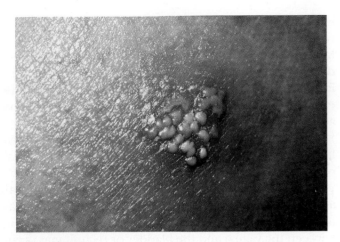

Figure 12-5
Herpes Simplex

lymph nodes and fever. The lesions heal spontaneously after 1-2 weeks. However, the virus remains in the body for the life of the patient, lying dormant in spinal cord ganglia.

A recurrence of herpes simplex at the same site as the original eruption can be triggered at any time by various physical or emotional stresses, including fever, sunburn, menses, and fatigue. Recurrent herpes simplex is usually milder than the primary attack and of shorter duration, and fever and lymph gland involvement seldom occur. Recurrences may come at intervals of days, weeks, months, or years; many patients never experience any recurrences at all.

In women with genital herpes, severely painful vulvar lesions are the rule, but when the cervix is the site of the eruption, it may go unnoticed. Anorectal lesions result from anal intercourse. Neonatal infection, acquired at birth by a child born to a mother with active genital herpes, often leads to disseminated disease with a high mortality rate.

Diagnosis of herpes simplex is usually obvious on direct examination. Confirmation may be obtained by means of a **Tzanck smear**, a stained preparation of material scraped or expressed from a lesion, which shows abnormal balloon cells with viral inclusion bodies. A **Pap smear** may also show these changes, but culture of the virus is much more specific and is the diagnostic procedure of choice. These tests are relatively insensitive, however, and cannot distinguish between herpes and other viral eruptions (chickenpox, herpes zoster).

Treatment of genital herpes with acyclovir, famciclovir, or valacyclovir shortens the period of clinical symptoms and of viral shedding, but does not eradicate the virus. Long-term prophylaxis with these agents has been helpful for some patients with frequent recurrences. Because genital herpes is a risk factor for cervical cancer, women with

a history of this disease are advised to have regular Pap smears throughout life. A woman who goes into labor with active genital herpes is delivered by cesarean section to prevent transmission of infection to the newborn.

Genital Warts. A wart is a benign skin tumor induced by infection with the **human papillomavirus (HPV)**. Genital warts (venereal warts), occurring on the skin and mucous membranes of the genitals and anus, are spread almost exclusively through sexual contact. Perianal spread may result from anal intercourse but is often due to migration of virus from the patient's own genital lesions. Genital warts are highly contagious: 60-90% of sexual partners of persons with genital warts also have genital warts. They are the most common viral STD, and their incidence is increasing. Genital warts are more likely to develop during pregnancy and in persons with impaired immunity.

In men genital warts usually appear on the penis, occasionally within the urethra or about the anus. In women genital warts typically affect the labia and perianal skin but may involve the vaginal lining and cervix. The principal symptom of genital warts is their visible presence. Itching and vaginal discharge may occur, and warts sometimes ulcerate or become infected with skin bacteria.

HPV types 6 and 11 cause the classical genital wart known as **condyloma acuminatum** (plural, **condylomata acuminata**). This is a slender, often finger-shaped growth with a narrow attachment to the skin, a tapered tip, and a somewhat rough texture. HPV types 16 and 18 cause flat warts rather than classical condylomata acuminata. These latter viral types are associated with a high risk of dysplasia or cancer in affected genital skin or mucous membranes, which may progress to invasive carcinoma of the cervix.

Genital warts can usually be diagnosed by simple inspection, but many cases of latent infection are only recognized on Pap smear or cervical biopsy. A standard procedure for identifying genital warts and other lesions of the cervix is **colposcopy**, an inspection of the cervix with a low-power binocular microscope. In both sexes, visualization of small, flat, or atypical warts is enhanced by prior application of 5% acetic acid (white vinegar) for a few minutes to the area of skin or mucous membrane to be examined. Acetic acid causes blanching (acetowhitening) in typical HPV lesions. This procedure is not highly specific, but at least it helps the examiner to decide which lesions should be biopsied. Screening tests based on molecular biology can confirm the presence of HPV and identify its type. HPV screening is often performed at the same time as a routine Pap smear to enhance the diagnostic value of the smear.

A wide variety of methods are used to treat genital warts, including surgical excision, electrodesiccation, cryosurgery, and laser ablation; application of liquid nitrogen, corrosive chemicals (trichlorocetic acid, dichlorocetic acid), or antimitotics (podophyllin, 5-FU); and intralesional injection of interferon. The choice of treatment depends on the site, character, and extent of involvement. Currently liquid nitrogen is favored for most lesions. Regardless of the method used, several treatments are usually needed to eliminate all warts, and rates of recurrence or treatment failure with all methods are substantial. A vaccine against HPV, licensed in 2006, provides excellent protection against several viral types, including 16 and 18.

Pelvic Inflammatory Disease (PID), Salpingitis, Endometritis.
Acute or chronic bacterial infection of the uterus and tubes.

Causes: Sexually transmitted infection with *Neisseria gonorrhoeae* or *Chlamydia trachomatis* ascending from the lower genital tract; infection with other organisms (streptococci, *Haemophilus influenzae*) may be blood borne. Risk factors include **nulliparity** (never having borne a viable child), nonwhite race, smoking, and sexual contact with many partners.

History: Pelvic pain, chills, fever, menstrual irregularities, purulent vaginal discharge, dyspareunia. Acute symptoms are more likely to occur during menses. With **Fitz-Hugh–Curtis syndrome**, right upper quadrant pain.

Physical Examination: Fever, abdominal tenderness; marked tenderness on manipulation of cervix and palpation of adnexa. Right upper quadrant tenderness in Fitz-Hugh–Curtis syndrome.

Diagnostic Tests: The white blood cell count is variably elevated. Smear and culture of material obtained from the cervix (or from the cul-de-sac by culdoscopy) may identify the infecting organism. Pelvic ultrasound and laparoscopy are used to refine the diagnosis.

Course: In about 25% of patients, the condition becomes recurrent or chronic even after treatment, with pelvic pain, infertility, and increased risk of ectopic pregnancy. Complications of PID include tubo-ovarian abscess with danger of rupture into the peritoneal cavity, and Fitz-Hugh–Curtis syndrome, a localized peritonitis in the right upper quadrant.

Treatment: Hospitalization, intravenous antibiotics (cefoxitin, clindamycin). For milder disease, outpatient treatment with oral antibiotics may suffice. Surgical drainage of abscesses; for severe disease, hysterectomy with bilateral salpingo-oophorectomy.

Carcinoma of the Cervix.
A slowly growing, invasive carcinoma of the uterine cervix, predominantly of squamous cell origin.

Causes: Squamous cell carcinoma of the cervix develops as a consequence of **cervical dysplasia**, which in turn is caused in a majority of cases by cervical infection with **human papillomavirus** (genital wart virus), particularly types 16, 18, and 31. The progression from dysplasia to invasive carcinoma typically takes 5-10 years. Peak incidence of cervical carcinoma occurs in the late 30s. Risk factors for cervical carcinoma are smoking, prolonged use of oral contraceptives, sexual contact with many partners, and HIV infection.

History: Irregular vaginal bleeding or spotting, particularly after intercourse; abnormal vaginal discharge; bowel or bladder pain or dysfunction.

Physical Examination: Cervical ulceration. With advanced disease, evidence of pelvic invasion or metastasis; a **fistula** (abnormal passage or communication) between the vagina and the bladder or rectum may occur.

Diagnostic Tests: Premalignant cellular changes can be detected early by routine Pap smear. As mentioned in the discussion of genital warts, HPV typing, performed either simultaneously with a routine Pap smear or as a followup to an abnormal smear, can confirm the presence of the virus and identify its type. About 20% of women with **ASC-US** (abnormal squamous cells of undetermined significance) eventually develop squamous intraepithelial lesions or invasive carcinoma. Detection of cellular dysplasia (low-grade squamous intraepithelial lesion, **LGSIL**, or high-grade squamous intraepithelial lesion, **HGSIL**) calls for followup in the form of colposcopy, cervical biopsy, and possibly surgical or laser excision of a cone of cervical tissue including the entire squamocolumnar junction. These provide precise information about the type and stage of disease.

Course: Severe bleeding may occur from ulceration and erosion of the cervix and surrounding tissues. Extension can lead to bilateral ureteral obstruction, with resultant kidney failure, or to rectovaginal or vesicovaginal fistula. The 5-year survival rate with treatment is about 60%.

Treatment: Early removal of localized disease by conization or, preferably, hysterectomy. In advanced disease, radiation is an alternative to radical surgery. A vaccine now available against HPV, which is particularly active against viral types associated with a high risk of malignant change, can be expected to reduce the incidence of cervical cancer markedly during the coming decades.

Vaginitis, Vulvovaginitis.
Inflammation of the vagina and vulva, generally due to infection and manifested by vaginal discharge and vulvar itching or pain. Most cases are due to one of three organisms:

Vaginal candidosis: *Candida albicans*, a yeastlike fungus, frequently causes vulvar pruritus and a thick white curdy discharge. Infection is more common in diabetes mellitus and pregnancy and in women taking oral contraceptives or broad-spectrum antibiotics.

Examination shows intense erythema of the vulva and curdy white material in the vaginal vault. A wet preparation of this material in potassium hydroxide examined microscopically identifies the causative organism. Culture may also be performed. Treatment is with topical antifungal medicines (miconazole, terconazole, clotrimazole) in vaginal suppositories, creams, or ointments, or with oral fluconazole in a single dose. Recurrences are common.

Trichomonas vaginitis: *Trichomonas vaginalis* is a sexually transmitted protozoan parasite that causes vulvar itching and vaginal discharge. Vaginal examination shows erythema, particularly of the cervix (**"strawberry cervix"**), and a watery, frothy, malodorous yellowish-brown discharge. Wet preparation of vaginal discharge shows motile protozoa. Treatment is with oral metronidazole for the patient and all sexual partners. (Symptoms in men are usually absent; dysuria and urethral discharge may occur.)

Bacterial vaginosis: *Gardnerella vaginalis* is at least one of the organisms involved in **bacterial vaginosis**, a mixed vaginal infection that causes a thin grayish discharge with a foul fishy odor but not much vulvar irritation or itching. Microscopic examination of discharge material shows **clue cells** (epithelial cells heavily studded with bacteria). This condition is associated with increased risk of premature labor and preterm birth. Treatment is with oral or vaginal metronidazole or clindamycin.

Fibrocystic Disease (or Condition) of the Breast (Cystic Mastitis, Mammary Dysplasia).
Formation of benign but painful cysts in the breasts (Figure 12-6).

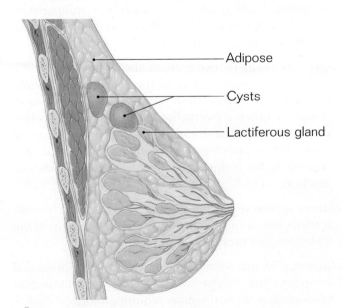

Cause: Probably inappropriate response of breast tissue to ovarian hormones. The condition affects as many as one third of all women between the ages of 25 and 50. The theory that caffeine (from coffee, tea, and chocolate) exacerbates symptoms remains unproven.

History: One or more lumps in the breast, typically painful and tender, and more so just before the onset of menses. Lumps are frequently multiple and may change markedly in size within a period of 2-3 days. Lumps typically disappear eventually, but meanwhile others often develop.

Physical Examination: One or more fluctuant, usually tender masses in one or both breasts. Occasionally nipple discharge is noted.

Diagnostic Tests: Needle aspiration of a cyst usually leads to its disappearance. Biopsy material obtained by fine-needle aspiration or other method from a solid or cystic mass helps to rule out malignant change. Biopsy may show **hyperplasia** of epithelial tissues, associated with an increased risk of malignant tumor of the breast. Mammography and ultrasound examinations may help to distinguish cysts from solid tumors.

Course: Fibrocystic disease tends to persist, with remissions and exacerbations, until menopause, and then to resolve completely and permanently. Forms of fibrocystic disease associated with proliferation of epithelial elements carry a slightly higher risk of progression to carcinoma of the breast.

Treatment: Analgesics, education, close observation for persisting or dominant lump, which may prove to be a solid tumor requiring further observation. For severe disease, danazol and, rarely, mastectomy may be advised.

Breast Cancer.
A malignant tumor of the female breast, arising most frequently from ductal epithelium (Figure 12-7). The commonest cancer in women, and the second commonest cause of cancer death (after lung cancer) in women. One in eight or nine women will develop breast cancer.

Cause: Women who have no children, or whose first pregnancy occurs late in the childbearing years, are at increased risk of breast cancer. So are women who have a family history of breast cancer, particularly cancer occurring at an early age in one or more female relatives, which may be associated with the BRCA1 or BRCA2 oncogene. The risk of breast cancer is increased by estrogen replacement therapy after menopause.

History: A solitary, firm, nontender mass in the breast, usually discovered by the patient accidentally or during breast self-examination. (All women over 20 should practice breast self-examination monthly.) Sixty percent occur in the upper outer quadrant of the breast. Occasionally nipple discharge is the presenting symptom. With advancing disease, swelling and local pain. Bone pain, weight

Figure 12-6
Fibrocystic Breast Disease, Adipose Tissue

Adipose

Cysts

Lactiferous gland

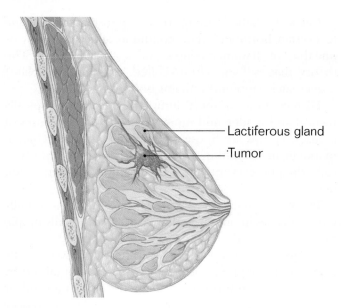

Figure 12-7
Breast Cancer: Tumor Growing Within a Milk Gland

loss, and jaundice are symptoms of systemic spread through metastasis.

Physical Examination: There may be enlargement or abnormal contour of one breast on inspection. The tumor is felt as a hard, ill-defined, nontender solitary mass. There may be skin or nipple retraction, fixation of the tumor to the underlying chest wall or the overlying skin, and signs of local inflammation (swelling, redness, ulceration). Axillary lymph nodes may be found enlarged if cancer cells have spread to them.

Diagnostic: Mammography (a specialized x-ray procedure) can identify changes indicative of breast cancer (calcification, mass, or both) as much as two years before a tumor becomes palpable, and is therefore a valuable screening procedure for asymptomatic women over 40, and for younger women believed to be at increased risk because of a family history of early-onset breast cancer or presence of BRCA 1 or 2 as detected by genetic testing. Ultrasound examination can supply valuable additional information. Biopsy is required for confirmation of malignancy and precise identification of tumor type. A biopsy can be obtained through the skin by either a large-needle or fine-needle technique. **Excisional biopsy** (removal of the tumor followed by frozen-section examination before closure of the surgical site) is the method usually chosen when clinical and mammographic evidence supports a diagnosis of cancer.

Course: An untreated breast cancer typically enlarges, invades surrounding and underlying tissues, and causes extensive cutaneous ulceration. Breast cancers spread to axillary and mediastinal lymph nodes, liver, bone, and brain. For a solitary localized tumor, the five-year survival

rate is 95% and the ten-year survival rate is 90%. The figures for disease that has become systemic before treatment is instituted are 5% and 2%, respectively. Five-year and even 10-year rates do not adequately reflect the long-term mortality of breast cancer, which is eventually the cause of death in most patients except when cancer is discovered very early by screening procedures.

Treatment: The basic treatment of breast cancer is surgical removal of the tumor. Various further procedures, including **radical mastectomy** (removal of the entire breast as well as surrounding and underlying tissues and axillary lymph nodes) may be appropriate with certain types and stages of cancer. Both radiation treatments and chemotherapy are usually administered after surgery. Radiation is not usually needed after radical mastectomy, but the procedure is mutilating and psychologically devastating. In metastatic disease, elimination of estrogen stimulation through either oophorectomy (removal of the ovaries) or administration of tamoxifen, a chemical anti-estrogen, delays progression of disease and mitigates symptoms.

Diagnostic and Surgical Procedures

amniocentesis A procedure to withdraw amniotic fluid through a needle from the uterus of a pregnant woman (Figure 12-8). The fetal cells and chemicals in the fluid are studied to identify fetal abnormalities.

basal body temperature Daily determination of oral temperature on arising is useful in confirming and dating ovulation. Daily graphing of basal body temperature will show a rise of 0.75 to 1.0°F (0.2 to 0.5°C) approximately one day after ovulation.

biopsy Removal of tissue from the cervix, the endometrium, or another part of the reproductive system for histologic examination to identify infection, neoplasm, or other abnormality. Cervical biopsy is colposcopically directed and may involve removal of plugs of tissue with a punch-type instrument or removal of a cone of tissue including the entire squamocolumnar junction.

cesarean section (C-section) Removal of the fetus (usually term or near-term) surgically though an incision in the abdomen and uterus.

colposcopy Examination of the cervix with an illuminated low-power microscope, which facilitates identification of suspicious cervical lesions requiring biopsy.

conization of the cervix Removal of a cone of tissue from the cervix for microscopic examination.

culdoscopy Endoscopic inspection of the cul-de-sac (pouch of Douglas), the lowermost part of the peritoneal cavity, which lies between the uterus and the rectum. The instrument is introduced vaginally under anesthesia.

dilatation and curettage (D&C) Scraping of the endometrium, after stretching of the cervix with graded dilators, to obtain specimen material for the diagnosis of endometrial disease. This procedure, performed under anesthesia (general, spinal, or intravenous), is also used therapeutically for various endometrial disorders.

hysterectomy Surgical removal of the uterus.

hysterosalpingogram A test to assess infertility in which radiopaque dye is injected into the uterus and fallopian tubes, and x-rays are taken to show if the tubes are patent (clear) or obstructed.

laparoscopy Inspection of pelvic viscera through a laparoscope, a tubular instrument with illumination and magnification, inserted through a small incision in the abdominal wall. Minor surgical procedures can be performed through the instrument (Figure 12-9).

mammogram X-ray of the breasts. Used as a screening test in large numbers of women, particularly those over age 40, to detect breast carcinomas.

Marshall-Marchetti-Krantz (MMK) procedure An operation for urinary stress incontinence, performed retropubically.

oophorectomy Surgical removal of an ovary.

salpingectomy Surgical removal of a uterine tube.

sonogram See *ultrasound*.

tubal ligation Surgical division of the uterine tubes to obtain sterility.

ultrasound The use of sound waves to assess tumors of the ovaries, uterus, breast, as well as the fetus in a pregnant woman.

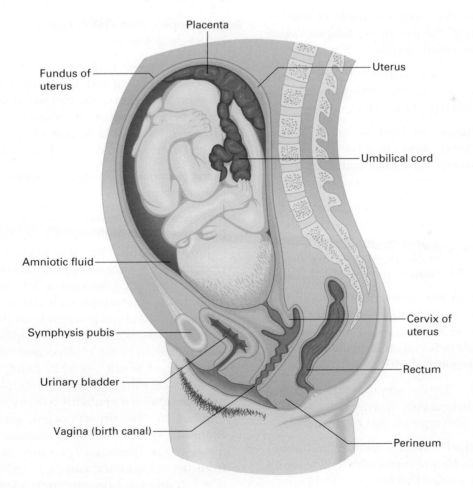

Placenta

Fundus of uterus

Uterus

Umbilical cord

Amniotic fluid

Symphysis pubis

Cervix of uterus

Urinary bladder

Rectum

Vagina (birth canal)

Perineum

Figure 12-8
Anatomy of Pregnancy

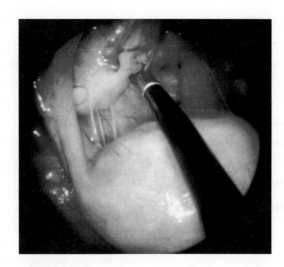

Figure 12-9
Removal of Adhesions Between the Uterus and
Ovary During Laparoscopic Procedure

Laboratory Procedures

beta HCG See *HCG*.

Candida albicans A yeastlike fungus capable of causing superficial infection in the mouth (thrush) or vagina and on the skin. Also called monilia.

Chlamydia trachomatis A gram-negative intracellular bacterium that causes sexually transmitted infections of the genital tract and other types of infection.

chocolate agar A culture medium containing blood which, when autoclaved, turns chocolate brown. It is used to culture *Neisseria gonorrhoeae* and *Haemophilus influenzae*.

Coombs test, direct A test to determine whether the patient's red blood cells have become coated with an antiglobulin. The test is positive in newborns with hemolytic disease due to Rh incompatibility and in others with acquired hemolytic disease.

Coombs test, indirect A test to determine whether the patient's serum contains antiglobulin to red blood cells. This test is positive in the mother of an infant with hemolytic disease due to Rh incompatibility and in others with acquired hemolytic disease.

dark-field microscopy A microscopic technique using special lighting that makes it easier to identify *Treponema pallidum*, the organism that causes syphilis.

estradiol The principal estrogen (female hormone) secreted by the ovary. Measurement of its level in serum gives an estimate of ovarian function.

FSH (follicle-stimulating hormone) A hormone secreted by the anterior pituitary gland that stimulates ovulation in women and spermatogenesis in men. Measurement of serum FSH is part of the evaluation of a patient for infertility or gonadal dysfunction.

FTA (fluorescent treponemal antibody) test An indirect immunofluorescence test, highly specific for syphilis.

Gardnerella vaginalis A gram-negative organism, formerly called *Haemophilus vaginalis,* which causes bacterial vaginosis.

HCG, hCG (human chorionic gonadotropin) A hormone produced by the placenta and detected in various blood and urine tests for pregnancy. A more specific test detects only the beta subunit of this hormone, hence the term beta-HCG.

Haemophilus vaginalis Older name for *Gardnerella vaginalis.*

herpes simplex virus (HSV) type 1 The herpesvirus that causes cold sores, pharyngitis, conjunctivitis, and some skin infections.

herpes simplex virus (HSV) type 2 The herpesvirus that causes genital herpes.

luteinizing hormone (LH) A hormone produced by the anterior pituitary gland. In women it stimulates ovulation and formation of the corpus luteum, and in men it stimulates production of androgens in the testicle. Measurement of LH is part of the evaluation of a patient for infertility or gonadal dysfunction.

Neisseria gonorrhoeae The gram-negative diplococcus that causes gonorrhea.

Pap (Papanicolaou) smear Removal of superficial cells from the vagina and cervix for cytologic examination, to judge hormonal effect and to identify abnormal cell changes due to inflammation, infection, dysplasia, or actual malignancy. Specimens are taken from three areas: 1) the vaginal vault, with a flat wooden spatula; 2) the squamocolumnar junction (transition line between the squamous epithelium of the vagina and the columnar epithelium of the endocervical canal), with a specially shaped wooden spatula (Ayre spatula); 3) the endocervical canal, with a bristle brush to ensure sampling of columnar epithelial cells. Interpretation of the Pap smear, usually reported according to the **Bethesda system**, includes assessment of the adequacy of the specimen (presence of columnar cells from the endocervical canal); detection of hormonal effect (estrogen, progesterone); identification of inflammatory or degenerative changes in cells; and identification of dysplastic or malignant changes in cells. Often infections (candida, trichomonas, herpes simplex, human papillomavirus) can also be reliably detected.

pregnancy test   See *HCG.*

RPR (rapid plasma reagin) Test for antibody to *Treponema pallidum.* Used in the diagnosis of syphilis.

semen analysis Examination of semen to determine the number, shape, and motility of spermatozoa as a part of an infertility evaluation.

smear and culture Microbiologic study of secretions or other materials from the cervix, vagina, urethra, rectum, or from superficial lesions, to identify causes of infection.

spinnbarkeit When the estrogen level is high but the progesterone level is low (the conditions existing just before and just after ovulation), a specimen of cervical mucus can be drawn out into strings or strands several centimeters in length. This property is called **spinnbarkeit** (German, "ability to be drawn out into a string"). When both estrogen and progesterone are present in large amounts, cervical mucus loses this property, and attempts to draw it out into a string fail.

spirochete A spiral-shaped bacterium. The organisms that cause syphilis and Lyme disease are spirochetes.

STD screen Sexually transmitted diseases screen.

STS (serologic test for syphilis) A general term referring to any test used to identify syphilis by a serologic method.

Thayer-Martin agar A culture medium containing denatured blood and antibiotics, intended to facilitate the growth of *Neisseria gonorrhoeae.*

TPI (*Treponema pallidum* immobilization) A diagnostic test for syphilis.

Treponema pallidum The spirochete that causes syphilis.

Trichomonas vaginalis A protozoan parasite that causes vaginitis.

Tzanck smear A stained smear of material from a cutaneous or mucosal lesion, intended to identify changes due to viral infection from herpes simplex or varicella.

VDRL (Venereal Disease Research Laboratory) A serologic test for syphilis.

yeast A one-celled fungus; often used interchangeably with *Candida albicans.*

Pharmacology

Drugs used to treat women with obstetric and gynecologic problems include drugs for infertility and vaginal infections, drugs that stimulate or suppress labor contractions, drugs that correct menstrual disorders and endometriosis, estrogen replacement therapy, and prophylactically prescribed birth control agents. Few drugs are prescribed during pregnancy, particularly during the first trimester, due to the increased risk of birth defects. However, antibiotics for infections and drugs to maintain good health (such as insulin or heart medications), as well as prenatal vitamins, iron, and folic acid, are given.

Ovulation-stimulating drugs for infertility.
These drugs block estrogen receptors on the ovary so estrogen cannot enter. The ovary responds to the lack of estrogen by signaling the pituitary gland that estrogen levels are low, and then the pituitary gland secretes luteinizing hormone (LH) and follicle-stimulating hormone (FSH). These hormones stimulate a nonovulating ovary to develop an ovarian follicle and release mature eggs. These drugs also aid in the formation of the corpus luteum, which secretes progesterone to maintain the pregnancy if the egg is fertilized.

Ovulation-stimulating drugs are appropriate for patients with anovulation (failure to ovulate), but are not appropriate for patients with infertility due to blocked uterine tubes or other mechanical problems that require surgical intervention.

> choriogonadotropin alfa (Ovidrel)
> clomiphene (Clomid, Serophene)
> follitropin alfa (Gonal-F)
> follitropin beta (Follistim)
> human chorionic gonadotropin (HCG or hCG)
>   (A.P.L., Pregnyl, Profasi)
> menotropins (Humegon, Pergonal, Repronex)
> sermorelin (Geref)
> urofollitropin (Fertinex, Metrodin)

Note. Clomid can be used alone, but menotropins and urofollitropin must be given concurrently with HCG to achieve a complete therapeutic effect.

Uterine relaxants.
Premature or preterm labor and delivery greatly increase morbidity and mortality in infants. Premature labor contractions can be inhibited by using uterine-relaxing drugs that act on beta$_2$ receptors in the smooth muscle of the uterus. These drugs are known as **tocolytics** (from the Greek words *tokos* "childbirth," and *lysis* "to release"). The relaxant ritodrine (Yutopar) decreases both the frequency and strength of contractions.

Uterine stimulants. Women in labor may be given a uterine stimulant if their uterine contractions are too weak to effect delivery (uterine inertia) or if complications such as preeclampsia or diabetes necessitate induction of labor. Normally, oxytocin (Pitocin), produced by the pituitary gland, stimulates the uterus by binding to special oxytocin receptors in the uterine muscle. Oxytocin as a drug increases both the frequency and strength of uterine contractions.

Oxytocin is not indicated when prolonged labor is due to cephalopelvic disproportion—the baby's skull is too large to fit through the mother's pelvic outlet.

> hexoprenaline (Delaprem)
> oxytocin (Pitocin, Syntocinon)

Labor is composed of uterine contractions as well as cervical dilatation (widening) and effacement (thinning). When the cervix does not dilate and thin, dinoprostone (Cervidil, Prepidil) may be applied topically to the cervix to ripen it.

Postpartum bleeding is due to uterine relaxation, which results in increased bleeding at the site of placental separation. Drugs used to treat postpartum bleeding include:

> carboprost (Hemabate)
> ergonovine (Ergotrate)
> methylergonovine (Methergine)
> oxytocin (Pitocin, Syntocinon)

Drugs used to treat endometriosis. Endometriosis develops when tissue from the uterus implants within the pelvic cavity and on the ovaries and other organs. It remains sensitive to hormonal influences, shedding blood when the uterus begins menstruation. Endometriosis causes pelvic pain, inflammation, and cyst formation. After hormonal drugs suppress the menstrual cycle for several months, endometrial implants may atrophy. Hormonal drugs used to treat endometriosis include:

> danazol (Danocrine)
> goserelin (Zoladex)
> leuprolide (Lupron Depot)
> nafarelin (Synarel)
> norethindrone (Aygestin)

Oral contraceptives. Birth control pills exert a hormonal influence to prevent pregnancy and are 95% effective if taken as directed. Most oral contraceptives contain a combination of estrogen and progestin that is taken for 21 days. During the final seven days of the 28-day menstrual cycle, the patient may take no tablets, seven sugar-filled tablets, and seven sugar tablets with iron (Fe). Other oral contraceptives contain only progestin.

Combination oral contraceptives that contain both estrogen and progestin are divided into three basic groups according to the relative amounts of progestin and estrogen provided during each day of the menstrual cycle. These three basic groups of combination oral contraceptives include monophasics, biphasics, and triphasics.

Monophasic oral contraceptives provide fixed amounts of progestin and estrogen in each tablet for each day of the 21-day period. The amounts of progestin and estrogen are designated by two numbers in the trade name of the drug. Example: Norinyl 1+50 contains 1 mg of progestin and 50 mg of estrogen in each tablet. Because an increased incidence of side effects (particularly thrombophlebitis) has been associated with higher estrogen dosages, a physician may elect to prescribe Norinyl 1+35, which contains 1 mg of progestin and just 35 mg of estrogen in each tablet.

Demulen 1/50	Demulen 1/35
Loestrin 1.5/30	Loestrin 1/20
Norinyl 1+50	Norinyl 1+35
Ortho-Novum 1/50	Ortho-Novum 1/35

Lunelle provides a fixed amount of progestin and estrogen in a once-monthly injection. Ortho Evra is a transdermal patch drug that provides a fixed amount of progestin and estrogen. NuvaRing provides a fixed amount of progestin and estrogen in a vaginal ring.

Biphasic oral contraceptives provide a fixed amount of estrogen in every tablet for each day of the 21-day period; the amount of progestin is fixed in the first half of the cycle but then increases in the second half of the cycle. This change is designated by two numbers following the trade name. Example: Ortho-Novum 10/11 provides 0.5 mg of progestin and 35 mg of estrogen in each tablet for the first 10 days; for the final 11 days, each tablet contains 1 mg of progestin and 35 mg of estrogen.

Triphasic oral contraceptives provide a fixed amount or slightly varying amount of estrogen for each day of the 21-day time period, while the amount of progestin increases or varies throughout that time. This is designated, at least in the case of Ortho-Novum, by the numbers 7/7/7 which show that the amount of progestin increases every 7 days. Other drugs in this category have the prefix *tri-* in their trade names to indicate the three phases of different dosages of progestin in the 21 days.

> Cyclessa
> Estrostep Fe, Estrostep 21
> Ortho-Novum 7/7/7
> Ortho-Tri-Cyclen

Tri-Levlen
Tri-Norinyl
Triphasil
Trivora-28

Contraceptives that contain only progestin are slightly less effective in preventing pregnancy than combination contraceptives, particularly if the patient forgets to take even one daily tablet. However, the risks (particularly thrombophlebitis) and other side effects of estrogen therapy due to combination oral contraceptives are avoided. Progestin-only contraceptives are taken orally, given by injection, implanted under the skin, or inserted into the uterus.

medroxyprogesterone (Depo-Provera)
Micronor
Mirena
Nor-QD
Ovrette
Progestasert

Two progestin-only drugs are taken in two doses after intercourse to prevent pregnancy: Plan B and Preven.

Drugs used to treat irregular menstruation.

Primary hypothalamic amenorrhea, the absence of menstruation due to decreased levels of gonadotropin-releasing hormone (GnRH), may be treated with a drug that stimulates the release of luteinizing hormone (LH) and follicle-stimulating hormone (FSH) from the pituitary gland. A special pump is needed to administer the drug IV in pulses that mimic the natural release of GnRH from the pituitary gland. Example: gonadorelin (Lutrepulse).

Amenorrhea and abnormal uterine bleeding may also be treated with progesterone-like drugs that act directly on the tissues of the endometrium to restore a normal menstrual cycle.

hydroxyprogesterone (Hylutin)
medroxyprogesterone (Amen, Cycrin, Provera)
norethindrone (Aygestin)
progesterone (Crinone)

Combination estrogen/progestin drugs used to treat irregular menstruation include Premphase and Prempro.

Spotlight on

Kits and Caboodle

by Judith Marshall

I had been sitting in the doctor's waiting room for over an hour. The phones rang incessantly with that electronic warbling toodle-toodle-toodle. A sound system jangled hard rock. Three secretaries at the carousel-like desk tried to chew gum and calm the patients at the same time. I was as unhappy as a squalling infant on a well-baby visit. Finally, one of the secretaries screeched my name, "JU-DEE, JU-DEE, JU-DEE. The doctor is ready for you." They all think they are Cary Grant. Not a quiet "Mrs. Marshall" with a smile, but that odious nickname. "Oh, what's the use," I thought, "at least the waiting is over."

No, it wasn't. They got me with the old beauty shop trick. When the operator is running late, someone shampoos the patron, who then waits some more, under a soggy, dripping towel. The doctor's office is worse. I was deposited in a cold, barren examining room, to sit shivering in a paper dress.

I waited another 20 minutes, staring at the stirrups and contemplating the sort of weapon they would make. The doctor bounded in with a cheery, "How are we today?" "We are

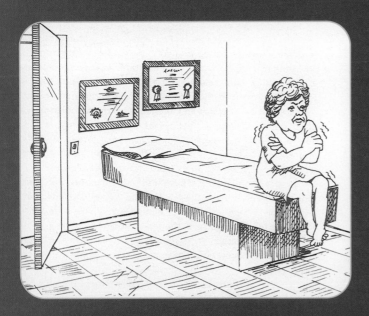

furious," I replied and told him why. He mumbled something about delays in surgery. "You're not a surgeon, Henry," I said. "All you've cut in fifteen years is roses from that garden of yours. But you are doing more overbooking than the airlines." A thorough annual physical examination was conducted in silence.

A few days later, one of the secretaries stopped filing her nails long enough to send me a letter. The Pap test specimen did not have enough cells. It was just a technical problem with the slide, and would I just pop in soon and have the test redone?

No wonder do-it-yourself medicine is flourishing. The diagnostic home testing kits must have been invented by people who sat around in paper dresses freezing their tail feathers. The manufacturers' incentive includes a market of over $300 million.

The educated consumer has come a long way from eating garlic and applying potato poultices (apologies to my grandmother), even if the chicken soup still works. Many people are fascinated by space travel, nuclear energy, and CAT scanners. I am more excited about Pampers, tampons, Velcro closures, and anything made with Gore-Tex. Women are always mopping something up. I adore those little twisty things that close bread wrappers and dog cookie bags. I went wild over the yellow stickies for scribbling (known by the pompous name of removable self-stick notes). Kiss your paper clips goodbye and join the 21st century.

The frustration with traditional healthcare delivery systems and the ferocious cost in time and money led me to the shiny local drugstore, a wonderland of self-help tools. The first thing I bought was a pill splitter for six dollars. Why nick my precious pinkies, pulverize the pills, or have them shatter all over the floor? Then I bought a fancy blood pressure tester. It is lightweight, compact, and has batteries and a digital clock. I will take it to transcription, and after the chief of orthopedics finishes his usual screaming, we can all take our pressure and monitor and adjust our medication, although some of my colleagues long to monitor and adjust the mouth of the chief of orthopedics. He has not been the same since his malpractice insurance increase.

There were two ovulation prediction tests on the shelf costing from $25 to $40 with 85-99% accuracy. The happy consumer knows when magic time is approaching, not afterward. All right, this is not romance with roses and champagne, but for over four million couples with fertility problems, it is a shot at heaven. When a lot of us were trying to keep our spouses out of the 1961 military draft (Vietnam was really heating up), all we had was a ridiculous chart and a roulette game with a thermometer I could never read anyway. The next thing I knew I was on a bus for visiting day at Fort Knox. I think a gypsy, wearing a kerchief and golden earrings, could have made a better set of predictions with a pack of cards.

The new thermometers are fabulous. One has the exact temperature visible in huge green digital numbers, instantaneously. This sure beats sitting on a squirming, screaming child whose forehead is hot, trying to keep a standard thermometer in place in any orifice handy. Ditto the crabby husband who can locate the break in 8,000 miles of pipe but can't find the underside of his tongue for a few minutes. In the future I predict human beings will have a built-in pop-up thermometer, just like a turkey. (Where to implant it?) As soon as the body temperature reaches 100°F, bingo!

There are tests to determine pregnancy, quickly and effectively. There is a privacy and an immediacy to these top sellers, and a blessing for rabbits everywhere. Women don't need

surprises or guesswork. They need fast, reliable, straightforward positives or negatives. The drug companies seem to have more faith in a woman's sense and ability to perform a test than the doctor who purses his lips and says, "Why not settle down and relax, Janie dear; it's probably just your nerves. If these so-called symptoms persist, call me in two weeks. You are just like your mother, so high-strung. Don't waste your money on a silly lab gimmick to use at home. It's much too complex for that pretty little mind of yours."

Alas, just when science discovers birth control pills and penicillin, "safe sex" remains elusive. AIDS, chlamydia, and herpes fester in our highly mobile, less inhibited population. "What a wonderful anniversary, my darling. I love you madly, but before we get cozy by the fire, let's step into the bathroom so I can run a few tests."

While there is nothing as effective as an actual blood-drawing kit, science is working on it. The blood glucose monitoring kits help diabetics every day, and don't the dieters just whoop with joy when those Ketostix turn purple! Early colon cancer, our national obsession, now can be tested on the Hemoccult card and routinely mailed back to the doctor's office. This leads me to speculate on the ever-increasing amounts of what the post office is delivering in addition to the junk mail.

I want to buy a program for my computer with questions and answers found on the routine history and physical. The system would utilize the information and apply the appropriate diagnosis, a magnificent Compusearch to call my own, or we could name it "Narcissus." The machine would spit out an FDA-approved prescription, I could take the scrip to the pharmacist and fulfill my destiny. "Consumer, heal thyself." Think of it, a hypochondriac's paradise.

Where does all this leave the beleaguered physician, besides setting broken bones, applying leeches, and staying out of surgical malpractice cases? I asked Belkin what he thought. "Self-help methods are great, Mrs. M. I got rid of my medical transcriptionist. All I do now is dictate, plug the tape into a computer, and it prints out perfect dictation. Eliminates the middle person. You see, I bought this new kit. . . ."

Source: Judith Marshall, *Medicate Me*, illustrated by Cindy Stevens

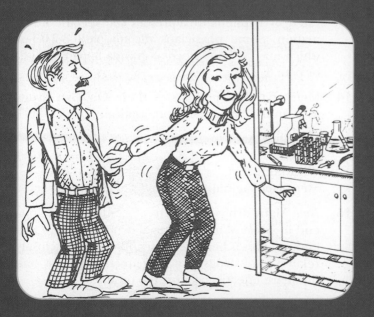

TRANSCRIPTION**TIPS**

1. Memorize these hard-to-spell Ob/Gyn terms.

   cornua, cornual
   cul-de-sac (hyphens mandatory)
   cystosarcoma phyllodes
   endometriosis
   menarche
   menstruation (*not* menestration)

2. *Pap smear* is an acceptable brief form for *Papanicolaou smear*.

3. The term *adnexa* refers to the uterine tubes and ovaries. The term is plural and takes a plural verb. ("The adnexa are unremarkable.")

4. The abbreviation *VBAC* (acronym for *vaginal birth after cesarean section*) is often pronounced "vee-back."

5. Both *hystero-* and *metro-* come from Greek words meaning *uterus*.

6. The slang term *primip* (sounds like "prime-ip") should be transcribed as *primipara* and *multip* as *multipara*.

7. The terms *gravida* and *para* are used to describe a woman's reproductive history. The pregnant uterus is said to be a *gravid* uterus.

8. The term *parous* (*not* "Paris") describes a woman who has given birth either vaginally or by cesarean section after the 20th week of gestation; *parity* is the number of such deliveries.

9. *Gravida*, followed by a number, refers to the number of pregnancies the patient has had, including ectopics, hydatidiform moles, abortions (either spontaneous or surgical), and normal pregnancies.

10. *Para*, followed by a number, refers to the number of deliveries after the 20th week of gestation (live or stillbirth, single or multiple, vaginal or cesarean) and does not correspond to the number of infants. A woman who has had only one pregnancy—even if she delivers twins or quintuplets—is still gravida 1, para 1. If she had an ectopic pregnancy and an abortion (less than 20 weeks'

gestation) prior to a delivery, she will be gravida 3, para 1.

11. *Para* may be expressed as a single number, or it may be a four-digit number, with each digit representing a particular type of birth. The first number indicates term infants; the second, premature infants; the third, abortions or miscarriages; and the fourth, the number of living children. Both of the following examples refer to the same patient.

    The patient is gravida 6, para 3 (6 pregnancies, 3 live births).

    The patient is gravida 6, para 2-1-0-3 (6 pregnancies, 2 term infants, 1 premature infant, 0 miscarriages = 3 live births).

12. Another example: A woman who is para 0-3-0-2 could have had three separate pregnancies resulting in premature deliveries, of which two children are now living, or she could have had triplets in one delivery with two living children, or even one premature and one twin premature delivery with two living children. Confused? Remember it this way. **FPAL** (Florida Power and Light): **F**ull-term deliveries, **P**remature (preterm) infants, **A**bortions, and **L**iving children.

13. Another method of documenting obstetrical history is an index called **GPMAL**. The letters refer to **G**ravida, **P**ara, **M**ultiple births, **A**bortions, and **L**ive births, and are expressed in numbers separated by hyphens to represent the specific information. Some physicians dictate para 3-2-0-1-2, which may be transcribed as gravida 3, para 2-0-1-2, or para 3, 2-0-1-2.

14. Memorize the spellings of these Ob/Gyn drugs with unusual internal capitalization.

    MICRhoGAM
    RhoGAM
    WinRho SDF
    MetroGel-Vaginal

15. *Note*: Many drugs used to treat candidal infections end in *-azole*. Many antifungal drugs also have this ending. This is because yeast and fungi are closely related, and drugs that are effective against one often are effective against the other.

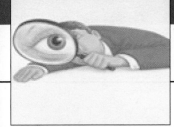

Proofreading Skills

Instructions: In the paragraphs below, circle the errors. Identify misspelled and missing medical and English words and punctuation errors, and write the correct words and punctuation in the numbered spaces opposite the text.

1   FINAL DIAGNOSIS   1 _____

2   1. Intrauterine pregnancy, deliverd.   2 delivered _____

3   2. Paraurethral tear.   3 _____

4   4 _____

5   HISTORY AND PHYSICAL   5 _____

6   This is a 27 year old secundigravida at term with blood   6 _____

7   type A-positive who had a pregnancy complicated   7 _____

8   except for some first trimester bleeding. She was admit-   8 _____

9   ted after 5 hours of good labor and was brought to the   9 _____

10   delivry room complete and pushing with membranes   10 _____

11   still intact. Spontaneous rupture of membranes ocurred   11 _____

12   only one minute prior to delivery. The delivery was very   12 _____

13   rapid, though well controlled, and resulted in a   13 _____

14   superficial paraurethral and labial tear which did not   14 _____

15   reqire suturing. No episiotomy was required. The   15 _____

16   infant was suctioned well on the perineum. Blood loss   16 _____

17   was minimal, and both mother and infant were stabel   17 _____

18   following delivery.   18 _____

19   19 _____

20   HOSPITAL COURSE   20 _____

21   Large urterine clots were expressed the first postpartum   21 _____

22   day, and the initial postpartum CBC reveeled a white   22 _____

23   count of 18.5 with 55 segs, 17 bands, and 23 lymphs.   23 _____

24   24 _____

25   The patient remained afebrile with a temp of 98.6 but   25 _____

26   had minimal uterine tenderness, and in light of the   26 _____

27   elevated white count, she was begun on ampicillin   27 _____

28   500 mg q.i.d. for a 10-day course. She was dischraged in   28 _____

29   stabel condition. Activity and diet as toleratd.   29 _____

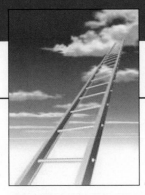

SkillsChallenge

Medical Terminology Matching Exercise

Instructions: Match the definitions in Column A with the terms in Column B.

Column A

1. ___ uterus
2. ___ incision made in perineum prior to delivery
3. ___ woman in her first pregnancy
4. ___ gradual end of menses
5. ___ (uterine) tubes
6. ___ vagina
7. ___ ovary
8. ___ fibroid cyst of uterus
9. ___ female
10. ___ onset of menstruation
11. ___ implantation of fertilized egg in uterine tube
12. ___ premature separation of placenta from uterine wall

Column B

A. menopause
B. menarche
C. colpo-
D. episiotomy
E. gyneco-
F. primigravida
G. leiomyoma
H. hystero-
I. abruptio placentae
J. oophor-
K. ectopic pregnancy
L. salpingo-

Drug Matching Exercise

Instructions: Match the drug names in Column A with the drug category in Column B. *Note*: Drug categories are used more than once.

Column A

1. ___ Demulen
2. ___ Pergonal
3. ___ Ortho-Novum
4. ___ ritodrine
5. ___ Monistat
6. ___ oxytocin
7. ___ Clomid
8. ___ Norinyl
9. ___ Gyne-Lotrimin
10. ___ Pitocin
11. ___ Loestrin

Column B

A. Stimulates ovulation
B. Prevents uterine contractions
C. Stimulates uterine contractions
D. Oral contraceptive
E. Treats vaginal yeast infections
F. Uterine relaxants

Abbreviations Exercise

Instructions: Define the following Ob/Gyn abbreviations. Then memorize both abbreviations and definitions to increase your speed and accuracy in transcribing Ob/Gyn dictation.

ASC-US _____
D&C _____
EDC _____
FSH _____
GC _____
HCG _____
HGSIL _____
IUD _____
LGSIL _____
LH _____
LMP _____
NSVD _____
PID _____
PMS _____
STD _____
TAH-BSO _____
TVH _____
VBAC _____

Soundalikes Exercise

Instructions: Circle the correct term from the soundalikes in parentheses in the following sentences.

1. Cesarean section was planned because the baby was in a (breach, breech) presentation.

2. Pelvic examination revealed a (Paris, parous) os and (cervical, surgical) adenosis.

3. On (colposcopy, culdoscopy) the vulva and vagina were seen to be normal.

4. There was no free fluid or blood found in the cul-de-sac on (colposcopy, culdoscopy).

5. The patient had production of (claustrum, colostrum) immediately following delivery.

6. On examination of the breasts, there were no (discrete, discreet) nodules.

7. Examination of this 65-year-old woman reveals an absent uterus and an (atopic, atrophic, ectopic) vagina.

8. Following delivery of the 9-pound infant, the patient had a large (fissure, fistula) of the (perineal, peroneal, peritoneal) body.

9. The baby was delivered and laid momentarily on the mother's (perineum, peritoneum).

10. This grand multipara came in with complaints of "brown stuff" coming from her vagina. On examination, a rectovaginal (fissure, fistula) was found.

11. Following a Stamey urethral suspension, the patient developed a vesicovaginal (fissure, fistula).

12. The uterus was closed and placed back in the (perineum, peritoneum), and (perineal, peroneal, peritoneal) closure was accomplished with 0 Vicryl.

13. Exploration of the uterus with forceps resulted in no tissue, and (general, gentle) suction curettage was then done, yielding minimal tissue.

14. Examination of the urethra revealed a small growth, probably a urethral (furuncle, caruncle, carbuncle).

15. After the right fallopian tube was isolated, a small (knuckle, nuchal) was picked up between (loops, loupes) of suture and excised.

16. The (lochial, local) discharge subsided after the first week postpartum.

17. The infant exhibited severe caput (molding, moulding) following a lengthy delivery.

18. Multiple uterine (myelomas, myomas) were noted upon examination of the uterine fundus.

19. The baby was delivered from the (vertex, vortex) position.

Word Root and Suffix Matching Exercise

Instructions: Combine the following word roots with suffixes to form words that match the definitions below. Fill in the blanks with the medical words that you construct.

Word Root	Suffix
dys-	-itis
hystero-	-ology
gyneco-	-otomy
salpingo-	-oscopy
episio-	-ectomy
cervi-	-rrhea
meno-	
colpo-	

A. The study of the female reproductive tract

_____

B. Surgical incision into the perineum prior to childbirth

_____

C. Inflammation of the cervix

_____

D. Surgical removal of the fallopian tube

_____

E. Using a scope to visualize the vagina

_____

F. Surgical removal of the uterus

_____

G. Difficult or painful menstruation
   (*Tip:* Use 2 word roots and 1 suffix.)

_____

Dictation Exercises

Prior to transcribing the dictations, complete these activities.

1. **Using Chapter 3, Style Guide**

   a. When, according to the Style Guide, do you expand brief forms?

   b. Review the guidelines for transcribing obstetrical terms. How would you transcribe "gravida six para six oh oh six," "G one P one"?

   c. What does the Style Guide say about punctuation within units of measure. For example, how would you transcribe "five feet six inches" or "six pounds four ounces"?

   d. According to the Style Guide, what is the proper way to make numbers plural? For example, how would you transcribe "pulse in the eighties"?

   e. Review the Numbers section of the Style Guide. How should you transcribe units of measure that accompany a numeral? What is the abbreviation for *gram, grams*?

   f. What can you do to avoid starting a sentence with a numeral?

   g. What are the recommendations in the Style Guide for transcribing ordinal numbers (first, second, third)?

   h. What part of speech is *followup*? What part of speech is *follow up*? What contextual clues may help you determine which to use?

   i. What is the symbol for percent? When is the symbol used as opposed to spelling out the word?

   j. According to the Style Guide, when it is not appropriate to use *x* for the word *times*?

   k. What are the Style Guide recommendations regarding the transcription of abbreviations?

   l. What are the style guidelines for transcribing possessive eponyms?

   m. Review the style guidelines under Capitalization for classifications and stages. How do you transcribe a "grade two over six murmur"?

   n. What is the correct abbreviation for *liters* and *milliliters*?

   o. Review the error-prone abbreviation list. What should you transcribe in place of a dictated *q.d.*?

   p. What are the style guidelines regarding the use of the ampersand (*&*)?

   q. How should possessive adjectives related to time be handled, for example, "two weeks time" or "one weeks supply"?

   r. What does the Style Guide say about expressing ranges of numbers?

   s. After dictating an admission or preoperative diagnosis, the dictator says "same" for the discharge or postoperative diagnosis. What should you do?

   t. Review the list of slang terms; how should *H&H* be transcribed? What should you do if *DC'd* is dictated?

   u. If a sentence starts with 1% Xylocaine or 0.25% Marcaine, what is the simplest way to avoid beginning the sentence with a numeral?

   v. If a dictator says "one-half percent," "one-quarter percent," or "two and a half centimeters," how should you transcribe these? (*Note*: See Metric units in the Style Guide.)

2. **Problem Solving**
   This activity is to help you prepare ahead of time for some of the problems you'll encounter in the dictations. Some of these items may not have a definitive answer but are intended to simply get you thinking about how to handle a variety of situations that are common in transcription. If nothing else, they will help you recognize a problem when you encounter it in the dictations.

   a. The doctor dictates an abbreviation that is difficult to understand. Is it *DE, BE, BNE, DNE, D&E, B&E*? What can you do to confirm that you have transcribed the correct abbreviation? What if you can't be sure—what should you do?

   b. What letters (consonants) may sound like *V* when not clearly enunciated? Which letters might sound like *N*? You think you're hearing *BIN, PIN, VIN*, but you're not sure which one it is. How do you determine which is the correct abbreviation?

   c. Say *admitted and taken to* aloud. First, say it slowly. Then, say it fast. Notice how the *d* sound at the end of *admitted* can get attached to the beginning of the word *and* that follows? Say it again fast. Does it almost sound as if there's another syllable or word between *and* and *taken*, like *anduhtaken* or *andendtaken*? This illustrates a common problem that occurs when transcriptionists have difficulty deciphering garbled or unclear dictation. Think about this problem and consider ways that you might be able to distinguish real sounds from non-sounds or spurious sounds when you're transcribing. Anticipating and identifying the problem is half the battle!

   d. A very common problem for students and practitioners alike is that dictators will often dictate an adjective without the accompanying noun. For example, instead of *Alzheimer disease*, a dictator might say *Alzheimer's*; instead of *peroneal nerve*, just *peroneal*; instead of *rectus muscle*, just *rectus*. It's rare to be able to find an adjective in the alphabetic listing in a medical dictionary because the adjectives are generally included only under the nouns they modify. If you don't know what noun is being referred to because it wasn't dictated, how can you find the adjective spelling and know that you are correctly hearing the term?

3. **Preparatory Research**

    Any information requested in these questions not readily available in your textbook (including the appendix) or required references can easily be found using Internet search engines such as Google or on-line medical dictionaries.

    a. What is the prefix meaning *before*? What medical term containing that prefix means *before birth*?

    b. Why is an alpha-fetoprotein test performed? When is the optimal time for performing this test?

    c. Define and note the spelling of the following terms: *menses, menorrhagia, dysmenorrhea*.

    d. What is a *myomectomy*?

    e. Research *endometrial ablation*. Why is the procedure performed? What are the different techniques that can be used for endometrial ablation?

    f. What is the obstetrical use for the seaweed *Laminaria*?

    g. Define *leiomyomata uteri*.

    h. What is the significance of a mother being Rh negative when the baby (or the baby's father) is not also Rh negative? How is an Rh-negative mother treated when there's a mismatch with the baby's blood?

    i. What does it mean when a physician says that a therapy or procedure is elective?

    j. What laboratory tests are done to check a patient's blood clotting time?

    k. On an abdominal exam, what is meant by *guarding* and *rebound*?

    l. What is meant by the expression *retained products of conception*?

    m. Define *follicular carcinoma* of the thyroid gland.

    n. Define *paracentesis*. For what reasons is this procedure performed?

    o. Define *mesenteric caking*. This may take some creativity; *cake* or *caking* will not be in your medical dictionary. (*Hint: Omental caking* is a related term.)

    p. Define the following: *exquisitely, introitus, candidiasis*.

    q. What are the indications for a *nonstress test* and *amniotic fluid index* determination in pregnancy? How are these tests performed?

    r. Define *oligohydramnios*. What complications of pregnancy are associated with this condition?

    s. Define the following terms: *vulvar intraepithelial neoplasia, fourchette*.

    t. Which is the correct adjectival form of vulva—vulvar or vulval? Defend your answer.

    u. What is the plural form of *condyloma*?

    v. How does Provera help control vaginal bleeding? What happens if a patient abruptly stops taking Provera?

    w. For what purpose is a *Jackson-Pratt* drain used? Define *epithelialization*. Define *ileostomy*. What would an *enterostomal therapy nursing* department do?

    x. For what purpose is a CA 125 laboratory test obtained? Is an elevated CA 125 level always indicative of cancer?

    y. Define *hydrosalpinx*. What is an *obturator*?

    z. If curettage is performed by scraping the endometrial cavity, what exactly is *suction curettage*?

    aa. Define *hyperplasia*. What implications, if any, does hyperplasia (whether it be of the endometrial or breast tissue or any other tissue) have in terms of a patient's future health? How does *hyperplasia* differ from *neoplasia*?

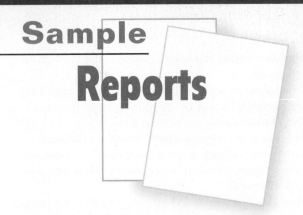

Sample
Reports

Sample obstetrics/gynecology reports appear on the following pages, illustrating a variety of reports. Fictional names are provided for illustration of proper format, and no resemblance to actual persons is intended. Sample transcripts were prepared according to the *AAMT Book of Style*, where possible.

Chart Note

CZAJKOWSKI, LAURA
17 June XXXX

SUBJECTIVE
Comes in today for annual exam. Menses are regular without intermenstrual bleeding. Her galactorrhea is unchanged. She continues to take bromocriptine 2.5 mg p.o. b.i.d. She takes chlorthalidone 50 mg daily and also daily potassium supplement. When seen a year ago she felt fatigued. Blood work at that time showed her to be hypokalemic. She resumed a potassium supplement at that time and felt much better. She has no headaches. She had some vaginal itching and discharge off and on during the summer but currently doesn't have any. She has never had a mammogram.

OBJECTIVE
Breasts without masses. There is bilateral galactorrhea. There was no axillary adenopathy. Abdomen soft and nontender. Pelvic: External genitalia are normal. Vagina rugous with a small amount of yellow discharge. Cervix clean. Uterus anterior, mobile, nontender, normal in size, shape, and consistency. Adnexa clear, nontender. Rectovaginal exam confirms. Pap smear was obtained. Wet smear is unremarkable.

ASSESSMENT
1. Long history of galactorrhea. Prolactins have been well controlled on Parlodel, as have her menses.
2. Has taken chlorthalidone daily for many years. This is for fluid retention.

PLAN
1. Parlodel 2.5 mg p.o. b.i.d. is renewed for a year.
2. Chlorthalidone 50 mg daily and potassium supplement 1 daily are renewed.
3. Serum prolactin and serum potassium levels are obtained.

FB:hpi

Operative Report

RUSSELL, KATHLEEN
#121359
Date of Operation: July 20, XXXX

PREOPERATIVE DIAGNOSIS
1. Intrauterine pregnancy, 40 weeks.
2. Arrest of descent with 3 hours pushing in 2nd stage. Failed trial of vacuum.
3. Chorioamnionitis.

POSTOPERATIVE DIAGNOSIS
1. Intrauterine pregnancy, 40 weeks.
2. Arrest of descent with 3 hours pushing in 2nd stage. Failed trial of vacuum.
3. Chorioamnionitis.

PROCEDURE
Primary low transverse cesarean section.

ANESTHESIA
Continuous lumbar epidural.

PROCEDURE
The patient became exhausted after approximately 3 hours of pushing in the 2nd stage, with descent of the vertex to +2 in the occipitotransverse (OT) position. She had been on cefotetan since developing a fever during the 2nd stage. After discussion of concerns and alternatives, it was decided to proceed with a trial of vacuum. She had a Foley catheter in place. Fetal heart tones were monitored continuously during the procedure and were stable. With placement of the vacuum over the occiput, there was absolutely no descent with two attempts at extraction with patient's efforts to push during a contraction. Attempts to continue a vaginal delivery were halted, the Pitocin augmentation was discontinued, and the intrauterine pressure catheter was removed. She was taken to the operating room after full informed consent was obtained. The epidural was adjusted for abdominal surgical analgesia.

The patient was prepped and draped in the usual manner for an abdominal procedure. A low transverse skin incision was made with a scalpel, and through a Pfannenstiel approach the peritoneum exposed and entered relatively high, with care being taken to avoid underlying bowel. The incision was extended superiorly and then inferiorly, with care being taken to avoid the bladder. Palpation revealed the vertex to be well down into the pelvis. The anterior leaf of the broad ligament was incised and the incision extended laterally in both directions and a bladder flap formed by a combination of sharp and blunt dissection. This was held out of the way with the bladder retractors, and the uterine incision was made in the midline with a scalpel. This was extended in both directions by gentle blunt traction. The vertex was found to be OT, +2 station, and well wedged into the pelvis and was removed from the pelvis with some difficulty. Once it had been elevated, the delivery of the head was accomplished with ease. Because of light meconium, the mouth and nares were suctioned on the perineum thoroughly. The shoulders and remainder of the baby were delivered without difficulty, the cord clamped and cut, and the neonate handed off to the waiting pediatrician. A segment of cord was obtained for cord blood gases. The 9 pound 5 ounce female was delivered at 0211 on July 20 and had Apgars of 9 and 9 and urinalysis with pH of 7.319.

The placenta was delivered by manual traction. A small amount of additional membrane was swept free from the anterior surface of the uterus. The uterus responded somewhat slowly to a dilute solution of Pitocin running intravenously. Inspection of the uterine incision revealed slight extension on the right and an active arterial bleeder at the left extent. This was clamped. The incision was closed with a continuous #1 chromic locking suture, beginning in the right extent of the

(continued)

RUSSELL, KATHLEEN
#121359
Date of Operation: July 20, XXXX
Page 2

incision, and was hemostatic. The second layer was a #1 chromic in a Lembert imbricating fashion. Because of a persistent bleeder at the left edge, interrupted figure-of-8 of #1 chromic was placed. Additional small bleeders were coagulated with the Bovie. The bladder flap was left open.

The uterus had been delivered after the placenta was delivered. The ovaries were both noted to be quite prominent, with decidual changes. The findings were otherwise unremarkable. The uterus was returned to the peritoneal cavity. The gutters were evacuated of a moderate amount of blood. The incision was again inspected and found to be hemostatic. The parietal peritoneum was closed with a continuous 0 chromic suture. The subfascial area was hemostatic. The fascia was closed with an 0 Vicryl beginning at each lateral margin, periodically locked and meeting in the midline. The subcutaneous tissue was irrigated and reapproximated loosely with three 3-0 Vicryl subcutaneous sutures. The skin was closed with staples. Dressing consisted of a large Band-Aid.

The Foley catheter was draining concentrated clear urine following the procedure. Pathologic specimen was the placenta for evaluation of likely chorioamnionitis. Sponge and needle counts were correct.

ESTIMATED BLOOD LOSS
1000 cc.

VALERIE RAHANIOTIS, MD

VR:hpi
d: 7/20/XXXX
t: 7/21/XXXX

History and Physical Examination

CROSCILL, MARLENE
#092431
Admitted: 5 May XXXX

CHIEF COMPLAINT
Uterine prolapse.

HISTORY OF PRESENT ILLNESS
This is a 64-year-old woman who is gravida 4, para 4, referred because of a large cystocele and uterine prolapse. The patient states that when she is on her feet, a bulge comes out of the vagina between her legs. She was found to have a large cystocele and a 2nd degree uterine prolapse, the cervix protruding through the os even with the patient lying down and when she strains. She does not have any significant problem with urinary tract control. She enters at this time for vaginal hysterectomy and anterior and posterior (A&P) repair.

PAST HISTORY
Her general health has been reasonably good. She is taking Lanoxin 0.25 mg, 1/2 tablet per day.

PHYSICAL EXAMINATION
GENERAL: A well-developed, well-nourished, slender white female at 131 pounds. Blood pressure was 130/70.
EARS: Negative.
EYES: Pupils small, react well to light. Sclerae clear.
MOUTH: I believe the patient has dentures. The throat is clear. The tonsils are absent.
NECK: Supple. No masses felt.
BREASTS: Quite good turgor for her age. No masses are felt.
LUNGS: Clear to percussion and auscultation (P&A).
HEART: Regular rhythm, no murmurs.
ABDOMEN: Soft and nontender.
GYN EXAM: There is relaxation. When the patient strains, the bladder bulges down and out and the cervix comes out through the introitus.
RECTAL: Negative. No intrinsic masses. Moderate rectocele.
EXTREMITIES: No significant deformities are noted. No edema. Reflexes are physiologic.

IMPRESSION
Second-degree uterine prolapse; cystocele with some rectocele.

PLAN
Vaginal hysterectomy, anterior repair, and possibly posterior repair at the same time.

PAUL LEI, MD

PL:hpi
D&T: 5/5/XXXX

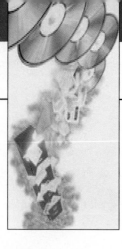

Transcription Practice

Key Words

The following terms appear in the obstetrics/gynecology dictations. Before beginning the medical transcription practice for Chapter 12, look up each term below in a medical or English dictionary and write out a short definition.

ablation
adnexal mass
candidiasis
C-section delivery
condyloma acuminatum
   (pl. condylomata
   acuminata)
D&C
ductal hyperplasia of breast

dysmenorrhea
endometrial carcinoma
fetal demise
hydrosalpinx
hypermenorrhea
ileostomy
leiomyoma uteri
lymph node dissection
menorrhagia (for ablation)

needle biopsy of breast
oligohydramnios
ovarian cancer
pelvic pain post TAB
perianal condylomata
polycystic ovarian syndrome
rectovaginal fistula

term intrauterine
   pregnancy
total abdominal hysterec-
   tomy and bilateral
   salpingo-oophorectomy
vaginal bleeding
vaginal candidiasis
VIN

After completing all the readings and exercises in Chapter 12, transcribe the obstetrics/gynecology dictations. Proofread your transcribed documents carefully, listening to the dictation while you read your transcripts.

Transcribe (*not* retype) the same reports again without referring to your previous transcription attempt. Initially, you may need to transcribe some reports more than twice before you can produce an error-free document. Your ultimate goal is to produce an error-free document the first time.

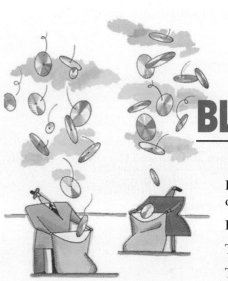

BLOOPERS

Incorrect	Correct
Periods of vaginal spotting with crabs.	Periods of vaginal spotting with cramps.
Postpartum bladder acne.	Postpartum bladder atony.
Theological test for syphilis.	Serological test for syphilis.
This Grandma Kipperus was given a sterno vaginal examination.	This grand multiparous was given a sterile vaginal examination.
The patient has had three current events.	The patient has had three term infants.
Endometrial cavity was exploded open with forceps.	Endometrial cavity was explored with open forceps.
Patient is a prime rib.	Patient is a primip.
Pelvic: Introitus, marital and tight.	Pelvic: Introitus, marital in type.
Perineum firm, ice cold.	Perineum firm, os closed.
Grabba two paira tools.	Gravida 2, para 2.
Pabst beer.	Pap smear.

Chapter 13

Orthopedics

Chapter Outline

Learning Objectives

- Describe the structure and function of the musculoskeletal system.
- Spell and define common orthopedic terms.
- Identify types of questions a physician might ask about the musculoskeletal system during the review of systems.
- Describe common features a physician looks for on examination of the back and extremities.
- Identify common diseases of the musculo-skeletal system. Describe their typical cause, course, and treatment options.

- Identify and define diagnostic and surgical procedures of the musculoskeletal system.
- List common orthopedic laboratory tests and procedures.
- Identify and describe common orthopedic drugs and their uses.
- Demonstrate knowledge of anatomical, medical, pharmacological, adjectival, and soundalike terms by accurately completing the exercises in this chapter.

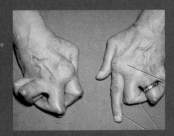
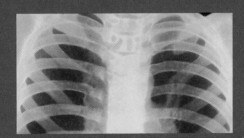
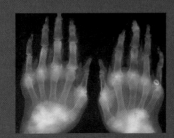

Transcribing Orthopedic Dictation

The musculoskeletal system comprises those structures that lend support and mobility to the body and that enable us to perform voluntary actions: bones, cartilage, muscles, and associated connective tissue structures (tendons, ligaments) (Figures 13-1, 13-2, 13-3).

Anatomy in Brief

Bone is a type of tissue in which a framework or matrix of organic (protein) fibers is reinforced by deposits of calcium and phosphorus salts, which provide strength and rigidity. Bone is not inert material. It has a rich blood supply, it can heal after severe injury, and its calcium content is in equilibrium with the calcium level of the blood. Most bones are covered by a dense sheet of connective tissue called **periosteum**. Each of the long bones of the extremities is divided into a **diaphysis** (shaft), an **epiphysis** (enlarged, knobby end) and a **metaphysis** (between the diaphysis and the epiphysis). **Long bones**, and some others, are hollow and contain bone marrow in their cavities. **Bone marrow** is the site of production of red blood cells, white blood cells, and platelets.

Cartilage is a noncalcified connective tissue similar to bone. In most joints, the contacting surfaces of the bones are covered by protective layers of cartilage. Some weight-bearing joints (intervertebral joints, knees) contain thick cushions of tougher cartilage (**fibrocartilage**). Cartilage also provides semirigid support for the nose, the external ear, the larynx, and the trachea and bronchi.

Muscle is a unique type of tissue that has the property of contracting (shortening) under appropriate stimulation, usually neural. The respiratory, digestive, and urinary tracts contain **smooth muscle**, which is **innervated** by (receives its nerve supply from) the autonomic nervous system and is not subject to voluntary control. The muscle of the heart is also not subject to voluntary control.

The anatomic description of each **voluntary muscle** includes mention of its shape and position, its origin (bone or other structure that serves to anchor it), insertion (bone or other structure that is moved or stabilized by the muscle), action, blood supply, and innervation. Each muscle is supplied by a nerve containing **motor fibers** (to transmit impulses from the brain and spinal cord) and **sensory fibers** (for **proprioception**, that is, perception of position and movement). Each motor nerve is attached to its muscle at a motor end-plate, where nerve impulses trigger contraction of muscle fibers.

While some muscles are attached directly to the periosteum of the bones that serve as their origin and insertion, most muscles are modified at one or both ends and equipped with **connective tissue** bands that serve for attachment to muscle. A narrow cordlike band is called a **tendon**; a broad sheetlike connection is called an **aponeurosis**. Some tendons (for example, those at the wrist and ankle) pass through tubular sheaths that act somewhat like pulleys to control direction of pull and reduce local friction. The subcutaneous tissue overlying some bony prominences (shoulder, heel) contains one or more **bursas** (purse-like cushions containing a little fluid to protect underlying surfaces and reduce friction).

A **joint** is the site at which two bones **articulate** (connect, generally in an arrangement whereby one or both can move with respect to the other). As mentioned above, the ends of bones forming a joint are usually protected by **articular cartilage** and sometimes by heavier fibrocartilage cushions (intervertebral disks, menisci of knees). The entire joint is surrounded by a capsule of **synovial membrane**, a delicate, highly vascular connective tissue that secretes a lubricating fluid in small amounts. A **ligament** is a band of inelastic connective tissue extending across the joint from one bone to the other to limit both the direction and the extent of motion at the joint. Most joints have several ligaments (the knee has 12).

Terminology Review

AK amputation Above-the-knee amputation.

ankylosis Immobility and consolidation of a joint due to disease, injury, or surgical procedure.

apophysis Bony outgrowth.

avascular necrosis Death of tissue due to loss of blood supply.

BK amputation Below-knee amputation.

bone wax Gel-like material that is exactly like wax that you would use in the kitchen. It has the ability to seal little pores in the bone that are exuding blood.

bridging Formation of a bridge from one bone to another by abnormal calcium deposition, as in osteoarthritis.

callus formation An unorganized meshwork of woven bone, which is formed following fracture of a bone and is normally replaced by hard adult bone.

cervical Pertaining to the neck.

crepitus Rubbing or grating sound.

eburnation Increased density of articular ends of bone.

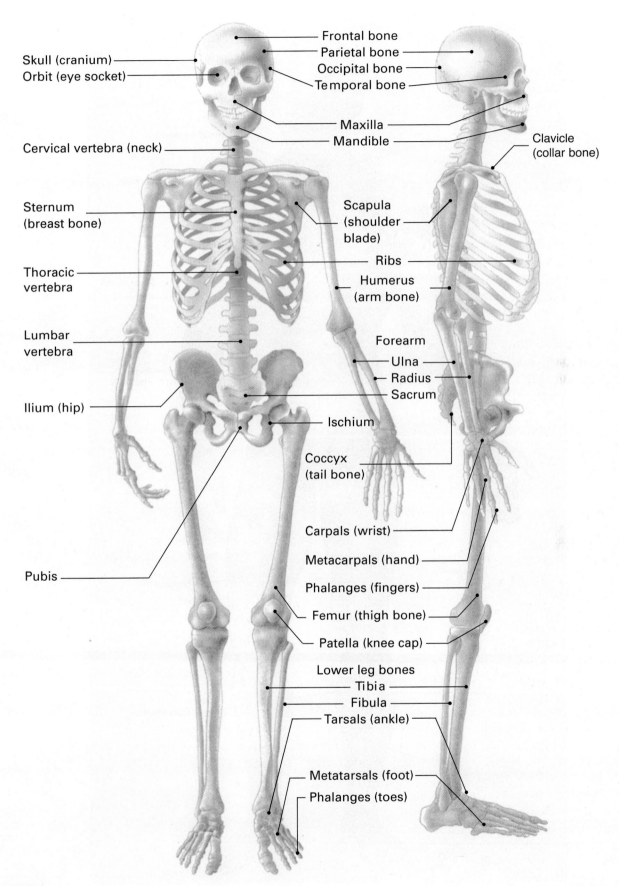

Frontal bone
Parietal bone
Skull (cranium)
Orbit (eye socket)
Occipital bone
Temporal bone

Maxilla
Mandible

Cervical vertebra (neck)

Clavicle
(collar bone)

Sternum
(breast bone)

Scapula
(shoulder
blade)

Ribs

Thoracic
vertebra

Humerus
(arm bone)

Forearm

Lumbar
vertebra

Ulna
Radius
Sacrum

Ilium (hip)

Ischium

Coccyx
(tail bone)

Pubis

Carpals (wrist)

Metacarpals (hand)

Phalanges (fingers)

Femur (thigh bone)

Patella (knee cap)

Lower leg bones
Tibia
Fibula
Tarsals (ankle)

Metatarsals (foot)

Phalanges (toes)

Figure 13-1
The Skeletal Bones

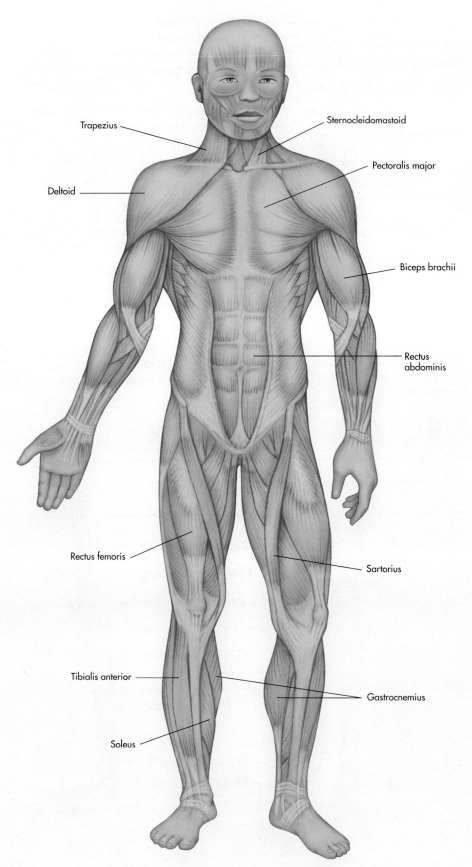

Trapezius

Sternocleidomastoid

Pectoralis major

Deltoid

Biceps brachii

Rectus abdominis

Rectus femoris

Sartorius

Tibialis anterior

Gastrocnemius

Soleus

Figure 13-2
Muscles, Anterior View

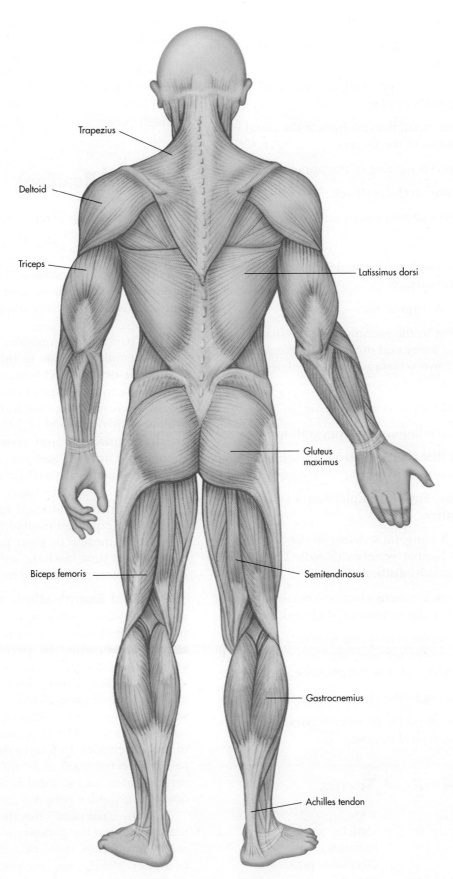

Figure 13-3
Muscles, Posterior View

epiphysis The expanded articular end of a long bone.

extra-articular Affecting or pertaining to structures other than joints.

fixation device A plate, pin, nail, or screw used to hold fracture fragments in place.

Heberden nodes Small firm nodules at the distal interphalangeal joints of the fingers.

kyphosis Forward hunching of the upper spine.

lumbar Pertaining to the midback.

NSAID Nonsteroidal anti-inflammatory drug.

osseous Bony.

osteophytes, osteophyte formation Outgrowths of bone from the surface.

rasp, raspatory A surgical file.

sacral Pertaining to the sacrum, a wedge-shaped mass of bone at the lower end of the spine that represents the fusion of five vertebrae and articulates with the pelvic bones.

scoliosis Lateral curvature of the spine.

sounds Clicking, popping, rubbing, grating.

spline Flat nail that is placed across a fracture or bone osteotomy to hold it in place.

spondylolisthesis Forward displacement of one vertebra over another.

spondylolysis A congenital defect in the pars interarticularis of a lumbar vertebra (usually L5) that predisposes to spondylolisthesis.

TENS unit Transcutaneous electrical nerve stimulator, a device used in the treatment of chronic pain.

test To locate specific orthopedic tests in a medical dictionary, look under *test, sign, maneuver,* or under the name of the test itself listed alphabetically.

thoracic Pertaining to the chest.

tophi Nodular deposits of urate crystals with local inflammation, typical in gout.

Lay and Medical Terms

ankle bone	talus
collar bone	clavicle
breast bone	sternum
elbow	olecranon process
finger bone, toe bone	phalanx
heel	calcaneus
kneecap	patella
seat bone	ischium
shin bone	tibia
shoulder blade	scapula
slipped disk	herniated nucleus pulposus
tail bone	coccyx
thigh bone	femur

Medical Readings

History and Physical Examination

by John H. Dirckx, M.D.

Review of Systems. The subject is questioned about prior diagnosis of, and treatment for, any fractures or dislocations, severe sprains, bursitis, tendinitis, or arthritis.

Most painful inflammatory conditions of the back and extremities are due to injury—either a single violent event or repeated strains of overuse. Hence the interviewer will attempt to elicit a history of trauma or unusual activities (moving furniture, sudden excessive athletic activity, change of job). Less likely possibilities are local infection and systemic disorders such as rheumatoid arthritis and gout. As with pain anywhere, an effort is made to establish a complete profile of back or extremity pain by learning its exact location, radiation, severity, intermittency, aggravating or mitigating factors, and effect on normal function. A patient complaining of muscle or joint pain will be asked about concomitant heat, swelling, stiffness, or spasm, and the effects of rest, exercise, and medicines.

Physical Examination. A full orthopedic examination requires considerable cooperation from the patient in assuming various positions and performing various movements. In performing the orthopedic examination, the physician looks for any developmental or traumatic deformities not previously noted and any evidence of generalized conditions such as muscle wasting or weakness, stiffness, or tremors. The terms *varus* and *valgus* refer to abnormal deviations in joints of the extremities. In a varus deformity, the bone distal to the affected joint is deviated inward; hence genu varum means *bowleg*. *Valgus* is outward deviation of the distal bone; hence *genu valgum* means *knock-knee*.

The physician puts joints through a passive range of motion and has the patient put them through an active range of motion, with or without resistance by the examiner. Muscles are assessed for development, bilateral symmetry, strength, tone, and spasm or tenderness. Bones are assessed for deformity, masses, or tenderness.

A **joint** is not simply the place where two bones are hooked together but a complex structure with highly specialized tissues, subject to many injuries and diseases. The physician examines joints for swelling, stiffness, thickening of synovial membranes, fluid, tenderness, and instability. The range of movement in a joint can be quantified with a **goniometer**, a simple device consisting of two arms connected at a movable joint, with a scale that reads in degrees of rotation.

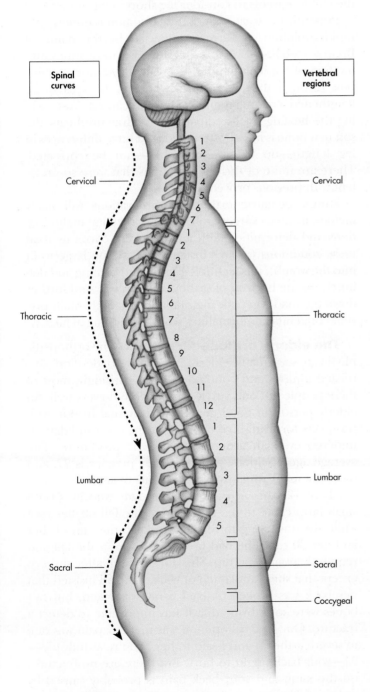

Spinal curves

Vertebral regions

Cervical
Thoracic
Lumbar
Sacral

Cervical
Thoracic
Lumbar
Sacral
Coccygeal

Figure 13-4
Spinal Curves, Vertebral Regions

In examining an injured extremity, the physician notes any swelling, deformity, cutaneous trauma, ecchymosis, or hematoma formation. The age of subcutaneous hemorrhage can be judged by its color. Muscular and skeletal structures are palpated for tenderness, spasm, deformity, or discontinuity, and active and passive ranges of motion are checked. Joints are palpated for crepitus or effusion and tested by manipulation for ligamentous laxity. The circulation and sensation of the part are also carefully evaluated.

The back (see Figure 13-4) is examined first with the subject standing and facing away from the examiner. Any spinal curvature or developmental deformities are noted, as well as any surgical scars. The heights of the iliac crests are compared as a rough test of leg length equality. The spinous processes of the vertebrae, the sacroiliac joints, and the sciatic notches are assessed by palpation for tenderness, the muscles for tenderness and spasm. The examiner notes the range of spinal movements as the subject bends forward, backward, and to the sides. The subject then lies supine (face up) on the examining table, and the physician tests for disorders of the sacroiliac and hip joints and for sciatic nerve irritation by manipulation of the lower extremities.

The neck is not simply a column for supporting the head. Through it pass all nerve connections between brain and body, all inspired oxygen and exhaled carbon dioxide, all swallowed food and drink, and all blood supply to the brain, which consumes 25% of the body's oxygen intake. Because subtle abnormalities of the neck can herald life-threatening developments, the region is carefully assessed.

The neck is subject to many musculoskeletal injuries and disorders, some of which can affect its configuration and mobility in obvious ways. The examiner tests neck mobility by gently grasping the subject's head and putting it through a range of movements, noting any restrictions due to joint stiffness, muscle spasm, or pain.

A Doctor's View

Orthopedic Practice and Surgery

by Michael A. Ellis, M.D.

Modern orthopedics can be defined as the medical discipline that deals with problems of bones, joints, and muscles. The specialty of orthopedics originally evolved to help crippled children—to correct their deformities, to make them straight. The word *orthopedic* literally means "straight child"—from the Greek *ortho-* (*straight*) and *pais* (child).

One of the most interesting facets of orthopedics is that it is a medical discipline subject to great change—change for the better, which is why I find the practice of orthopedics exciting and enjoyable. An orthopedic physician who sees ambulatory patients or outpatients in the office will recommend surgery only about one in 20 times. This average increases, of course, for the orthopedist whose caseload includes trauma victims. In a general orthopedic practice, approximately one half of patients require emergency surgery for trauma, infections, or tumors. The rest are cases in which surgery is done electively, after nonsurgical approaches to the problem are unsuccessful.

Treatment of children. A general orthopedist, whose training is about 20% in pediatric orthopedics, frequently encounters children with orthopedic difficulties. The worst of these are noticeable at birth and include such problems as clubfoot and congenital dislocation of the hip. In addition, birth trauma may result in orthopedic complications, particularly fractured clavicles.

Babies with fractures require little treatment. Their blood circulation is so efficient that one can almost see the healing process taking place. For instance, clavicular fractures occur frequently at birth but heal within four or five days, and without the use of an immobilizer. Unfortunately, our blood circulation gets steadily worse from the day of birth until we die, so that a fracture requiring only a few days to heal in a child may take six to eight weeks to heal in an adult.

Tradition once mandated that a child with clubfoot (a condition in which the foot is bent downward and inward) would receive no treatment until walking age. Frankly, the rationale for this was the blind hope that the foot would improve on its own. Even as recently as 20 years ago, treatment of clubfoot was delayed until the child was a year old, requiring an average of four operations between ages one and 15 years. Usually these attempts were unsuccessful, leaving the patient with a fused foot that would not bend normally.

Today it is recognized that surgical intervention for clubfoot should be carried out at an early age. By the time the infant is three months old, the physician is able to assess whether cast technique or nonsurgical methods will be effective in the treatment of clubfoot. If nonsurgical treatment is unsuccessful by age three months, surgery is carried out. The procedure is not performed on the newborn because the stress of anesthesia and surgery is considered detrimental and is better tolerated when the infant is older.

Children with a congenital discrepancy in leg lengths present an entirely different challenge to the orthopedic surgeon. In the past, the usual method of leg length equalization was time-consuming, debilitating, and required frequent hospitalization that often necessitated withdrawing the child from school for approximately two years. The surgery consisted of shortening the longer leg by cutting a

segment out of it. Or, if the child was still growing, staples were placed across the epiphyseal growth plate to slow the growth of that leg until the legs equalized in length.

These procedures were arduous and fraught with complications, including interruption of the blood or nerve supply to the leg. The surgery was so debilitating that it was performed only when leg length discrepancy was severe enough that amputation was the only alternative. And today, when tallness is considered a positive rather than a negative social trait, physicians cannot convince a child or the child's parents to consider leg shortening surgery.

Presently the treatment of this condition is undergoing rapid evolution. A Russian physician by the name of Ilizarov ("eh-líz-a-rov") has developed a most innovative method of leg lengthening. It involves inserting metallic pins through the leg above and below the area to be lengthened, creating a surgical fracture, and then stretching the healing fracture apart. As the fracture heals, the soft new bone is literally stretched, and huge differences in leg length—up to several inches—can be corrected. There are none of the complications that were so prevalent with previous procedures.

Future pediatric orthopedic innovations will likely include in utero surgery to correct congenital malformations and deformities. Although we can't currently treat these conditions (today's instruments are too large to fit into the womb), this technology is up and coming and definitely on the horizon of orthopedic surgery. And further down the road is genetic manipulation that will totally prevent congenital abnormalities from developing at all.

The elderly orthopedic patient. The orthopedic physician sees many elderly patients who develop age-related injuries and conditions. Yet surprisingly, most of these people not only survive surgery but do very well. An elderly person in good general and mental health, with prospects for living five or more years, is a candidate to undergo even an arduous orthopedic procedure. The average age of elderly patients in my practice is 77, and there are many who are over 100 years of age!

About 12 years ago a 94-year-old lady who lives on a small farm came to see me because she fell off her roof while she was trying to repair it to keep the rain off her and her 30 cats. She had broken her hip in the fall and required an artificial hip. She did very well after surgery, except that she complained of back pain and insisted that her back was broken. A back x-ray was taken, but her bones were so arthritic that it was impossible to detect a fracture. Our medical opinion was that her pain was due to severe arthritis, and I said to her, "You're awfully old—94—your back ought to hurt! But there are no fractures on the x-ray, and your back pain is probably caused by arthritis." Her reply was, "Oh no, Dr. Sonny" (her name for me, since I was just 38 at the time), "I know my back is broken." Three months later we took a followup x-ray, and there was the fracture!

The most prevalent surgical problem of the aged is that of stress fractures due to osteoporosis (thin and brittle bones). Older people, especially women, are not accustomed to falling; they do not employ their bodies in an agile way to prevent fractures when they fall. Complications and fractures resulting from falls are a staple of life for the aging person, especially the woman with osteoporosis.

A fallacy often repeated is that patients with osteoporotic fractures heal slowly. In actual fact, their fractures heal nearly as rapidly as those of a 30-year-old; the rate of healing for both is about the same. It is the quality of healing that is different. While the young patient heals with strong bone, the osteoporotic patient heals with bone of poor quality.

Osteoporosis is demonstrated on x-ray by bone volume loss of 50% or more. By adding up the millimeters of thickness of the bone cortices (the outer bone coatings), the sum of the two cortices should at least be equal to the diameter of the intramedullary canal. If the sum of the two cortices is one third or less the diameter of the intramedullary canal, severe osteoporosis is present. The experienced orthopedist will know at a glance if advanced osteoporosis is present on x-ray.

In addition to osteoporosis and fractures, elderly patients present with a wide variety of other orthopedic problems. Degenerative arthritis of the joints is a common presenting complaint of the elderly. In the mid-1950s, older people with hip fractures were simply put to bed—and nearly every person died within three months from pneumonia or other complications of forced bed rest, including the mental disorientation that older people experience when they are subjected to major stress.

Today, the ultimate orthopedic solution is to replace the joint, and joint replacement surgery has evolved to the point where hip, knee, elbow, and wrist joints can be replaced with quite satisfactory results. Even very elderly patients opt for joint replacement surgery when the prospect of regaining mobility and independence is offered. The death rate in orthopedic surgery of the elderly is surprisingly low—about 2%, which is actually comparable to the risk from a stroke or coronary. These statistics support the opinion that aggressive treatment for severe orthopedic problems is better than marginal treatment or no treatment.

Total hip replacement. When artificial hip surgery first came into vogue, there was only one brand of prosthesis—an artificial hip invented by Dr. Charnley of England and manufactured of stainless steel in Switzerland. Today there are many choices in hip prostheses, and the best ones are made of titanium rather than stainless steel. Titanium is durable, lighter, and its flexibility is more like that of real bone. (A metal apparatus that is rigid and cannot deflect will work its way loose or break the bone.)

Hemophilia. Why would a hemophiliac be under the care of an orthopedic surgeon? Blood contains enzymes that break down cartilage and impair the generation of lubricating material by the synovium. By the age of five, a hemophiliac child will have experienced thousands of bleeds into the joints, leading to destruction of the joints by the late teen years or early adulthood.

The high motion and weightbearing joints are the first to degenerate, beginning with the knees and usually followed by elbows, ankles, and hips. As the joints become deformed and contracted, the patient is left with only partial movement and characteristic body posture—walking on the toes with knees, elbows, and hips bent.

Osteogenesis imperfecta. More rare than hemophilia, osteogenesis imperfecta is a genetically transmitted disease of collagenous tissue that leads to fractures and disfigurement early in life. Patients with osteogenesis imperfecta are said to have "blue eyes and brittle bones." Collagen tissue in the eye is so deficient that light is able to penetrate the sclerae, revealing underlying blue veins, and thus the whites of the eyes appear blue. These patients have so many fractures that their bones often curve and shorten by the time they are young adults.

Treatment for osteogenesis imperfecta requires intramedullary rodding with multiple osteotomies—in lay terms, a "shish kebab" operation. The curved bone is rebroken in multiple places, a rod is inserted down the middle, and the bones are allowed to heal in a straightened position.

Ollier disease. Ollier disease is a rare hereditary disorder in which there is defective conversion of cartilage within bones during childhood. Bones become weakened and are subject to frequent fracturing, and there may be visible lumps of cartilage that interfere with joint fusion. A child with this condition may have dozens of these lumpy tumors, and, unfortunately, surgical removal is not a practical consideration.

Sports medicine. Sports medicine is simply good medicine applied to people who play sports. That it has become a subspecialty is inappropriate, I believe, since there are no new or different treatments offered to the sports individual that are not offered to any other orthopedic patient.

When I was the team physician for the Baltimore Bullets, a professional basketball team, I used the same medical treatment for the professional athletes as I did for my nonathlete patients. The basic difference lay not in the treatment but rather in the patient. The athlete is usually in better overall physical condition, is more motivated in getting through treatment, and in setting post-treatment goals.

Neurosurgery. In nonmetropolitan areas, spinal surgery frequently falls under the care of the orthopedist. Conversely, in larger hospitals and medical centers, neurosurgeons characteristically do all spinal surgery except for fusions and fracture repairs. I personally do fracture repairs with rods and grafts and do spinal fusions on those patients who have deteriorating disk disease. I leave the actual treatment of nerves and nerve roots to the neurosurgeons.

Orthopedics is an exciting medical and surgical specialty in an era of evolution. It is a discipline which offers much more today than it did 20 years ago, and 20 years from now will offer much more than it can today. For me, that is exciting to contemplate.

Common Diseases

Muscular Dystrophy. This term includes a number of inherited disorders of voluntary muscle tissue having various clinical features. Some begin in infancy and others in middle age; some cause death within a few years and others progress slowly and have little impact on lifestyle or life expectancy. Progressive muscular weakness and wasting of muscle tissue are features of most types of muscular dystrophy. In some types, enlargement of affected muscles (**pseudohypertrophy**) occurs. Some are associated with mental retardation or other defects. Diagnosis is made by history (including family history), physical examination, electromyography, muscle biopsy, and detection of elevated serum creatine kinase. Prenatal diagnosis is possible. Treatment is purely supportive and consists of physical therapy and regular exercise.

Scoliosis. Lateral curvature of the spine in the erect position, due to malalignment of vertebrae (Figure 13-5). Two types are recognized. **Structural scoliosis** affects the vertebrae primarily. It may be caused by bone, nerve, or muscle disease, but in 90% of cases the cause is unknown. In most of these cases a genetic cause is likely. This type of scoliosis is both commoner and more severe in women. Onset is around the age of puberty. **Nonstructural scoliosis** occurs as a result of abnormality or disease other than in the affected vertebrae. Many cases are due to significant discrepancy in leg length, which brings about a compensatory curve in the upper spine to keep the head and shoulders level.

In both types of scoliosis, there is usually some rotational deformity of the spine in addition to lateral curvature. Generally there are no symptoms at first, and

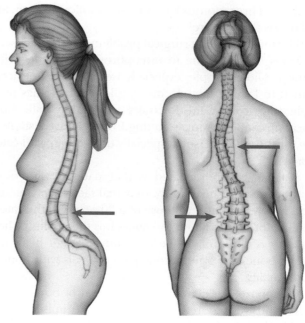

Figure 13-5
Scoliosis

detection is made on routine physical examination, chest x-ray, or school screening. Direct inspection of the back often fails to disclose mild scoliosis, especially in overweight patients. When a person with scoliosis bends forward from the waist, one side of the thorax appears more prominent than the other because of the rotatory component of the deformity. X-ray examination and measurement of the curvature is needed for precise diagnosis.

A curvature of more than 20° is considered significant, particularly because it is likely to progress. When significant scoliosis is detected before the mid-teens, vigorous efforts are made to correct it before spinal growth ceases. Correction is by bracing or casting. In severe or neglected cases, surgical fusion of the spine may be indicated. Untreated scoliosis may lead to severe deformity and disability, even compromise of cardiac and pulmonary function.

Legg-Calvé-Perthes Disease. Avascular necrosis of the head of the femur, occurring in children near the middle or end of the first decade of life. Symptoms are hip pain and limping. Imaging studies including radionuclide scan can show altered physical and chemical properties of the affected part of the femur. Spontaneous healing occurs after two or three years, but may leave the child with a badly deformed femoral head and serious hip joint malfunction. Treatment is by splinting or casting to keep the hip in abduction during weightbearing, and occasionally surgery.

Tendinitis (Tenosynovitis). Inflammation of a tendon or, more precisely, of a tendon sheath. The cause is usually repetitive or extreme strain on the tendon, as in an occupational or athletic setting. The symptoms are pain on active or passive movement of the part, localized tenderness over the tendon, and sometimes swelling and **crepitus** (grating, grinding, or crunching sounds) with movement. Disability may be severe, but spontaneous resolution usually occurs if the inciting activity can be stopped.

Treatment is with analgesics and anti-inflammatory agents, wrapping or splinting, and local heat. Injection of adrenal corticosteroid into the site of inflammation often yields prompt if temporary relief, but repeated injections may lead to complications, including rupture of the tendon.

Bursitis. Inflammation of a **bursa**, usually due to local trauma, often repetitive (kneeling on concrete, working overhead). Inflammation can also result from local infection or as an extension from an inflamed joint. Onset is typically sudden; initial symptoms are sharply localized pain and tenderness and often pronounced swelling, with **fluctuancy** (the sensation of contained fluid on palpation) due to accumulation of inflammatory fluid within the affected bursa. The diagnosis is usually evident from the history and physical examination.

If infection is suspected, the bursa must be aspirated and the fluid examined by smear and culture for pathogenic microorganisms. Treatment options include rest, immobilization if necessary, local heat, nonsteroidal anti-inflammatory drugs, local corticosteroid injections, and antibiotics for infection if present.

Common sites of bursitis are subdeltoid (near the point of the shoulder), olecranon (near the point of the elbow), prepatellar (overlying the patella; housemaid's knee), popliteal (**Baker cyst**; fluctuant swelling of the bursa behind the knee joint, which communicates with the joint space, as a result of local trauma or disease), and calcaneal (near the point of the heel).

Fibromyalgia Syndrome. A syndrome of chronic musculoskeletal pain accompanied by weakness, fatigue, and sleep disorders.

Cause: Unknown. The condition occurs almost exclusively in adult women with onset before age 50. Depression and viral infection have been proposed as underlying causes in some cases. The disorder sometimes occurs in hypothyroidism.

History: Chronic widespread aching and stiffness, typically bilaterally symmetrical and involving particularly the neck, shoulders, back, and hips, which is aggravated by use of affected muscles. Usually there are associated fatigue, a sense of weakness or inability to perform certain movements, paresthesia, difficulty sleeping, and headaches.

Physical Examination: Trigger points: sharply localized and extremely tender points, particularly in the neck and back, and often bilaterally symmetric. Some of these points may correspond to sites of pain and others may be painless until palpated. Otherwise examination is normal. There is no fever or local swelling or redness, and joints are not involved.

Diagnostic Tests: Complete blood count, erythrocyte sedimentation rate, and imaging studies yield uniformly normal results.

Course: The condition tends to be chronic, with moderate to severe disability, but symptoms can usually be mitigated by treatment. Symptoms do not progress, and objective signs of disease never develop.

Treatment: Education, exercise, physical therapy. Psychoactive medicines such as amitriptyline and chlorpromazine occasionally help.

Herniated Disk (Herniated Nucleus Pulposus, HNP; Slipped Disk). Extrusion of the soft center of an **intervertebral disk**, with symptoms due to pressure on adjacent spinal nerves.

Cause: *Predisposing cause.* Degeneration of the intervertebral disk due to aging or other pathologic process. *Precipitating cause.* Lifting or straining that puts unusual force on the disk.

History: Pain in the back or extremities, often of sudden onset and associated with lifting or straining. The pain may radiate along the course of an extremity like an electric shock and may be associated with paresthesia and hypesthesia. Movement or coughing may aggravate pain. Bowel or bladder function may be affected.

Physical Examination: There may be tenderness at the site of herniation. Neurologic examination may show impairment of deep tendon reflexes due to compression of dorsal nerve roots.

Diagnostic Tests: CT and myelography (x-ray of spine with contrast medium injected into the subarachnoid space) may show bulging or displacement of a disk. MRI is a more sensitive technique for showing herniation.

Course: Prolonged disability may occur if the condition is left untreated, although milder cases may often be asymptomatic.

Treatment: Bed rest, analgesics, and muscle relaxants usually provide symptomatic relief. With radiologic evidence of severe or progressive disease or significant neurologic impairment, **laminectomy** (cutting through the posterior arch of one or more vertebrae) and removal of herniated disk material are indicated.

Torn Meniscus. The **menisci** are crescent- or C-shaped pads of fibrocartilage within the knee joint, one medial and one lateral, that cushion shocks between the femur and the tibia. Injury to a meniscus is common and usually results from twisting the knee joint with the foot planted, often in an athletic setting. The patient hears a pop and feels sudden severe pain. Swelling develops soon, and the knee may lock or buckle with weightbearing. The medial meniscus is torn 10 times as often as the lateral meniscus. Meniscal tears do not heal. A piece broken off a meniscus remains in the joint as a **loose body** and may impair mobility.

Examination shows effusion of fluid into the joint space, crepitus, and a positive **McMurray test**: extension of the knee from full flexion with the leg and foot externally rotated causes an audible or palpable snap in medial meniscus tear; extension with the leg and foot internally rotated causes a snap in lateral meniscus tear. Treatment is with ice, elevation, a bulky compression dressing, and crutches, with attention to maintaining mobility and muscle strength and tone in the **quadriceps muscle** (the large four-headed muscle on the front of the thigh that extends the knee joint). Mild tears may eventually become asymptomatic. For persistent symptoms, **arthroscopic** (but occasionally open) **surgery** is required, with removal of loose fragments and reshaping of remaining cartilage.

Patellofemoral Syndrome. Pain in the knee, occurring most often in active teenagers or young adults, due to abnormal friction between the patella (kneecap) and the groove on the femur in which it slides. Any disturbance in the normal alignment or tracking of the patella in its groove, such as may result from uneven pull by the four heads of the quadriceps muscle, can cause chronic trauma to the back of the patella, with resultant **degenerative changes** (roughening, fraying, even complete loss of cartilage), known collectively as **chondromalacia patellae**. The principal symptom is pain with walking, especially on stairs, and with squatting.

Physical examination shows tenderness on manipulation of the patella and sometimes swelling and crepitus. X-rays are negative. Some cases resolve spontaneously with rest and anti-inflammatory medicines. **Quadriceps exercises** (repeatedly bringing the knee into full extension, with tensing of the muscles of the front of the thigh) often help to correct muscle imbalances. Shaving the roughened posterior surface of the patella arthroscopically may relieve pain. If tracking of the patella in its groove on the anterior femur is grossly deviant, surgical transplantation of the patellar tendon may be needed.

Osteoporosis. A disorder in which the density of bone is inadequate for its normal supporting function (Figure 13-6).

Causes: Resorption of calcium from bone to maintain serum calcium level, a complex phenomenon involving parathyroid hormone, intestinal and renal function, activity level, and dietary intake of calcium, phosphorus, and vitamin D. Postmenopausal deficiency of estrogen increases sensitivity of bone to factors that promote calcium loss; 80% of patients are postmenopausal women. Other causes include genetic disorders (cystic fibrosis, Marfan syndrome, osteogenesis imperfecta), endocrine disorders (diabetes mellitus, Cushing syndrome, thyrotoxicosis, hyperparathyroidism), prolonged amenorrhea in female athletes, and reduced level of mobility and physical activity because of illness, injury, or lifestyle. Asian or Caucasian race, underweight, dietary calcium deficiency, alcohol use, and cigarette smoking are all risk factors.

History: Backache, reduction of stature, **kyphosis** (forward hunching of the upper spine), **pathologic fractures** (fractures for which underlying abnormality of bone are partly responsible).

Physical Examination: Unremarkable except for features noted above.

Diagnostic Tests: X-ray examination shows bone deformity or fractures but does not reliably demonstrate minor degrees of demineralization. Bone density is more accurately assessed by CT scan, single-photon absorptiometry (SPA), dual-energy x-ray absorptiometry (DEXA), or ultrasound.

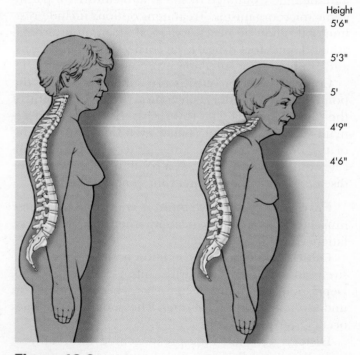

Figure 13-6
Spinal Changes Caused by Osteoporosis, Shown at 60 and 70 Years Old

Course: Osteoporosis is responsible for 50% of fractures occurring in women over age 50. Compression fractures of the vertebrae and traumatic fractures of the wrist and femoral neck are most common. Gradual collapse of vertebrae causes loss of body height and senile kyphosis. The one-year mortality after hip fracture is about 20%.

Treatment: Administration of calcium along with vitamin D and calcitonin (orally or nasally). Bisphosphonates (alendronate, etidronate) and the selective estrogen receptor modulator raloxifene improve resistance of bone to enzymatic breakdown. Men with reduced androgen levels are treated with testosterone. Physical therapy, increased mobility.

Osteomyelitis. Bacterial infection of bone.

Cause: Infection with staphylococci, streptococci, or other organisms. Bacteria may be introduced directly into bone tissue (gunshot wound, surgery, compound fracture) (Figure 13-7) or migrate there from adjacent soft tissue infection (sinusitis, deep abscess) or a remote source (systemic infections such as typhoid or tuberculosis, bacteremia in IV drug abusers). Osteomyelitis due to *Salmonella* frequently occurs as a complication of sickle cell disease and other inherited hemoglobin abnormalities.

History: Gradual or sudden onset of bone pain, fever, and chills.

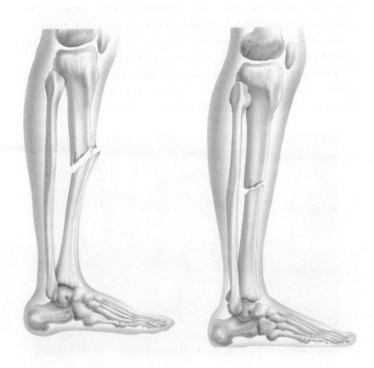

Figure 13-7
Open (Compound) Fracture, left; **Closed (Simple) Fracture**, right

Physical Examination: Fever, tenderness of site of infection. In severe infection there may be signs of toxemia.

Diagnostic Tests: The erythrocyte sedimentation rate is elevated. Causative organisms can be cultured from material aspirated from infected bone or from the blood. Serologic studies can identify infection due to *Salmonella*. X-ray or, preferably, CT and MRI studies show local swelling, decalcification, and eventually erosive destruction of bone.

Course: Without prompt treatment, infection may become chronic. Bone destruction can lead to severe deformity and disability.

Treatment: Rest, immobilization, analgesics. Antibiotics based on culture findings. Surgical drainage of the infection site. Severe or advanced disease may require radical surgical excision of infected bone (**saucerization**). Physical therapy as needed.

Arthritis. Inflammation of one or more joints. Arthritis is not just one disease but a group of many (perhaps over 200) that have joint inflammation as a common feature.

Degenerative Joint Disease (DJD; Osteoarthritis). A joint disorder characterized by degeneration of articular cartilage (Figure 13-8).

Cause: Unknown. Familial factors may be operative. Cartilage protecting articular surfaces of bones degenerates, allowing bony surfaces to touch and erode each other. Hypertrophy of bone at the affected site adds to symptoms. Onset of symptoms is typically in early middle-age. Trauma, overweight, and the presence of other orthopedic disorders in the area of the affected joint may precipitate or accelerate symptoms.

History: Gradual onset of pain and stiffness in joints, particularly the intervertebral joints, hips, and knees; pain is aggravated by activity and relieved by rest.

Physical Examination: Stiffness, crepitus, and occasional swelling of affected joints. **Heberden nodes** (small firm nodules at the distal interphalangeal joints of the fingers) may be present.

Diagnostic Tests: X-rays show narrowing of joint spaces due to destruction and wearing away of cartilage; increased density (**eburnation**) of articular ends of bone due to mutual compaction after loss of protective cartilage; and hypertrophy of bone near the joint, with formation of **osteophytes** (outgrowths of bone from the surface) variously described as beaking, lipping, and **bridging** (forming a bridge from one bone to the other).

Course: Progressive pain and stiffening of joints, with eventual deformity and disability, may occur.

Treatment: Rest, physical therapy, prescribed exercise programs, correction of underlying causes if possible, weight reduction in overweight patients, mild analgesics

Skull

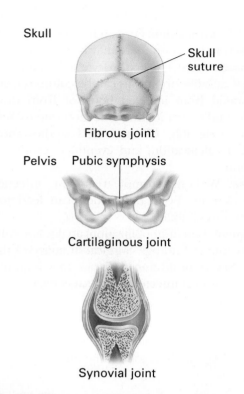

Skull suture

Fibrous joint

Pelvis Pubic symphysis

Cartilaginous joint

Synovial joint

Figure 13-8
Types of Joints

(acetaminophen). Surgical replacement of the hip or knee joint reduces pain and improves mobility.

Gout. A systemic disease with joint symptoms due to deposition of **urate crystals** (Figure 13-9).

Causes: Elevation of serum uric acid due to overproduction, impaired excretion, or both. Some forms of gout are hereditary. Signs and symptoms of gout can be precipitated by certain drugs (thiazide diuretics, nicotinic acid, low-dose aspirin), malignancies of blood-forming tissues and other disorders characterized by rapid breakdown of cellular nucleic acid, renal disease, hypothyroidism, and lead poisoning (saturnine gout). Nearly all patients are men over 40.

History: Recurrent acute episodes of severe pain, tenderness, and swelling, usually affecting a single joint, often occurring at night, and separated by symptom-free intervals. The first metatarsophalangeal joint is most often affected. After the acute episode, itching and scaling of the skin overlying the affected joint. Eventual development of nodules in soft tissues.

Physical Examination: Redness, swelling, and exquisite tenderness of the affected joint. **Tophi** (nodular deposits of urate crystals with local inflammation) may appear in cartilage (the outer ear), in tissues around joints (subcutaneous tissue, tendons), or at other sites.

Diagnostic Tests: The serum uric acid level is generally elevated, as well as the erythrocyte sedimentation rate. Microscopic examination of material aspirated from affected joints or tophi shows urate crystals. In chronic disease, x-rays may show tophi in bone as punched out (**radiolucent**) areas.

Course: Without treatment an acute attack can last for days or weeks. Chronic disease may lead to joint destruction, deformity, and disability. Uric acid kidney stones are a common complication. With advanced disease, renal failure may occur.

Treatment: An acute attack of gout is promptly aborted by nonsteroidal anti-inflammatory agents or corticosteroid. Rest and immobilization may also be important in shortening the attack. Options for prophylactic treatment between attacks include drugs that inhibit uric acid production (allopurinol) or increase its excretion (probenecid). Colchicine can also be used. Abstinence from certain foods (liver, sweetbreads, anchovies) and alcohol is usually recommended, but the impact of dietary restrictions is minimal in a patient taking adequate doses of prophylactic medicine.

Rheumatoid Arthritis. A chronic systemic disease causing inflammatory changes in many tissues, particularly joint membranes.

Cause: Formation of antibody to one's own tissues, particularly synovial membranes. About 1-2% of the population are affected, and the disease is three times more common in women. It tends to run in families. Onset is typically between 20 and 40 and may be triggered by emotional or physical stress, surgery, or childbirth.

History: Gradual onset of pain, stiffness, and warmth in joints, particularly smaller joints (proximal interphalangeal and metacarpophalangeal joints, wrists, knees,

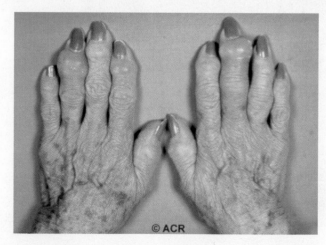

Figure 13-9
Gout of the Interphalangeal Joints

ankles, and toes). Stiffness is worse in the morning (**"jelling"**). Malaise, fever, and weight loss may accompany the onset of the disease.

Physical Examination: Tenderness, warmth, stiffness of affected joints. Enlargement and deformity of joints, including ulnar deviation of finger joints, may occur late. About 20% of patients have subcutaneous nodules over bony prominences on extremities.

Diagnostic Tests: The erythrocyte sedimentation rate is elevated. A mild anemia is common, and platelets may be increased. Testing for rheumatoid arthritis (RA) factor is positive in about 75% of patients, and for antinuclear antibody in about 20%. Serum protein studies may detect an increase in immune globulin. X-rays are normal early in the disease but eventually show osteoporosis of bone near affected joints, erosion of joint surfaces, and narrowing of joint spaces.

Course: In as many as one half of all patients, symptoms remit largely or completely within two years. Patients in whom symptoms continue may have intermittent or persistent pain and stiffness, with increasing deformity and fusion of affected joints. Extra-articular manifestations include pericarditis, pleurisy with effusion, lymphadenopathy, splenomegaly, vasculitis, dry mouth and eyes (**Sjögren syndrome**), and peripheral nerve entrapment problems such as **carpal tunnel syndrome**.

Treatment: The standard treatment is aspirin (ASA), but other nonsteroidal anti-inflammatory drugs (NSAIDs) may also be used. In refractory cases other drugs may prove useful, including immunosuppressants (azathioprine, cyclosporine, methotrexate), antimalarials, gold salts, and adrenal corticosteroids. All of these drugs have problematic side effects or toxicities. Physical therapy is important in maintaining mobility. Surgery may be needed to correct severe deformity.

Lupus Erythematosus (LE). A chronic inflammatory disorder of connective tissue due to formation of antibody to nucleoprotein.

Cause: Unknown. Ninety percent of patients are young women. Antinuclear antibody and anti-DNA antibody are found in the serum.

History: Gradual or abrupt onset of widely varying symptoms: joint pain, butterfly rash over the cheeks, discoid lesions and other skin changes (purpura, alopecia), fever, chest pain, mood changes and other psychiatric symptoms.

Physical Examination: Fever, signs of swelling and inflammation in joints, malar "butterfly" eruption, lymphadenopathy, splenomegaly, pericardial or pleural friction rub heard on auscultation.

Diagnostic Tests: The erythrocyte sedimentation rate is elevated, white blood cells (particularly lymphocytes) and platelets are decreased. Tests based on detection of abnormal antibodies (LE cell preparation, antinuclear antibody, anti-DNA antibody) are often positive. Serologic test for syphilis may be falsely positive. Urinalysis may show proteinuria, red blood cells, and casts.

Course: The disease is chronic and relapsing, with spontaneous remissions and exacerbations. With treatment the 10-year survival rate is about 95%. Most patients eventually develop kidney disease (lupus nephritis), and death is usually due to renal failure.

Treatment: Nonsteroidal anti-inflammatory drugs (NSAIDs) and general supportive measures may suffice to control symptoms. Antimalarial drugs (hydroxychloroquine and others), adrenal corticosteroids, and immunosuppressive drugs (azathioprine, cyclophosphamide) are useful in more severe cases.

Laboratory Procedures

alkaline phosphatase An enzyme whose level in the serum is often increased in bone disease and obstructive liver disease. The slang "alk phos" should be expanded.

ANA (antinuclear antibody) An antibody detected by immunofluorescence in patients with rheumatoid arthritis, lupus erythematosus, and other autoimmune diseases.

erythrocyte sedimentation rate (ESR, sed rate) The rate at which red blood cells settle to the bottom of a specimen of whole blood that has been treated with anticoagulant. The rate is expressed in millimeters per hour (mm/h), as measured in a standard glass column. Elevation of the sedimentation rate occurs in various inflammatory and malignant diseases but is diagnostic of none. An acceptable brief form is *sed rate*.

LE cell prep Lupus erythematosus cell test.

RA test Rheumatoid arthritis test. See *rheumatoid factor*.

rheumatoid factor (RF) An antibody present in the serum of patients with rheumatoid arthritis and other autoimmune disorders.

sed rate See *erythrocyte sedimentation rate*.

uric acid, serum A breakdown product of purine metabolism, increased in gout and other disorders.

Diagnostic and Surgical Procedures

anterior drawer test With the patient supine, the injured knee is bent to 90 degrees. The physician then grasps the upper end of the tibia and pulls it anteriorly. Excessive movement means the anterior cruciate ligament within the knee joint is damaged or torn.

arthroscopy A surgical procedure which involves an incision into a joint and the insertion of an arthroscope to view the structures inside the joint.

bone scan A nuclear imaging test which, following the intravenous administration of radioisotope, uses a scanning device to detect areas of abnormal uptake in the bones to identify fractures.

crossed (or contralateral) straight leg raising With the patient supine, the unaffected leg is held straight and flexed at the hip. If sciatica is present, the patient will experience pain in the opposite, affected side.

densitometry Determination of variations in density (for example, bone density) by comparison with that of another material or with a certain standard. See *dual photon densitometry*.

dual photon densitometry A quantitative assessment of a patient's bone density, and comparison with normal ranges for persons of the same age and sex.

EMG (electromyogram) Test to determine the response pattern of muscles when stimulated by an electrical impulse from a needle electrode inserted into the muscle.

imaging studies Including x-ray, the most common and least expensive diagnostic tool for assessing bone structure and integrity. Also called *radiograph, film, roentgenogram, roentgenograph*. *MRI, CT scan*, and *nuclear medicine studies* are also used for diagnostic purposes.

Lachman test Similar to the anterior drawer test, but performed with the patient's knee flexed only to 15-20°. Also used to evaluate anterior cruciate ligament stability.

laminectomy Surgical cutting through the posterior arch of one or more vertebrae and removal of herniated disk material.

Lasègue sign or test See *straight leg raising*.

McMurray test or sign Extension of the knee from full flexion with the leg and foot externally rotated causes an audible or palpable snap in medial meniscus tear; extension with the leg and foot internally rotated causes a snap in lateral meniscus tear.

open reduction, internal fixation (ORIF) A surgical procedure to correct a fracture that requires alignment and fixation with a plate, pin, or screw.

pivot-shift test With the patient supine, the foot is held in the physician's hand. The physician then turns the foot inward while pushing on the outside of the knee with the opposite hand, at the same time flexing and extending the patient's leg. This test is also used to evaluate anterior cruciate ligament stability.

quadriceps exercises Repeatedly bringing the knee into full extension, with tensing of the muscles of the front of the thigh.

saucerization Radical surgical excision of infected bone.

straight leg raising With the patient supine, the leg is elevated with the knee straight to the point where pain is experienced in the back or leg itself, or dorsiflexion of the foot causes an increase in pain. This test is done to determine if nerve root irritation is present. Also known as *Lasègue sign* or *test*.

Pharmacology

Orthopedic conditions such as arthritis (rheumatoid and osteoarthritis), bursitis, tendinitis, gout, and muscle spasms are treated with aspirin, nonsteroidal anti-inflammatory drugs (NSAIDs), gold salts, and muscle relaxants, among others. Acute musculoskeletal conditions such as strains, sprains, and "pulled muscles" are treated with analgesics and anti-inflammatory drugs. The physician may also elect to prescribe a skeletal muscle relaxant.

Drugs used to treat osteoarthritis reduce pain and inflammation. These drugs include salicylates (such as aspirin), nonsteroidal anti-inflammatory drugs (NSAIDs), and COX-2 inhibitors. In addition, corticosteroids may be used. None of these drugs, however, can reverse the cartilage and bone damage that has already occurred in the joint.

Salicylic acid compounds. The oldest drug used to treat arthritis is aspirin. Aspirin is also known as *acetylsalicylic acid*, abbreviated *ASA*. It has anti-inflammatory, analgesic, and antipyretic actions. Salicylates (salicylic acid compounds) include:

> aspirin (Arthritis Foundation Pain Reliever, Ecotrin, Empirin, Extended Release Bayer 8-Hour Caplets, Norwich Extra-Strength)
> choline salicylate (Arthropan)
> choline salicylate/magnesium salicylate (Trilisate)
> diflunisal (Dolobid)
> salsalate (Disalcid)

Because salicylate drugs such as aspirin are irritating to the stomach, and long-term therapy with such drugs has been shown to cause peptic ulcers, some manufacturers have taken precautions to reduce this irritation. Ecotrin is manufactured as an enteric-coated tablet that does not dissolve in stomach acid; it dissolves only when it comes in contact with the higher pH environment of the duodenum.

Aspirin is often combined with an antacid to raise the pH of the stomach, inhibit the action of pepsin, and neutralize stomach acid, all of which prevent the formation of peptic ulcers during aspirin therapy.

> Arthritis Pain Formula
> Ascriptin, Ascriptin A/D, Ascriptin Extra Strength
> Bayer Buffered Aspirin, Bayer Plus Extra Strength
> Bufferin, Tri-Buffered Bufferin
> Cama Arthritis Pain Reliever

Acetaminophen. Although acetaminophen is an analgesic like aspirin, it lacks the ability to inhibit the production of prostaglandins and has no anti-inflammatory action. However, the American College of Rheumatology recommends using acetaminophen to treat osteoarthritis because it has fewer side effects compared to NSAIDS.

> acetaminophen
> Aspirin Free Anacin Maximum Strength
> Panadol
> Tylenol
> Tylenol Arthritis
> Tylenol Arthritis Extended Relief
> Tylenol Extra Strength
> Tylenol Regular Strength

NSAIDs ("en´sayds" or "en´seds") (**nonsteroidal anti-inflammatory drugs**) inhibit the production of prostaglandins for an anti-inflammatory effect, and they also relieve pain directly (analgesic effect). NSAIDs have less of a tendency than aspirin to cause stomach irritation or peptic ulcers. Their structure is similar enough to aspirin that patients allergic to aspirin should not take NSAIDs. NSAIDs include:

> diclofenac (Cataflam, Voltaren, Voltaren-XR)
> etodolac (Lodine, Lodine XL)
> fenoprofen (Nalfon Pulvules)
> flurbiprofen (Ansaid)
> ibuprofen (Advil, Advil Liqui-Gels, Haltran, Motrin, Motrin IB)
> indomethacin (Indocin, Indocin SR)
> ketoprofen (Orudis, Orudis KT, Oruvail)
> meclofenamate (Meclomen)
> meloxicam (Mobic)
> nabumetone (Relafen)
> naproxen (Aleve, Anaprox, Anaprox DS, Naprelan, EC-Naprosyn, Naprosyn)
> oxaprozin (Daypro)
> piroxicam (Feldene)
> sulindac (Clinoril)

Arthrotec contains an NSAID (diclofenac) combined with a synthetic prostaglandin (misoprostol) that protects the gastric mucosa and prevents the formation of peptic ulcers.

COX-2 inhibitors, which also belong to the larger category of NSAIDs, selectively inhibit the enzyme cyclooxygenase-2 (COX-2) to decrease the production of prostaglandins and relieve pain.

> celecoxib (Celebrex)

Corticosteroids, which are produced naturally in the adrenal cortex, have a powerful anti-inflammatory effect and are given orally to treat acute episodes of osteoarthritis associated with inflammation of the synovial membrane. Because of the side effects associated with prolonged oral use, corticosteroid drugs are used only to treat acute exacerbations.

> betamethasone (Celestone Soluspan)
> dexamethasone (Dalalone, Dalalone D.P., Dalalone L.A., Decadron, Decadron-LA, Hexadrol)
> hydrocortisone (Hydrocortone)
> methylprednisolone (Depo-Medrol, Depopred-40, Depopred-80)
> prednisolone (Hydeltrasol, Key-Pred 25, Key-Pred 50, Key-Pred-SP, Predalone 50, Prednisol TBA)
> triamcinolone (Aristocort Forte, Aristospan Intra-articular, Kenalog-40)

Hyaluronic acid is secreted by the synovial membrane of a joint and helps to maintain the lubricating quality of the synovial fluid. These drugs, derivatives of hyaluronic acid, are injected into the joints of patients with osteoarthritis:

> hyaluronic acid derivative (Hyalgan, Synvisc)
> sodium hyaluronate (Supartz)

Gold salts contain actual gold (from 29 to 50% of the total drug) in capsules or in solution for injection; they are used to treat active rheumatoid arthritis. Rheumatoid arthritis is an autoimmune disease in which the patient's own macrophages attack and damage cartilage. Gold salts inhibit the activity of macrophages but cannot reverse past damage.

> auranofin (Ridaura)
> aurothioglucose (Solganal)
> gold sodium thiomalate (Myochrysine)

Unlike other antiarthritis drugs, gold salts are never prescribed for osteoarthritis, as this disease is caused by degenerative wear and tear, not by an immune response. NSAIDs are the first line of treatment for rheumatoid arthritis, but if these fail, gold salts may be added to the treatment regimen. Plaquenil (hydroxychloroquine) is also effective in treating rheumatoid arthritis, as well as anakinra (Kineret), which is human interleukin-1 produced through recombinant DNA technology.

Osteoporosis drugs. Osteoporosis is a thinning of the bone due to demineralization.

Osteoporosis is much more common in women than in men, and most common in postmenopausal women. As estrogen levels decrease in menopause, the rate of bone formation decreases but the rate of bone breakdown remains constant, causing the bones to slowly and progressively thin. Additional risk factors for osteoporosis include Caucasian or Asian race, slender build, smoking, and alcohol abuse.

Osteoporosis is prevented or treated by supplementing calcium, and increasing exercise (to stimulate bone growth). Estrogen taken orally or administered through a transdermal patch reverses postmenopausal bone loss but increases the risk of cardiovascular disease, thromboembolism, and certain cancers.

The hormone **calcitonin** is normally produced by the thyroid gland and regulates calcium and the rate of bone resorption (breakdown). Miacalcin, an analog of human calcitonin derived from salmon, is given by injection or nasal spray to inhibit calcium loss in osteoporosis.

These drugs decrease the rate of bone resorption by inhibiting osteoclasts (cells that break down bone).

> alendronate (Fosamax)
> etidronate (Didronel)
> pamidronate (Aredia)
> risedronate (Actonel)

Evista (raloxifene) belongs to the class of drugs known as selective estrogen receptor modulators (SERMs) and activates estrogen receptors to decrease the rate of bone resorption.

Skeletal muscle relaxants. Skeletal muscle relaxants specifically relieve muscle spasm and stiffness. These drugs are also prescribed for patients with multiple sclerosis, cerebral palsy, stroke, and spinal cord injury who have muscle spasticity. Most of these drugs also have a sedative effect.

> carisoprodol (Soma)
> chlorphenesin (Maolate)
> chlorzoxazone (Paraflex, Parafon Forte DSC)
> cyclobenzaprine (Flexeril)
> diazepam (Valium)
> metaxalone (Skelaxin)
> methocarbamol (Robaxin, Robaxin-750)
> orphenadrine (Norflex)

These skeletal muscle relaxants are used to treat severe muscle spasticity in patients with multiple sclerosis, cerebral palsy, stroke, or spinal cord injury.

> baclofen (Lioresal)
> dantrolene (Dantrium)
> tizanidine (Zanaflex)

Combination skeletal muscle relaxants include Norgesic (orphenadrine and aspirin), Robaxisal (methocarbamol and aspirin), Soma Compound (carisoprodol and aspirin), and Soma Compound with Codeine (carisoprodol, aspirin, codeine).

Drugs used to treat gout. Gout is caused by a metabolic defect that allows uric acid to accumulate in the blood. The kidneys are unable to excrete the excess uric acid, and it crystallizes within the joints, causing pain and inflammation.

Drugs used to treat gout act either by increasing the excretion of uric acid in the urine or by inhibiting enzymes that produce uric acid in the blood.

> allopurinol (Zyloprim)
> colchicine
> potassium citrate/sodium citrate (Polycitra, Polycitra-LC)
> probenecid (Benemid)
> sulfinpyrazone (Anturane)

In addition, certain NSAIDs have been found to be of particular benefit in treating gout.

> indomethacin (Indocin, Indocin SR)
> naproxen (Aleve, Anaprox, Anaprox DS, EC-Naprosyn, Naprosyn)
> sulindac (Clinoril)

Drugs used to treat phantom limb pain. After an amputation, most patients experience pain that seems to come from the amputated limb. Nerve impulses coming from just above the area of amputation are interpreted by the brain as being from the missing limb. This pain diminishes over time but is treated with tricyclic antidepressants that have been found to be effective in treating different types of pain.

> amitriptyline (Elavil)
> amoxapine (Asendin)
> desipramine (Norpramin)
> doxepin (Sinequan, Sinequan Concentrate)
> imipramine (Tofranil, Tofranil-PM)
> nortriptyline (Aventyl, Aventyl Pulvules, Pamelor)
> protriptyline (Vivactil)

TRANSCRIPTION**TIPS**

1. There are several soundalike terms related to the musculoskeletal system. Memorize the terms and their meanings so that you can select the appropriate term for a correct transcript.

   peroneal (pertaining to the fibula)
   perineal (pertaining to the area between the genitalia and anus)
   peritoneal (cavity located within the abdomen)

   humeral (pertaining to the humerus, an arm bone)
   humoral (pertaining to immunity from antibodies in the blood)
   humerus (arm bone)
   humorous (funny)

   ilium (hip bone)
   ileum (part of the small intestine)

   malleolus (bony prominence on either side of ankle)
   malleus (bone of middle ear)

2. Orthopedists commonly dictate "a-b-duction" and "a-d-duction." These are not slang terms. The dictator is simply spelling the first two letters of the term and then pronouncing the rest as a word. This is done in order to assist the transcriptionist in differentiating between the two terms.

3. Several nouns pertaining to the musculoskeletal system change their spelling when forming derivatives.

   femur becomes *femora* or *femurs* (noun) and *femoral* (adjective)
   foramen becomes *foramina* (noun) and *foraminal* (adjective)
   tendon becomes *tendinitis*
   fascia lata becomes *tensor fasciae latae*

4. Paget disease of the bone is different from Paget disease of the breast and the related Paget disease of the vulva and perianal region, although they are spelled the same.

5. *Weightbearing, weight bearing, weight-bearing*—which is the correct spelling? Consulting a dictionary will not provide the answer. We have followed the rationale of *Vera Pyle's Current Medical Terminology*, 10th ed., in *MTF&P* transcript keys: "The trend in language is to combine words without hyphens after compound nouns become common. . . . It seems simpler and cleaner to make *weightbearing* and *nonweightbearing* single words." *Webster's 11th Collegiate Dictionary*, *Webster's Unabridged*, *Dorland's 30th*, and *Stedman's 28th*, unfortunately, do not list any form of *weightbearing*, which is commonly used in orthopedic and neurology medical reports. *The Oxford English Dictionary* alone gives *weight-bearing* (with hyphen) as the proper form for both noun and adjective, as well as *non-weight-bearing* (with hyphens).

6. The following terms have more than one acceptable spelling: *orthopedics, orthopaedics; orthopedist, orthopaedist; disk, disc.*

   Note. Orthopaedic is from the Greek and is found in British and Canadian references. Unless specified by the dictating physician, the *a* in the diphthong *ae* should be omitted. *Exceptions:* The official name of the American Academy of Orthopaedic Surgeons, as well as some orthopedic groups and hospitals.

7. Memorize the unusual spellings of these orthopedic terms:

   psoas muscle (silent *p*)
   bony (*not* boney)

8. The names of several gold salts contain *au*, the chemical symbol for gold: *au*ranofin, Rid*au*ra, *au*rothioglucose.

9. *Flexeril* (a muscle relaxant) is often misspelled as *Flexoril* because of association with the flexor muscles and tendons.

10. Transcribe these slang terms correctly when encountered in dictation:

Slang	Translation
K wire	Kirschner wire
tib-fib	tibia-fibula (noun) *or* tibiofibular (adjective)

10. Physicians frequently mispronounce *tensor fasciae latae* as if it were spelled "tensor fascia lata" and *chondromalacia patellae* as if it were spelled "chondromalacia patella." Note the correct spellings.

11. Some structures have two (or more) names that may be used interchangeably, even in the same dictation:

    calcaneus = os calcis
    navicular bone = scaphoid bone
    (bony) pelvis = innominate bone = os coxae
    talus = astragalus
    xiphoid cartilage = ensiform cartilage

Spotlight on

Transcribing Orthopedic Dictation

by Carolyn Cadigan

The transcription of orthopedic dictation is not unlike the transcription of other medical specialties—some love it, others don't. But once you have mastered the terminology of bones, muscles, tendons, ligaments, and surgical instruments (many of which sound as if they belong in carpentry), you may find that you have also developed a unique sense of humor. Orthopedic transcriptionists look forward to rainy days (arthritis complaints) and icy and snowy days (accidents, strained muscles). They count the number of injuries while watching sports events.

Colorful terminology. Orthopedic terminology is relatively constant: the names of the bones, muscles, tendons, and ligaments do not change, names of fractures and sprains remain basically the same, and orthopedic instrument names remain relatively constant. The most significant changes occur when new orthopedic appliances are developed and when doctors themselves coin and create new terminology for specific purposes.

Orthopedic terminology tends to be descriptive. Should a patient present with a complaint of a painful knee, it is common to hear the physician dictate the following: *snap, crack, pop, clink, clunk, grind, tear, catch,* and *giving way.* And from the list of instruments used in orthopedic procedures, one would think the surgeon was building a house instead of repairing or replacing a joint: screws, washers, rods, plates, burs, drills, rasps, saws, chisels, tamps, clamps, and cement. On a followup postoperative office visit, it is not unusual for the physician to dictate that the patient is able to bend, flex, lift, A-B-duct (abduct), A-D-duct (adduct), and perform the normal activities of daily living.

Assessment and treatment. The orthopedist carries out a physical examination that may differ from the patient's expectations. The orthopedist does not usually listen to the patient's lungs or take the pulse, but may ask the patient to sit, stand, walk, squat, cross legs, and bend forward.

What can a physician determine from such tests? From bending forward, scoliosis; from a hairy patch on a child's spine, spina bifida or myelomeningocele; from heel and toe walking, Achilles tendon involvement; from holding the hands in an inverted prayer position, carpal tunnel syndrome.

Orthopedic tests. To locate specific orthopedic tests in a medical dictionary, look under *test, sign,* and *maneuver,* or under the name of the test itself listed alphabetically.

Occasionally the orthopedist will order x-rays of the involved site in an attempt to determine or verify the presence of a tear, rupture, fracture, dislocation, or foreign body. X-rays may include AP, PA, oblique, and lateral projections, as well as such exotic-sounding views as sunrise, sunset, tunnel, and coned-down.

Treatment modalities used in orthopedic cases vary widely but are generally conservative. Before recommending surgery, the orthopedist usually tries any one of a number of conservative treatments—splints, casts, supports, physical therapy, exercises, heat or ice applications, dressings (such as Unna boot), braces (such as cowhorn, Milwaukee, DonJoy), and shoes (such as open toe, straight last, reverse last).

Resources. As with any other specialty, orthopedists have their own language—words and phrases and abbreviations which are specific to orthopedics. In addition to a number of helpful orthopedic references, I have come to rely heavily upon the patient's chart as well as the surgical and central supply departments of the hospital for information on orthopedic devices. The handwritten operating room record, which is prepared on every patient having surgery, lists all instruments used during the procedure, including the names of orthopedic pins, rods, prosthetic devices, and so on. Surgical components frequently arrive in the central supply and surgical departments direct from the manufacturer, with the name of the company and the product boldly printed on the outside of the box. In addition, the physical therapy/rehabilitation department of the hospital can provide you with the names of braces, supports, exercises, and other terms.

Remember to keep your own personal dictionary as you go along. You will find that in time you rely on it more than other reference books, if the entries you make are thoroughly checked for accuracy before you write them in.

Transcribing orthopedic dictation. A great many orthopedic terms are difficult to confirm in reference books. For example, when an orthopedist dictates on a fractured lateral malleolus, the transcriptionist may not have a clue as to what part of the body is involved since this structure is not listed under the heading *bone* in a medical dictionary. What the transcriptionist does find is that *malleolus* is listed under its own heading alphabetically, defined as a rounded prominence on either side of the ankle. (Do not confuse *malleolus,* the ankle bone, with *malleus,* one of the bones in the middle ear, also known as the *hammer.*)

The same problem occurs when *scapholunate* is dictated. This term is not listed under *bone,* and a further search reveals that, although both *scaphoid* and *lunate* are listed separately under *bone,* the transcriptionist is referred to the Latin forms of each word for a definition. A check under the heading *os* reveals *os scaphoideum* (scaphoid) is the most lateral carpal (wrist) bone, and that *os lunatum* is the lunate bone. Therefore, a scapholunate dissociation is an abnormal separation between the scaphoid and lunate bones of the wrist.

Terminology involving the muscular system may present a challenge as well. When the phrase *vastus lateralis* is dictated, how does the transcriptionist know where to look?

It is important to know that medical dictionaries usually have both an English and a Latin listing for certain anatomic structures. For example, a specific muscle may be found under the listing *muscle* as well as under *musculus*. And in the case of *vastus lateralis*, which is obviously Latin, the transcriptionist would search under *musculus* (Latin) as opposed to *muscle* (English) to locate the definition.

For tendons, there are also two listings: *tendo* (Latin) and *tendon* (English). However, there are many more tendons in the body than are listed in the dictionaries. To find e*xtensor carpi radialis longus tendon* (not listed under *tendon*), the transcriptionist does a bit of detective work. The word *tendon* is the first clue. Although this phrase is not actually listed under *tendon*, the definition of a tendon is a cord which attaches a muscle to a bone. The transcriptionist would then know to look under the listing for *muscle*, or in this case *musculus*, because the phrase is in Latin.

Anatomic review. Transcribing dictation on the spine can be difficult and therefore time-consuming if one does not know the terminology. The first step is to become familiar with the basic makeup of the spinal column: the cervical spine (C1 through C7), the thoracic spine (T1 through T12), the lumbar spine (L1 through L5), and the sacral spine (S1 through S5). It is common to hear reference made to the L6 vertebra, which is identified as either lumbarization of S1 or the sacralization of L5. Additionally, some physicians dictate *D spine* for *dorsal (thoracic) spine*.

There are different ways to transcribe vertebrae and their identifying numbers. Many references join the vertebra and number without a hyphen (for example, T12) and use a hyphen for vertebral interspaces (L5-S1). However, in some settings, the transcriptionists have been instructed to use hyphens between the vertebra and the number, e.g., L-4; and to use hyphens and slashes for vertebral interspaces, e.g., L-5/S-1.

In hip surgery, the transcriptionist may encounter terms such as *femoral prosthesis, acetabular component, Knowles pinning,* and *figure-4 position*. An orthopedic reference book will help the transcriptionist identify *Knowles* as the brand name of a type of pin used in setting hip fractures. The definition of *figure-4 position* is more difficult to locate. Imagine

yourself lying on your left side. Now bring your right ankle up until it is resting on your left knee. This is the *figure-4 position*.

Another interesting term is *triple diapering,* which is used in the treatment of congenitally dislocated hips of newborn infants if the defect is detected at a very early age. The application of three layers of diapers holds the infant's thighs in external rotation to properly seat the femoral heads back into the acetabular cups.

The language of knee surgery can be most descriptive. On examining the knee joint during arthroscopy, the physician may describe *parrot-beak tear, bucket-handle tear, crabmeat-like appearance, horseshoe appearance, choppy-sea sign, spongy appearance,* and *medial shelf* or *lateral shelf*. Along with this descriptive terminology, the physician will also use anatomical and medical words such as *meniscus, chondromalacia, Gerdy tubercle,* and the *master knot of Henry*.

Some of the above terms are difficult to locate. *Gerdy tubercle* can be found under *Gerdy* but not under *tubercle*. The *master knot of Henry* is not listed under *master knot* but is listed as the *ligament of Henry* in one reference. In this instance, the support of another transcriptionist or the physician is of the greatest help in providing verification.

Orthopedic abbreviations. When it comes to orthopedic abbreviations, one can quickly get lost within the first sentence without a good reference book and a personal list of abbreviations. For example, "The patient presented with a chief complaint of MTA and ITT." Here the transcriptionist is given no clues. Once the transcriptionist discovers that *MTA* and *ITT* stand for *metatarsus adductus* and *internal tibial torsion,* respectively, the next step is to insert these definitions into a personal dictionary so that they will be readily available the next time.

Another example: "The patient was scheduled for AAA (or 3-A or triple A) procedure." Many reference sources define the abbreviation *AAA* as *abdominal aortic aneurysm*. This definition would not be appropriate for a scheduled orthopedic surgery. By asking another transcriptionist or the physician, or by consulting the patient's chart, the transcriptionist will see that the patient is scheduled for a diagnostic arthroscopy, operative arthroscopy, and possible operative arthrotomy.

A final word. If you cannot interpret an orthopedic term in the dictation, and have carefully researched it in all the available resources, leave a blank temporarily and continue with the transcription. Chances are that the physician will dictate the word again later, and it will be clearer, and then you can fill in the blank.

Source: *The SUM Program Orthopedic Transcription Unit*

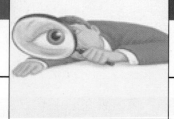

Proofreading Skills

Instructions: In the paragraphs below, circle the errors. Identify misspelled and missing medical and English words and punctuation errors, and write the correct words and punctuation in the numbered spaces opposite the text.

1 The patient comes to the clnc today because of
2 problems with recurrent bursitus. What's troubling
3 him at this time is recurrent tindonitis to the left arm
4 (this has been injected successfully with cortisone on
5 multiple occasions) as well as intermittent problems
6 of left hip pain which also seems to be tendinitis/
7 bursitis in nature.
8
9 EXAMINATION
10 The patietn has a marked trigger point on the lateral
11 epicondyle. His hip is asymptomatic at this time, and
12 exam is benine.
13
14 After discussing the different posibilities, I elected to
15 try conservative theraphy. Tennis elbow armband is
16 placed to the right arm. He is begun on Anaprox DS
17 on a trial basis. If this gives adequate releif I would
18 have him use it on a p.r.n. basis. If he continues to
19 have signifcant pain would recomend return to clinic
20 for trigger-point injection.

1 clinic _____
2 _____
3 _____
4 _____
5 _____
6 _____
7 _____
8 _____
9 _____
10 _____
11 _____
12 _____
13 _____
14 _____
15 _____
16 _____
17 _____
18 _____
19 _____
20 _____

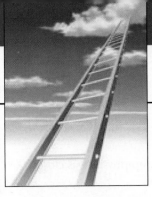

SkillsChallenge

Fill-in Exercise: The Bones

Instructions: The numbered blanks correspond to the numbers in the narrative paragraphs. Fill in the blanks with the correct entry from the word list following the paragraphs.

Beginning with the toes, or (1), one proceeds along the foot, encountering the bones of the midfoot (2) and bones of the ankle (3), to the heel bone, or (4), and then to the ankle bone, or (5).

Next, moving proximally, the (6) and (7) are located in the leg, followed by the kneecap, or (8), and then the (9) in the thigh. The ball of the femur, also known as the (10), fits snugly in the (11), or socket, in the pelvic bone. The lower part of the pelvic bone, including the seat bones, is called the (12), while the upper part that flares widely and is called the "hip bone" is the (13).

Moving up the spinal column, which is composed of (14) and (15), one encounters the ribs. There are 12 pairs of ribs, of which 7 pairs are joined at the front of the body to the breast bone, or (16). Superior to the manubrium and the first ribs is the (17), or collarbone. As the clavicle continues across the shoulder joint, it joins the shoulder blade, or (18).

From the shoulder joint, moving distally down the arm, the bones encountered include the (19), then the elbow, or (20), then the two bones of the forearm—the (21) and (22), to the (23) in the wrist, the (24) in the midhand, and finally to the fingers, or (25).

acetabulum	metacarpals
calcaneus	metatarsals
carpals	olecranon process
clavicle	patella
femoral head	phalanges (2)
femur	radius
fibula	scapula
humerus	sternum
ilium	tarsals
intervertebral disk	tibia
ischium	ulna
malleolus	vertebrae

1. _____
2. _____
3. _____
4. _____
5. _____
6. _____
7. _____
8. _____
9. _____
10. _____
11. _____
12. _____
13. _____
14. _____
15. _____
16. _____
17. _____
18. _____
19. _____
20. _____
21. _____
22. _____
23. _____
24. _____
25. _____

Adjectives Exercise

Adjectives are formed from nouns by adding adjectival suffixes such as *-ac*, *-al*, *-ar*, *-ary*, *-eal*, *-ed*, *-ent*, *-iac*, *-ial*, *-ic*, *-ical*, *-ive*, *-lar*, *-oid*, *-ous*, *-tic*, and *-tous*. In addition, some adjectives have a different form entirely from the noun, which may be either Latin or Greek in origin.

Instructions: Test your knowledge of adjectives by writing the adjectival form of the following orthopedic words. Consult a medical dictionary to select the correct adjectival ending as necessary.

1. muscle _____
2. bone _____
3. spine _____
4. vertebra _____
5. cartilage _____
6. rib _____
7. pelvis _____
8. humerus _____
9. radius _____
10. ulna _____
11. clavicle _____
12. femur _____
13. tibia _____
14. fibula _____
15. patella _____
16. malleolus _____
17. phalanx _____
18. ligament _____
19. tendon _____
20. arthritis _____

Soundalikes Exercise

Instructions: Circle the correct term from the soundalikes in parentheses in the following sentences.

1. On the x-ray, the bony (apophysis, epiphysis) was closed in this precocious 12-year-old child.

2. The patient shattered the calcaneal (apophysis, epiphysis) when he jumped from the roof and landed on his feet.

3. The seventh (cervical, surgical) vertebra was fractured when the patient dived into the river and hit a submerged rock.

4. The humerus was fractured in its upper portion just at the (cervical, surgical) neck.

5. The child's right femoral (diaphysis, diastasis, diathesis) measured 13 cm; the left measured 11.5 cm.

6. On strength testing, the (flexor, flexure) muscles of the right forearm were weaker than the left.

7. The patient had a (callous, callus) on his (heal, heel).

8. The thenar (eminence, imminence) was not visualized on the x-ray.

9. The ischium and (ileum, ilium) were shattered, the hip totally dislocated.

10. The remainder of the median nerve dissection was done under (loop, loupe) magnification.

11. The (metacarpal, metatarsal) bones of the patient's right hand were slightly calcified.

12. The left second (metacarpal, metatarsal) was fractured and the toe deviated to the right.

13. On x-ray the line between the epiphysis and (metaphysis, metastasis) was not visible.

14. (Osteal, Ostial) density was thin and the bone porous in this postmenopausal woman.

15. (Axis, Obvious, Osseous) overgrowth of the (pen, pin) in the hip was noted.

16. The pain started in the buttock and traveled along the peroneal nerve down into the patient's left (side, thigh).

17. The cowboy had a pronounced genu (valgum, varum) deformity.

18. The child was knock-kneed, genu (valgum, varum), and pigeon-toed, metatarsus (abductus, adductus).

Abbreviations Exercise

Common abbreviations may be transcribed as dictated in the body of a report. Uncommon abbreviations must be spelled out, with the abbreviation appearing in parentheses after the translation. All abbreviations (except laboratory test names) must be spelled out in the Diagnosis or Impression section of any report.

Instructions: Define the following orthopedic abbreviations. Then memorize both abbreviations and definitions to increase your speed and accuracy in transcribing orthopedic dictation.

AAA _____

AK amputation _____

BK amputation _____

C1-C7 _____

T1-T12 _____

L1-L5 _____

CTD _____

CTS _____

DTR _____

EMG _____

HNP _____

NSAID _____

ORIF _____

PIP _____

RF _____

RSI _____

TENS unit _____

VMO _____

Medical Terminology Matching Exercise

Instructions: Match each definition in Column A with its term in Column B.

Column A

1. ___ lateral curvature of spine
2. ___ dorsal curvature of thoracic spine
3. ___ connects bone to bone
4. ___ refers to ankle bone
5. ___ overstretching of muscle
6. ___ fibula
7. ___ joint
8. ___ anterior curvature of lumbar spine
9. ___ decreased bone density
10. ___ bacterial infection of bone
11. ___ degeneration of joint and cartilage
12. ___ referring to bone
13. ___ incomplete dislocation
14. ___ referring to lower back
15. ___ connects bone to muscle
16. ___ rib
17. ___ malignant bone tumor

Column B

A. osteoarthritis

B. arthro-

C. kypho-

D. tendon

E. lordo-

F. osteosarcoma

G. lumbo-

H. strain

I. osteo-

J. scolio-

K. osteomyelitis

L. ligament

M. peroneo-

N. osteoporosis

O. costo-

P. subluxation

Q. malleolo-

Dictation Exercises

Prior to transcribing the dictations, complete these activities.

1. Using Chapter 3, Style Guide

a. When, according to the Style Guide, do you expand brief forms and abbreviations?

b. What are the Style Guide recommendations concerning the transcription of dictated contractions (he's, don't, I've, etc.)?

c. Review the section in the Style Guide on Formats. What does it say about adding headings not dictated?

d. Read the first paragraph under General Information and the section on Editing. Ask your instructor for additional guidelines on how much editing you're allowed to do.

e. When, according to the Style Guide, should you flag a report? Ask your instructor what procedure you should follow to indicate that you have identified a discrepancy or contradiction.

f. What does the Style Guide say about abbreviating English units of measure (pounds, inches, feet)?

g What does the Style Guide say about using symbols, such as the degree (°) symbol, for temperature and angles? Will a file with degree symbols transmit electronically?

h. Consult your acceptable Brief Forms and Medical Slang list. Is *rehab* an acceptable brief form?

i. How should ordinal numbers (second, third, fourth) be transcribed, according to the Style Guide?

j. Read the section in the Style Guide on Capitalization. What does it say about capitalizing proper names (eponyms, geographic place names, etc.)?

k. Read the section in the Style Guide on Symbols. When it is appropriate to use the plus (+) sign?

l. According to the Style Guide, is it ever appropriate to abbreviate English units of measure in a medical report?

m. What is the correct way to transcribe vertebral interspaces—with a hyphen or a slash (C5/6 or C5-6)?

n. Read the section in the Style Guide on Hyphens and compound adjectives.

o. What is the simplest way to avoid beginning a sentence with a numeral when the sentence starts with "one percent lidocaine"?

p. What is the correct way to transcribe metric fractions? For example, if "one quarter percent Marcaine" is dictated, how would you transcribe it?

q. How do you transcribe a numerical ratio, such as a "fifty-fifty mixture"?

2. Problem Solving

This activity is to help you prepare ahead of time for some of the problems you'll encounter in the dictations. Some of these items may not have a definitive answer but are intended to simply get you thinking about how to handle a variety of situations that are common in transcription. If nothing else, they will help you recognize a problem when you encounter it in the dictations.

a. Transcriptionists must be alert to the contextual meaning of the report they're transcribing—no "in through the ears and out through the fingers" for a good MT. The words must pass through the brain and be interpreted first. An experienced MT can spot discrepancies and contradictions and sometimes decipher terms that were difficult to hear at the beginning of a report because the terms are repeated (or there is more information) later in the report. This is a skill that takes time to develop, and it is difficult for students who are trying to learn so many things at once. Until you learn this skill so that you can do this in "real time," what other things might you do that will help you to spot discrepancies and problems within a report?

b. There is a *left-right* discrepancy within a report that you transcribe. How would you handle this?

c. An abbreviation used within a report can be expanded in more than one way. How do you determine which expansion is correct? What do you do if you cannot determine which expansion is correct?

d. There are many errors that a spelling checker does not catch, perhaps the most common being homophones or soundalikes. Even the best, most experienced MT can "zone out" and transcribe something like *heal* for *heel.* Describe some ways in which you might develop habits that help you avoid making errors like this.

e. On a physical exam, the dictator says "height five four." How would you transcribe this? Should you add the omitted units of measure?

f. You're transcribing a dictator who consistently omits connecting words (*and* and *or*) and leaves off the adverb endings *(-ly)* of words as well. Do you just sigh and transcribe as dictated or do you edit to make the report grammatically correct and read more smoothly?

g. One of your goals as a student should be to work on ear training—picking up sounds that may be difficult to distinguish and making sense of them. As you proofread your transcription against the answer keys or when your instructor returns your graded transcripts, make note of the vocabulary errors you made, even those "little" errors that may only involve word endings like *-en*, *-ed*, *-s*, and *-ly*. Word endings like *-ened* can be especially troubling. Go back and listen again to all the words you missed until you can hear the words correctly. Analyze why you didn't hear the terms correctly the first time, and over time develop strategies for avoiding the same types of errors in the future.

3. **Preparatory Research**

Any information requested in these questions not readily available in your textbook (including the appendix) or required references can easily be found using Internet search engines such as Google or online medical dictionaries.

a. Define *adventitious* (lung sounds).
b. Review the bones of the wrist.
c. How is the intensity of pain scored?
d. What is the volar aspect of the wrist?
e. How is a differential diagnosis different from the final diagnosis?
f. Define *drawer sign*. Define *emanating*.
g. What is the difference between *incidence* and *incidents*?
h. What is the difference between a cortical cancellous bone graft and a vascularized bone graft?
i. Define *exquisitely*.
j. What is the plural of *calcaneus*?
k. What is the medical term for *inflammation of the fascia*? (*Note*: Watch the spelling; this one is tricky.)
l. Review the anatomy of the ankle and leg. Which muscle is known by the abbreviation *EHL*? Define *syndesmosis*.
m. What is the correct expansion for the *DIP* joint of the finger? What is a *traumatic amputation*?
n. Define *radiculopathy*. Define *conversant*.
o. Research the techniques involved in *microdiskectomy* of the cervical spine.
p. Research types of fractures that occur at the ankle. Make a list. Note the ones that are hardest to spell and pronounce! Make note of the anatomical structures involved in the fractures. (*Note*: You can put "ankle fracture types," without the quotation marks, in Google.)
q. Define *mortise* (as in ankle mortise). What is the adjectival form of *syndesmosis*?
r. Review the anatomy (bones and joints) of the fingers. What is the correct expansion for *PIP*?
s. Research the procedures *open reduction and external fixation* and *open reduction and internal fixation*. What are their abbreviations?
t. What is a *herniated disk* (of the spine)? Research the anatomy and techniques used for cervical spine fusion.
u. What suffix can be added to a variety of directional terms that alters the term to mean in the direction of *x* (*x* being the base word)?
v. What is the abbreviation for *millimeters of mercury*?
w. What is an Esmarch bandage used for? What is a *ganglion cyst*?
x. What is the *MCP joint* (in the hand)?
y. Research types of bandages used in surgery. Make a list.
z. What is the difference between a *frozen section* and a *permanent section* (in pathology). Which is more likely to be performed on a ganglion cyst?

Sample Reports

Sample orthopedic reports appear on the following pages, illustrating a variety of reports. Fictional names are provided for illustration of proper format, and no resemblance to actual persons is intended. Sample transcripts were prepared according to the *AAMT Book of Style*, where possible.

Operative Report

HALVERSEN, JORDAN
#052562
Date of Operation: 9/25/XXXX

PREOPERATIVE DIAGNOSIS
1. Left knee medial collateral ligament tear.
2. Anterior cruciate ligament tear.
3. Possible meniscus tear.

POSTOPERATIVE DIAGNOSIS
1. Left knee medial collateral ligament tear.
2. Anterior cruciate ligament tear.
3. Possible meniscus tear.

PROCEDURES
1. Exam under anesthesia.
2. Diagnostic arthroscopy.
3. Debridement, anterior cruciate ligament stump.
4. Repair, lateral meniscus, arthroscopically.

ESTIMATED BLOOD LOSS
Minimal.

TOURNIQUET TIME
Two hours.

INDICATIONS
This is a 38-year-old white male who sustained an injury to his left knee 3 days prior to admission when he was jumping from a boat onto a dock and had an external rotation injury with his foot planted. On clinical examination, he was noted to have increased valgus stress at the end point, slightly increased Lachman; however, the patient was quite guarded on exam. In addition, he had a hemarthrosis. It was felt that he would benefit from exam under anesthesia and diagnostic arthroscopy and repair of structures as necessary.

(continued)

HALVERSEN, JORDAN
#052562
Page 2

PROCEDURE
The patient was taken to the operating room, placed in a supine position on the operating room table, and turned in the left lateral decubitus position where an epidural anesthetic was placed. Once this had taken effect, the patient's left leg was examined under anesthesia and noted to have an increased valgus laxity with end point, a positive Lachman test, and positive pivot-shift test.

The patient's left lower extremity was then prepped and draped in the normal fashion, exsanguinated, and the tourniquet applied to 350 mmHg. The knee was then insufflated with fluid, a large trocar placed in the medial suprapatellar pouch, and two parapatellar portholes, one lateral and one medial, just above joint line were made. The knee was thoroughly irrigated with fluid using the arthroscopic sheath, and then using the 25° 0.5-mm arthroscope, visualization of the joint was begun. Beginning in the suprapatellar pouch, there was no significant abnormality noted or loose bodies. The undersurface of the patella showed some mild wear laterally. It was noted to ride in the femoral groove in a centrally directed fashion without deviation. Exam of the medial joint revealed a medial plica which was not fibrous or inflamed. Exam of the medial gutter revealed no loose bodies. Exam of the medial joint line revealed the meniscus to be intact, being probed in its entirety, and good femoral and tibial articular cartilage noted.

The meniscus was well visualized due to the medial collateral ligament injury. The deep collateral ligament was visualized and noted to be stretched but not completely torn. The posterior horn of the medial meniscus was examined through the notch using a 70° scope, and no evidence of meniscal tear was noted.

Examination of the notch revealed the anterior cruciate ligament to be completely avulsed from its femoral attachment. The remaining tendon was debrided using the automated shaver. Attention was then turned to the lateral joint line, where the posterior horn of the lateral meniscus was torn in its periphery. The remainder of the meniscus was noted to be intact. The popliteus tendon was visualized and noted to be intact. The femoral and tibial articular cartilage was noted to be intact. Exam of the lateral gutter revealed no loose bodies or abnormalities.

Attention was then turned to the lateral meniscus where, using a meniscal shaver, the tear was debrided. Using the arthroscope, the posterior horn of the lateral meniscus was then sutured with two mattress-type sutures of nonabsorbable 2-0 material. This was accomplished, making a 2-inch lateral incision in order to visualize the posterolateral joint, including the fascia lata distally. The sutures were then tied over the posterolateral capsule, and visualization with the arthroscope revealed the meniscus to be in excellent position and stable. Once this was accomplished, the wound was thoroughly irrigated. The subcutaneous tissue was closed using 3-0 Vicryl suture in an interrupted fashion and the skin with a 3-0 nylon running stitch. The knee was irrigated with copious fluid and closed using 4-0 nylon suture in an interrupted fashion. A sterile compressive dressing was applied. The patient was placed in TED hose and Watco brace, setting the brace between 40° and 60° of free motion. He was then taken to the recovery room in stable condition. The instrument, sponge, and needle counts were correct.

STEVEN RALSTON, MD

SR:hpi
d: 9/25/XXXX
t: 9/26/XXXX

WERNER, MURIEL
#89810
Date of Operation: 7/14/XXXX

PREOPERATIVE DIAGNOSES
1. Chronic ankle pain, left.
2. Status post left Brostrom procedure and subtalar debridement.

POSTOPERATIVE DIAGNOSES
1. Chronic ankle pain, left.
2. Status post left Brostrom procedure and subtalar debridement.
3. Chronic synovitis of the left ankle with scarring.
4. Posterolateral osteochondral lesion of the talus.

PROCEDURE
Left ankle arthroscopy with extensive debridement of scar tissue and curettage and debridement of posterolateral talar osteochondral lesion.

TOURNIQUET TIME
72 minutes.

INDICATIONS
The patient is a 52-year-old female status post a left Brostrom procedure and subtalar debridement who complains of persistent discomfort in her posterior ankle joint which was relieved by Marcaine injections. She is brought to the operating room for a surgical debridement procedure.

The patient was taken to the operating room and after adequate general anesthesia was obtained, stress x-rays were performed of the ankle which showed no instability. She was given 1 g IV Ancef. The leg was placed in a leg holder and prepped and draped in the usual sterile fashion. External distraction was used. Anterolateral and anteromedial portals were used. A 2.7-mm Storz arthroscope was placed in the anteromedial portal and an outflow cannula in the anterolateral. It was difficult to see at first because of a significant amount of scar tissue in the anterior part of the ankle joint, which was debrided using a 2.9-mm full radius shaver. Upon visualization of the ankle joint, there was a significant amount of synovitis and scar tissue in the anterior portion of the medial gutter and a moderate amount in the anterior portion of the anterolateral gutter. There was a moderate amount of scar tissue and synovitis in both the posteromedial and posterolateral ankle joint. Upon probing, there was an area of extremely soft cartilage over the posterolateral talus consistent with an osteochondral lesion. This lesion was debrided with a curette and a shaver, and a grasper was used to remove the fragments.

We had some difficulty visualizing from the anteromedial portal. In order to complete the procedure, a posterolateral portal was made and the arthroscope placed in the anterolateral portal and the shaver in the posterolateral portal. All of the scar tissue was debrided and afterwards the osteochondral lesion had a firm bleeding cancellous bed. Of note, this was done with the tourniquet inflated to 250 mmHg. Upon completing the procedure, there was also no evidence of any loose bodies in the joint. The tourniquet was released. The incision was closed with 3-0 nylon. At that point 0.5% plain Marcaine was injected into the joint. A compressive Jones dressing was applied.

NEAL KRAUS, MD

NK:hpi
d: 7/14/XXXX
t: 7/15/XXXX

Discharge Summary

GONZALES, JUANITA
#081948
Admitted: 8/25/XXXX
Discharged: 8/26/XXXX

ADMITTING DIAGNOSIS
Tensor fasciae latae syndrome, left thigh.

DISCHARGE DIAGNOSIS
Tensor fasciae latae syndrome, left thigh.

OPERATION PERFORMED
Excision, trochanteric bursa, and division, fascia lata, left thigh.

HISTORY
The patient has had difficulty since June or July and has had a variety of treatments, including physiotherapy and local injections, none of which produced any substantial or ongoing relief.

PHYSICAL EXAMINATION
There was restricted range of motion in the left hip.

LABORATORY WORK
The patient had a slightly elevated uric acid at 6.9 and a slightly elevated cholesterol of 212.

The pathology specimen was unreported at the time of discharge. Segments of the trochanteric bursa were sent to the laboratory for evaluation.

HOSPITAL COURSE
On the day of admission, the patient was admitted for a 23-hour-day case, and the hip was opened through a rather extensive lateral incision down to the greater trochanteric bursa. This was excised together with an oblique incision distally through the tensor fasciae latae, actually distally and proximally. The subcutaneous tissues other than the fascia were closed together with an intracuticular stitch in the skin. The patient had more pain than anticipated and was hospitalized.

CONDITION ON DISCHARGE
At the time of discharge, the patient was ambulatory on crutches. She did, however, have a low-grade temperature but had no clinical symptoms. The wound appeared entirely satisfactory.

POSTOPERATIVE PLAN
The patient should be on crutches, increasing her weightbearing gradually.

J. STEPHEN FOX, MD

JSF:hpi
d: 8/25/XXXX
t: 8/27/XXXX

Operative Report

REINEKE, KARL
#711406
Date of Operation: 7/14/XXXX

PREOPERATIVE DIAGNOSIS
Anterior knee pain, left knee.

POSTOPERATIVE DIAGNOSES
1. Anterior knee pain, left knee.
2. Mild Outerbridge grade II focal chondromalacia trochleae.

PROCEDURE
Diagnostic arthroscopy, left knee, and debridement of articular cartilage.

ANESTHESIA
Spinal.

FINDINGS
1. Normal patella.
2. Large medial parapatellar plica.
3. Focal chondromalacia, femoral trochlea.
4. Normal medial joint space.
5. Intact anterior cruciate ligament (ACL).
6. Normal lateral joint space.

DISPOSITION
Stable to recovery room.

INDICATIONS
The patient is a 40-year-old white male with anterior knee pain. He failed conservative treatment and was scheduled for diagnostic arthroscopy as well as possible lateral release due to patellar tilt seen on sunrise views.

The patient was brought to the operating room and underwent induction of spinal anesthesia without difficulty. His left lower extremity was prepped and draped in the outstretched position on the table. A tourniquet was placed but not inflated for the procedure.

A superior medial portal site was chosen and a knife was used to incise the skin only. Then a blunt trocar with a blunt tip pillow was passed through the incision into the knee joint itself. The scope was advanced through the trocar sleeve into the knee. Once its articular position was verified, the knee was infiltrated with sterile normal saline. Then a small knife wound was made in the lateral parapatellar tendon and an outflow trocar was placed. Examination from the superior medial portal showed that the patella appeared to track nearly anatomically and engage the trochlear groove appropriately. There was no noticeable excessive tilt. There was no striking out on the lateral portion of the femoral condyle noted. There was no deviation of the patella as it entered into the trochlear groove.

After examination from the superior portion was completed, the scope was removed from the superior medial portal and the outflow was changed from the lateral parapatellar portal to the superior medial portal. The scope was then introduced through the trocar, which had been passed into the lateral parapatellar tendon portal. A systematic diagnostic arthroscopy of the knee was then carried out which showed clear gutters both medially and laterally, intact medial and lateral joint spaces, and an intact ACL.

(continued)

398

REINEKE, KARL
#711406
Date of Operation: 7/14/XXXX
Page 2

Next our attention was turned to a large plica that did not appear to strike the medial femoral condyle but had a continuation distally and inferiorly that looked slightly inflamed and may have been interfering with patellar motion. This was debrided with a Dyonics lime green shaver. The small 5 x 7 mm focal trochlear lesion was also debrided. Following this, knee motion was again checked and patellar tracking from the inferior portal again showed near-anatomic alignment of the patella with the femoral trochlea. The knee was copiously irrigated. Antibiotic solution was instilled and then expressed through the trocar. All trocars were removed. Steri-Strips were placed over the portal sites, and the knee was sterilely dressed. The patient tolerated the procedure well and was transferred to the recovery room in satisfactory condition.

MARIO SANTUCCI, MD

MS:hpi
d: 7/14/XXXX
t: 7/14/XXXX

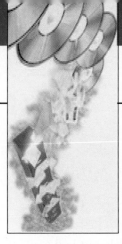

Transcription Practice

Key Words

The following terms appear in the orthopedic dictations. Before beginning the medical transcription practice for Chapter 13, look up each term below in a medical or English dictionary and write out a short definition.

bone grafting	ganglion cyst excision
calcaneus (pl. calcanei)	herniated disk
cervical disk and spur	laceration
Cloward fusion	lumbar strain
contusion	Maisonneuve-type ankle
CVA tenderness	injury
delayed scaphoid union	microdiskectomy
DIP joint	neuromata
EHL muscle	nonunion of scaphoid
fibular shaft fracture	ORIF
fusion and plating	palmar mass

phalanx reconstitution	stress fracture
PIP joint	syndesmosis
plantar fasciitis	syndesmotic screws
radial ulnar styloid	total hip replacement
radiculopathy	traumatic amputation of
revascularization	finger
scaphoid nonunion	trimalleolar ankle fracture
sciatica	vascularized bone graft
screw placement	

After completing all the readings and exercises in Chapter 13, transcribe the orthopedic dictation. Proofread your transcribed documents carefully, listening to the dictation while you read your transcripts.

Transcribe (*not* retype) the same reports again without referring to your previous transcription attempt. Initially, you may need to transcribe some reports more than twice before you can produce an error-free document. Your ultimate goal is to produce an error-free document the first time.

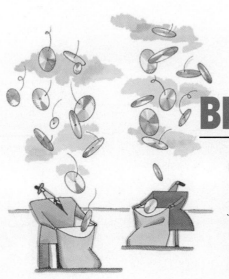

BLOOPERS

Incorrect	Correct
Rectal exam showed hyperactive ankle jerks.	Peripheral exam showed hyperactive ankle jerks.
No evidence of fracture or osseous mythology.	No evidence of fracture or osseous pathology.
Treated with Parafon #4 tape.	Treated with Parafon Forte.
There is full range of emotion.	There is full range of motion.
C5 disconnectomy.	C5 diskectomy.
General conditioning to unembalmed extremities.	General conditioning to uninvolved extremities.
The knee is swollen, tender, red, and warped.	The knee is swollen, tender, red, and warm.
Foot is cold with a purple shoe.	Foot is cold with a purplish hue.
Status post blown knee amputation.	Status post below-knee amputation.
There is pain on the platter aspect.	There is pain on the plantar aspect.
Long legged pants were removed.	Long leg cast was removed.

Chapter 14

Neurology

Chapter Outline

Transcribing Neurology Dictation
Anatomy in Brief
Terminology Review
Lay and Medical Terms
Medical Readings
History and Physical Examination
Common Diseases
Diagnostic and Surgical Procedures

Laboratory Procedures
Pharmacology
Transcription Tips
Spotlight
Proofreading Skills
Skills Challenge
Sample Reports
Transcription Practice
Bloopers

Learning Objectives

- Describe the structure and function of the nervous system.
- Spell and define common neurology terms.
- Identify types of questions a physician might ask about the nervous system during the review of systems.
- Describe common features a physician looks for on neurologic examination.
- Identify common diseases of the nervous system. Describe their typical cause, course, and treatment options.

- Identify and define diagnostic and surgical procedures of the nervous system.
- List common neurologic laboratory tests and procedures.
- Identify and describe common neurologic drugs and their uses.
- Demonstrate knowledge of anatomical, medical, pharmacological, adjectival, and soundalike terms by accurately completing the exercises in this chapter.

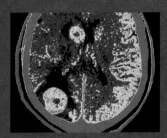
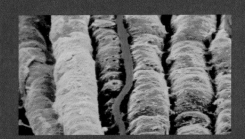
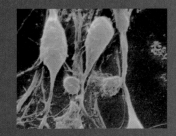

Transcribing Neurology Dictation

The **nervous system** (Figure 14-1) is an exceedingly complex arrangement of nerve cells and their fibers that extends throughout the body and receives, processes, and interprets sensory stimuli; initiates and coordinates voluntary muscular movement; regulates autonomic processes such as heartbeat, vascular constriction and dilatation, bronchiolar caliber, sweating, and gastrointestinal secretion and motility; carries out complex mental functions and operations including memory and recall of past events, recognition of persons and objects, abstract reasoning and practical problem solving, judgment, and language production and comprehension; and is the seat of mood and emotions.

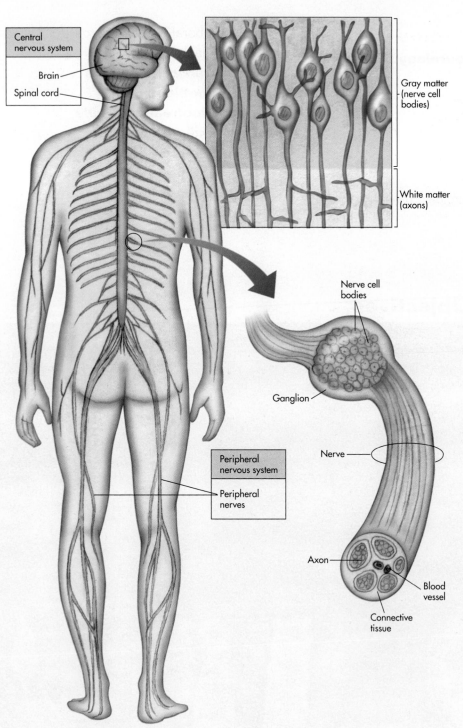

Central
nervous system

Brain

Spinal cord

Gray matter
(nerve cell
bodies)

White matter
(axons)

Nerve cell
bodies

Ganglion

Nerve

Peripheral
nervous system

Peripheral
nerves

Axon

Blood
vessel

Connective
tissue

Figure 14-1
The Nervous System

Anatomy in Brief

All nerve tissue is made up of **nerve cells** and their processes. Although nerve cells vary widely in structure and function, all conform to a basic pattern. Each nerve cell (**neuron**) consists of a cell body containing a nucleus; one or more short treelike processes called **dendrites**; and a single long straight process, the **axon**. Dendrites conduct nerve impulses toward the cell body, and are therefore called **afferent processes**; axons conduct impulses away from the cell and are therefore called efferent processes. The point of contact between processes of two different cells is called a **synapse**. Chemical substances called neurotransmitters are produced in infinitesimal quantities at nerve endings and serve to transmit nerve impulses, either stimulating or inhibiting, across the synapse.

The axons of some nerve cells are enveloped in a thin layer of fatty white material called **myelin**. The **myelin sheath** serves as an electrical insulator. Nerve tissue consisting of many myelinated fibers is called **white matter**; tissue consisting chiefly of nerve cell bodies is called **gray matter**.

The nervous system is divided into two major sections: the **central nervous system**, consisting of the brain and spinal cord; and the **peripheral nervous system**, consisting of the peripheral motor and sensory nerves and the **autonomic nervous system**. The **brain** (Figure 14-2), which entirely fills the cranial cavity, is traditionally broken down into major parts on the basis of gross anatomic features:

The **cerebrum**, made up of two symmetric hemispheres and concerned with the higher mental processes; its surface, the **cerebral cortex**, is thrown into deep convolutions like the kernel of a walnut. The convexities (raised areas) are called **gyri**, and the grooves between them are called **sulci**. Deeper grooves (**fissures**) divide each hemisphere into four lobes: **frontal**, **temporal**, **parietal**, and **occipital**.

The **cerebellum** lies behind the cerebrum and looks like a smaller version of it, as its name implies. Its principal function is coordination of voluntary motor activity.

Four structures—diencephalon, mesencephalon or midbrain, pons, and medulla oblongata—compose, from front to back, the **ventral surface of the brain**; the last three make up the **brain stem**. The medulla continues below the skull as the **spinal cord**.

The brain and spinal cord are covered by three protective membranes called **meninges**. The outer membrane, the **dura mater**, is in contact with the bony interior of the skull and spinal column. Within the dura is the delicate **arachnoid membrane**, and within that is the **pia mater**, which lies on the surface of the brain and spinal cord.

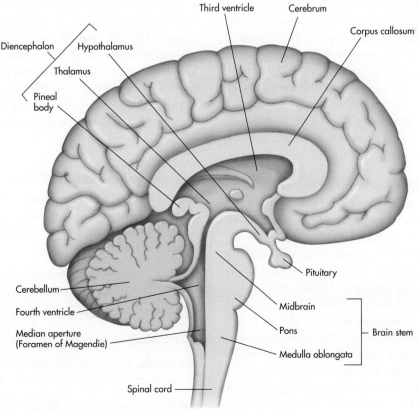

Figure 14-2
The Major Divisions of the Brain

Within the cerebrum and the diencephalon is a system of communicating hollow chambers (the two **lateral ventricles**, the **third ventricle**, and the **fourth ventricle**) (Figure 14-2). **Cerebrospinal fluid** (CSF) is a watery medium that is both formed and reabsorbed within the skull and serves primarily as a shock absorber. It surrounds the brain and spinal cord in the subarachnoid space and also fills the ventricular system and the hollow central canal of the spinal cord.

Twelve pairs of cranial nerves (traditionally represented by Roman numerals) emerge from the ventral surface of the brain and brain stem and serve important sensory and motor functions, chiefly within the head. These are described in detail later.

The **spinal cord** is made up largely of axons of nerve cells, some with cell bodies in the brain (carrying motor impulses to various spinal segments) and others with cell bodies in the cord itself (carrying sensory impulses from spinal segments to various brain centers). Whereas the visible surface of the cerebral cortex is made up of gray matter (cell bodies), with white matter inside, in the spinal cord the white matter, consisting of ascending and descending myelinated nerve fibers, is on the outside, and the gray matter is within.

The **peripheral nervous system** comprises all nerve tissue outside the brain and spinal cord. Its two major divisions are the **spinal nerves** and the **autonomic nervous system**. Spinal nerves are those that originate in the spinal cord and pass between pairs of vertebrae to supply the body with sensation and voluntary motor power. There are 31 sets of spinal nerves, one arising from each spinal segment; these segments correspond closely to the cervical, thoracic, lumbar, and (fused) sacral vertebrae.

Each spinal segment gives off a pair of nerve roots on each side: a **dorsal (sensory) root** and a **ventral (motor) root**. Each dorsal root has a visible node or swelling (**ganglion**) containing cell bodies of sensory nerves. The dorsal and ventral roots fuse to form **segmental nerves**, which pass forward around the body and give off branches to all external surfaces and internal structures, particularly muscles of the trunk and extremities.

Each visible and named peripheral nerve is a bundle of thousands of myelinated axons of motor neurons whose cell bodies lie in the brain and spinal cord, and of dendrites of sensory nerves, whose cell bodies are located in the dorsal root ganglia. **Motor nerves** send signals to voluntary muscles throughout the body. **Sensory nerves** carry impulses from sensory structures in the skin that respond to pain, pressure, light touch, hot, and cold; from visceral sensors that respond to pressure or stretching and pain; and from proprioceptive sensors in voluntary muscles that signal the brain as to their position, tension, and movement.

The **autonomic nervous system** is a purely motor system concerned with automatic or involuntary activities or processes, such as heart rate and digestion. The bodily effects of emotion (tachycardia, sweating, pallor, sense of constriction in the chest) largely result from the actions of the autonomic nervous system.

Nerves of the sympathetic or thoracolumbar division arise from a series of ganglia lying along each side of the thoracic and lumbar segments of the spinal cord, but outside the spinal column. These communicate with the spinal cord and with one another by both myelinated and nonmyelinated fibers. The **sympathetic nervous system** is concerned with the so-called fight or flight response mediated by **epinephrine** and **norepinephrine**. Nerves of the sympathetic division are distributed to the eye, where they cause pupillary dilatation; the heart, where they increase the pulse rate; the lungs, where they cause bronchodilation; and the skin, where they constrict blood vessels, stimulate secretion of sweat, and cause erection of hairs.

The **parasympathetic** or **craniosacral** division of the autonomic nervous system provides motor innervation to cranial, thoracic, abdominal, and pelvic viscera, generally of an opposite nature to sympathetic innervation. That is, parasympathetic activity occurs chiefly during periods of rest or quiet, and is associated with cardiac rate and with such physiologic processes as gastrointestinal secretion and motility and sexual activity.

Parasympathetic nerves arise only from the brain and from sacral segments of the spinal cord. Three cranial nerves (III, VII, and IX) send parasympathetic fibers to structures in the head (iris, ciliary body, salivary glands; a fourth (X) sends fibers to thoracic, abdominal, and pelvic viscera (heart, lungs, digestive system). Parasympathetic nerves from sacral segments of the spinal cord supply the urinary tract and reproductive system.

Terminology Review

altered level of consciousness Varying from slight drowsiness or inattentiveness, to confusion and disorientation, to deep coma from which the subject cannot be aroused by any stimulus.

absence ("absáhnce") **seizure** (petit mal) Brief loss of attention and perception.

amnesia Loss of memory, recent, remote, or total.

anencephaly Absence of cerebral hemispheres.

anesthesia Total loss of sensation on one or more parts of the body surface.

aphasia Impairment of the ability to communicate through spoken or written language, or to understand spoken or written language, or both.

ataxia Impairment of complex movements due to loss of proprioceptive impulses from the muscles of the trunk or limbs.

athetosis Slow, writhing, involuntary movements of the face or limbs.

Babinski reflex Consists of dorsiflexion of the great toe and flaring of the other toes in response to stroking the sole of the foot toward the toes; an indication of disease or injury affecting a corticospinal tract. A normal reflex is downgoing, except in newborns and infants, in which the normal Babinski reflex is upgoing.

causalgia Burning or stinging due to irritation or inflammation of nerves.

Chaddock reflex Extension of the great toe elicited by tapping the ankle behind the lateral malleolus, a sign of disease or injury of a corticospinal tract.

chorea Rapid, jerky, purposeless involuntary movements of one or several muscle groups.

complex seizure Impaired alertness or unconsciousness; sometimes with psychic symptoms or automatisms.

deep tendon reflexes Also called *muscle stretch reflexes*; occur in response to sudden stretching of a muscle, usually induced by tapping a tendon with a rubber-headed reflex hammer. Tendon reflexes are tested in several muscles of the upper and lower extremities, with comparison of the two sides.

dementia Deterioration of mental function.

dysequilibrium Loss of balance sense; tendency to fall without support.

flaccidity Absence of muscle tone and absence of reflexes.

generalized seizure A seizure in which the entire cerebral cortex is involved.

grand mal seizure See *tonic-clonic.*

headache Local or generalized, intermittent or constant; can result from infection, neoplasm, or hemorrhage within the cranium, obstruction to the flow of cerebrospinal fluid, trauma, or migraine.

hydranencephaly A more severe form of microcephaly, with very little cerebral cortex remaining.

hypesthesia Partial loss of sensation on one or more parts of the body surface.

incoordination Jerkiness and awkwardness in activities requiring smooth coordination of several muscles.

intention tremor Tremor occurring only during voluntary movement.

microcephaly Abnormally small, maldeveloped cerebral hemispheres, typically associated with mental and motor retardation.

myoclonic seizures Repeated shocklike, often violent contractions in one or more muscle groups.

paralysis Complete loss of muscular function.

paresis Muscle weakness.

paresthesia A sense of tingling or prickling ("pins and needles") on a part of the body surface. The lay term "numbness" is applied indiscriminately to hypesthesia, anesthesia, and paresthesia.

partial seizure Seizure in which only part of one cerebral cortex is involved.

pathologic reflexes Present only in neurological disorders, such as Babinski reflex or Chaddock reflex.

petit mal seizure (absence seizure) Characterized by brief loss of attention and perception.

Phalen sign Reproduction of pain or paresthesia in carpal tunnel syndrome when both wrists are flexed with the hands firmly pressing one another back-to-back for 60 seconds.

porencephaly One or more cysts or cavities in a cerebral hemisphere communicating with the ventricular system. There may be little or no neurologic impairment.

postictal state After awakening from seizure, subject is drowsy and amnesic for a variable period.

reflex A muscular contraction occurring in response to a sensory stimulus.

resting tremor Tremor occurring only when the affected muscles are not being used for purposeful activity.

seizures Sudden, transitory impairment of central nervous system function, with or without loss of consciousness, and with or without local or generalized tonic and clonic contractions of voluntary muscles.

simple seizure No unconsciousness; local twitching or jerking; perception of flashing lights or other abnormal sensory phenomena.

spasm Sustained contraction, usually painful, of a muscle.

spasticity Tight muscles with resistance to manipulation and hyperactive reflexes.

spina bifida A failure of closure of one or more vertebrae in the posterior midline, which may be associated with bulging of meninges (**meningocele**) or of spinal cord and meninges (**meningomyelocele**) (Figure 14-3).

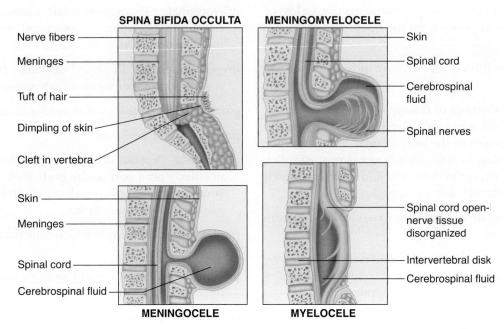

Figure 14-3
Forms of Spina Bifida

status epilepticus Series of grand mal seizures without waking intervals.

superficial reflexes Muscle contractions in response to stroking the skin; those of the abdominal wall are tested as part of a complete neurologic examination.

syncope (fainting) Sudden loss of consciousness, usually transitory, due to circulatory or neurologic abnormality, including central nervous system intoxication or injury, but frequently the result of strong emotion in the absence of organic disease.

tic A rapid involuntary muscle twitch, typically recurrent and stereotyped, affecting one or several body areas.

Tinel sign Shocklike pain when the volar aspect of the wrist is tapped; indicative of carpal tunnel syndrome.

tonic-clonic seizure In the tonic phase the victim becomes rigid, often cries out, loses consciousness, falls, stops breathing. In the clonic phase there is generalized muscular jerking; may bite tongue or lips, may be incontinent of urine or stool.

tremor(s) Shaking of parts of the body supplied by voluntary muscles, principally the arms, forearms, and hands.

vertigo A subjective sense of spinning. Dysequilibrium and vertigo sometimes occur together, and both are indiscriminately referred to as dizziness by the laity.

Lay and Medical Terms

fainting	syncope
fit, convulsion	seizure; epileptic seizure
numbness	hypesthesia, anesthesia, or paresthesia
pins and needles	sense of tingling or prickling
spinal tap	lumbar puncture
stroke	cerebrovascular accident (CVA)
water on the brain	hydrocephalus

Medical Readings

History and Physical Examination

by John H. Dirckx, M.D.

Review of Systems. The subject is questioned about prior diagnosis of, and treatment for, seizures, brain concussion, brain tumor, stroke, paralysis, and neuritis.

Symptoms suggestive of **central nervous system disease** are severe or unusual headache; unexplained drowsiness or dysequilibrium; confusion; disorientation; sudden deterioration of memory, judgment, or emotional stability; tremors; incoordination; disorders of speech; weakness, clumsiness, paralysis, or spasticity of the extremities; and seizures. Often, detailed information on these points must be obtained from someone other than the patient. In obtaining a full picture of any of these symptoms, the interviewer asks whether it is constant, intermittent, or progressive; to what extent it impairs normal function; and whether any cause can be suggested for the symptom, such as a recent or remote injury or use of alcohol or drugs.

In gathering data about **syncopal episodes** or seizures, the physician will try to learn from an observer whether the patient displayed any warning signs of distress, cried out, fell, lost consciousness completely or only became confused; whether there was local or general twitching or writhing of the extremities; whether the patient was incontinent of urine during the seizure; and how long after the seizure any weakness, drowsiness, or confusion remained.

Peripheral nerve disorders are suggested by numbness, paresthesia (a tingling or "pins and needles" sensation), weakness, or paralysis in an extremity. The pain of peripheral neuritis is often described as stinging or burning and often seems to shoot along or just under the surface like an electric shock. The diagnostician inquires whether symptoms are brought on or aggravated by fatigue, certain activities or positions, or a cold or damp environment, and whether there has been exposure to toxic drugs or chemicals.

Physical Examination. The examination of the central and peripheral nervous systems, like that of the heart, consists almost exclusively of tests of function. Many of these tests require the cooperation of the patient. However, the more urgent the need for a neurologic exam, the less capable the patient may be of cooperating. The extreme example is the comatose patient, whose life may depend on prompt and accurate diagnosis but who cannot cooperate at all. The basic neurologic examination is augmented by special procedures as history and findings direct.

Most parts of the neurologic examination are carried out on a regional basis and interspersed with examinations of other systems. In analyzing and recording findings, however, the physician classifies them according to anatomic and functional divisions of the nervous system. The central nervous system (CNS) comprises the brain and spinal cord; the peripheral nervous system, the cranial and spinal nerves. Peripheral nerve fibers are either motor (efferent) fibers carrying impulses to muscles, or sensory (afferent) fibers carrying impulses to the spinal cord or brain stem. Both kinds of fibers are often combined in a single nerve trunk.

The physician tests sensory functions by stimulating appropriate receptors and noting the subject's responses. Motor functions are tested by observing the subject's ability to perform certain actions. Even in an unconscious patient, testing the deep tendon reflexes enables the examiner to assess the integrity of the

spinal reflex arcs, which consist of both sensory (stretch receptor) and motor nerve fibers. But evaluation of complex voluntary movements and muscle coordination requires the conscious collaboration of the patient.

If the patient is stuporous or unconscious, the physician tries to determine the degree of central nervous system depression by noting the size and reactivity of the pupils, the rate and rhythm of breathing, the response to noxious stimuli such as loud noises and firm pressure over bony prominences, and the presence of certain primitive reflexes such as the corneal and gag reflex. In the doll's eye maneuver, the examiner rotates the patient's head from side to side and notes the effect on eye position. Normally the eyes rotate in a direction opposite to that in which the head is moved, tending to maintain the same direction of gaze (oculocephalic reflex). Failure of the eyes to rotate around their own vertical axes during this maneuver indicates brain stem damage.

Cranial Nerves. The twelve pairs of cranial nerves (traditionally represented by Roman numerals) (see Figure 14-4) emanate from the brain stem and pass to structures in the head and neck. They serve important sensory and motor functions, chiefly within the head. The cranial nerves are assessed individually by the following maneuvers:

I. **Olfactory:** Testing sense of smell. This assessment is often omitted, hence the frequent expression, "Cranial nerves II through XII are intact." It can be evaluated by asking the subject to identify common substances (soap, tobacco) by their odors.

II. **Optic:** Testing the subject's vision with standard eye charts. Checking peripheral vision and visual fields by simple techniques. Examination of the ocular fundi with an ophthalmoscope.

III. **Oculomotor:** Testing ocular movements; observing for strabismus, nystagmus, and drooping of eyelids. Testing the ability of the pupil to constrict when stimulated by light and when focused on a near object.

IV. **Trochlear:** Extraocular movements already assessed.

V. **Trigeminal:** Sensitivity to light touch (wisp of cotton or fine brush) and pain (sterile needle) are tested over the skin of the face. The blink reflex to touching the cornea with cotton is also tested. The integrity of motor branches to the muscles of mastication is tested by having the subject open the mouth wide and then clench the teeth together.

VI. **Abducens:** Extraocular muscles already assessed.

VII. **Facial:** Testing muscles of facial expression by having the subject wrinkle the forehead, close the eyes tightly, retract the lips so as to show the teeth, and purse the lips as for whistling. Taste on the anterior two thirds (front

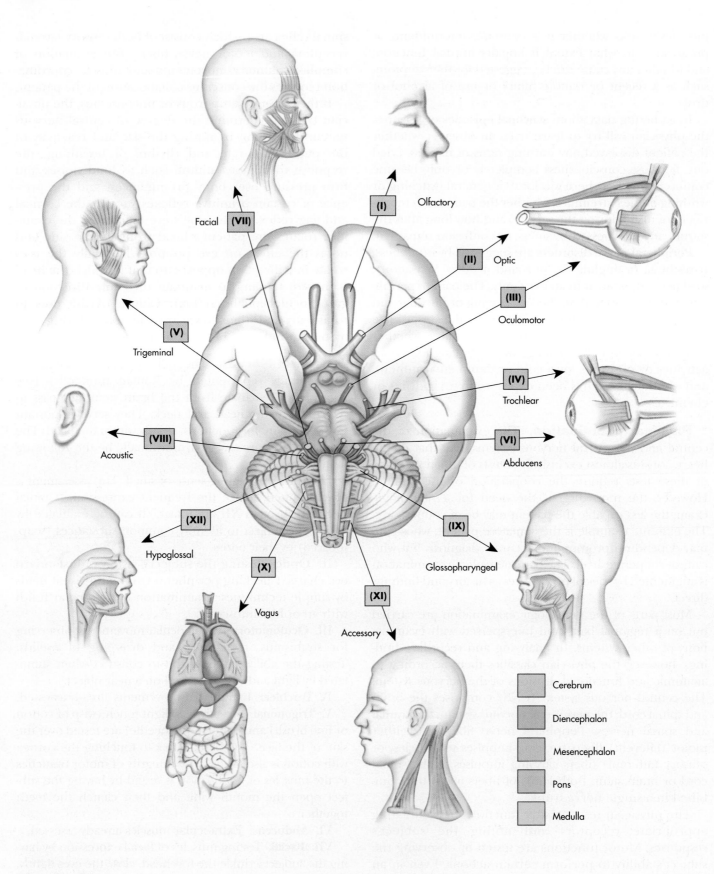

Figure 14-4
The Relationship of the Twelve Cranial Nerves to Specific Regions of the Brain

part) of the tongue may be tested by touching the tongue with a drop of salt or sugar solution or vinegar.

VIII. **Vestibulocochlear**: Hearing and equilibrium. Cold caloric test: when ice water is poured into the ear canal, a normal vestibular apparatus causes nystagmus with the quick component to the opposite side. Hearing is tested in each ear separately.

IX. **Glossopharyngeal**: With impairment of innervation to one side of the palate, the uvula deviates to the normal side, particularly during the gag reflex. Swallowing is affected by impairment of either the ninth or the tenth cranial nerve.

X. **Vagus**: The subject's ability to speak and to swallow is observed.

XI. **Accessory**: The subject's ability to push against the examiner's hand with each side of the chin indicates integrity of the nerve supply to the sternocleidomastoid and trapezius muscles.

XII. **Hypoglossal**: The examiner notes the symmetry of development of the tongue muscles at rest and the symmetry of movement when the tongue is protruded. Impairment of a hypoglossal nerve causes deviation of the tongue to the affected side.

Spinal Nerve Examination. Sensory innervation of the skin is assessed by the subject's ability to recognize **light touch** (wisp of cotton), **pain** (sterile needle), **hot and cold** (test tubes of hot and cold water) on various parts of the body surface. Examination may include tests of **stereognosis** (ability to recognize an object by handling it), **vibratory sense** (ability to sense the vibration of a tuning fork when the stem is placed on a bone near the surface, such as the elbow or the shin), **two-point discrimination** (ability to distinguish two points close together on the skin).

Proprioception is tested by having the subject report whether a toe or finger is moved up or down by the examiner, and by observation of stance and gait. The **Romberg test** (having the subject stand with feet together and eyes open, then eyes closed) assesses position sense in the trunk and legs.

Motor innervation is tested by observation of muscle development, tone, and voluntary movement in the trunk and limbs, with comparison of the two sides. The examiner notes any wasting, paralysis, spasm or rigidity, or involuntary movements (tremors, tics, chorea, athetosis). Coordination is tested by having the subject perform **rapid alternating movements** with the hands or feet. The **finger-to-nose** and **heel-to-shin tests** and **tandem walking** are other ways of judging coordination.

Reflexes: A reflex is a muscular contraction occurring in response to a sensory stimulus, such as tapping the patellar tendon. All the nerve cells and fibers involved in a reflex are located in a spinal cord segment, and its sensory and motor roots form a so-called **reflex arc**; the brain is not involved.

Muscle stretch (deep tendon) reflexes occur in response to sudden stretching of a muscle, usually induced by tapping a tendon with a rubber-headed reflex hammer. Tendon reflexes are tested in several muscles of the upper and lower extremities, with comparison of the two sides.

Superficial (cutaneous) reflexes are muscle contractions in response to stroking the skin; those of the abdominal wall are tested as part of a complete neurologic examination.

Pathologic reflexes are present only in neurologic disorders. The **Babinski reflex** consists of dorsiflexion of the great toe and flaring of the other toes in response to stroking of the sole of the foot toward the toes. The **Chaddock reflex** is the same response to tapping the lateral aspect of the ankle. These and similar pathologic reflexes, along with spastic paralysis and rigidity, indicate an **upper motor neuron lesion**—interruption of motor tracts from the cerebral cortex to the spinal segment involved, without impairment of the reflex arc. Flaccid paralysis, absence of normal and abnormal reflexes, and muscle wasting indicate a **lower motor neuron lesion**—interruption of motor tracts from spinal cord to muscle.

Common Diseases

Congenital Hydrocephalus. Enlargement of the head by excessive fluid pressure within the ventricular system, evident at birth or within the first few weeks of life.

Causes: Obstruction to the normal outflow of cerebrospinal fluid from the ventricular system due to a congenital defect, often the result of maternal infection (toxoplasmosis, rubella, cytomegalovirus, syphilis).

Physical Examination: Abnormally large circumference of the head at birth, or disproportionate increase in head size during early infancy.

Diagnostic Tests: CT scan and ultrasonography confirm ventricular enlargement and may indicate the site of obstruction.

Course: Without treatment, progressive enlargement of the ventricular system can be expected, with damage to the cerebral hemispheres and other intracranial structures.

Treatment: Surgical insertion of a shunt from the obstructed ventricular system to the right atrium of the heart or to the peritoneal cavity (Figure 14-5).

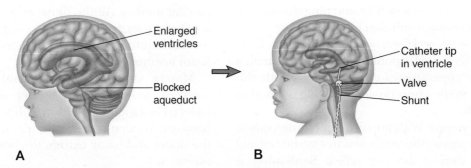

Figure 14-5
A) Hydrocephalus; B) Excess Cerebrospinal Fluid Drained by a Shunt

Multiple Sclerosis (MS). A chronic sensory and motor disorder of variable presentation, due to loss of myelin from nerve cells in the central nervous system.

Cause: Patchy deterioration of the myelin sheaths of nerve tracts in the brain and spinal cord and in the optic nerve leads to deterioration of nerve function. The cause is unknown; genetic, infectious, and autoimmune factors have been suggested. Onset is usually between the ages of 20 and 40. The incidence is higher in women and in cooler latitudes. Disease is sometimes apparently precipitated by fatigue, emotional stress, pregnancy, or viral respiratory infection.

History: Irregular, intermittent or progressive impairment of sensory or motor function: hypesthesia, paresthesia, visual disturbances, disorders of equilibrium; muscular weakness, spasticity, or unsteadiness; tremors, nystagmus, diplopia, disturbances of swallowing or bladder function.

Physical Examination: Findings on neurologic examination are typically diffuse and highly variable: hypesthesia or anesthesia, irregularly distributed muscle weakness with spasticity and hyperactive deep tendon reflexes, Babinski reflex, impaired superficial abdominal reflexes, ataxia, uncoordinated (scanning) speech, tremors, nystagmus, temporal pallor of the optic disks followed by optic atrophy, visual field defects, emotional lability.

Diagnostic Tests: The spinal fluid may show moderate lymphocytosis and elevation of the immune globulins, including oligoclonal IgG globulins (antibody to myelin) not found in serum. The electroencephalogram may show nonspecific abnormalities. MRI of the brain and spinal cord shows multiple patchy lesions. Visual evoked potential testing may corroborate the diagnosis.

Course: The disease is highly unpredictable. Four patterns are distinguished: relapsing remitting, primary progressive, secondary progressive, and progressive relapsing. Presenting symptoms often remit for months or years. Typically the disease progresses gradually, with remissions and exacerbations, and eventually produces some disability. Relapses may be triggered by excessive fatigue.

Treatment: Increased rest, particularly during periods of heightened symptoms. Adrenocortical steroids often mitigate neurologic impairment, particularly during acute relapses. Physical therapy and muscle relaxants are helpful in dealing with muscle weakness and spasm. Immunotherapy, plasmapheresis, and synthetic myelin protein are among treatments currently being evaluated. Psychotherapy or counseling may be necessary.

Guillain-Barré Syndrome. A chronic inflammation of peripheral nerves, causing muscle weakness or paralysis.

Cause: Formation of autoantibody to myelin, with resultant segmental demyelination of peripheral nerve fibers, usually reversible. Precipitating causes: acute infection (influenza, infectious mononucleosis, varicellazoster), myocardial infarction, certain vaccines, surgery.

History: Progressive, symmetric muscle weakness in both arms and legs, paresthesia, hypesthesia, and pain, coming on 1-4 weeks after the precipitating event. The cranial nerves may be involved. Loss of bladder control and respiratory paralysis may occur.

Physical Examination: Peripheral sensation is impaired, and deep tendon reflexes are diminished or absent. The pulse and blood pressure may be elevated.

Diagnostic Tests: The spinal fluid contains elevated protein but normal cell counts.

Course: The case fatality rate is about 5%. About 65% of patients who recover have minor neurologic impairment and 10% remain severely disabled.

Treatment: Physical therapy; cardiac monitoring and pulse oximetry, with mechanical ventilation as needed. Intravenous immune globulin. Plasmapheresis to remove antibody from serum.

Amyotrophic Lateral Sclerosis (Lou Gehrig Disease). Progressive paralysis and wasting of muscles due to degeneration of motor neurons.

Cause: Unknown. There is a genetic predisposition, and men are affected more than women by a ratio of 3:1.

Viral or autoimmune factors cannot be excluded. Possible precipitating factors include trauma, extreme stress or fatigue, viral respiratory infection, and myocardial infarction.

History: Onset, between the ages of 30 and 50, of weakness and wasting of voluntary muscles, particularly those in the hands and feet. **Fasciculations** (repeated twitching of small groups of voluntary muscle fibers) may precede any other symptoms. Eventually, with brain stem involvement, difficulty in speaking, eating, and even breathing. Depression commonly occurs with progressive deterioration.

Physical Examination: Muscle weakness and atrophy, visible fasciculations, evidence of cranial and spinal motor nerve malfunction without sensory impairment. Hyperactive deep tendon reflexes, spasticity, and rigidity indicate upper motor neuron degeneration.

Diagnostic Tests: Electromyography and muscle biopsy confirm loss of motor nerve supply to affected areas.

Course: Usually the disease is steadily progressive and death occurs in 2-5 years.

Treatment: Purely supportive; physical therapy, muscle relaxants; nasogastric tube or gastrostomy feedings, tracheotomy and respirator as needed.

Parkinsonism (Parkinson Disease, Paralysis Agitans). A chronic, progressive neurologic disorder causing muscle tremor and rigidity.

Cause: Unknown. Neurologic symptoms are due to deterioration and dopamine depletion in certain brain nuclei (corpus striatum, globus pallidus, substantia nigra). It is more common in men and onset is usually between 45 and 65. Certain toxic chemicals (carbon disulfide, carbon monoxide), drugs (chlorpromazine, haloperidol, and other neuroleptic drugs), and a history of encephalitis can induce parkinsonian symptoms.

History: Resting tremor, initially in one extremity, that is exacerbated by emotional stress and reduced during voluntary motion. Stiffness, rigidity, and **bradykinesia** (slowness of movement) commonly occur, with postural instability and gait disorders.

Physical Examination: Immobile, masklike face, with infrequent blinking. Reduced automatic movements such as swinging the arms while walking. Hyperactive deep tendon reflexes and resistance to passive movement of joints, often with **"cogwheel" rigidity**. A flexed posture, a shuffling and seemingly hurried (festinating) gait, and difficulty in standing from a sitting position are typical. Seborrhea (excessive secretion of sebum) on the scalp and face and excessive drooling are also often seen. The handwriting becomes smaller (**micrographia**). There may be mild deterioration of mental function.

Course: Typically progressive, with death in about 10 years.

Treatment: Drug treatment is helpful in advanced disease: amantadine, anticholinergics (trihexyphenidyl, ethopropazine), levodopa and carbidopa, bromocriptine, and selegiline. Surgical removal of degenerating brain tissue may be a good choice in younger patients. Physical and speech therapy and counseling are important for most patients.

Encephalitis. Inflammation of the brain due to viral infection.

Cause: Most cases of encephalitis are due to viruses transmitted by mosquitoes (Eastern and Western equine encephalitis, Japanese B encephalitis) or ticks. Numerous other viruses (coxsackievirus, herpes simplex virus, mumps virus, HIV) can cause encephalitis.

History: Abrupt onset of fever and headache, with muscle weakness or paralysis, restlessness, personality or behavioral changes, delirium, seizures, and lethargy perhaps progressing to coma.

Physical Examination: Fever, depressed level of consciousness, signs of meningeal irritation, evidence of focal or diffuse neurologic damage including tremors, paralysis, hyperreactive reflexes, and pathologic reflexes.

Diagnostic Tests: Serologic studies can identify the causative virus. The CSF shows increase of pressure, protein, and cells. Abnormal findings on electroencephalogram (EEG) are nonspecific.

Course: Most cases resolve without sequelae after a few weeks, but many are followed by residual paralysis, seizures, and parkinsonism.

Treatment: Largely supportive. Physical therapy; attention to nutrition and hydration. Drug therapy as needed to provide sedation, relieve fever and headache, and control convulsions. Herpes simplex encephalitis responds to acyclovir. In severe disease, adrenal corticosteroids may reduce cerebral edema and inflammation.

Meningitis. Infection of the meninges, with neurologic and systemic effects.

Causes: Infection with bacteria (*Staphylococcus*, pneumococcus, meningococcus, *Haemophilus influenzae*, *Escherichia coli*, *Mycobacterium tuberculosis*), viruses (mumps virus, coxsackievirus, herpes simplex virus), fungi, or protozoans. Causative organisms may be introduced by a penetrating head wound, spread locally from infections of the ears or sinuses, or reach the meninges through the bloodstream from remote sites (pneumonia, endocarditis). Symptoms vary considerably with the etiologic agent; signs and symptoms are milder in viral than in bacterial meningitis and the prognosis more favorable. Meningitis due to meningococcus (*Neisseria meningitidis*) is a rapidly progressive and highly lethal disease, particularly because the meningococcus causes a severe toxemia that can lead to shock and death, even in the absence of signs of meningitis.

History: Abrupt onset of fever, headache, and vomiting. Painful stiffness of the neck and back muscles, visual disturbances, and irritability, twitching, or seizures. Clouding of the sensorium, delirium, and coma may follow rapidly.

Physical Examination: Fever, depressed level of consciousness. Signs of meningeal irritation include **nuchal rigidity** (stiffness of the neck, with inability to touch the chin to the chest), painful stiffness of other muscles, hyperreflexia, **Kernig sign** (inability to extend the knee when the thigh is flexed), **Brudzinski sign** (passive flexion of the neck causes active flexion of the hip and knee). In an infant, bulging of the fontanelles.

Diagnostic Tests: Lumbar puncture shows elevated pressure. The CSF may be purulent. White blood cells and protein are elevated. In bacterial meningitis, CSF glucose is low. Smear and culture of the fluid identify bacterial agents. In viral (aseptic) meningitis the fluid is clear and the glucose is normal; viral culture may identify the cause.

Course: Without treatment, viral meningitis nearly always resolves without sequelae, and bacterial meningitis nearly always proves fatal, particularly in children and the elderly. Meningococcemia, which may occur with or without meningitis, causes a petechial rash and profound and fulminant systemic abnormalities, including widespread hemorrhages and vascular collapse, sometimes due to adrenal hemorrhage (**Waterhouse-Friderichsen syndrome**). Patients who have recovered from meningitis may have residual mental retardation, paralysis, or seizures.

Treatment: Meningitis is an emergency. Hospitalization and administration of intravenous antibiotics are routine. Antibiotics are started even before reports of CSF studies are available, and discontinued or changed on the basis of these studies. Antibiotics are usually continued for three weeks or longer. Supportive care, including physical therapy, attention to nutrition and hydration, artificial ventilation, and measures to control fever, reverse shock, and reduce intracranial pressure, is vitally important. Asymptomatic persons who have been closely exposed to a patient with meningococcal meningitis receive prophylactic rifampin or ciprofloxacin to terminate the carrier state. A vaccine active against some strains of meningococcus is available.

West Nile Virus Disease. An infection of wild crows and jays transmitted by several species of mosquito. Human infection, first recognized in the U.S. as recently as 1999, has now spread throughout most of the contiguous states.

Although human infection is usually subclinical, encephalitis, meningitis, and paralytic syndromes may occur, especially in the elderly, in whom the mortality rate is significant. Adults who recover from the disease often have residual neurologic, muscular, or psychiatric impairment.

Transmission by blood transfusion and organ transplantation has occurred, but person-to-person transmission by mosquitoes is not recognized. The highest incidence of human infections occurs during the mosquito season (late spring, summer, and early fall).

Treatment is strictly symptomatic and supportive. Elimination of mosquito breeding places and use of insect repellent are strongly recommended as preventive measures.

Migraine Headache. Recurring severe unilateral headache with neurologic concomitants.

Cause: Unknown. Head pain is apparently related to constriction, dilatation, and throbbing of meningeal and other vessels. Chemical factors (release of vasodilator substances, depletion of plasma serotonin) probably play a part. The disease runs in families and is more common in young women, affecting about 15% of adult women in the U.S. Oral contraceptives may bring on headaches in susceptible women.

History: Recurring episodes of severe unilateral throbbing headache accompanied by nausea, vomiting, photophobia, intolerance to noise, and sometimes neurologic symptoms (diplopia, transient local anesthesia or paralysis). In **migraine with aura**, the patient experiences a warning symptom (aura) before the headache begins. Most often this consists of seeing flashes or zigzags of light in both eyes, usually with transitory visual field defects (**scintillating scotomas**).

In **migraine without aura**, the headache may be less severe and more generalized. Headaches typically last for many hours and may be severely incapacitating. Often complete relief is not obtained until after sleep. In susceptible persons, a migraine headache may be triggered by emotional stress, fatigue, menstruation, skipping a meal, certain foods (chocolate, prepared foods containing nitrates), or alcohol.

Physical Examination: Essentially normal during attacks, and entirely so between attacks.

Diagnostic Tests: Chiefly of use in ruling out more serious disorders; no specific findings.

Course: The disorder often begins in childhood and continues for many years. Depending on the presence of triggering factors, headaches may occur daily or at intervals of months or years.

Treatment: Mild analgesics sometimes help; nonsteroidal anti-inflammatory drugs (aspirin, ibuprofen, naproxen), especially when combined with caffeine, provide adequate relief for many patients. Selective serotonin receptor agonists (sumatriptan, rizatriptan, zolmitriptan) orally or by injection can abort a headache at any stage of its development. For patients who have extremely frequent headaches (one or more a week), prophylactic treatment usually provides good control. Prophylactic drugs include beta-adrenergic blocking agents (propranolol, atenolol) and others (amitriptyline).

Epilepsy. A neurologic disorder in which the patient experiences recurrent seizures consisting of transient disturbances of cerebral function due to paroxysmal neuronal discharge.

Causes: Seizure disorders, especially those first causing symptoms in childhood, are often idiopathic (without demonstrable cause). Seizures can be induced by cerebral trauma, infection, vascular disease, neoplasms, degenerative diseases (Alzheimer disease), drugs and chemical poisons, metabolic disorders (renal failure, hypoglycemia), and, in children, high fever. In persons with idiopathic epilepsy, seizures may be triggered by physical or emotional stress, lack of sleep, fever, drugs, alcohol, alcohol withdrawal, menstruation, or flashing lights.

Symptoms: Seizures are classified on the basis of overt presentation:

Partial (only part of one cerebral cortex is involved).

Simple (no unconsciousness): Local twitching or jerking; perception of flashing lights or other abnormal sensory phenomena.

Complex (impaired alertness or unconsciousness): Sometimes with psychic symptoms or automatisms.

Generalized (entire cerebral cortex involved).

Absence (petit mal): Brief loss of attention and perception.

Tonic-clonic (grand mal): In the tonic phase the victim becomes rigid, often cries out, loses consciousness, falls, stops breathing. In the clonic phase the victim has generalized muscular jerking, may bite the tongue or lips, may be incontinent of urine or stool. In the postictal state, after awakening, the subject is drowsy and amnesic for a variable period.

Myoclonic: Repeated shocklike, often violent contractions in one or more muscle groups.

Status epilepticus: Series of grand mal seizures without waking intervals.

Physical Examination: Between seizures there is no detectable abnormality. Signs of neurologic disease may be found in secondary epilepsy.

Diagnostic Tests: The electroencephalogram generally shows focal abnormalities in the rate, rhythm, or relative intensity of cerebral cortical rhythms, allowing diagnosis and classification of epilepsy. Laboratory studies and CT scan or MRI may be performed to rule out treatable causes of epilepsy.

Treatment: In idiopathic epilepsy, long-term treatment with anticonvulsant medicine (phenytoin, carbamazepine, valproic acid, phenobarbital, ethosuximide, and others) provides excellent control for most patients. Blood levels of medicine may require monitoring to ensure optimum dosage. Avoidance of triggering factors is important. For intractable cases, surgical treatment is sometimes successful.

Bell Palsy. Weakness or paralysis of muscles on one side of the face (Figure 14-6) caused by inflammation or compression of the seventh cranial nerve (facial nerve) as it passes through the bony facial canal and emerges at the stylomastoid foramen behind the ear. The cause is unknown, but exposure to cold and herpes simplex virus infection have been suggested. Onset of symptoms is often accompanied by pain below or behind the ear.

Onset of facial weakness is usually abrupt, producing a characteristic asymmetry of the face and diminished ability or inability to close the eyes, smile, or purse the lips. Speech and eating may be slightly disturbed. There may be impairment of hearing and taste on the tip of the tongue.

The diagnosis is clinically evident, but electromyography and nerve conduction velocity studies may give indications of prognosis. More than half of cases resolve spontaneously in a few days to a few weeks, but residual weakness and asymmetry of the face, occasionally severe, may be permanent. A systemic corticosteroid is usually prescribed.

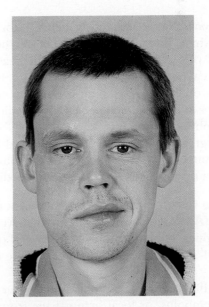

Figure 14-6
Patient with Bell Palsy

Transient Ischemic Attack (TIA). Sudden onset of neurologic symptoms that resolve completely within 24 hours.

Cause: Transient interruption of blood supply to some part of the brain. Common causes include blockage by an embolus (from an infected heart valve, mural thrombus, or sloughed arteriosclerotic plaque) and reduction in blood supply due to the combined effects of arterial disease (arteritis, systemic lupus erythematosus) and reduced flow (hypotension; subclavian steal syndrome, in which blockage of a subclavian artery near its origin leads to reversal of blood flow in a vertebral artery to provide collateral flow beyond the obstruction, at the expense of brain tissue normally supplied by the vertebral artery).

History: Sudden onset of focal neurologic symptoms (weakness, numbness, unilateral loss of vision, diplopia, speech disturbances, vertigo, ataxia, falling) depending on site of circulatory impairment, resolving in less than 24 hours (usually in less than 4 hours).

Physical Examination: Flaccid weakness or paralysis, hyperreflexia, Babinski reflex, hypesthesia or anesthesia, depending on site of lesion. All neurologic signs resolve within 24 hours.

Diagnostic Tests: CT scan may be done to rule out hemorrhage. Arteriography, MR angiography, or carotid duplex ultrasonography may be used to assess the cerebral circulation. X-ray, laboratory, and electrocardiography or echocardiography may trace the underlying cause.

Course: By definition a TIA has no complications. Many patients, however, will eventually have one or more strokes.

Treatment: No treatment is needed for the acute episode, which has often resolved before the patient is seen by a physician. Depending on the reason for the attacks, treatment directed against future attacks may include carotid endarterectomy, control of cardiac or systemic disease, and use of anticoagulant medicines. Long-term prophylactic administration of drugs that inhibit platelet aggregation (aspirin, ticlopidine) reduces the risk of further attacks. Heparin and Coumadin may be needed if there is a major problem with thrombotic disease.

Stroke (Brain Attack, Cerebrovascular Accident, CVA).
Sudden onset of neurologic symptoms due to interruption of blood supply to some part of the brain (Figure 14-7). Stroke ranks third as a cause of death in the U.S.

Cause: Blockage of a cerebral artery by a clot (thrombosis) or embolus, or local hemorrhage from a cerebral vessel. Most cases are due to underlying vascular disease (arteriosclerosis, cerebral aneurysm, hypertension, diabetes mellitus, valvular heart disease).

History: Sudden onset of weakness, numbness or paralysis, usually on one side of the body, or other neurologic deficit (loss of vision, dizziness, difficulty speaking, confusion, loss of consciousness), depending on part of brain affected. Severe headache, vomiting, or seizures may also occur. Usually there is a history of cardiovascular disease, sometimes of preceding TIAs. Neurologic deficit may progress to coma and death.

Physical Examination: Evidence of neurologic deficit, depending on location and extent of brain tissue involved, and duration of circulatory impairment. Muscle weakness or paralysis, which may initially be flaccid but eventually becomes spastic, with rigidity, hyperreflexia, Babinski and other pathologic reflexes. Aphasia, confusion, delirium, coma.

Diagnostic Tests: CT scan of the head can show areas of hemorrhage or infarction. Magnetic resonance imaging may also be used, without contrast material. Lumbar puncture helps to distinguish hemorrhage (blood in fluid, elevated opening pressure) from thrombosis. Blood studies, electrocardiography, and other diagnostic procedures may be used to identify underlying disease.

Course: Many cases of stroke resolve without any residual symptoms. Paralysis, weakness, or dementia may worsen. Stroke may progress rapidly to a fatal termination when the damage is extensive.

Treatment: If neurologic impairment is progressive and hemorrhage has been ruled out, anticoagulants (IV heparin followed by oral Coumadin) are used during the acute phase. In selected cases, tissue plasminogen activator (tPA) is administered to dissolve a freshly formed thrombus. Vigorous supportive treatment (oxygen, parenteral nutrition, prevention of respiratory and urinary tract infection, prevention of bedsores) must be instituted early. Physical therapy is important to maintain mobility and achieve maximum rehabilitation as neurologic function returns. Braces or splints may be necessary to promote mobility despite weakness of certain muscle groups.

Polyneuritis.
A disease process involving a number of peripheral nerves.

Causes: Hereditary (Charcot-Marie-Tooth disease, Dejerine-Sottas disease, Friedreich ataxia), metabolic (diabetes mellitus, uremia), vitamin deficiency, alcoholism, drugs (INH, phenytoin), chemical poisons (lead, arsenic), autoimmunity (Guillain-Barré syndrome).

History: Hypesthesia, anesthesia, paresthesia, causalgia, weakness, muscle wasting involving various areas often in an irregular and shifting pattern.

Physical Examination: Reflexes diminished or absent; muscular atrophy.

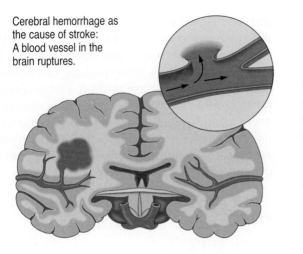

Cerebral hemorrhage as the cause of stroke: A blood vessel in the brain ruptures.

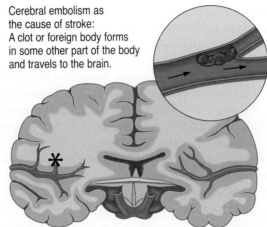

Cerebral embolism as the cause of stroke: A clot or foreign body forms in some other part of the body and travels to the brain.

STROKE

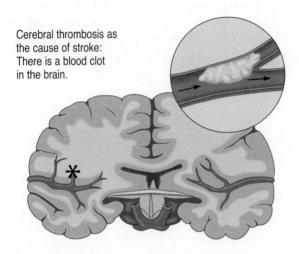

Cerebral thrombosis as the cause of stroke: There is a blood clot in the brain.

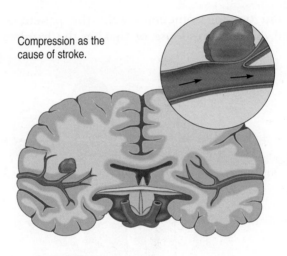

Compression as the cause of stroke.

Figure 14-7
Causes of Stroke

Diagnostic Tests: Electromyography and nerve conduction velocity tests confirm neural malfunction. Emphasis is on finding a systemic cause (diabetes mellitus, other metabolic diseases, lead poisoning).

Treatment: Removal or treatment of underlying cause, if possible.

Head Injuries. Blunt or penetrating wounds of the head can cause irreversible damage to the brain, and hemorrhage within the brain or between the brain and the skull. Such injuries are frequently lethal or result in permanent impairment of mental function.

Cerebral concussion is defined as a violent blow to the skull that causes brief unconsciousness but does no permanent damage to the brain or its supporting structures. In **cerebral contusion**, there is local injury to brain tissue, but again without lasting consequences. **Cerebral laceration** is a still more violent injury in which part of the brain is torn. The outcome is often death or severe permanent impairment (paralysis, seizures, dementia).

Intracranial hemorrhage can be extradural (also called epidural, between the outermost covering of the brain, the dura mater, and the skull), subdural (beneath the dura mater), subarachnoid (under the arachnoid membrane covering the brain), or intracerebral (within the substance of the brain). **Extradural hemorrhage** usually results from arterial bleeding and often proves rapidly fatal. **Subdural hemorrhage** is often venous, with chronic signs and symptoms (gradually progressing headache, stupor, personality change, or neurologic impairment). **Subarachnoid hemorrhage** is less often due to trauma than to rupture of a congenital aneurysm (abnormal bulge or weakness in a cerebral artery, present from birth). Any intracranial hemorrhage is life-threatening because of the danger of irreversible damage from compression of brain tissue within the rigid, nonexpanding skull. The treatment of head injury demands prompt and decisive action to conserve brain tissue and arrest hemorrhage.

Carpal Tunnel Syndrome (CTS). Pain, tingling, and hypesthesia or anesthesia in the **thenar** (the fleshy part of the palm proximal to the thumb and index finger), with weakness and eventual atrophy in muscles of the thenar supplied by the **median nerve**, as a result of compression of this nerve on the volar aspect of the wrist where it passes through the carpal tunnel, formed by wrist bones and the nonyielding carpal ligament (Figure 14-8). Many cases are induced by repetitive wrist flexion, as in jobs or hobbies. The incidence is increased during pregnancy and among persons with certain systemic diseases (diabetes mellitus, hypothyroidism, rheumatoid arthritis).

Pain and tingling sometimes wake the patient at night and elicit the response of shaking the hand to restore normal feeling. **Tinel sign** (shocklike pain when the volar aspect of the wrist is tapped) and **Phalen sign** (reproduction of pain or paresthesia when both wrists are flexed with the hands firmly pressing one another back-to-back for 60 seconds) are positive. Electromyography and nerve conduction velocity studies can confirm the site of nerve compression. Treatment is by removal of known underlying causes; splinting, at least at night; physical therapy; local injection of corticosteroid; and often surgical division of the carpal ligament.

Diagnostic and Surgical Procedures

angiography May be used to show cranial vasculature with injected contrast medium. In digital subtraction angiography, x-ray images of the head with and without contrast medium are processed by a computer, which

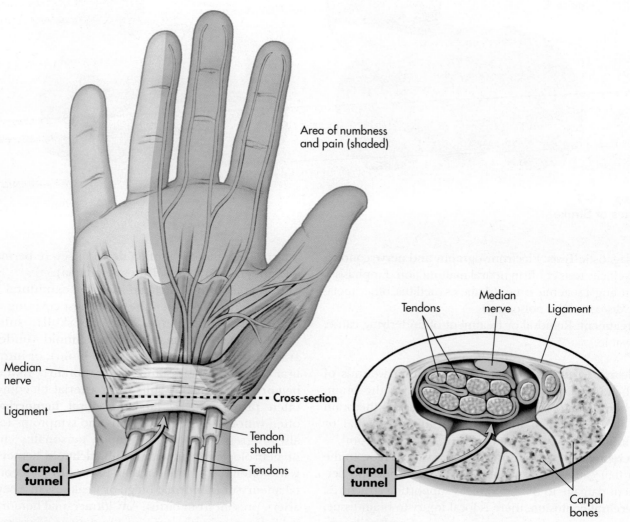

Area of numbness and pain (shaded)

Median nerve

Ligament

Cross-section

Tendon sheath

Tendons

Carpal tunnel

Tendons

Median nerve

Ligament

Carpal tunnel

Carpal bones

Figure 14-8
Carpal Tunnel Syndrome

deletes all shadows common to both films (skull bones, soft tissue profiles and interfaces), leaving only the vascular system visible.

brain scan An examination based on the distribution of a radioactive isotope injected systemically in brain tissue.

craniotomy Surgical incision into the cranium, which necessitates drilling or sawing through the bone of the skull.

craniectomy Surgical removal of part of the bone of the skull.

electroencephalography (EEG) Measurement and recording of electrical activity from several sites simultaneously. Electrodes are attached with fine needles to standard sites on the scalp, and the record is made on a strip of moving paper. Tracings are usually made after administration of a short-acting sedative (with the subject asleep, if possible). The effects of hyperventilation and of photic stimulation (exposure to a flashing light) are recorded also. The EEG is particularly useful in identifying and classifying seizure disorders.

electrophysiologic studies Measurement of electrical activity in nerves and muscles. Electromyography (EMG) involves insertion of fine needle electrodes into voluntary muscles. Nerve conduction velocity (NCV) is measured by timing the passage of nerve impulses between a stimulating and a recording electrode, which are a precisely measured distance apart.

finger-to-nose test The patient extends the arms outward laterally, closes the eyes, and tries to touch the finger to the nose. Tests coordination.

heel-to-shin test With the patient standing straight, the heel of one foot is placed against the shin of the opposing leg. Tests coordination.

hot and cold testing Assessing the subject's ability to recognize hot and cold (via test tubes of hot and cold water) on various parts of the body surface (a sensory examination).

imaging studies CT scan (with or without intravenous injection of contrast medium), MRI, and standard x-ray views of the skull.

light touch test Assessing the subject's ability to recognize a wisp of cotton drawn across the skin on various parts of the body surface (a sensory examination).

lumbar puncture (LP) Withdrawal of a specimen of cerebrospinal fluid from the subarachnoid space by inserting a needle between two vertebrae (usually L4 and L5) at the lower end of the spinal cord (Figure 14-9). A **manometer** (graduated glass tube) is used to measure the pressure of the fluid at the beginning of the procedure (**opening pressure**) and the end (**closing pressure**). Specimens of fluid are examined microscopically (stained smear) for cells (neutrophils and lymphocytes) and pathogenic microorganisms; chemically for glucose, protein, and other substances; by culture for bacterial pathogens; and, if indicated, serologically for evidence of syphilis, Lyme disease, or other infections, and by cytologic techniques for malignant cells. Normal CSF is water clear. **Xanthochromia** (yellowness) of the fluid suggests recent but not current hemorrhage. Frank blood in the specimen may indicate subarachnoid hemorrhage but may also be due to local injury by the needle (**traumatic tap**).

myelography Visualization of the spinal canal (the tubular enclosure of the spinal cord formed collectively by the vertebrae) by x-ray with contrast medium introduced into the subarachnoid space by lumbar puncture.

pain test Assessing the subject's ability to recognize a prick from a sterile needle on various parts of the body surface (a sensory examination).

proprioception test Tested by having the subject report whether a toe or finger is moved up or down by the examiner.

rapidly alternating movements test A test for coordination, this test has the patient perform rapid alternating movements of the hands or feet.

Romberg test Has the subject stand with feet together and eyes open, then eyes closed, to assess position sense in the trunk and legs.

spinal tap See *lumbar puncture*.

stereognosis test Test of the patient's ability to recognize an object by handling it.

surgical drainage of an abscess Usually preceded by antibiotic therapy, a craniotomy is performed and the abscess drained.

tandem walking test Tests the subject's ability to walk with one foot in front of the other in a straight line. A coordination test, often used by police officers to assess drivers for substance abuse.

two-point discrimination test Test of the patient's ability to distinguish two points close together on the skin.

vibratory sense test Test of the patient's ability to sense the vibration of a tuning fork when the stem is placed on a bone near the surface, such as the elbow or the shin.

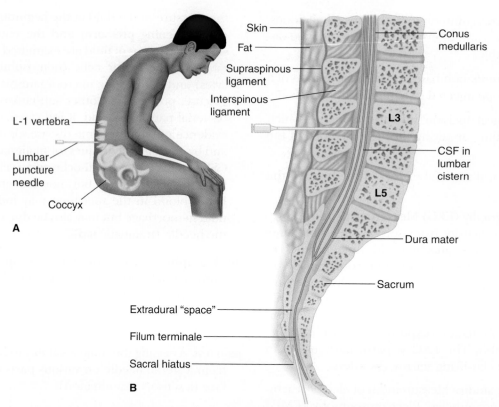

Skin
Fat
Supraspinous ligament
Interspinous ligament
Conus medullaris
L3
CSF in lumbar cistern
L5
L-1 vertebra
Lumbar puncture needle
Coccyx
Dura mater
Sacrum
Extradural "space"
Filum terminale
Sacral hiatus

A

B

Figure 14-9
A) Lumbar Puncture or Spinal Tap; B) Section of the Vertebral Column Showing the Spinal Cord and Membranes. Lumbar puncture needles are shown at L3-4 and in the sacral hiatus.

Laboratory Procedures

CSF (cerebrospinal fluid) The fluid medium of the central nervous system (brain and spinal cord), which can be sampled by lumbar puncture (spinal tap) for chemical testing, cell counts, and culture.

Pharmacology

Epilepsy drugs. Drugs used to treat epilepsy are known as anticonvulsants because epilepsy is characterized by seizures or convulsions. Barbiturates are sedative drugs, some of which also possess an anticonvulsant action. Barbiturates are controlled substance drugs (Schedule IV) that inhibit conduction of nerve impulses coming into the cortex of the brain and depress motor areas of the brain.

> mephobarbital (Mebaral)
> phenobarbital (Luminal, Solfoton)

Hydantoins act on the cell membrane of neurons in the cortex of the brain. These drugs affect the flow of sodium in and out of the cell, thereby preventing the neuron from depolarizing and repolarizing (i.e., sending out an impulse) too rapidly or repeatedly.

> ethotoin (Peganone)
> mephenytoin (Mesantoin)
> phenytoin (Dilantin Infatabs, Dilantin Kapseals, Dilantin-125)

Succinimides depress the cortex and raise the seizure threshold.

> ethosuximide (Zarontin)
> methsuximide (Celontin Kapseals)
> phensuximide (Milontin Kapseals)

Benzodiazepine drugs act on several different types of receptors throughout the body to affect memory, emotion, and muscles. They exert an anticonvulsant effect on receptors in the brainstem.

These are controlled substance drugs (Schedule IV).

> clonazepam (Klonopin)
> clorazepate (Tranxene, Tranxene-SD, Tranxene-SD Half Strength, Tranxene-T)
> diazepam (Diazepam Intensol, Valium)

The mechanism of action of these antiepileptic drugs varies.

> acetazolamide (Diamox)
> carbamazepine (Atretol, Carbatrol, Epitol,
>   Tegretol, Tegretol-XR)
> clobazam (Frisium)
> felbamate (Felbatol)
> fosphenytoin (Cerebyx)
> gabapentin (Neurontin)
> lamotrigine (Lamictal, Lamictal Chewable
>   Dispersible Tablet)
> primidone (Mysoline)
> valproic acid (Depacon, Depakene, Depakote ER)

No one drug has therapeutic effects against all types of seizures. Some drugs that are effective for controlling one type of seizure may actually provoke another type.

Parkinson disease drugs. Drug therapy for Parkinson disease is divided into two main categories: drugs that increase or enhance the action of dopamine in the brain, and drugs that inhibit the action of acetylcholine. All of these drugs act to restore the natural balance between dopamine and acetylcholine. Drugs that increase the amount of dopamine, enhance its action in the brain, or directly stimulate dopamine receptors include:

> amantadine (Symmetrel)
> bromocriptine (Parlodel, Parlodel Snap Tabs)
> carbidopa (Lodosyn)
> levodopa (L-dopa, Larodopa)
> pergolide mesylate (Permax)
> pramipexole (Mirapex)
> ropinirole (Requip)
> selegiline (Carbex, Eldepryl)

Drugs that inhibit the action of acetylcholine in the brain are called anticholinergic drugs and include:

> benztropine (Cogentin)
> biperiden (Akineton)
> diphenhydramine (Benadryl)
> procyclidine (Kemadrin)
> trihexyphenidyl (Artane, Artane Sequels)

Combination drugs used to treat Parkinson disease include the various dosage forms of Sinemet, which indicate the milligrams of carbidopa per milligram of levodopa: Sinemet 10-100, Sinemet 25-100, Sinemet 25-250. The FDA has also approved the use of the orphan drugs apomorphine, NeuroCell-PD, and Spheramine to treat Parkinson disease.

Dopamine-receptor agonists bind with dopamine receptors in the brain to activate them. These drugs include pramipexole (Mirapex) and ropinirole (Requip). None of the drugs prescribed can cure Parkinson disease. In fact, over time, tolerance to the drugs' therapeutic effects can develop. Larger doses are then required to maintain control of parkinsonian symptoms, producing more side effects. When doses can no longer be increased or side effects become intolerable, the physician will gradually withdraw all medication, placing the patient on a "drug holiday" for a few days. When therapy is again initiated, the patient will respond to lower doses of antiparkinsonian drugs.

Insomnia drugs. Drugs used to induce sleep are termed hypnotics after *hypnos*, the Greek word for *sleep*.

> acecarbromal (Paxarel)
> chloral hydrate (Aquachloral Supprettes)
> estazolam (ProSom)
> eszopiclone (Lunesta)
> flurazepam (Dalmane)
> glutethimide (Doriden)
> lorazepam (Ativan)
> quazepam (Doral)
> temazepam (Restoril)
> triazolam (Halcion)
> zaleplon (Sonata)
> zolpidem (Ambien, Ambien CR)

Over-the-counter (OTC) sleep aids commonly contain the antihistamine diphenhydramine. These sleep aids use the antihistamine's side effects of drowsiness as the therapeutic effect to treat insomnia.

> Bufferin AF Nite Time
> Compoz Nighttime Sleep Aid
> Excedrin P.M., Excedrin P.M. Liquigels
> Nytol
> Sominex
> Extra Strength Tylenol PM
> Sominex, Sominex Pain Relief

TRANSCRIPTION**TIPS**

1. The term *disk* represents the preferred spelling in both *Dorland's* and *Stedman's* medical dictionaries; the alternative acceptable spelling is *disc*.

2. The term *diskectomy* is spelled only with a *k*.

3. Do not confuse the abbreviation *CNS* (central nervous system) with *C&S* (culture and sensitivity). It is preferable to spell out the latter term in transcription.

4. The French term *absence* ("ab sáhnce") is used to describe seizures that were formerly known as *petit mal* ("petty mahl").

5. The generic names of benzodiazepines typically end in *-azepam*, *-azolam*, or some variant (*-azam*, *-azepate*, *-azepoxide*).

6. Spelling tips:

foramen (singular)	foramina (plural)
neural foramen	neural foramina
foraminotomy	*not* foramenotomy

7. Do not confuse *mater* and *matter*.

   dura mater (one *f*) (rhymes with "later")
   white matter (two *f*s) (rhymes with "fatter")

Spotlight on

Neurology Dictation

by *John H. Dirckx, M.D.*

The **Glasgow Coma Scale** is a widely used measure of consciousness. It is a standardized system for assessing response to stimuli in a neurologically impaired individual. Reactions are given a numerical value in three categories: eye opening, verbal responsiveness, and motor responsiveness. The three scores are then added together. The lowest values are the worst clinical scores.

Best motor response (upper extremity)

6 obeys commands
5 localizes pain
4 withdraws from stimulus
3 abnormal flexing
2 extensor response
1 none

Best verbal response

5 oriented (makes sentences)
4 confused speech (words)
3 gibberish (vocal sounds)
2 incomprehensible sounds
1 none

Eye opening

4 spontaneous
3 to speech
2 to pain
1 none

Source: *Human Diseases*

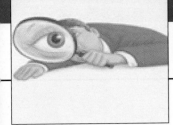

Proofreading Skills

Instructions: In the paragraphs below, circle the errors. Identify misspelled and missing medical and English words and punctuation errors, and write the correct words and punctuation in the numbered spaces opposite the text.

1 PROVISIONAL DIAGNOSIS	1 _____
2 Acute bacteral meningitis.	2 <u>bacterial</u> _____
3	3 _____
4 BRIEF HISTORY	4 _____
5 The patient is a 4-year-old male with a 5-day history of	5 _____
6 nausea vomiting temperature elevation, increasing	6 _____
7 lethargy. He was seen and evaluated in the office on the	7 _____
8 day of admission and brought to the emergency	8 _____
9 department for lumbar puncture. His revealed cloudy	9 _____
10 fluid. Also, a CBC was consistent with a bacterial	10 _____
11 process.	11 _____
12	12 _____
13 PHYSICAL EXAMINATION	13 _____
14 Blood pressure 92/64, pulse 100, respirations 24,	14 _____
15 temp 100.8. HEENT revealed marked stiffness of the	15 _____
16 neck with nuchal rigidity. Positive Brudzinski, Kernig	16 _____
17 signs. Chest was clear. Heart regular rhythm. Abdomen	17 _____
18 was soft. Neuro: The patient was fairly lethargic and did	18 _____
19 not respond appropriately to painful stimuli.	19 _____
20	20 _____
21 LABORATORY DATA	21 _____
22 Lumbar puncture revealed normal pressure. CSF	22 _____
23 protein 67. WBC 7,040 with 98% polys 2% lymphs,	23 _____
24 210 RBCs. Gram stain postive for gram-negative cocci.	24 _____
25 CSF glucose 26, serum glucose 96. CBC revealed WBC	25 _____
26 of 21.9 with 70 segs, 13 bands, 14 lymphs. Hemoglobin	26 _____
27 11.6, hematocrit 35.1.	27 _____
28	28 _____
29 PLAN	29 _____
30 Patient to be admitted emergently with probable	30 _____
31 meningitis.	31 _____

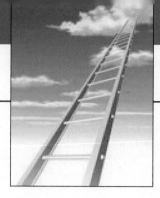

SkillsChallenge

Fill-in Exercise: Central Nervous System

Instructions: The numbered blanks correspond to the numbers in the narrative paragraphs. Fill in the blanks with the correct entry from the word list following the paragraphs.

The (1), or CNS, is the largest division of the nervous system and consists of the brain and spinal cord. The peripheral nervous system consists of 12 pairs of (2) and 31 pairs of spinal nerves. The spinal (3), into which the spinal nerves enter, is protected by the spinal column, consisting of seven (4) vertebrae, twelve (5) vertebrae, five (6) vertebrae, and five (7) vertebrae. The end of the spinal cord is called the (8) because the ending group of nerves resembles the hair of a horse's tail.

There are three protective layers of membrane that surround the spinal cord and brain. The outermost layer, which is the thickest, is called the (9); the middle layer is the arachnoid membrane; and the innermost layer, which is thin and contains many blood vessels, is called the (10).

The brain itself is divided into several parts. The largest division is the (11), which is further divided into lobes: the (12) lobe in the forehead region, whose functions include memory and perception; the (13) lobe under the temporal bone of the skull, whose functions include hearing and understanding speech; the parietal lobe; and the (14) lobe at the base of the skull, whose functions include vision. Other parts of the brain include the thalamus; the (15), which regulates body temperature; and the (16), which contains centers that automatically regulate breathing and heart rate; the (17), which connects the cerebrum to the cerebellum; and the (18), which is concerned with coordination of voluntary movements.

In the center and between the various lobes of the cerebrum are the (19), cavities filled with cerebrospinal fluid.

1. _____
2. _____
3. _____
4. _____
5. _____
6. _____
7. _____
8. _____
9. _____
10. _____
11. _____
12. _____

13. _____
14. _____
15. _____
16. _____
17. _____
18. _____
19. _____

cauda equina	lumbar
central nervous system	medulla oblongata
cerebellum	occipital
cerebrum	pia mater
cervical	pons
cranial	sacral
cord	temporal
dura mater	thoracic
frontal	ventricles
hypothalamus	

Adjectives Exercise

Adjectives are formed from nouns by adding adjectival suffixes such as *-ac, -al, -ar, -ary, -eal, -ed, -ent, -iac, -ial, -ic, -ical, -ive, -lar, -oid, -ous, -tic*, and *-tous*. In addition, some adjectives have a different form entirely from the noun, which may be either Latin or Greek in origin.

Instructions: Test your knowledge of adjectives by writing the adjectival form of the neurology words. Consult a medical dictionary to select the correct adjectival ending as necessary.

1. nerve _____
2. spine _____
3. cranium _____
4. cerebrum _____
5. cerebellum _____
6. meninges _____
7. paraplegia _____
8. hydrocephalus _____
9. epilepsy _____
10. ventricle _____
11. arachnoid _____
12. anulus _____

Abbreviations Exercise

Common abbreviations may be transcribed as dictated in the body of a report. Uncommon abbreviations must be spelled out, with the abbreviations appearing in parentheses after the translation. All abbreviations (except laboratory test names) must be spelled out in the Diagnosis or Impression section of any report.

Instructions: Define the following neurology abbreviations. Then memorize both the abbreviations and the definitions to increase your speed and accuracy in transcribing neurology dictation.

CNS   _____

CSF   _____

CVA   _____

EEG   _____

EMG   _____

LP   _____

MS   _____

NCV   _____

TIA   _____

tPA   _____

Medical Terminology Matching Exercise

Instructions: Match the definitions in Column A with the terms in Column B.

Column A	Column B
1. ___ clefts in surface of the brain	**A.** concussion
2. ___ painful sensation	**B.** encephalo-
3. ___ brain	**C.** sulci
4. ___ nerve	**D.** dura mater
5. ___ paralysis of lower body	**E.** neuro-
6. ___ malignant brain tumor	**F.** paresthesia
7. ___ brief loss of consciousness after head injury	**G.** radiculo-
8. ___ largest division of the brain	**H.** paraplegia
9. ___ numbness, tingling	**I.** multiple sclerosis
10. ___ caused by demyelination of nerves	**J.** -algia
11. ___ shows neurofibrillary tangles in brain on autopsy	**K.** syncope
12. ___ spinal nerve root	**L.** Alzheimer disease
13. ___ outermost meningeal layer	**M.** cerebrum
14. ___ fainting	**N.** astrocytoma

Word Root and Suffix-Matching Exercise

Instructions: Combine the following word roots with suffixes to form words that match the definitions below. Fill in the blanks with the medical words that you construct.

Word Root	Suffix
meningo-	-gram
encephalo-	-oma
myelo-	-plegia
neuro-	-itis
para-	-opathy
quadri-	

A. paralysis affecting both legs

_____

B. inflammation of the brain

_____

C. disease condition of the nerves

_____

D. inflammation of a nerve

_____

E. paralysis affecting all four extremities

_____

F. inflammation of the membranes surrounding the brain

_____

G. tumor arising from the meninges

_____

H. record of a study of the spinal column using contrast medium

_____

I. disease condition of the brain

_____

Soundalikes Exercise

Instructions: Circle the correct term from the soundalikes in parentheses in the following sentences.

1. Following the stroke, the patient had (dysphagia, dysphasia, dysplasia), so that we had to administer medicines by the intravenous route.

2. Due to the patient's (dysphagia, dysphasia, dysplasia), we were unable to get a complete history, but his neighbor said he was found on the floor in a pool of urine, (conscience, conscious) but confused.

3. (Accept, Except) for a slight weakness in the left arm, the patient had no residual symptoms of stroke.

4. This patient with Huntington disease has continuous (corneal, choreal, chorial) movements.

5. There was blood mixed with cerebrospinal fluid coming from the basilar (cistern, system).

6. The patient's headaches were preceded by an (aura, ora) consisting of wavy, colored lines.

7. The patient was observed to have a (concussion, convulsion) by the paramedics, who inserted a mouth gag to keep him from biting his tongue.

8. The parents were warned of the signs and symptoms of (concussion, convulsion) following a head injury and told if the patient became excessively sleepy to return.

9. The patient was not (conscience, conscious) when the EMTs arrived.

10. A seizure (diaphysis, diastasis, diathesis) of uncertain origin was diagnosed.

11. The ventricular (cistern, system) is well demonstrated on the MRI scan, and there appear to be no impingements or hemorrhages.

12. The (facial, fascial, faucial) sheath was picked up and the nerves examined.

13. This poststroke patient has an ataxic (gait, gate).

14. With high fever, elevated white count, and (knuckle, nuchal) rigidity, meningitis is almost a certainty in this young male.

15. The patient was unresponsive to (noxious, nocuous) stimuli.

16. The neural (sheet, sheath) was inflamed and compressed.

17. On MRI scan of the brain, a (cellar, sellar) tumor was suspected.

18. A (fecal, thecal) injection of morphine failed to relieve the patient's intense pain.

19. A (facial, fascial, faucial) (tic, tick) involving almost continuous winking of the left eye was seen.

Dictation Exercise

Prior to transcribing the dictations, complete these activities.

1. **Using Chapter 3, Style Guide**

   a. When, according to the Style Guide, do you expand brief forms and abbreviations?

   b. In the section on Compound Adjectives, compound modifiers in a series, what does the Style Guide say about suspensive hyphens? Give an example of a suspensive hyphen use.

   c. What is the recommended style for possessive eponyms?

   d. What is the purpose of the semicolon in a series of items that would normally be punctuated with commas?

   e. How should English fractions be transcribed? If the patient smokes "one and a half packs of cigarettes," how should it be transcribed?

   f. Review the list of slang and acceptable brief forms. Are *mets* and *coags* acceptable?

   g. Is it acceptable to insert subjects, helping verbs, prepositions, and articles when not dictated?

   h. How should metric fractions be transcribed? If the physician says "two and a half milligrams" or "half percent Marcaine," how would you transcribe the dictation?

   i. How do you transcribe plural numbers ("forties to fifties," for example)?

   j. What symbol is used for the word *over* between two numbers ("two over three")?

   k. How should dictated contractions (*I've, he's*, etc.) be transcribed?

   l. The physician dictates a redundant expression, such as "4 a.m. in the morning." What should you transcribe?

   m. What should you do if the doctor dictates "same" for a diagnosis?

   n. What do you do if a sentence begins with a numeral?

   o. If a dictator says that a patient is "5 foot tall," how should you transcribe it?

   p. Read the fourth paragraph in the section on Spelling about combining anatomical and directional terms. If you cannot determine whether the physician is saying *frontoparietal* or *frontal-parietal*, how do you decide which to transcribe?

2. Problem Solving

a. *ENG* and *EMG* are two very different studies, but they sound much alike when dictated. What can you do to make sure you don't transcribe the incorrect abbreviation?

b. The doctor dictates a plural form of a medical term that appears to have no plural form. How would you handle this?

c. How is a *pull test* performed? (*Hint*: It's used to evaluate Parkinson disease.)

d. The doctor uses a term to describe spells that a patient is having, but you cannot confirm the term you're hearing in any dictionary. It's not even in **www. onelook.com**. The spells involve a sensation as if the patient is going to pass out or lose consciousness, but the patient does not actually become unconscious. How can you determine how the term is spelled, and if asked to define it, how would you define it when you cannot find it in a dictionary? (*Hint*: Remember your medical terminology study of prefixes, suffixes, and root words.)

e. The dictator uses an abbreviation in the diagnosis at the beginning of the report that can be translated, literally, several different ways. What do you do?

f. When is it appropriate to use quotation marks in a medical report?

g. The physician does not dictate the unit of measure for a given drug dosage (for example, he dictates "Accupril 40 a day"). How should you handle this situation?

h. Should numbers one through nine be transcribed as numerals (1 through 9) or spelled out?

i. A physician dictates two starkly contradictory statements in succession without so much as a hesitation or indication that he is making a correction. What should you do?

j. Physicians sometimes try to help out MTs by changing the pronunciation of a term to correlate with the spelling or they may spell part or all of a term. For example, physicians might emphasize the short *a* sound (as in *hat*) on the word *affect* and say "ee-fekt" for *effect* used as a verb. They may also say "a-b-duct" for *abduct* and "a-d-duct" for *adduct*. Students who are not expecting this may not find it so helpful and spend hours looking for the spelling "adeduct." Keep this in mind and keep notes on the ways in which physicians alter their dictation in an effort to "help."

k. A physician spells a term for you; should you transcribe as dictated? If not, what should you do? If you find that the physician misspelled the term, should you tell the physician the correct spelling?

l. Read the section in the Style Guide on editing. Some physicians, especially disorganized ones, need more editing than others. Ask your instructor how much editing and "cleaning up" is recommended.

3. Preparatory Research

a. What types of studies are used to diagnose carpal tunnel syndrome?

b. Define *diaphoresis, paresthesia.*

c. What kinds of conditions can be evaluated or diagnosed with an EEG?

d. What is a *tilt table test* and what is it used for?

e. Define *vertebrobasilar insufficiency.*

f. Define *titrate* and *abate.*

g. What is *DigiTrace*? What is a *trough level* (of a drug)? Define *idiopathic.*

h. What are the signs and symptoms of multiple sclerosis? How is it treated?

i. What is *rosacea*?

j. What are *neutralizing antibodies*?

k. What is an *IVC filter* and what is it used for?

l. Define the following: *transverse myelitis, paresthesia, vertigo, dysarthria, ataxic.*

m. Define the following: *supranuclear palsy, mask facies.*

n. What are the indications for Aricept and Mirapex?

o. Define the following: *alleviate, orthostatic.*

p. Research *normal-pressure hydrocephalus*. What causes it, what are the symptoms, how is it treated?

q. Define the following: *titrate, herald.*

r. Define the following: *migratory, normocephalic, exudates, papilledema.*

s. Research *nerve conduction study*. List key terms and reasons for such a study.

t. Define the following: *polyneuropathy, demyelinating.*

u. Review the anatomy of the hand and wrist. See if you can find a sample report on-line for carpal tunnel decompression.

v. Find on-line lists of surgical bandages and dressings. Bookmark the best list.

w. Define the following: *investing fascia, reapproximate, tourniquet, Webril.*

x. What is a *somatosensory evoked potential* study?

y. What is a *subacute subdural hematoma*? What are the treatment options for this condition?

z. What is a *ventriculopleural shunt*? For what conditions might such a shunt have been placed?

aa. Define the following: *manometer, pneumothorax, extubate, migrate.*

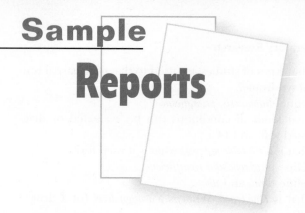

Sample Reports

Sample neurology reports appear on the following pages, illustrating a variety of reports. Fictional names are provided for illustration of proper format, and no resemblance to actual persons is intended. Sample transcripts were prepared according to the *AAMT Book of Style*, where possible.

Chart Note

RICE, DONNA
Age 74
June 20, XXXX

This very pleasant 74-year-old woman has rather advanced parkinsonism, present for many years. It is affecting her daily living to a great degree. She has difficulty dressing, has frequent falls occasionally related to freezing or to festination, but also occurring without any apparent cause. She has marked hesitancy on changing direction and unsteadiness with fatigue. She has a minor problem with sialorrhea, eating, and swallowing. She is able to maintain her personal hygiene without any difficulty. She has had some symptoms of depression along with her Parkinson disease.

On neurologic exam she did have mild to moderate impairment in cognition and short-term memory, although she is oriented x3. She has a mild tremor, worse in the left arm than the right. She has rigidity in the upper extremities. She has marked poverty of movement, with long delays in initiating movement and frequent freezing. She has a moderately flexed posture and cannot straighten to command. She has postural instability. Her speech is mildly dysarthric. She has paucity of spontaneous facial expression. Her gait is characterized by shuffling strides with festination in propulsion. She does not need assistance with gait. She can arise from a chair with difficulty only after multiple attempts. She has micrographia. Deep tendon reflexes are symmetrical, and toes are downgoing. Cranial nerves are unremarkable.

She has been on Sinemet 25/100 t.i.d. for the last 6 years or so. She will be going on vacation soon, and I would not attempt to add a second antiparkinsonian medication. However, I have asked her to increase her Sinemet dose to q.i.d. We will see how she does with Sinemet and plan to add bromocriptine 1 mg per day when she returns.

PW:hpi

Operative Report

MARTINEZ, OLIVIA
#998877
03/25/XXXX

PREOPERATIVE DIAGNOSIS
Herniated nucleus pulposus, L5-S1.

POSTOPERATIVE DIAGNOSIS
Herniated nucleus pulposus, L5-S1.

OPERATION PERFORMED
Microdiskectomy of L5-S1.

PROCEDURE
After a satisfactory level of general endotracheal anesthesia was obtained, the patient was rolled prone on the Relton-Hall frame, and her back was prepared and draped in a routine manner. A midline skin incision was made about 2 inches long, a little longer than usual because of her obesity. The subcutaneous tissues were dissected down to the fascia. A deep retractor was necessary simply to retract the fat down to the fascia. An incision was made along the fascia. A towel clip was placed on the L5 spinous process confirmed by x-ray. The Grossman retractor was utilized to retract the paraspinous muscles on the left side. A microscope was draped out and brought into place.

The ligamentum flavum was excised. The medial aspect of the pedicle was exposed. A laminectomy was continued inferiorly because it was recognized preoperatively that the extrusion of disk material extended inferiorly into the spinal canal. The S1 nerve root was clearly identified and gently retracted medially. It was found to be under a great deal of tension. The anulus was tented up, an incision was made into the anulus, and a large amount of disk material that was herniated centrally was removed. The anulus was incised inferiorly enough to expose some inferior extrusion of disk. When all the centrally herniated disk material was removed, the canal was probed with a Murphy ball. The more caudal portion of the sacral canal was explored. There appeared to be a fragment of disk scarred up, or at least adherent to the dura ventrally. This was teased free with a blunt hook, and a massive fragment of herniated disk material was serially gently freed up with a blunt hook and gently pulled with a pituitary microrongeur, which seemed to free this massive fragment of disk material in its entirety. The spinal canal was probed with a Murphy ball, and no further free material could be identified. The wound was vigorously irrigated.

Dissection had been somewhat slow and tedious to assure freeing up the caudally herniated disk extrusion. Consequently the blood loss was 500 mL. Hemostasis, however, was satisfactorily achieved with gentle tamponade with Gelfoam and cottonoids. One epidural vein laterally in the canal did require electrocautery. There were excellent dural pulsations at the completion of the case. There seemed to be adequate epidural fat to cover the exposed nerve root, so no free fat graft was taken. Because of the blood loss during the case and the patient's obesity and anticipated oozing, it was elected to place a deep medium Hemovac drain that was brought out through the fascia and through a separate stab wound in the skin.

The midline fascial closure was made with 0 Vicryl, subcutaneous tissue with 2-0 Vicryl, and skin closure was made with a running subcuticular undyed 3-0 Dexon. Steri-Strips were applied. A sterile dressing was placed, and the patient was returned to the recovery room in satisfactory condition.

PAUL WHITEHEAD, MD

PW:hpi
d&t: 3/25/XXXX7

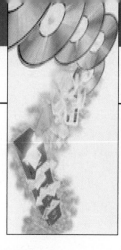

Transcription Practice

Key Words

The following terms appear in the neurology dictations. Before beginning the medical transcription practice for Chapter 14, look up each term below in a medical or English dictionary and write out a short definition.

altered awareness and
    functioning
balance
brain ischemia
brain metastases
carpal tunnel repair
cognitive decline
craniotomy
epilepsy
gait impairment
hydrocephalus
idiopathic epilepsy
multiple sclerosis

nerve conduction study
ocular migraine
Parkinson disease
polyneuropathy
seizure
spells
shunt revision
spinal tap
subdural hematoma
supranuclear palsy
transverse myelitis
ventriculopleural shunt
    malfunction

After completing all the readings and exercises in Chapter 14, transcribe the neurology dictation. Proofread your transcribed documents carefully, listening to the dictation while you read your transcripts.

Transcribe (*not* retype) the same reports again without referring to your previous transcription attempt. Initially, you may need to transcribe some reports more than twice before you can produce an error-free document. Your ultimate goal is to produce an error-free document the first time.

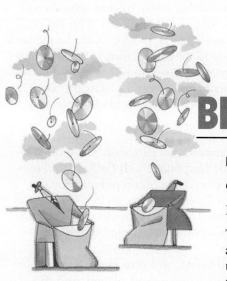

BLOOPERS

Incorrect	Correct
Grandma fissures.	Grand mal seizures.
Impressive neurosis.	Depressive neurosis.
The facial nerve functioned normally at the conclusion of the case and was taken to the recovery room in satisfactory condition.	The facial nerve functioned normally at the conclusion of the case, and the patient was taken to the recovery room in satisfactory condition.
Because of increasing lethargy and inappropriate behavior, she was brought to the emergency department for evaluation by her son.	Because of increasing lethargy and inappropriate behavior, she was brought by her son to the emergency department.
Five years ago the patient had a subarachnoid hemorrhoid.	Five years ago the patient had a subarachoid hemorrhage.
Finger-to-nose and nose-to-nose coordination tests were normal.	Finger-to-nose and heel-to-shin coordination tests were normal.

Chapter 15

Psychiatry

Chapter Outline

Transcribing Psychiatric Dictation
Terminology Review
Lay and Medical Terms
Medical Readings
History and Physical Examination
A Doctor's View
Common Diseases
Diagnostic and Therapeutic Procedures

Pharmacology
Spotlight
Transcription Tips
Proofreading Skills
Skills Challenge
Sample Reports
Transcription Practice
Bloopers

Learning Objectives

- Spell and define common psychiatric terms.
- Identify types of questions a physician might ask about mental health symptoms during the review of systems.
- Identify common psychiatric diseases. Describe their typical cause, course, and treatment options.
- Identify and define psychiatric diagnostic procedures.

- List common psychiatric laboratory tests and procedures.
- Identify and describe common psychiatric drugs and their uses.
- Demonstrate knowledge of anatomical, medical, pharmacological, adjectival, and soundalike terms by accurately completing the exercises in this chapter.

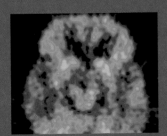
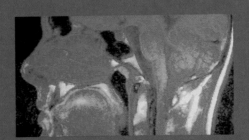
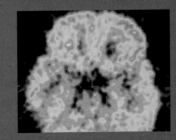

Transcribing Psychiatric Dictation

Disorders of perception, mood, and behavior have always been placed in a separate category from other illnesses, by both physicians and laity. Except for a few conditions obviously caused by organic disease or injury of the central nervous system (alcoholic dementia, inability to speak after head injury or a stroke), mental illnesses were long thought to result from failure of normal personality development, inadequate adaptation to life stresses, acquired distortions of thought processes, and other vague and intangible factors. The specialty of psychiatry came into being as a field concentrating on disturbances of mood and thought for which no organic basis could be found.

Within the past few decades, psychiatric theory has undergone remarkable changes in orientation. With important exceptions, most modern psychologists and psychiatrists believe that all mental disorders are due to **structural**, **chemical**, or **electrical abnormalities** in the brain. This idea is supported by abundant evidence from diverse sources. Genetic studies show that many mental disorders run in families, and some have actually been traced to specific chromosomal abnormalities.

Biochemical research has established a correlation between the distribution of neurotransmitters such as **serotonin**, **dopamine**, and **norepinephrine** in the central nervous system and certain disorders of **cognition**, **mood**, and **behavior**. A chemical basis has been found for the way in which many drugs help in mental disorders, and new drugs designed with specific chemical goals have attained their object of providing improved control of anxiety, depression, and other common disorders. Although **drug therapy** may still be considered an adjunct to counseling and other forms of psychotherapy, for many disorders it is currently the most rapid, effective, and predictable mode of treatment.

Terminology Review

affect One's prevailing mood or emotional state, pleasant or unpleasant, particularly as perceived by the examiner: basic emotional state, and emotional content of responses to examiner (apathetic, blunted, depressed, elated, euphoric, flat, inappropriate, labile).

amnesia Loss of memory.

aversion therapy A form of behavior therapy that associates an objectionable or undesirable pattern of behavior with an unpleasant experience or consequence, so as to reduce or extinguish the behavior.

behavior (behavioral) therapy Any type of psychotherapy that focuses on the alteration or correction of undesirable behavior, including such responses to external stimuli as anxiety, depression, and physical symptoms of emotion (tachycardia, muscle tension, sweating). Behavior therapy uses conditioning, muscle relaxation techniques, meditation, breathing retraining, biofeedback, guided learning, and other methods.

client The recipient of psychotherapy; a term preferred to "patient" when the therapist is not a physician.

client-centered therapy A form of psychotherapy in which the client is encouraged, with a minimum of direction by the therapist, to discover the sources of distressing mental symptoms and means of resolving them.

cognitive therapy A form of psychotherapy based on promoting the client's rational understanding of the source of distressing emotions, thought patterns, and undesirable behaviors, and correction of these by adoption of more mature, balanced, and realistic attitudes.

compensation (overcompensation) A mechanism by which one covers up a defect or weakness by exaggerating or overdeveloping some other property or faculty.

confabulation Invention of stories about one's past, often bizarre and complex, to fill in gaps left by amnesia; a typical feature of Korsakoff syndrome in chronic alcoholics.

cyclothymia Abnormal lability of mood, which varies between excitement and depression without becoming severe enough to be called bipolar disorder.

delusion A distorted belief or perception, such as thinking that one is a famous historical figure (Jesus, Napoleon) or that one is the object of persecution.

denial A mechanism by which one refuses to believe, remember, or accept an unpleasant fact or circumstance, such as a past painful experience or the fact of being ill.

Diagnostic and Statistical Manual of Mental Disorders (DSM) A description and classification of mental disorders based on objective categories. Recognized as a diagnostic standard and widely used for reporting, coding, and statistical purposes, *DSM* is published by the American Psychiatric Association. The current (fourth) edition (*DSM-IV*) appeared in 1994. See *multiaxial assessment*.

dysphoria A general feeling of mental or emotional discomfort.

dysthymia A depressed mood, usually chronic or recurrent, that is not severe enough to be called major depression.

eating disorders See *anorexia nervosa* and *bulimia nervosa* under Common Diseases.

encephalopathy Any organic disease or damage of the brain, particularly the cerebral cortex, that causes impairment of mental or physical functioning; often due to degenerative diseases (Alzheimer disease, Creutzfeldt-Jakob disease) or chemical intoxications (alcohol, lead).

family therapy Psychotherapy that treats the family as a unit and seeks to promote understanding and correction of pathologic attitudes and relationships among members of the unit.

group therapy Psychotherapy administered to several persons at once, making use of sharing of perceptions, experiences, and feelings, group dynamics, and mutual understanding and support.

guilt A sense of having done wrong, of having failed to meet one's own or others' expectations or standards, or of being inferior or inadequate; as used in psychiatry and psychoanalysis, guilt is a distinct concept from moral guilt, which arises from deliberate violation of ethical principles or civil law.

hallucination A sensory experience, usually auditory or visual, without any physical basis—for example, seeing snakes floating in the air or hearing voices urging one to do something.

hypnosis A technique by which the therapist places the client into a sleeplike trance in which outside stimuli are reduced to a minimum, the subconscious is more directly accessible, and the client is more susceptible to the influence of the therapist's suggestions and advice.

identification A mental process whereby one takes on the properties or actions of another with whom an emotional tie exists (a boy walking and talking like his father; a woman dressing and behaving like a movie idol).

libido Sexual desire or drive; often, more generally, the totality of pleasure-directed energy or activity.

mechanism (also defense mechanism, ego-defensive mechanism, mental mechanism, unconscious mechanism) An automatic, unconscious mental process whereby repressed emotions (painful feelings, sexual urges) generate new beliefs or attitudes to protect the ego from a sense of guilt, inadequacy, or other negative feelings. See *compensation, identification, projection, rationalization, repression, sublimation.*

multiaxial assessment As outlined in *DSM-IV*, provides for a comprehensive diagnostic formulation of mental illness that includes consideration of five distinct domains or axes. Axes I and II refer to formal psychiatric diagnoses, including the presenting complaint or chief problem as well as other conditions that may be a focus of clinical attention. Axis I covers all such diagnoses except personality disorders and mental retardation, which are included in Axis II. Axis III comprises nonpsychiatric medical diagnoses, such as neurologic disease, infections, tumors, and diabetes mellitus. Axis IV focuses on psychosocial and environmental problems, including those related to family and other interpersonal relationships, education, employment, housing, finances, access to healthcare, and interaction with the legal system. In Axis V the clinician records a global assessment of functioning.

narcissism Extreme self-love; excessive preoccupation with oneself and one's own concerns and needs, to the exclusion of normal emotional ties with others.

neurosis A mental disorder in which the patient experiences, and gives evidence of, emotional distress, but remains in touch with reality at all times.

neurotransmitter A normal chemical substance produced in minute quantities by nerve tissue and involved in the transmission of electrical impulses from one nerve cell to another. The effect of a neurotransmitter may be to stimulate or inhibit the nerve cell on which it acts. Well-known neurotransmitters include acetylcholine, dopamine, epinephrine, gamma-aminobutyric acid (GABA), norepinephrine, and serotonin.

pharmacotherapy Treatment of disease with drugs, as contrasted with methods such as counseling, diet, and surgery.

play therapy A form of psychotherapy used with children, in which structured or unstructured play settings with dolls and other toys enable the therapist to identify and correct false or unhealthy attitudes and behavior patterns.

projection A mechanism whereby one unconsciously attributes one's own thoughts and attitudes (usually negative or unpleasant) to others as a means of dealing with a sense of guilt or inadequacy.

psyche A vague term roughly equivalent to "mind."

psychiatry The branch of medicine concerned with the diagnosis and treatment of mental disorders; all psychiatrists are physicians.

psychoanalysis A school of clinical psychology founded by Sigmund Freud and based on lengthy, searching analysis of the patient's mental life, including particularly the content of the subconscious, which can be made manifest by hypnosis, dream interpretation, free association (nondirected reflections voiced by the patient), and other methods. Many psychiatrists are psychoanalysts, but not all psychoanalysts are psychiatrists (physicians).

psychodrama A type of group therapy in which clients resolve conflicts and distressing emotional states by acting out their fantasies and fears in the setting of a dramatic performance before an audience of fellow clients.

psychology Broadly, the study of all mental processes and functions (perception, memory, judgment, learning ability, mood, social interaction, communication, and others). Clinical psychology is a professional discipline concerned with the nonmedical treatment of mental disorders. A clinical psychologist ordinarily does not hold a medical degree.

psychosis A mental disorder in which, in addition to emotional distress, the patient experiences a break with reality, manifested by delusions, hallucinations, and grossly bizarre or socially inappropriate behavior.

psychotherapy Any method or technique, except the administration of medicines, used in the treatment of mental disorders.

rational therapy A form of treatment in which mental disorders, which are thought to result from misinformation, wrong belief systems, and distorted logic, are improved by the therapist's use of direct, positive teaching and advice.

rationalization A mental process of justifying some act or omission through logical reasoning or argumentation, usually as a means of reducing feelings of guilt or inadequacy.

reality testing An individual's ability to perceive reality as it is, not as distorted by abnormal thought processes, disorders of perception, delusions, or hallucinations.

repression The mental process of thrusting out of consciousness impulses or desires that are perceived as incompatible with one's own standards or sense of fitness, and that therefore generate unpleasant emotions; repressed material occupies a large part of the subconscious.

subconscious (mind) Elements of one's personality (feelings, attitudes, prejudices, desires, behavior patterns) of which one is unaware; a general and somewhat vague term including but not always identical to what Freud called the unconscious (*Unbewusstsein*).

suicidal ideation Thoughts of committing suicide as a relief from mental distress, without actual attempts at suicide.

sublimation Diversion of sexual energy or impulses into higher or more socially acceptable activities.

therapist One who treats; in mental health, anyone administering psychotherapy.

transference The development, on the part of the client, of an emotional bond (positive or negative) with the therapist.

Lay and Medical Terms

fear	phobia
manic depressive	bipolar disorder
mood	affect

Medical Readings

History and Physical Examination

by John H. Dirckx, M.D.

Review of Systems. The psychiatric part of the Review of Systems is often omitted. The psychiatric history is even more intimate and sensitive, if possible, than the sexual history. A person with severe psychiatric impairment makes a most unreliable historian. For example, there is usually not much point in asking someone about a history of hallucinations or delusions, for these terms are used only by persons who are convinced of the unreality of the experiences.

A person with even a mild mood or personality disorder frequently resists talking about it. Hence part or all of the psychiatric history may have to be obtained from the patient's family or friends or from medical records.

At times it is hard to distinguish between psychiatric history-taking and psychiatric examination, since both make use of the same basic tool—interviewing the patient. When the patient's chief complaint is not psychiatric, inquiries about past or present mental illness or emotional disturbance are more clearly historical in intent. The interviewer asks about any prior diagnosis of mental, emotional, or nervous illness (anxiety, depression, social phobia, panic attacks, obsessive-compulsive disorder, bipolar disorder, schizophrenia, alcoholism, drug addiction) and treatments used, including counseling, group therapy, drug therapy, hospitalization, and electroshock.

A general notion of the subject's mental and emotional health history can be obtained by inquiring about family and marital harmony, school performance, job stability and satisfaction, social contacts, sleep pattern, drug and alcohol use, and general sense of well-being, self-esteem, and purpose in life.

Mental Status Examination. The formal mental status examination (Figure 15-1) consists of the following parts:

Appearance: Dress, grooming, makeup, hair care, jewelry or other adornments; slovenly, unkempt, bizarre, mismatched, or incongruous garments or adornments.

Sensorium: Responsiveness to visual, auditory, and tactile stimuli; alertness, attention span; ability to recognize and classify objects.

Activity and Behavior: Gait, posture, level of motor activity, speech; bizarre or compulsive actions, mannerisms, or posturings.

Mood (Affect): Basic emotional state, and emotional content of responses to examiner (apathetic, blunted, depressed, elated, euphoric, flat, inappropriate, labile).

Thought Content: Unconventional thoughts, fantasies, phobias, obsessive ideas, delusions, hallucinations, poverty of imagination.

Intellectual Function: Speed, coherence, and relevance of abstract reasoning; mental arithmetic, interpretation of idioms ("time on your hands") and proverbs ("a rolling stone gathers no moss").

Orientation: Awareness of time (time of day, day of week, date, season, year), place (state, city, exact present location), person (ability to identify self, relatives, friends).

Memory: Recall of recent and remote events; general information ("How many cents in a quarter? Who is the president?").

Judgment: Competence in analyzing situations, solving problems, taking practical action ("What would you do if the house across the street caught fire?").

Insight: The patient's awareness of being ill or impaired, and a recognition of the nature and implications of the illness.

Orientation, memory, and judgment are often called the organic triad because they are commonly affected in organic dementia. In addition to relatively unstructured interviewing, the subject may be given various formal, standardized tests of intelligence and personality.

There is a certain overlapping of material between parts of the mental status examination. Some of the observations pertain to the field of neurology rather than psychiatry. In addition to the mental status examination outlined above, the patient may be asked to complete one or more formal standardized tests of intelligence and personality.

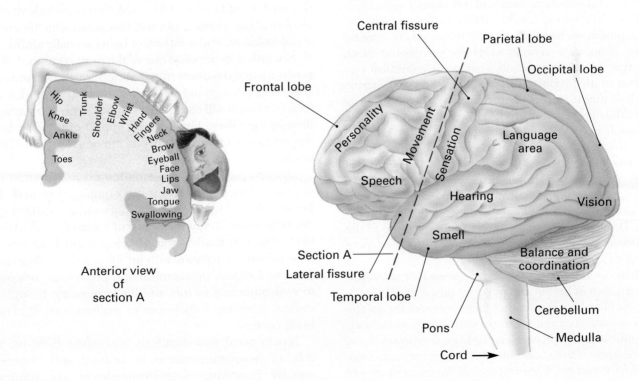

Figure 15-1
The Brain, Lateral View

...

Drug *Addiction*

Many drugs, particularly those used to treat pain, anxiety, and depression, can temporarily induce pleasant emotional states, varying from carefree serenity to euphoria and exhilaration. Even when such a feeling is not part of the intended therapeutic effect of the drug, it can exercise such an appeal that the patient becomes *habituated* to the drug—that is, craves another dose as soon as the effect of the previous dose begins to wear off.

Narcotic analgesics, barbiturates, amphetamines, and benzodiazepine tranquilizers are among the prescription drugs most commonly associated with habituation, but habituation to alcohol, caffeine, and nicotine is even more prevalent. The nature of habituation is not fully understood. There appears to be a genetic tendency to alcoholism and perhaps to some other types of drug habituation.

Some habituating drugs also produce physical *dependence*. That means that after repeated dosing, the body adapts neurologically or biochemically in such a way that withdrawal of the drug can induce physical symptoms such as diaphoresis, restlessness, dysphoria, and even seizures. The development of withdrawal symptoms reinforces the craving due to psychological habituation. In fact, the victim of drug dependence may keep repeating doses not so much to get "high" over and over as just to reverse withdrawal symptoms and feel normal again.

Drug habituation can be further complicated by the development of *tolerance*—that is, the need to increase dosage continually in order to achieve the desired effect. One type of tolerance occurs when a drug stimulates an increase in the production of a cytochrome P-450 enzyme that is involved in its own breakdown. The more drug taken, the more enzyme produced; and the more enzyme, the less drug effect from a given dose.

Addiction is variously defined; some have advised abandonment of the term (as well as of *drug abuse*) because of acquired judgmental connotations. The usual meaning of addiction is a severe, disabling preoccupation with the use of a drug involving habituation, dependence, and tolerance. Drug addicts, like alcoholics, often drop out of the workforce and out of society, and some are driven to crime in order to feed their habits.

Many drugs that were formerly approved for use in this country, such as heroin and phencyclidine ("angel dust"), are now illegal because of their high potential for habituation or addiction, and the use of some other agents, such as amphetamines and cocaine, has been sharply restricted for the same reason. Cocaine is a potent coronary vasoconstrictor and has been responsible for many deaths of young persons from acute myocardial infarction.

John H. Dirckx, M.D.
Perspectives on the Medical Transcription Profession

A Doctor's View

Depression

by John H. Dirckx, M.D.

We all experience periods of sadness or grief in response to losses, disappointments, or failure to attain specific goals or wishes. The diagnosis of "major" or "clinical" depression, however, implies a more severe and lasting degree of distress and disability than these normal low tides in our emotional life.

The criteria for a major depressive episode include either a marked reduction of interest or pleasure in virtually all activities, or a depressed mood, or both, most or all of the time, for at least two weeks. In addition, three or more of the following must be present: gain or loss of weight, increased or decreased sleep, increased or decreased level of psychomotor activity, fatigue, feelings of guilt or worthlessness, diminished ability to concentrate, and recurring thoughts of death or suicide. Chronic depression that is not severe enough to meet the criteria for major depression is called dysthymia.

The first episode of depression typically occurs before the age of 40. Recurrences are common, and later episodes tend to be more frequent, more severe, and more lasting. Besides being more common in women, the disease runs in families. Other risk factors include drug or alcohol abuse, chronic physical illness, stressful life events, social isolation, and a history of being sexually abused.

Not only is **depression** one of the most commonly diagnosed mental disorders in our society today, but undoubtedly many cases go unrecognized. About 10% of men and 25% of women will experience clinical depression at some time in their lives. The negative impact of the disease on the economy of this country is estimated at $16 billion yearly.

Modern psychiatry is moving toward the position that virtually all mental disorders are organically caused. The familial clustering of many disorders and the striking gender differences in the incidence of some of them make it likely that the tendency to develop them is genetically determined. In persons with an inherited predisposition to mental illness, biochemical and physiologic responses to environmental factors and life stresses are thought to induce persisting imbalances or malfunctions in certain brain centers.

Biochemical investigations have shed light on the role of neurotransmitters in normal and abnormal mental function. Neurotransmitters are naturally occurring chemical substances that, when released at nerve endings, stimulate or inhibit the function of adjacent nerve cells.

Two neurotransmitters, dopamine and serotonin, are thought to play roles in the genesis of depressive disease. **Dopamine** is the chemical precursor of norepinephrine, the hormone that acts on alpha- and beta-adrenergic receptors in the sympathetic nervous system and is the body's principal vasoconstrictor agent. Dopamine, which itself has vasoconstrictor activity, acts as a neurotransmitter or regulator in the CNS. Dopamine appears to be deficient or inactive in certain parts of the limbic system in patients with depression.

Serotonin, also called 5-hydroxytryptamine or 5HT, has an even broader range of functions. Formed in chromaffin cells of the central nervous system, peripheral neurons, the gastrointestinal mucosa, and the pineal gland, it constricts blood vessels, inhibits gastric secretion, stimulates smooth muscle, promotes the release of pituitary hormones, and serves as a precursor of the pineal hormone melatonin (which regulates the sleep-wakefulness cycle), besides acting as a neurotransmitter in the CNS.

Depression appears to be closely linked to the action of serotonin at synapses in the limbic system. It may reflect abnormalities in the sensitivity of receptors to serotonin, or in the feedback system that normally regulates serotonin production and release, or both. Besides having low levels of CNS serotonin, persons with major depression also have elevated levels of serum cortisol which are not suppressed by the administration of dexamethasone, a synthetic corticosteroid.

A number of highly effective drugs are available to treat depression. These include the older tricyclic compounds (amitriptyline, imipramine), the selective serotonin reuptake inhibitors (SSRIs or serotoninergics) (escitalopram, fluoxetine, sertraline), monoamine oxidase inhibitors (pargyline, phenelzine), and other agents (bupropion, nefazodone, trazodone, venlafaxine).

Many patients experience troublesome side effects (drowsiness, headaches, dry mouth, disturbances of gastrointestinal or sexual function). Some of these tend to diminish or disappear with continued use, but about 15% of patients discontinue antidepressant medicine because of side effects. Hence the total pharmacologic profiles of these drugs need to be taken into consideration in individualizing treatment. Patients taking monoamine oxidase inhibitors (MAOIs) must carefully avoid many medicines (decongestants, antihistamines, antihypertensives), foods (cheese, sausage, chocolate), caffeine, and alcohol because of the risk of fatal hypertensive crisis.

The neurotransmitters dopamine and norepinephrine belong to the monoamines class. Monoamine oxidase is a naturally occurring enzyme that breaks down these substances immediately after they have exerted their effects. By blocking this breakdown, MAOIs boost levels of dopamine and norepinephrine at critical sites.

Insomnia

Insomnia has been defined as the inability to sleep long enough or deeply enough at night to maintain optimum central nervous system (CNS) health and function during the day. Since sleep requirements vary markedly from person to person, no quantitative definition (so many minutes or hours in such-and-such a stage of sleep) is feasible. Moreover, the diagnosis of insomnia is generally based on the patient's own observations, and extensive studies have shown that these observations are often unreliable.

Insomnia is regarded as a significant and widespread public health problem. The prevalence of chronic insomnia (defined as inadequate sleep at least three nights a week for at least one month) may be as high as 15% in the general population. Besides leading to daytime drowsiness, difficulty concentrating, impairment of memory, irritability, and restlessness or anxiety, insomnia is believed to be responsible for much poor job performance and many industrial and automobile accidents.

Insomnia is not a single disorder but rather a symptom with numerous possible causes. Various patterns of sleep disturbance occur. Difficulty in falling asleep (prolonged sleep latency) can result from mental preoccupation, emotional upset (anxiety, anger), ingestion of a large meal or use of CNS stimulants (caffeine, nicotine, or various medicines) shortly before bedtime, physical distress (pain, nausea), symptoms aggravated by recumbency (cough, gastroesophageal reflux, orthopnea), or disruption of the sleep-wake rhythm (jet lag, shift work, daytime napping).

Another type of insomnia, which consists of failure to attain sleep stages 3 and 4, with frequent awakenings during the night, can also be due to emotionally induced restlessness or to physical factors such as chronic musculoskeletal problems (osteoarthritis, fibromyalgia) and nocturia due to urinary tract disease.

A third type, called terminal insomnia, isn't as serious as it sounds. This refers to awakening in the early morning (two to three hours before intended rising time) with inability to fall back asleep. Terminal insomnia is a cardinal feature of clinical depression but may occur in other conditions as well.

Alleviating insomnia begins logically with an attempt to find and eliminate its cause. Treatment of physical or emotional illness or correction of an unhealthful lifestyle may lead to improvement in sleep. Many medicines (decongestants, antidepressants, antihypertensives, nicotine patches prescribed to facilitate smoking cessation, even some antibiotics) can delay the onset of sleep or impair its quality. Changing medicines or dosage times may restore a healthy sleep pattern.

John H. Dirckx, M.D.
Perspectives on the Medical Transcription Profession

Typically it takes 4-6 weeks for full control of depression to be achieved. Antidepressant therapy is ordinarily continued for at least one year after symptoms improve. Counseling and other forms of psychotherapy may be useful in hastening remission and reducing the risk of relapse.

In **seasonal affective disorder (SAD)**, exposure to high-intensity light for 1-3 hours a day has been shown to abolish symptoms in many patients. While advocates of the cognitive theory of depression may use drug treatment to relieve symptoms, they emphasize other therapeutic strategies: avoidance of depressing people, places, or situations; correction of drug or alcohol problems; improved socialization; assignment of gradually more challenging daily tasks; search for pleasurable activities; and correction of distorted or maladaptive thinking patterns. For severe depression that does not respond to either drug or cognitive-behavioral therapy, electroshock therapy is sometimes beneficial.

Common Diseases

Anxiety Disorders. A group of mental disorders characterized by chronic worry or fear. **Anxiety disorders** are the most common ones seen by psychiatrists; often anxiety accompanies other disorders (depression, schizophrenia).

Cause: Probably a malfunction in the part of the brain called the reticular formation. This system regulates sleep and wakefulness as well as many autonomic and endocrine functions. Persons with chronic anxiety have abnormal levels of certain neurotransmitters (norepinephrine, serotonin, gamma-aminobutyric acid) in brain tissue.

History: Persisting or recurring feelings of apprehension, uneasiness, worry, or fear (with or without a clearly defined object) that is out of proportion to any actual danger or threat. The sense of dread may become so absorbing as to distract the patient's attention from personal, social, and occupational activities. Anxiety may be triggered by a wide variety of settings and circumstances. Besides the mental condition of constant worry or dread, the patient usually experiences physical signs of autonomic and endocrine response: heightened muscle tension, rapid pulse, hyperventilation, sweating, insomnia, problems with appetite and sexual function. *DSM-IV* lists specific criteria for 14 anxiety disorders. Five of these are described here.

Generalized Anxiety Disorder. An abiding state of excessive, distressing, and disabling worry about a number of issues, associated with restlessness, muscle tension, irritability, abnormal fatigue, and insomnia. The condition is twice as common in women and often accompanies depression.

Social Phobia. The most common anxiety disorder. A phobia is an irrational fear of some object or situation, with resulting efforts to avoid it. While recognizing that the fear is unfounded or out of proportion to any actual danger, the victim of a phobia is unable to overcome it. The victim of social phobia experiences an exaggerated and persistent fear of embarrassment or humiliation in a social setting, or when appearing or performing in public. This can lead to severe social, educational, or occupational disability. Many persons with this disorder also suffer from depression or alcoholism.

Agoraphobia. An intense fear of being alone or being in a public place from which escape might be difficult, or help unavailable, in case of sudden incapacitation (such as passing out or having a heart attack). Victims of agoraphobia avoid open spaces, crowded enclosures such as stores or churches, tunnels, elevators, and public transportation.

Panic Disorder. Recurring sudden spontaneous attacks of intense anxiety, lasting minutes or hours, and accompanied by marked physical symptoms such as chest pain, tachycardia, dyspnea or choking, sweating, faintness, tremors, and tingling in the extremities. Because of the type and severity of physical symptoms, panic disorder is sometimes mistaken for a heart attack or other life-threatening emergency by both the victim and others, including physicians. Although either agoraphobia or panic disorder can occur by itself, the two are often associated in the same patient.

Obsessive-Compulsive Disorder (OCD). A chronic anxiety disorder in which the patient suffers from both obsessions and compulsions. An obsession is a recurring or persisting idea, thought, or image that is perceived as intrusive, distracting, and repugnant, but that the victim is unable to ignore or suppress. Examples are recurring thoughts of harming oneself or others; fear of contamination or infections; and worry about losing or throwing away something that is or may later become important. A compulsion is an urge to repeat a ritualistic or stereotyped form of behavior that is recognized by the victim as irrational but that cannot be omitted without an increase of anxiety. Examples include excessive, repetitive handwashing; rigid attention to order or symmetry; repeated checking of locks, switches, or clocks; and performance of everyday actions in a ritualized fashion.

Treatment: The treatment of an anxiety disorder depends on the exact nature of the disorder, its source, and its symptoms. Individual or group psychotherapy can provide emotional support, help the patient to gain insight into the nature of the problem, encourage psychic growth and maturation, and teach positive attitudes and goal-directed behavior. Most anxiety disorders respond well to short-term or long-term drug treatment. Agents that reduce the level of uneasiness and worry are called **anxiolytics**. Most of the anxiolytics in current use belong to the benzodiazepine class (alprazolam, oxazepam). Certain drugs used in the treatment of depression (fluoxetine, fluvoxamine) are useful in obsessive-compulsive disorder. Paroxetine is beneficial in social anxiety disorder and panic disorder. Beta-adrenergic blocking agents such as propranolol can control the autonomic component of performance anxiety, social anxiety disorder, and panic disorder (tachycardia, sweaty palms, tremors).

Bipolar Disorder (Manic-Depressive Disorder). A type of depressive illness in which the patient's mood oscillates between depression and mania.

Cause: Apparently a malfunction of the limbic system. Susceptibility to this disorder has been traced to a gene on chromosome 18. Half of patients have at least one parent with an affective disorder.

History: Alternations of mood between **mania** and **clinical depression**, with variable intervals of normal mood in between. A manic episode is a period of abnormal elevation of mood, irritability, or restlessness that lasts at least one week and is accompanied by some or all of the following: inflated self-esteem, hyperactivity, **flight of ideas**, abnormal talkativeness or **pressured speech** (rapid, strained speech as if the subject's mouth can't keep up with the flow of thoughts), reduced need for sleep, short attention span, and reckless behavior. Unlike anxiety and simple depression, bipolar disorder may include a loss of touch with reality; that is, it may be a true psychosis. During either the manic or the depressive phase, the patient may experience delusions or hallucinations, or may display grossly bizarre behavior.

Treatment: Drug therapy with lithium salts, carbamazepine, or valproic acid usually controls the manic phase of bipolar disorder and helps to prevent recurrences of mania. **Tranquilizers** and **antidepressants** may also be used. Mania generally causes severe impairment of social and occupational functioning and may require hospitalization.

Schizophrenia. A chronic or recurring **psychosis** due to a disorder of thought processes.

Cause: Susceptibility to schizophrenia is probably inherited as a complex of variations affecting several genes. Neurophysiologic studies have shown abnormally small size of the part of the brain called the thalamus, as well as changes in signal intensity in adjacent white matter.

History: Gradual onset, usually before age 40, of cognitive malfunctions—disturbances of perception and thinking characterized by **delusions, hallucinations**, gross distortion of mental function, or all of these. These basic features of schizophrenia are usually accompanied by reduced energy level, flat or depressed affect, **anhedonia** (inability to experience pleasure from normally pleasurable activities), and **abulia** (diminished ability to make decisions). Virtually all patients display impoverished thought content, social withdrawal, and impairment of occupational functioning. Even with intensive psychotherapy and drug treatment, about 25% of persons with schizophrenia require custodial or institutional care. Schizophrenia is divided, on the basis of dominant clinical manifestations, into the following types:

- **disorganized (hebephrenic) schizophrenia:** severe breakdown of mental function and incongruous or silly behavior.
- **paranoid schizophrenia:** prominent delusions of persecution or grandeur, often reinforced by hallucinations.
- **catatonic schizophrenia:** statue-like posturing, rigidity, or stupor.
- **undifferentiated schizophrenia:** without defining features.
- **residual schizophrenia:** history of schizophrenia but only mild, nonpsychotic residual impairment of mental function.

Treatment: Psychotherapy is inconsistently effective in helping patients overcome disordered thinking and improving social functioning. The modern treatment of schizophrenia depends heavily on the use of drugs known as **neuroleptics** or **antipsychotics**. The older members of this class belong to the group known chemically as **phenothiazines** (chlorpromazine, fluphenazine, trifluoperazine).

Patients treated with these drugs frequently develop **parkinsonian symptoms**, including tremors, rigidity, and **akathisia** (extreme restlessness, inability to remain seated). These may be adequately controlled with drugs used to treat parkinsonism (benztropine, trihexyphenidyl). A few suffer from **tardive dyskinesia**, an irreversible neurologic disorder causing twitching and writhing movements, particularly in the lips and tongue. Neuroleptics in other classes (clozapine, haloperidol, risperidone) are useful alternatives but have their own side effects. Fluphenazine and haloperidol can be given as long-acting injections to patients who have trouble complying with daily oral medicine regimens.

Alzheimer Dementia. Chronic, progressive deterioration of mental function (Figure 15-2).

Cause: Degeneration of cortical neurons typically beginning in middle life, usually due to inherited abnormality of brain chemistry but sometimes acquired.

History: Usually gradual onset of steady deterioration in certain mental functions: short-term memory loss,

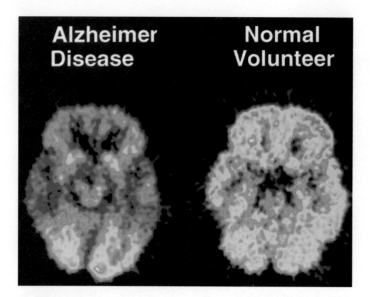

Figure 15-2
PET Scan Comparing the Metabolic Activity Levels of a Normal Brain and the Brain of an Alzheimer Sufferer.
Red and yellow colors indicate high activity levels, while blue colors represent low activity levels.

inability to understand spoken or written language and to express oneself in speech and writing, diminished or distorted sensory perception, inability to perform purposeful actions, personality changes with irritability and depression, deterioration of impulse control.

Course: Dementia is irreversible and progressive, usually culminating in death within 5-10 years.

Treatment: Acetylcholinesterase inhibitors (donepezil, galantamine, rivastigmine, tacrine) produce improvement in cognitive function. Anxiolytics, neuroleptics, and antidepressants may be used to control disorders of mood and behavior. Behavioral therapy is sometimes successful in reinforcing acceptable behavior and extinguishing unacceptable behavior. A comfortable, secure environment (preferably home, unless the patient is too disruptive or the burden of care too taxing for the family), with familiar faces and a simple, steady routine, provide a setting in which the patient's impairments are least distressing and disabling. Support and counsel for the family are of major importance.

Attention-Deficit Hyperactivity Disorder (ADHD). A chronic behavioral disorder, most striking in children, involving hyperactivity, short attention span, and impulsiveness.

Cause: The disease runs in families, and about 25% of patients have at least one parent who is similarly affected. It is three to eight times more common in boys. Magnetic resonance imaging has shown abnormalities in the corpus callosum, the band of fibers connecting the two cerebral hemispheres. The theory that sugar and food colorings or other additives trigger hyperactivity is entirely without scientific support.

History: Often there is evidence of behavioral disturbance in infancy, and the full-blown disorder is typically recognizable by the age of six. The three cardinal features of ADHD are **inattentiveness** (short attention span, distractibility, inability to complete tasks undertaken, difficulty in following directions, tendency to lose personal articles, disregard for personal safety), **impulsiveness** (blurting out one's thoughts without adequate reflection, butting in front of others in waiting lines), and **hyperactivity** (restlessness, fidgeting, or squirming instead of sitting or standing still, excessive talking). Children with this disorder have a high incidence of academic failure, conflict with parents, teachers, and law enforcement officials, antisocial behavior, and substance abuse.

Treatment: Central nervous system stimulants (dextroamphetamine, methylphenidate, and pemoline) are usually successful in enhancing learning ability and improving social functioning. These medicines are taken early in the day so as to avoid nighttime insomnia. When improvement in academic achievement is the chief goal of treatment, the patient may be given "drug holidays" on weekends and during school vacations.

Anorexia Nervosa. A compulsive reduction of body weight to an unhealthful level by rigorous dieting, often supplemented by strenuous exercise, self-induced vomiting, or the use of diuretics or laxatives (Figure 15-3).

Most patients are women with perfectionistic, obsessional personalities and distorted body image (**body dysmorphic disorder**). Onset typically occurs at or just after puberty. Steady loss of subcutaneous fat and wasting of muscle mass can lead to severe emaciation. Chronic nutritional deficiency induces abnormalities in body chemistry and physiology including amenorrhea, bradycardia, hypotension, electrolyte imbalance, anemia, and dry skin with increased pigmentation and downy hair growth (lanugo).

Treatment often requires intensive counseling, pharmacotherapy, and even hospital confinement with intravenous alimentation.

Bulimia nervosa. A common behavioral disorder of young women characterized by recurrent episodes of binge eating.

The typical patient engages in uncontrollable gorging with high-carbohydrate food several times a week. Resulting anxiety about weight gain usually leads to self-induced vomiting or purging with laxatives. Unlike anorexia nervosa, this disorder is not usually associated with marked weight loss or amenorrhea.

Repeated vomiting may result in erosion of dental enamel, chronic throat irritation, or esophageal injury. Treatment includes counseling and pharmacotherapy.

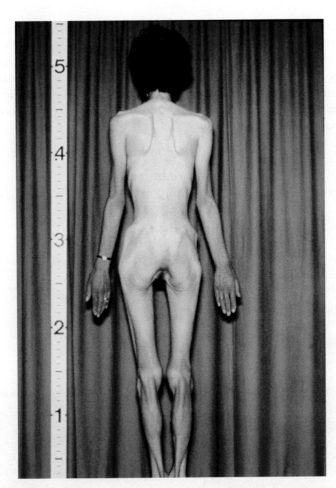

Figure 15-3
An Emaciated Young Woman with Anorexia Nervosa

Diagnostic and Therapeutic Procedures

electroconvulsive (electroshock) therapy Delivery of controlled electric shocks to the brain to alter electrochemical function, primarily in depression. The treatment, administered only by a physician, causes convulsions and loss of consciousness; the patient awakens in a state of disorientation. Several treatment sessions may be necessary before improvement is noted.

therapeutic blood level Tests the amount of measurable drug in the serum. Many drugs have optimum levels where they are most effective (therapeutic range).

Pharmacology

It is estimated that nearly 50% of all hospital admissions are in some way related to a mental health problem such as anxiety, depression, suicide, postpartum depression, psychosis, psychosomatic illness, attention-deficit hyperactivity disorder (ADHD), panic attacks, social phobias, obsessive-compulsive disorder (OCD), post-traumatic stress disorder (PTSD), drug addiction, or alcoholism. Drugs, as well as psychotherapy, behavior modification, or educational programs, are used to treat these diseases.

The treatment of neurosis involves the use of antianxiety drugs, also known as anxiolytic agents or minor tranquilizers. The term **minor tranquilizer** is somewhat of a misnomer in that it carries the connotation that this class of drugs is somehow less effective in treating symptoms than the **major tranquilizers** (used to treat psychosis), or that the minor tranquilizers are only major tranquilizers given at a lower dose. In fact, minor tranquilizers are completely unrelated chemically to major tranquilizers. They are extremely effective drugs of great importance with specific therapeutic action in treating neurosis.

Tranquilizers (anxiolytics). The benzodiazepines are by far the most commonly prescribed drugs for the treatment of anxiety and neurosis. They bind to several different types of receptor sites in the brain to provide sedation. They affect thought processes, they affect emotional behavior by their action in the limbic area of the brain, and they also decrease the muscle tension that comes with anxiety. All of the benzodiazepines are Schedule IV drugs.

>   alprazolam (Niravam, Xanax)
>   chlordiazepoxide (Librium, Reposans-10)
>   clonazepam (Klonopin)
>   clorazepate (Tranxene)
>   diazepam (Valium)
>   halazepam (Paxipam)
>   lorazepam (Ativan)
>   oxazepam (Serax)

Frequently prescribed antidepressant drugs, whose mechanisms of action vary, include:

>   buspirone (BuSpar)
>   doxepin (Sinequan)
>   escitalopram (Lexapro)
>   hydroxyzine (Atarax, Atarax 100, Vistaril)

meprobamate (Equanil, Miltown)
paroxetine (Paxil)
prochlorperazine (Compazine)
sertraline (Zoloft)
venlafaxine (Effexor)

Drugs used to treat psychosis. The symptoms of psychosis include a loss of touch with reality with resulting delusions, hallucinations, inappropriate mood, and bizarre behaviors. Psychotic symptomatology may be based in part on an overactivity of the neurotransmitter dopamine in the brain either from overproduction of dopamine or from hypersensitivity of dopamine receptors.

The treatment of psychosis involves the use of antipsychotic drugs, which are also known as major tranquilizers or neuroleptics. These drugs block dopamine receptors in many areas of the brain including the limbic system, which controls emotions. Antipsychotic drugs decrease psychotic symptoms of hostility, agitation, and paranoia without causing confusion or sedation. Unlike some antianxiety drugs, none of the antipsychotic drugs are addictive; they are not scheduled drugs or controlled substances.

Phenothiazine drugs used to treat psychosis include:

chlorpromazine (Thorazine)
fluphenazine (Permitil, Prolixin)
mesoridazine (Serentil)
perphenazine (Trilafon)
prochlorperazine (Compazine)
promazine (Sparine)
thioridazine (Mellaril)
trifluoperazine (Stelazine)

Spotlight on

Curve Balls

by Mary Ann and Elizabeth D'Onofrio

For the medical transcriptionist, the differences between general medical and psychiatric reports are more than mind over body. Psychiatry presents unique challenges requiring formats and knowledge not demanded by the other specialties. It is true that each specialty has its own unique tests, but psychiatry, and especially psychology, demands that the results be displayed in specific format. In addition, the content of many psychiatric reports is dotted with people and place names common to American culture, past and present.

General medical transcriptionists are ever so familiar with the ubiquitous laboratory data section of the discharge summary wherein multiple tests with their results are described by the physician dictator. These results, at least, can be transcribed in a narrative format. However, the transcriptionist who transcribes psychological evaluations must, for the most part, detail the results of the client/patient's tests in tabular form. Since each of these tests has its own unique set of parameters, varying at times in wording from psychologist to psychologist, the process of setting up the test results is tedious and laborious. A time-saving device for transcriptionists using word processors is the use of templates for this repetitive display of test data.

The unique demands of psychiatric transcription encompass challenges beyond those of format. The challenge goes so far as to leave the vocabulary of medicine altogether and enter the world of popular culture.

This is especially true in the area of chemical dependency. All medical transcriptionists are challenged to spell medications accurately, the psychiatric transcriptionist included. Transcriptionists in the field of cardiology are expected to know the correct spellings of such drugs as mexiletine and Streptase. Psychiatric transcriptionists, in turn, must know how to spell desipramine and Prozac; however, they may also be expected to spell *whippets*, *tooies*, or *sinsemilla*. It is common for psychiatrists and psychologists to include in their dictations vernacular renderings of the illicit drugs used by certain patients.

The impact of popular culture is also markedly apparent when one transcribes reports about adolescent patients. The environment in which patients live has direct influence on their personal development. And for the adolescent patient of today, the influences come predominantly from music, television, and video games. Transcriptionists working on reports in adolescent psychiatry, without children or grandchildren around to keep them "hip," would do well to have a television guide and the phone number of a local record store on hand.

In general medicine, the transcriptionist must know that when internists dictate "I and E okay," they mean "inspiration

Other antipsychotic drugs frequently prescribed include:

carbamazepine (Tegretol)
clonazepam (Klonopin)
clozapine (Clozaril)
fluoxetine (Prozac)
haloperidol (Haldol)
risperidone (Risperdal)
thiothixene (Navane)

Drugs for attention deficit disorder (ADD).

Drugs used to treat ADD include amphetamines and other related CNS-stimulating drugs. They have a paradoxical reverse effect in that they do not overstimulate but actually reduce impulsive behavior and lengthen the attention span.

Amphetamines used to treat ADD/ADHD are classified as Schedule II drugs. They have the highest potential for abuse and addiction of any drugs used medically.

amphetamine and dextroamphetamine (Adderall)
atomoxetine (Strattera)
dexmethylphenidate (Focalin)
dextroamphetamine (Dexedrine,
    Dexedrine Spansules, Dextrostat)
fluoxetine (Prozac, Prozac Weekly)
methamphetamine (Desoxyn)
methylphenidate (Concerta, Metadate CD,
    Metadate ER, Methylin, Ritalin, Ritalin-SR)

and expiration, satisfactory," *not* "INEOK." The psychiatric transcriptionist, however, may encounter a physician dictating that the patient's favorite rock group is "In Excess," which is correctly spelled "INXS." The correct spelling of a rock group's name may seem frivolous, but there is a great difference between "The patient claims to listen to simple minds, and in excess, every day," and "The patient claims to listen to Simple Minds and INXS every day." Rock groups are notorious for inventing unique spellings for their names, but even common names can require "expert" verification for accuracy. Paula is a common name, but when slurred by the dictator, the question of gender needs to be clarified. Such was the case when the music therapist spoke of singer Paula Abdul.

Video games, too, find their way into psychiatric transcription. Only the pop-culturally aware transcriptionist will know to supply the almost silent initial "n" in "Nintendo." Even older toys like "fooseball" can present a spelling challenge. The psychiatric transcriptionist may do well to keep the phone number of a local toy store on file, too.

Child psychology provides another challenge. One projective attitude test, the so-called "magician question," requires a child to imagine himself as a magician capable of turning family members into animals; the animals he designates reveal a lot about how he perceives his family. Exposed to the multimedia environment of today, children are very sophisticated in their knowledge of unusual animals. Suddenly the medical transcriptionist becomes a zoological transcriptionist. Exotic names we encountered in dictation recently included cockatiel, peccary, and lemur. A quality thesaurus on the bookshelf provides accurate spellings.

Maps are also an excellent resource to have on hand—old as well as current. Invariably, patients were born in cities other than the city of treatment. A map or place name atlas will give the transcriptionist, in general medicine or psychiatry, accurate spellings. Psychiatric transcriptionists may find that maps of Vietnam and Southeast Asia are especially helpful when veterans name the places where they have served.

Accurate medical reports are not only the goal of the medical transcriptionist, they are key to success in the field. The correct spellings of medications, operations, and instruments, to name a few, are of paramount importance to the verity of the legal document that is the medical report. In psychiatry and psychology, however, the pool of terminology floods over the borders of the merely medical and encompasses words and experiences from all walks of life. The challenge to the psychiatric transcriptionist is to maintain the field's high standards of accuracy in form and content by hitting the "curve balls" as well as the straight pitches.

Source: *Perspectives on the Medical Transcription Profession*

TRANSCRIPTION**TIPS**

1. The abbreviation *SAD* (seasonal affective disorder) should not be confused with the emotion of sadness.

2. Do not confuse *allusion* (an indirect reference) and *illusion* (an unreal or misleading image or perception).

   The patient made frequent *allusions* to childhood molestation by her father.
   He made *allusion* to a history of some kind of tropical disease.
   The patient was suffering from the *illusion* that there were insects crawling all over him.
   The patient suffered from *illusions* of being weightless and transparent.

3. Many words in this medical specialty begin with a silent *p*: psychiatry, psychiatrist, psychology, psychologist, psychoanalysis, psychogenic, psychomotor, psychoneurosis.

4. Transcribe the slang term *psych* as either *psychiatric* (adjective) or *psychiatry* (noun), selecting the meaning that is appropriate to the context of the report.

5. A common phrase in psychiatry is "the patient is oriented in three spheres," meaning the patient is oriented to time, person and place. This is the same as "oriented x3," which is pronounced "oriented times three."

6. The chief complaint in a psychiatric history is often quoted in the first person.

   Chief Complaint: "I'm here because I can't stop crying."

7. The antidepressant drug *Asendin* allows patients to *ascend* from the depths of depression; note, however, that the spelling of *Asendin* does not include the *c* in *ascend*.

8. Notice the difference in pronunciation between the following pairs of terms:

   psy **chi** a try   psy chi **at** ric
   psy **chol** o gy   psy cho **log** i cal

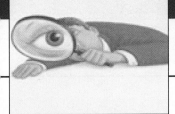

Proofreading Skills

Instructions: In the paragraphs below, circle the errors. Identify misspelled and missing medical and English words and punctuation errors, and write the correct words and punctuation in the numbered spaces opposite the text.

1 DISCHARGE SUMMARY	1 _____
2	2 _____
3 This intervenous drug user has a past psychiatric	3 _intravenous_____
4 history of illusions of grandeur, the history of which is	4 _____
5 well detailed from past admissions. He seemed	5 _____
6 cooperative but with a degree of suspiciousness which	6 _____
7 appeared to underlie all his behaviour.	7 _____
8	8 _____
9 He denied the use of Illicit Drugs but did admit to	9 _____
10 smoking four packs of cigarettes daily. He has been on	10 _____
11 his perscription anti-anxiety medication, Xanax, and	11 _____
12 reports that her symptoms have greatly improved.	12 _____
13	13 _____
14 On admission the patient exhibited the classic signs of	14 _____
15 depression: feelings of hopelessness helplessness and	15 _____
16 worthlessness. He also complained of irritability and	16 _____
17 easy fatigability. The patient was neatly groomed but	17 _____
18 exhibited a blank, empty stare and masklike facies. It	18 _____
19 was not unusual to expect that this schizophrenic	19 _____
20 patient, given his diagnosis, would exhibit bizarre	20 _____
21 behavior.	21 _____
22	22 _____
23 During the hospitalization, the patient's effect became	23 _____
24 more appropriate, although he still had some loose	24 _____
25 associations noted on mental status examination shortly	25 _____
26 preceding discharge. Today, for the first time, th patient	26 _____
27 demonstrated some insight by admitting that his beleifs	27 _____
28 may be delusional in nature, although his overall	28 _____
29 judgment remains questionable. He is discharged to be	29 _____
30 followed up in the office on Monday.	30 _____
31	31 _____
32 DIAGNOSIS	32 _____
33 Access I: Paranoia, chronic, severe, manifested by	33 _____
34 persistent fixed allusions.	34 _____

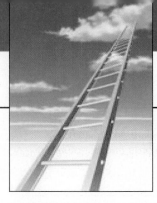

SkillsChallenge

Medical Terminology Matching Exercise

Instructions: Match the definitions in Column A with their terms in Column B.

Column A

1. ___ fear of particular objects or circumstances
2. ___ cycles of binge eating and vomiting
3. ___ inner feelings as expressed by facial features and voice
4. ___ M.D. with additional training in mental disorders
5. ___ feelings of anxiety and fear
6. ___ persistent idea that invades thought processes
7. ___ loss of touch with reality
8. ___ uncontrollable repetitious act
9. ___ also known as bipolar disorder because of mood swings between opposite poles
10. ___ usually has Ph.D in psychology

Column B

A. psychiatrist
B. manic-depressive
C. bulimia
D. obsession
E. psychologist
F. compulsion
G. affect
H. psychosis
I. neurosis
J. phobia

Abbreviations Exercise

Instructions: Define the following psychiatric abbreviations. Then memorize both abbreviations and definitions to increase your speed and accuracy in transcribing psychiatric dictation.

ADD _____

ADHD _____

CNS _____

DSM-IV _____

OCD _____

PTSD _____

Adjectives Exercise

Adjectives are formed from nouns by adding adjectival suffixes such as *-ac, -al, -ar, -ary, -eal, -ed, -ent, -iac, -ial, -ic, -ical, -ive, -lar, -oid, -ous, -tic,* and *-tous.* In addition, some adjectives have a different form entirely from the noun, which may be either Latin or Greek in origin.

Instructions: Test your knowledge of adjectives by writing the adjectival forms of the following psychiatric terms. Consult a medical dictionary to select the correct adjectival ending as necessary.

1. neurosis _____
2. psychosis _____
3. psychiatry _____
4. mania _____
5. compulsion _____
6. apathy _____
7. claustrophobia _____
8. paranoia _____
9. hypochondriasis _____
10. bulimia _____
11. autism _____
12. phobia _____

Dictation Exercises

Prior to transcribing the dictations, complete these activities.

1. **Using Chapter 3, Style Guide**

   a. When are quotation marks used in a medical report? Make note of when end punctuation goes inside quotations marks and when it goes outside.

   b. What are Style Guide recommendations for handling abbreviations in headings and in the body of the report?

   c. What is an acronym? How does it differ from an abbreviation?

   d. Review the section in the Style Guide on Flagging. Methods for flagging vary from employer to employer, so ask your instructor how you should handle flagging in class.

   e. When, according to the Style Guide, do you expand brief forms?

2. **Problem Solving**

   This activity is to help you prepare ahead of time for some of the problems you'll encounter in the dictations. Some of these items may not have a definitive answer but are intended to simply get you thinking about how to handle a variety of situations that are common in transcription. If nothing else, they will help you recognize a problem when you encounter it in the dictations.

   a. The physician dictates a medication that you cannot understand. You think if you saw the name of the drug, you'd be able to recognize it. The patient has depression as well as posttraumatic stress disorder. What can you do to decipher the name of the drug?

   b. If acronyms are pronounced like words but are really abbreviations, how can you know when the sound you're hearing is an acronym instead of an actual word?

   c. You cannot tell whether the physician is saying *peripatellar* or *parapatellar*. How would you resolve this problem?

   d. The dictator indicates that the patient had surgery on the knee but slurs over the type of surgery that was performed. There are very few contextual clues to help you decipher the term. What can you do now?

3. **Preparatory Research**

   Any information requested in these questions not readily available in your textbook (including the Appendix) or required references can easily be found using Internet search engines such as Google or on-line medical dictionaries.

   a. Research the WAIS and WAIS-R on-line and become familiar with the tests and subtests.

   b. What is *dysthymia?*

   c. Research *DSM-IV* coding for psychiatric diagnoses. What are the 5 categories or axes of psychiatric diagnoses under the *DSM-IV* system?

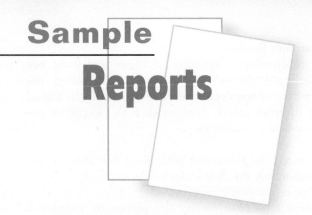

Sample Reports

Sample psychiatry reports appear on the following pages, illustrating a variety of reports. Fictional names are provided for illustration of proper format, and no resemblance to actual persons is intended. Sample transcripts were prepared according to the *AAMT Book of Style*, where possible.

Discharge Summary

ROUSCH, WANDA
Hospital #010347
Admitted: May 1, XXXX
Discharged: May 14, XXXX

CHIEF COMPLAINT
The patient was transferred from the emergency department where she was treated after deliberate suicide attempt on multiple medications.

HISTORY OF PRESENT PSYCHIATRIC ILLNESS
This was the first acute psychiatric hospitalization for this 45-year-old divorced white female, who was admitted to the locked unit on an involuntary commitment status for treatment of depression. The patient attempted suicide by taking an overdose of Asendin, lithium, Xanax, Elavil, and Zoloft. The patient was admitted with the following diagnoses: (1) Major depression with possible psychotic features. (2) Paranoid personality features. (3) Rule out subclinical dementia.

HOSPITAL COURSE
The patient was initially admitted to the locked psychiatric unit on May 1 and was started on Elavil 25 mg p.o. at bedtime and Ativan 1 mg p.o. h.s. p.r.n. insomnia. The patient received regular individual psychotherapy and various group psychotherapies that were available on the unit. After several days of stabilization in the locked psychiatric unit, she was transferred to the acute adult psychiatric unit, where psychiatric treatment continued.

The patient was seen in consultation by her family physician, as described above. Since the patient continued to complain of sleep difficulties, the dose of Elavil was increased to 75 mg, which she tolerated without any side effects. The patient was started on Zoloft on May 9, which she tolerated without side effects during her hospital stay. The dosage of Elavil was further increased to 100 mg p.o. at bedtime on May 10. The patient remained quite depressed, tearful, anxious, and insecure during her hospitalization, especially during the first 5 days. The patient was allowed to hold individual therapy sessions with her outpatient psychotherapist during the last 2-3 days of her hospitalization. Since the patient remained quite anxious, she was started on Librium 5 mg p.o. daily on May 11.

(continued)

ROUSCH, WANDA
Hospital #010347
Page 2

The patient was cooperative and compliant with all therapeutic assignments and expectations. She actively participated in individual and group therapy sessions and was able to bring up conflictual issues such as anger, dependency, and poor self-esteem, and was able to begin to deal with these issues effectively. The patient successfully completed the treatment program and was discharged on May 14.

Evaluation prior to discharge revealed that the patient did not have any acute suicidal ideation, intent, or plan. Her mood at the time of discharge was significantly less depressed, with appropriate affect. She denied any feelings of hopelessness or helplessness.

The patient was discharged with prescriptions for Eskalith CR 45 mg p.o. daily, dispense 20; Ogen 1.25 mg p.o. at bedtime, dispense 20; Synthroid 0.1 mg p.o. daily, dispense 20; Elavil 100 mg p.o. at bedtime, dispense 20; Zoloft 50 mg p.o. daily, dispense 20; Librium 5 mg p.o., dispense 20; and Bentyl 20 mg p.o., dispense 20, without refill. The patient had an appointment at the clinic the following day for outpatient followup. She was also strongly advised to obtain medical followup by her family medical doctor after discharge.

DISCHARGE DIAGNOSES
1. Major depression, severe, single episode.
2. Mixed personality disorder with schizoid, hostile-dependent, and passive-aggressive features.

MICHAEL KLIGMAN, MD

MK:hpi
D: 5/15/XXXX
T: 5/16/XXXX

Letter

June 25, XXXX

Department of Social Services
Disability Evaluation Division
1992 Golden Gate Boulevard, Suite 9
San Francisco, CA 94132

Re: RITH, RATHANY #123-45-6789

Dear Staff:

Thank you for referring to me the case of Ms. Rith for psychiatric evaluation. The patient was examined in psychiatric consultation on June 22 with the aid of an interpreter. No physical examination was given. No psychological testing was given. All past medical records provided were noted and reviewed.

HISTORY OF PRESENT ILLNESS
Ms. Rith is a 44-year-old Cambodian refugee. She lives in an apartment with her husband and three children. She describes feeling sick all the time, too weak and tired, dizzy and depressed, to do anything except "rest." Currently, she is taking a combination of five different medications under the care of two different physicians. She takes Proventil inhaler for relief of asthmalike symptoms, analgesics, decongestants, and two different forms of tricyclic antidepressants. She feels that the medications are helping her. She is not receiving any formal psychiatric treatment with or without medication.

MENTAL EXAMINATION
The patient is a clean, neatly dressed, well-groomed Asian female. She understands English and responds to questions before they are translated. There is no evidence of any ambulatory difficulties or speech impediments. There is no evidence or history of alcoholism or illicit drug use. She is oriented to time, place, persons, and events. There is no evidence of any delusion or hallucinations at the present time and no history of such in the past. There is no evidence of any paranoia such as feelings of being persecuted or plotted against. Thought content is generally well organized, coherent, and relevant, without flight of ideas or loose associations.

Depression is manifested by occasional crying periods, usually occurring every other day. There is fitful sleep. There are occasional nightmares. There is no suicidal ideation or history of any suicidal attempts. Energy level is described as poor, with description of fatigue with minimal exertion.

Memory for recent and remote events, she feels, is impaired. She cannot recall her Social Security number. She can recall her address and phone number. She can do simple arithmetic such as addition and subtraction between the sums of 1 and 10. General information and knowledge appear to be average.

It is my medical opinion that at Ms. Rith's current level of daily functioning, she has minimal difficulty in relating to others. In appearance she seems to have the ability to care for her personal needs. How much her interests, habits, and daily activities are constricted as a result of mental impairments is difficult to assess because it is my medical opinion that this represents a factitious disorder.

(continued)

Department of Social Services
Re: RITH, RATHANY
#123-45-6789
June 25, XXXX
Page 2

DIAGNOSIS

AXIS I
Factitious disorder, not otherwise specified. Rule out posttraumatic stress disorder.

AXIS II
Diagnosis deferred.

AXIS III
No known documented physical illness.

AXIS IV
Degree of psychosocial stressors cannot be evaluated.

AXIS V
Highest level of adaptive functioning cannot be evaluated because of the factitious disorder.

It is my medical opinion that Ms. Rith's impairments regarding her ability to carry out work-related activities cannot be assessed because of the factitious disorder.

Very truly yours,

KRISTINA HELFER, MD

KH:hpi

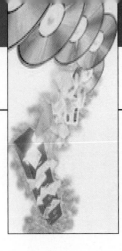

Transcription Practice

Key Words

The following terms appear in the psychiatry dictations. Before beginning the medical transcription practice for Chapter 15, look up each term below in a medical or English dictionary and write out a short definition.

CPM (continuous passive motion) machine
delusional disorder
dementia
depression
factitious disorder
hallucinations

PTSD (posttraumatic stress disorder)
WAIS (Wechsler Adult Intelligence Scale)
WAIS-R (Revised Wechsler Adult Intelligence Scale)
Wechsler Memory Scale

After completing all the readings and exercises in Chapter 15, transcribe the psychiatry dictation. Proofread your transcribed documents carefully, listening to the dictation while you read your transcripts.

Transcribe (*not* retype) the same reports again without referring to your previous transcription attempt. Initially, you may need to transcribe some reports more than twice before you can produce an error-free document. Your ultimate goal is to produce an error-free document the first time.

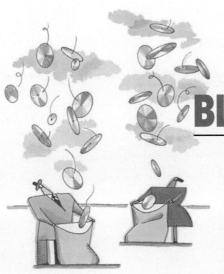

BLOOPERS

The patient said her husband took "downers" and she took "uppers" and the relationship didn't work out.

The husband brought the patient to the emergency department because she was unresponsive in bed.

The patient has visions of becoming an expert locksmith and then either having his own business or becoming a burglar. Because of his poor contact with reality, I have doubts that he could function in any of these fields.

He thinks he might have poor memory; however, he cannot remember any details.

It was our opinion that the patient could return to his usual work. The patient was not of the same opinion.

She said she had married the patient for better or for worse. However, she stated she did not expect that there would be so much worse.

Mr. Blank is a giant of a man who appears to be roughly 24 months' pregnant.

The patient says she had an ovary but it died.

The patient says he is already too screwed up to try drugs.

He states he is unable to lift anything heavier than a bottle of beer without causing pain.

Pathology

Chapter Outline

Learning Objectives

- Spell and define common pathology terms.
- Define *gross description, microscopic description, biopsy, autopsy.*
- Demonstrate knowledge of anatomical, medical, pharmacological, adjectival, and soundalike terms by accurately completing the exercises in this chapter.

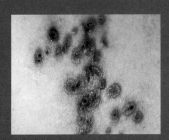
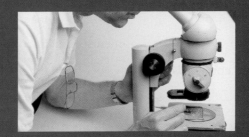
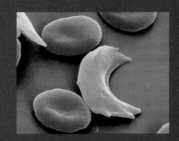

Transcribing Pathology Dictation

Pathology is the branch of medicine that studies the structural and functional changes produced in the living body by injury or disease. The practice of pathology is divided into three principal branches. *Anatomic pathology* is concerned with the gross and microscopic changes brought about in living human tissues by disease. *Clinical pathology* refers to the laboratory examination of bodily fluids and waste products such as blood, spinal fluid, urine, and feces. *Forensic pathology* involves the application of knowledge comprised by the other two branches to certain issues in both civil and criminal law. This chapter is concerned chiefly with basic practices and dictation pertaining to anatomic pathology.

When a surgical specimen or body is received by the pathologist, the gross examination is done first. Gross specimens are described by size, color, texture, and appearance. After a gross examination has been performed, the pathologist takes small samples of representative tissue (referred to as **sections**) and makes slides from the tissue for microscopic analysis. These slides are usually ready for viewing the following day. By examining these tissue sections through the microscope, the pathologist can perform a detailed cell structure analysis to determine the presence or absence of abnormalities.

In addition to analyzing **gross and microscopic specimens**, the pathologist is frequently called upon to perform a **frozen section**. The pathologist receives a tissue specimen that requires an immediate microscopic diagnosis. The pathologist quick-freezes the specimen, cuts it, stains it, analyzes it under a microscope, and renders a frozen section diagnosis. Because a specimen processed in this manner is not satisfactory for detailed cell analysis, **permanent sections** are taken as well for routine microscopic examination.

Terminology Review

adipocere A waxy substance that forms in a dead body after prolonged immersion.

anatomic pathology Concerned with the gross and microscopic changes brought about in living human tissues by disease.

benign Not malignant or recurrent.

carcinoma A malignant tumor arising from epithelial cells (Figure 16-1).

clinical pathology Refers to the laboratory examination of bodily fluids and waste products such as blood, spinal fluid, urine, and feces.

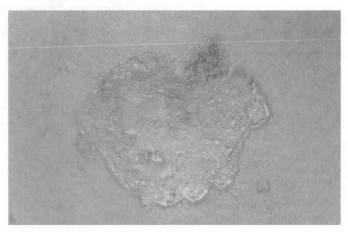

Figure 16-1
Basal Cell Carcinoma

cytology Study of cells that have been detached from a surface for microscopic study, such as a Pap smear.

diener The morgue attendant.

fixative A fluid used to arrest the process of decomposition that begins almost at once in devitalized tissue, to kill bacteria and fungi in or on the specimen, and to begin hardening the tissue to facilitate preparation for microscopic study.

forensic pathology Involves the application of clinical and anatomical pathology to certain issues in civil and criminal law.

gross description The pathologist's findings after examining a specimen with the naked eye.

H&E Hematoxylin and eosin, the most commonly used stain for microscopic analysis.

histology The division of anatomy concerned with the microscopic study of tissues.

livor mortis A purplish discoloration of the skin due to engorgement of capillaries that occurs shortly after death.

malignant Tending to become worse; having the properties of anaplasia, invasion, and metastasis. Carcinoma is an example of malignancy (Figure 16-2).

metastasis The spread of disease, especially malignant disease, to other sites in the body (Figure 16-3).

microscopic description The pathologist's findings upon examination of a specimen under the microscope.

post Short for *postmortem*.

rigor mortis Stiffening of the muscles that comes on within a few hours after death and passes off after another few hours.

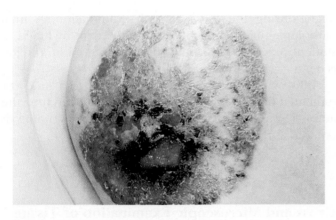

Figure 16-2
Paget Disease of the Breast: Infiltration of the Skin by Malignant Cells from an Intraductal Carcinoma

Lay and Medical Terms

belly button, navel	umbilicus
blood clot	thrombus

Medical Readings

Pathology Reports

The pathology report. The pathology report usually consists of three parts: the **gross description**, the **microscopic description**, and the **diagnosis**.

In most settings, the pathologist dictates several cases consisting of only gross specimens. The gross descriptions are transcribed and the pathologist reviews them for accuracy. When the microscopic descriptions have been dictated, the transcriptionist carefully matches each document with the appropriate patient and specimen, transcribing each microscopic description on the page of the corresponding gross description.

The tissue diagnosis should be dictated at the same time as the microscopic description. Some specimens (teeth, for example) do not require a microscopic diagnosis, and the dictation will consist only of a gross description and diagnosis.

Although some pathologists prefer to dictate their findings after the examination has taken place, many dictate as they perform the exam. A microphone rigged to a headset or lapel is remotely attached to dictation equipment, and a foot pedal controls the dictation unit. This arrangement leaves the dictator's hands free to perform

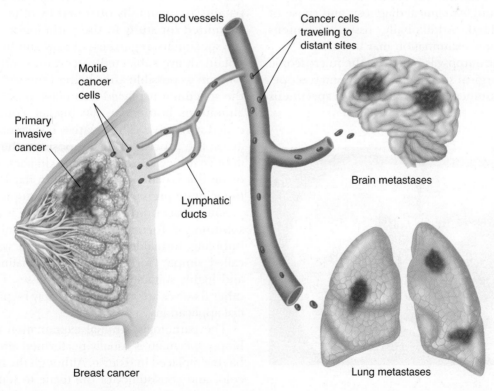

Figure 16-3
Invasion and Metastasis by Cancer Cells

the exam while simultaneously operating the dictation equipment.

The autopsy report. A gross autopsy report will typically include an external examination, an internal examination, a summary of findings, and one or more provisional diagnoses. Some pathologists also include a clinical history.

The external examination includes a systematic description of the decedent by body system, noting the presence or absence of clothing; the condition of eyes, teeth, skin, and appendages; the degree of decompositional change; the presence or absence of scars, wounds, or obvious trauma; and palpation of the usual anatomic landmarks.

The internal examination includes a detailed gross examination of all body cavities. The body is usually opened through a Y-shaped incision (literally in the shape of a *Y*), and the findings are described categorically by body system. These findings include a description of the endocrine, respiratory, cardiovascular, gastrointestinal, urogenital, and central nervous systems in their unaltered state, as well as a description of specific organs that have been removed for measurement and closer examination, including the lungs, heart, liver, spleen, pancreas, kidneys, and brain (Figure 16-4).

The results of available laboratory tests (for example, screening tests for drugs and alcohol) are often reported at the conclusion of the autopsy report, as are the provisional (tentative) and/or clinical diagnosis and cause of death, if determined. Additionally, tissue specimens taken for microscopic examination may be listed.

The microscopic autopsy is similar to the microscopic description of a surgical specimen. Using a microscope, the pathologist examines representative tissue specimens taken during the gross autopsy examination. A final pathologic diagnosis is then rendered. Not included in student practice transcripts but encountered on the job is demographic information.

Autopsy reports also include the date and time (or estimated time) of death, as well as the date and time the autopsy was performed. The pathologist's name is entered at the bottom of each report.

A Doctor's View

Gross and Microscopic Examination of Tissue

by John H. Dirckx, M.D.

The materials examined by an anatomic pathologist fall into two major classes: specimens taken from living patients, and autopsy specimens. At autopsy it is feasible to remove vital organs such as the heart and the liver in their entirety and subject them to thorough, destructive dissection. Specimens from living patients are necessarily limited in type and volume. Such specimens are either tissues or organs removed during surgical operations (Figures 16-5 and 16-6) or samples of material (biopsy specimens) removed from the living body for the purpose of examination.

Whereas the pathologist obtains and selects autopsy material for examination, specimens from the living patient are generally obtained by other physicians and submitted for study to the pathologist. Virtually all tissue specimens, regardless of how and by whom they are obtained, are subjected to certain routine procedures. As soon as possible after being removed from the body, the specimen is placed in a glass, plastic, fiberglass, or aluminum bottle, jar, or bucket containing a fluid called a **fixative**. The fixative has several purposes: to arrest the process of decomposition that begins almost at once in devitalized tissue, to kill bacteria and fungi in or on the specimen, and to begin hardening the tissue to facilitate preparation for microscopic study.

The most commonly used fixative is a 10% aqueous solution of **formalin**. Because formalin is made by bubbling formaldehyde gas through water, it is often called simply "formaldehyde." Formalin is inexpensive and highly suitable for most purposes. However, several other fixatives are available and may be preferred for special applications.

The pathologist's initial examination of a surgical or biopsy specimen is usually performed after the specimen has been placed in fixative. Although the fixative alters the color and consistency of the tissue to some extent, gross pathologic features can still generally be recognized. Occasionally specimens are brought directly from the

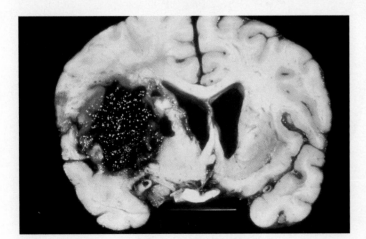

Figure 16-4
Cross Section of Brain Showing Cerebrovascular Accident (CVA)

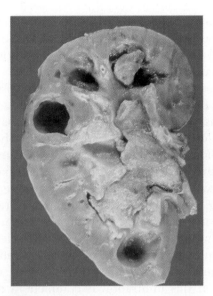

Figure 16-5
Sectioned Kidney with Calculi

operating room to the pathologist without being placed in preservative or fixative.

The pathologist performs the examination at a cutting board, which protects the top of the workbench from knife cuts and from the chemical action of fixatives. The specimens are handled with rubber gloves or with forceps, soaking up excess fluid with paper towels or other absorbent materials. Scalpels, razor blades, and scissors are used to open specimens for further examination and to trim them to the proper size for processing. One dimension, at least, of the trimmed specimen must be no more than 3-4 mm to allow penetration of processing chemicals. The trimmed pieces of tissue are placed in small flat round or oblong cassettes of perforated metal or plastic with lids of the same material, in which they will remain during the first stages of processing.

The pathologist dictates the findings during or immediately after the gross inspection and cutting of surgical specimens.

Identification of the specimen. The dictation always begins with basic identifying data: the patient's name as shown on the label of the container and on the laboratory requisition accompanying the specimen, and a general indication of what material has been submitted.

At every step in the handling of a specimen, care is taken to ensure that it is correctly identified. The container in which it is placed by the pathologist, surgeon, or operating room technician is labeled with the patient's name, the nature of the specimen, and often the date, the name of the person obtaining the specimen, and other information. Alternatively, a serial number or accession number may be assigned to the specimen container and the pertinent data kept in a register.

If only one specimen is taken during an operation, as in an appendectomy, it may be unnecessary to identify it other than by the patient's name. When anatomically indistinguishable specimens are submitted, such as abdominal lymph nodes taken from several areas and possibly containing metastatic malignancy, they must be kept carefully separated and distinguished as to their origins.

In removing a specimen, the surgeon may cut it to a certain shape to indicate its origin or its orientation in the patient's body. Orientation may also be indicated by placement of a suture (**surgical stitch**) at a certain place in the specimen, such as at the uppermost point of a tumor excised from the skin. In cutting autopsy specimens from paired organs such as the lungs and the kidneys, the pathologist may indicate by the shape of the specimen which side it came from—for example, triangular for left, square for right.

After identifying the specimen, the pathologist may include clinical information (patient's medical history) in dictation if this is available; often it is entered on the requisition.

Dimensions. The size of each specimen as submitted is usually determined and recorded in three planes in metric units (cm or mm). Solid organs or tumors may be weighed, if practicable, and the weight recorded in grams (g). The volume of any contained fluid (as in a cystic cavity) may be measured or (more often) estimated, and recorded in milliliters (mL) or cubic centimeters (cc).

Gross description. The pathologist then describes the physical features of the specimen, with particular attention to any abnormalities such as swelling, hemorrhage, scarring, or tumor (Figure 16-7). The description typically includes mention of the color, texture, and consistency of both the exterior and the cut surfaces of the specimen. Any well-defined abnormality (nodule, cyst, ulcer, perforation, scar, pigmentation) is measured as precisely as possible. Not only the exact size and location of any tumor, but also its relation to the margins of the surgical

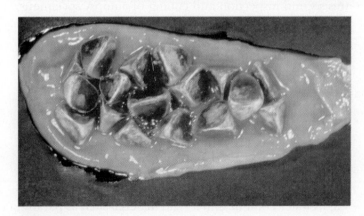

Figure 16-6
Gallbladder with Gallstones

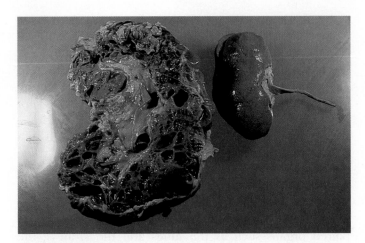

Figure 16-7
A Polycystic Kidney (on the left) **Compared to a Normal Kidney** (on the right)

specimen, must be carefully determined to document the adequacy of removal.

Microscopic examination of certain kinds of surgical specimens is routinely omitted unless the pathologist's gross examination shows abnormalities needing further study. Surgically removed tissues that are not usually sectioned for microscopic study include hernia sacs, blood clots, varicose veins, healthy bone (e.g., a section of rib removed for access to thoracic organs), and teeth. If microscopic examination will not be done, the pathologist dictates a diagnostic impression at the conclusion of the report on gross findings.

Because the tissue specimens taken by the pathologist in the autopsy room are generally too large to be handed over directly to a histology technician for preparation of microscope slides, these specimens are subjected to further examination and selective cutting in the pathology laboratory, just as with surgical specimens. Ordinarily, however, the pathologist does not dictate a report after this second inspection and cutting of autopsy specimens, since gross findings are included in the report of the autopsy.

The histopathology laboratory and the microscopic examination of tissue. The preparation of microscope slides from a gross tissue specimen is a complex and exacting process consisting of many steps, some of which are performed by automatic machinery.

The process actually begins when the specimen is placed in fixative. The fixative arrests decomposition and hardens tissue. Before the tissue can be cut into transparent sections, it is necessary to make it still harder by replacing its water content with a rigid material such as paraffin or cellulose. (Bone, however, is too hard for sectioning. A specimen containing bone must be decalcified with either

dilute acid, an ion exchange resin, or a chelating agent, or by electrolysis before it can be processed. The same is true of teeth and soft tissue specimens such as sclerotic arteries and scar tissue containing calcium.)

When the paraffin method is used, the tissue specimen is first dehydrated by immersion in a graded series of solutions of an organic solvent such as acetone, Cellosolve, ethyl alcohol, or isopropyl alcohol, which replaces the water. The dehydrated tissue is then immersed in a clearing agent such as xylene (xylol), benzene, cedarwood oil, or chloroform, which replaces the dehydrating agent and renders the tissue transparent. Certain agents (dioxane, tetrahydrofuran) can serve as both dehydrating and clearing agents. After clearing, the tissue is transferred to a bath of melted paraffin, which replaces the clearing agent and infiltrates the tissue spaces. When this infiltration is complete, a technician removes the specimen from the paraffin bath with warmed forceps and embeds it in a cube-shaped mold containing fresh melted paraffin.

When the mold has cooled, the result is a block of paraffin inside which the tissue is embedded with all its water replaced, and its empty spaces filled, by paraffin. This paraffin block is then trimmed to appropriate dimensions and cut on a microtome, a precision instrument on the order of an electric meat slicer, which makes transparent slices that are only about 5 micrometers (0.005 mm) thick. For technical reasons, sections are usually made by cutting across the broadest flat surface of the tissue specimen, unless the pathologist has given special instructions for an edge cut or **cross section**. Usually only one or two sections from each paraffin block are chosen to be made into slides. Sometimes **serial sections** (for example, every tenth or twentieth slice) are taken so as to provide the pathologist with a three-dimensional concept of a tissue or lesion.

Immediately after cutting, the paraffin sections are floated on a bath of warm water, which helps to smooth out wrinkles and curled edges. Each section is affixed to a separate microscope slide (a thin strip of clear glass about 1 x 3 inches) by means of a film of albumin solution or other suitable adhesive. The slides are identified with labels bearing names or numbers matching those of the containers in which the gross specimens were submitted.

Substances other than paraffin are sometimes used to infiltrate and embed tissue for sectioning. With Carbowax, which is water-soluble, the dehydration and clearing steps can be omitted. However, obtaining satisfactory sections with Carbowax demands a high degree of technical skill. Celloidin is a suspension of a cellulose derivative in a volatile solvent. Because infiltration and embedding with celloidin do not require heat, there is less distortion of tissue than with the paraffin and Carbowax methods. However, celloidin takes much more time; as much as a month may elapse between fixation and sectioning. Commercially available embedding media besides Carbowax include Epon, Paraplast, and Parlodion.

Microscopic examination of the slide at this stage would yield little information, because all of the tissue spaces are filled with the infiltrating medium. This must be removed and replaced with water or some other suitable fluid by a reversal of the procedures used in making the block. Once the infiltrating agent has been removed and the tissue section rehydrated, the slide is immersed in one or more coloring solutions called **stains**. These impart a more or less intense coloration to the tissues, which greatly facilitates microscopic examination.

Seldom is only a single color applied. Different stains have affinities for different components of tissue, depending on their chemical properties. Hence it is usual to apply at least two contrasting colors. The use of standard combinations of stains enables the pathologist to recognize normal and abnormal microscopic features of tissue consistently and confidently.

In practice, staining usually involves a number of steps besides immersion of the prepared slide in a coloring agent. First a **mordant** may be applied to render the tissue chemically more receptive to staining. Many fixatives have mordant properties. After the first stain has been applied, the slide is immersed in or washed with a **decolorizer**, which removes stain from all parts of the tissue to which it has not become chemically bound. The slide is then treated with a **counterstain** of a contrasting color, which is taken up by tissues decolorized in the preceding step. A **polychrome stain** is a mixture of two or more coloring agents in one solution. With a polychrome stain, differential staining of tissue components takes place even though the tissue is exposed to all of the coloring agents simultaneously. A **metachromatic stain** is one that changes color on becoming chemically bound to certain tissues.

By far the most commonly used combination of stains for routine histopathology work is **hematoxylin and eosin (H&E)**. Hematoxylin is a deep blue stain which imparts various shades of blue and purple to cell nuclei and other tissue components of slightly acidic nature. Eosin stains most of the other components pink to red. Many special stains and techniques are available to bring out certain features (nerve tissue, reticular fibers, lipid material, pathogenic microorganisms) that are not shown by routine stains. In submitting a tissue block to the histology technician, the pathologist may write instructions regarding the use of special stains. Some staining operations can be done by automatic machinery, but often part or all of the staining process is performed manually. Slides are placed vertically in tall narrow glass

Forensic *Transcription*

Forensic transcription is a possibility that most medical transcriptionists have never considered. Some transcriptionists who have considered it tell me that they are too squeamish to explore it further. And it is true—shotgun wounds and decapitations are not for the fainthearted. But for those who are steady of hand and strong of stomach, forensic medicine provides a window on the state of science.

Many transcriptionists have experience with clinical pathology, dermatopathology, and hospital autopsies. These areas and other experience with laboratory medicine provide excellent building blocks from which to launch a career in forensic transcription. There are, however, several important differences between the hospital autopsy and the forensic autopsy. These differences directly affect the type of transcription challenges you will encounter.

Most frequently, the cause of death is already known (or at least suspected) in the hospital autopsy. The hospital pathologist is attempting to document the progress and extent of that disease process, the effects of any therapy, and uncover any underlying disease process that may have played a part in the death of the patient.

The forensic pathologist is, as mandated by law, attempting to determine the true and accurate cause of death. Additionally, it falls to the forensic pathologist to correctly identify the decedent, and to determine the time and manner of death and whether the death was a natural death, an accident, a suicide, or a homicide. He or she may well have to testify to the veracity of findings in a court of law. Thus, forensic autopsies are frequently much more complex than are hospital autopsies.

What are some skills and traits that make for a successful forensic transcriptionist? Here are a few:

- Familiarity with laboratory medicine.
- Strong science background, preferably in anatomy, physiology, and chemistry.
- A sense of precision and detail, as many measurements are involved.
- A genuine sense of inquiry and interest in related disciplines such as ballistics, toxicology, accident reconstruction, police science, and so on.
- A willingness to tolerate variety—no two cases are ever the same.

Some avenues into forensic transcription are the civil service, coroner/medical examiners' offices, hospital pathology departments, and private autopsy services.

Sidney K. Moormeister, Ph.D.
Perspectives on the Medical Transcription Profession

containers called Coplin jars, which are filled with stain or other solutions.

After staining and drying, the tissue section on the slide is ordinarily protected with a cover slip, a very thin sheet of glass about 7/8 of an inch square. A film of balsam or other mounting medium is first placed over the tissue section, and the cover slip is gently dropped into place. The balsam eventually hardens around the edges, but under the cover slip it remains fluid indefinitely, preserving the section in a clear, homogeneous, refractile medium. Mounting media in common use are Apathy medium, (Canada) balsam, Clarite, and Permount.

In most laboratories, slides are available for the pathologist's examination 24-72 hours after the tissue is removed from the body. Processing is speeded and simplified by the use of automated machinery that dehydrates, clears, and infiltrates tissue during the night. The preceding day's specimens are then embedded, sectioned, and stained on the following morning.

The pathologist examines or "reads" slides with a light microscope, using various magnifications as needed. The standard magnifications are scanning power (X35-50), low power (X100), and high power (X450-500). The greater the magnification, the more the detail that can be distinguished, but the smaller the zone of tissue that can be viewed without moving the slide. After reviewing the slides, the pathologist dictates the microscopic findings and then states one or more diagnoses or diagnostic impressions.

Since gross and microscopic reports are dictated on different days, they are seldom transcribed at the same session. Ordinarily the gross report is transcribed on the top half of a standard surgical pathology form. This transcription is made available to the pathologist when the slides of the tissue are examined. The dictation of microscopic findings and diagnosis is then transcribed on the bottom half of the form, and the form is returned to the pathologist for review and signature.

Diagnostic and Surgical Procedures

autopsy The examination of a body after death, consisting of detailed visual observations of external body tissues and internal organs, and microscopic analyses of the internal organs and structures following tissue dissection. Also called *postmortem examination, necropsy, "post."*

biopsy A sample of tissue removed from a living patient and submitted for pathologic examination.

biopsy punch A cylindrical instrument used to obtain a plug of tissue for examination.

curettage A surgical scraping.

excisional biopsy The surgical removal of an entire tumor, lesion, or diseased organ from a living patient.

fine-needle aspiration A technique used to remove cells by suction from certain structures such as the prostate, subcutaneous lymph nodes and other neck masses, and breast masses.

incisional biopsy Refers to the surgical removal of part of a tumor, lesion, or diseased organ for pathologic study.

needle biopsy A needle is passed through the skin directly into the organ to be studied, and an inner cutting needle slices and removes a core of tissue.

shave biopsy A thin layer of skin consisting mostly or entirely of epidermis is removed with a blade held approximately parallel to the surface.

Laboratory Procedures

electron microscopy The study of specimens with an electron microscope.

frozen section Specimen that is quick-frozen so that it can be examined under the microscope.

permanent section Prepared, stained, and fixed specimen that is ready for microscopic examination.

smear Material spread thinly over a microscopic slide.

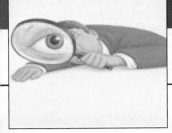

Proofreading Skills

Instructions: In the paragraphs below, circle the errors. Identify misspelled and missing medical and English words and punctuation errors, and write the correct words and punctuation in the numbered spaces opposite the text.

1 CLINICAL DATA
2 Left hilar mass, fine-needle aspirate; malignant cells
3 present consistant with poorly differentiated
4 carcinoma.
5
6 GROSS EXAMINATION
7 Four smear preprations stained with a Diff-Quik stain
8 are available for review along with sections of the cell
9 button and one slide wich contains two sections of the
10 cell button stained with H&E.
11
12 MICROSCOPIC EXAMINATION
13 The smear contains erythrocytes and a few scatered
14 benigne mononuclear cells. In the sections of the cell
15 button, fragments of a malignant neoplasm are
16 present. Malignancy is characterized by nests of highly
17 atypical cells with scant cytoplasm. The tissues are
18 moderately infiltrated wtih leukocytes. The cells nest
19 together, indicating carcinoma. In some areas the cells
20 have a slight increase in the amount of eosinophilic
21 fibrillar cytoplasm, which may represent squamous
22 differentiation, although this canot be identified with
23 certainty.

1 _____
2 _____
3 _consistent_____
4 _____
5 _____
6 _____
7 _____
8 _____
9 _____
10 _____
11 _____
12 _____
13 _____
14 _____
15 _____
16 _____
17 _____
18 _____
19 _____
20 _____
21 _____
22 _____
23 _____

Spotlight on

Transcriptionists Are People, Too

by Kathryn Stewart

Medical transcription is my profession. It's what I do, 7, 8, sometimes 11 or 12 hours a day. Having one's ears bombarded that long every day by one account of sickness after another isn't good for one's psyche unless there are also leisure-time activities to offset the strain of listening to so many different doctors with so many different accents and so many different speaking peculiarities.

One of my hobbies is writing. There are also days when I consider myself a feminist: Women Hold Up Half the Sky, and all that. Thus, when the assignment for a writing class I was taking was to go somewhere in Southern California I hadn't been before and write about it, I immediately thought of the Women's Building in Los Angeles. I'd wanted to go there for a long time but was shy enough to need an excuse. The class assignment was that excuse. Before I was able to get to L.A., however, something intervened. My trip was much shorter, though it was to a place I'd never been before.

One of my transcription clients was the pathologist of a small nearby hospital. I was in the lab to pick up the day's work when the pathologist came out of his office. "Hi, got a few minutes?" he asked. I nodded. "I'm just starting on the specimens from today's tabbies. Want to watch?" (TAB is an acronym for *therapeutic abortion*. No one could tell me why it had been corrupted to *tabby*. The medical world is not the most reverent of places. Too much sickness and death can desensitize a person.) I shrugged and followed the pathologist back into his cigar smoke-filled office.

I believe a woman's body is her own and should be free from regulation by any government, but I'm still more unsure than most of my feminist and liberal friends whether the body within the woman's body is also hers to do with as she would. Then there was the strictly physiological fact that watching specimens of any kind be cut up might make my stomach react, but my curiosity had to be satisfied.

Several containers the size and shape of large cottage cheese cartons sat on the black-tiled counter. Next to them was what looked like a small footstool (it turned out to be the dissecting bench) covered with paper towels, on top of which lay several scalpels, a pair of throwaway plastic gloves, and a metric ruler. The pathologist clipped a small mike to his tie, donned his gloves, switched on his dictating equipment, and opened the nearest container. The smell of formalin mixed with the stale cigar smoke. My stomach jumped in acknowledgment, but I knew I would stay.

"Well, this is what all that messing around comes to," he said, as he lifted the fetus from its cottage cheese carton and laid it on the table. I had seen pictures of babies in the womb before. I had seen premature babies in the hospital nursery. This specimen was similar to both, yet not quite the same as either. It was grayish-pink and mottled, and when the doctor pulled its legs or touched its head, it squeaked like a rubber toy.

He turned to me, one hand squeaking its head, and smiled. "Pink scalpel or blue?" I giggled, a high nervous sound, then asked if he could really tell what the fetus' sex was. "Of course," he said, taking it by its head and stretching its legs out. "See?" It squeaked again. I saw. "World's got too many women in it, anyway," he said, using the metric ruler to measure its length. He told me its crown-rump and crown-to-heel measurements, but I didn't remember them: My eyes were closed, and I was struggling to control the heat in my face.

"Now comes the fun part," the pathologist said, and I opened my eyes in time to watch the scalpel (not pink or blue, only shiny stainless steel) slit its way into the top of the rubber head and slide, squeaking, down and back, to the neck. I was determined to stay. He put a thumb on either side of the knife's path and opened it slightly. I could tell he was enjoying the moment of suspense, but I would stay. He pulled the sides apart slightly and looked at me. "Sex should be something done in a dark closet," he said. I turned toward the door.

"Leave it open, will you?" he called after me. "It's getting a little stuffy in here." He was chuckling as I walked away. I was thinking I should have gone to the Women's Building as I had originally intended.

Well, I thought as I pushed open the double doors and walked outside, at least I have something to write about. And maybe I can find a nice quiet ophthalmologist to replace this account.

I took a deep breath. The air smelled of a stage II alert.

Source: *Perspectives on the Medical Transcription Profession*

TRANSCRIPTION**TIPS**

1. Do not confuse the abbreviation *C&S* (culture and sensitivity) and *CNS* (central nervous system). It is preferable to spell out *C&S* in transcription.

2. Tissue specimens are often labeled as "block #1," "block #2," and so on. Do not confuse the terms for specimens with *en bloc* (pronounced "ahn block") which means "in a lump; as a whole."

   The specimen is submitted in its entirety as block #2.
   Block #1 is left common iliac node.

3. Note the proper forms of cross section (noun), cross-section (verb), and cross-sectional (adj.).

4. Do not confuse *livor* and *liver*, and do not confuse *rigor mortis* and *livor mortis*. Both are Latin terms, with *mortis* meaning *of death*. *Rigor mortis* refers to the stiffening of muscles that comes on a few hours after death. *Livor mortis* refers to the purplish discoloration of areas of the body closest to the ground.

5. All of the following terms are synonymous and interchangeable and may be transcribed as dictated.

   neutrophils
   polymorphonuclear leukocytes
   PMNs *or* polys
   segs
   segmented neutrophils

6. Avoid using slang terms in pathology reports or lists of laboratory values.

Slang	*Translate to read*
alk phos	alkaline phosphatase
bili	bilirubin
CA	carcinoma
crit	hematocrit
diff	differential
lytes	electrolytes
mets	metastases
tabby	TAB or therapeutic abortion

7. These brief forms are acceptable as dictated and need not be translated:

bands	band neutrophils
basos	basophils
blasts	very immature leukocytes
eos	eosinophils
lab	laboratory
lymphs	lymphocytes
monos	monocytes
polys	polymorphonuclear leukocytes
segs	segmented neutrophils
stabs	another name for *bands*, from the German word *Stab*, meaning *"stick, rod"*

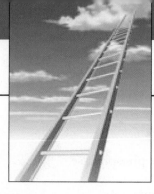

SkillsChallenge

Medical Terminology Matching Exercise

Instructions: Match the definitions in Column A with their terms in Column B.

Column A

1. ___ mass of cells misplaced during embryonic development
2. ___ material spread thinly over microscopic slide
3. ___ thickened
4. ___ malignancy still within original area of growth, not metastasized
5. ___ commonly used tissue fixative
6. ___ scraping with a sharp instrument to obtain cells for examination
7. ___ used to identify patient's body
8. ___ the cause of a disease
9. ___ container for holding tissue specimens
10. ___ open, unobstructed
11. ___ allows pathologist to make diagnosis while patient is still in the operating room
12. ___ without shape
13. ___ another name for an autopsy
14. ___ morgue attendant
15. ___ uses cylindrical instrument to obtain plug of tissue for examination
16. ___ crumbly

Column B

A. patent
B. toe tag
C. punch biopsy
D. formaldehyde
E. smear
F. curettage
G. diener
H. in situ
I. amorphous
J. etiology
K. friable
L. inspissated
M. rest
N. post
O. cassette
P. frozen section

Abbreviations Exercise

Instructions: Define the following laboratory and pathology abbreviations. Place an asterisk next to the ones that need not be expanded in medical transcripts, unless they appear in the diagnosis or impression section of a report.

1. ABGs _____
2. ACTH _____
3. AFI _____
4. ALT _____
5. ANA _____
6. AST _____
7. BMP _____
6. BNP _____
8. BUN _____
9. C&S _____
10. CBC _____
11. CEA _____
12. CPK _____
13. CSF _____
14. ELISA _____
15. ESR _____
16. FiO2 _____
17. H&E _____
18. HDL _____
19. LDH _____
20. O&P _____
21. PKU _____
22. RBCs _____
23. WBCs _____
24. wbc/hpf _____

Dictation Exercises

Prior to transcribing the dictations, complete these activities.

1. **Using Chapter 3, Style Guide**

   a. When, according to the Style Guide, do you expand brief forms and abbreviations?

   b. Should metric measurements used as adjectives be hyphenated?

   c. How are dimensions that incorporate the word *by* properly transcribed?

   d. When is it appropriate to use *x* when the word *times* is dictated?

   e. Review the list of acceptable slang and brief forms. Is *Pap* an acceptable brief form?

   f. What is the proper way to transcribe metric measurements that are less than 1 (for example, "point five centimeters").

   g. Review the Style Guide recommendations for classifications of cancer. How are Gleason scores transcribed?

   h. What does the Style Guide say about punctuating coordinate adjectives?

   i. What does the Style Guide say about numbering diagnoses?

   j. Check the rules for hyphens as they apply to the following terms: *well-differentiated adenocarcinoma* and *moderately well differentiated adenocarcinoma*.

2. **Problem Solving**

   Pathology dictation is very descriptive and colorful. Anatomical vocabulary, down to the cellular and microscopic level, is also pervasive. Find as many Internet resources as you can that offer explanations and photographs of biopsies, specimens, histology, microbiology, etc. Bookmark these sites.

3. **Preparatory Research**

   a. What is *formalin*?

   b. What is a *punch biopsy*?

   c. Define the following: *cohesive, grenz zone* (*Hint*: Look under *zone* in the dictionary.), *epidermal inclusion cyst, laminated, keratotic, lymphohistiocytic.*

   d. What is the adjectival form of *appendix*?

   e. Define *postcoital.* What is a colposcopic examination?

   f. What does the brief form *Pap* stand for?

   g. How are specimens prepared for microscopic examination?

   h. What is meant by *Cytospin* and *Nuclepore preparations*?

   i. Define the following: *adipose tissue, follicular hyperplasia, sinus histiocytosis.*

   j. What is meant by *well-differentiated adenocarcinoma*?

   k. Research the Gleason score method for staging of carcinoma.

   l. What are the plural forms of the following terms: *alveolus, lumen, bronchus, focus, nucleus, cortex, glomerulus, pelvis.*

   m. Define the following: *fibrinous exudate, columnar epithelium, disarray, vacuolated, neoplasm, malpighian body, sinusoids, interstitial tissue.*

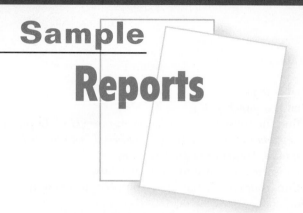

Sample Reports

Sample pathology reports appear on the following pages, illustrating a variety of reports. Fictional names are provided for illustration of proper format, and no resemblance to actual persons is intended. Sample transcripts were prepared according to the *AAMT Book of Style*, where possible.

Pathology Report

KNUDSEN, HEATHER
#122442

CLINICAL HISTORY
Thrombocytopenia.

MATERIAL SUBMITTED
Spleen.

GROSS DESCRIPTION
The specimen is labeled "spleen." Received in formalin is an 80-g spleen measuring 10.0 x 7.0 x 2.5 cm. The external capsule appears discretely lobulated and wrinkled purple-gray without evidence of lacerations or discolorations. A small amount of attached fatty tissue is present throughout the hilum. Upon sectioning the parenchyma appears glistening dark red, with pinpoint bulging follicles and unremarkable trabecular architecture. No areas suggestive of infarction or hemorrhage are grossly noted. Representative sections are submitted in four cassettes (A-D).

d&t: 11/05/XXXX

MICROSCOPIC EXAMINATION
Sections from the spleen reveal somewhat attenuated white pulp regions with only a rare small germinal center found. The sinuses are slightly congested with slight infiltration of neutrophils. Occasional plasma cells are also found. Small collections of 2 and 3 foamy histiocytes are found in some areas. A rare megakaryocyte is also present. There is no evidence of capsular fibrosis, granuloma formation, or malignancy in the tissue submitted.

DIAGNOSES
1. Spleen: Benign splenic tissue demonstrating mild sinus congestion together with small aggregates of foamy histiocytes.
2. No evidence of malignancy.

MICHELLE PANTZIRIS, MD

MP:hpi
d&t: 11/06/XXXX

KUENTZEL, ERIK
#060109
Expired: 11/23/XXXX

EXTERNAL EXAMINATION

The body is that of an adult white male. The body has been embalmed. The head is normocephalic. There is gray hair distributed over the scalp. The ears are without lesion. The nose is without lesion. The eyes have been capped. The mouth has been sealed. At the right base of the neck there is a sutured embalming wound. The chest is symmetric and stable. The abdomen is rounded. There is an old healed surgical wound between the umbilicus and the pubis in the midline. The scar expands as wide as 8 cm and is associated with a ventral hernia that measures approximately 15 cm x 12 cm x 8 cm. The upper extremities are without lesion. There is a yellow metal ring present on the fourth finger of the left hand. The lower extremities are well formed. The back is without lesion. The external genitalia are adult male. The penis is uncircumcised. The testicles are descended into the scrotum and are without masses. Along the left hip there is a 25 cm in length, recently healed surgical wound.

INTERNAL EXAMINATION

The body is opened by the usual Y-shaped incision, revealing approximately 5 cm of subcutaneous fat present at the level of the umbilicus. The ventral hernia sac is filled with yellow, clear, low-viscosity fluid. The walls of the hernia sac are shiny and trabeculated. The pleural spaces are without abnormal accumulations of fluid. Fibrous adhesions are not present. The peritoneal cavity is smooth and glistening. There are no abnormal accumulations of fluid. No significant fibrous adhesions are observed.

RESPIRATORY SYSTEM

The larynx is palpated in situ and is without lesion. The trachea is patent and without lesion. The major bronchi are well formed. The right and left lungs are heavy. The visceral pleura is smooth and glistening. Bilaterally the posterior aspects of both lungs are congested. At the lateral base of the right lower lobe there is a 3 cm in diameter white metastatic tumor mass. In the right upper lobe and in the left upper and lower lobes, there are numerous small metastatic white tumors, none exceeding 0.5 cm in diameter. The carinal lymph nodes are enlarged to approximately 3 cm in diameter and filled with gray tumor. The parenchyma of the lung reveals severe panlobular and centrilobular emphysema with extensive anthracotic pigmentation.

CARDIOVASCULAR SYSTEM

The pericardium is lightly adhesed to the surface of the heart. The pericardial space is obliterated by fibrinous adhesions. These are easily broken. The heart appears slightly enlarged, with dominance of the left ventricle. The myocardium is red and meaty. No evidence of scarring or past infarction is observed. The right atrium is well formed. The tricuspid valve is well formed and without lesion. The sinus and conus of the right ventricle are well formed. The right ventricular free wall measures up to 0.7 cm in thickness. The pulmonary valve is well formed. The pulmonary arteries fail to reveal blood clots. There are four pulmonary veins which return to the left atrium. The mitral valve is well formed. The left ventricle is well formed. The left ventricular free wall measures up to 2.1 cm in thickness. The aortic valve is without lesion. The coronary arteries are distributed over the heart in the usual fashion, and there is no significant atherosclerosis observed. The aorta runs the usual course and reveals only mild atherosclerosis. The great veins are without blood clot or other abnormality. The lymph nodes, right and left of the aorta, from the pelvic floor to the diaphragm, are markedly enlarged, up to 5 cm in diameter, white, and filled with tumor.

GASTROINTESTINAL SYSTEM

The esophagus runs the usual course and is without lesion. The stomach is well formed. The small intestine and large intestine are well formed. The appendix is present and without lesion.

(continued)

KUENTZEL, ERIK
#060109
Expired: 11/23/XXXX
Page 2

LIVER

The liver is of the expected size, shape, and position. Glisson capsule is smooth and glistening. The hepatic parenchyma is slightly buttery in character but shows no evidence of metastatic tumor and no evidence of cirrhosis. The gallbladder is present in the usual position and contains approximately 70 mL of greenish-black viscid bile. No stones are observed. The extrahepatic biliary ducts are of the expected caliber and run the usual course.

SPLEEN

The spleen is enlarged and weighs approximately 400 g. The splenic capsule is intact. The splenic parenchyma is red, meaty, and uniform. No metastatic tumor masses are observed.

PANCREAS

The pancreas is of the expected size, shape, and position and is without specific gross abnormality.

ADRENAL GLANDS

The adrenal glands are of the expected size, shape, and position. Both the cortices and medullae are well formed.

THYROID GLAND

The thyroid gland is palpated in situ and is without lesion.

UROGENITAL SYSTEM

The kidneys are of the expected size, shape, and position. The capsules are smooth and glistening and strip with ease. The renal parenchyma is well formed. The cortex is greater than 0.5 cm in thickness. The pelves and calices and pyramids are all well formed. The ureters run the usual course and are of the usual caliber. The bladder is contracted and trabeculated. The prostate appears to be about 20 g in weight and is gray and uniform.

CENTRAL NERVOUS SYSTEM

The central nervous system is not examined in this dissection.

PROVISIONAL ANATOMIC DIAGNOSES

1. Bilateral bronchopneumonia.
2. Malignant tumor of unknown primary with metastases to:
   a. Periaortic lymph nodes.
   b. Left and right lungs.
   c. Carinal lymph nodes.
3. Past history of bladder carcinoma.
4. Myocardial hypertrophy with left ventricular thickening.
5. Splenic hypertrophy.

KENNETH WONG, MD

KW:hpi
d: 11/25/XXXX
t: 11/26/XXXX

CAMPBELL, ALEXANDER
#111313
Expired: 10/14/XXXX

GROSS DESCRIPTION

EXTERNAL EXAMINATION
The body is that of a tall, somewhat obese Caucasian male who appears his stated age of 67 years. There is a white hypopigmented horizontal lesion located in the right mid abdomen, measuring up to 4 cm in maximal length. This may represent an old well-healed surgical scar. The patient has gray-brown hair in the normal distribution. The pupils are symmetric and measure 0.5 cm bilaterally. The face and neck are cyanotic. The chest appears symmetric. The abdomen is obese and distended. The extremities are symmetric and contain no obvious ulcerations.

INTERNAL EXAMINATION
A Y-shaped incision is made in the usual fashion, opening the thoracic and abdominal cavities. The pleural cavities and the pericardium contain no obvious adhesions or effusions. The abdominal cavity contains no ascites. There are no obvious abnormalities in the locations of the thoracic and abdominal organs.

Heart: The heart weighs 560 g. The epicardial surface is smooth and unremarkable. The coronary arteries show moderate atherosclerosis mainly involving the left anterior descending artery. Cross sections through the myometrium reveal no obvious focal scarring or recent infarct.

Gastrointestinal tract: The mucosal surfaces of the esophagus, stomach, small and large intestines are smooth and unremarkable.

Liver: The liver weighs 1500 g. The serosal surface contains one small white round discoloration on the superior surface of the right lobe measuring up to 0.3 cm in maximal dimension. Sectioning through the liver parenchyma reveals a somewhat nutmeg appearance. No obvious nodules or focal lesions are seen.

Spleen: The spleen weighs 380 g. The spleen parenchyma is markedly congested. However, no obvious nodules or focal lesions are seen.

Pancreas: The pancreas is of normal size and appearance. No obvious nodules or focal lesions are seen.

Kidneys: The right and left kidneys each weigh 210 g. The cortical surfaces of both kidneys are somewhat granular. Sectioning through the parenchyma reveals no obvious nodules or focal lesions.

Pelvic organs: The bladder mucosa is smooth and unremarkable. The prostate is somewhat nodular and irregular. Sectioning through the testes reveals no obvious nodules or focal lesions.

Vascular system: The distal aorta shows moderate atherosclerosis. No obvious thrombus formation is noted.

Bone marrow: The bone marrow is red and of normal consistency. No focal lesions are seen.

Nervous system: The formalin-fixed brain without dura mater weighs 1300 g (1220 g prior to fixation, 1289 g following draining of ventricular cerebrospinal fluid). The cerebellum weighs 138 g. The dura mater over the cerebral convexity is unremarkable. The superior sagittal sinus is patent and unremarkable. The cerebral hemispheres are symmetrical and show no edema or atrophy. No convolutional abnormality is recognized. The leptomeninx is thin and translucent.

(continued)

CAMPBELL, ALEXANDER
#111313
Expired: 10/14/XXXX
Page 2

The cranial nerves show no gross abnormality. The major cerebral arteries are well preserved and show moderate to marked atherosclerosis. The calvaria and dura are unremarkable. The cerebral hemispheres are symmetric and show no obvious edema or herniation.

GROSS IMPRESSION
Moderate to marked atherosclerosis of the cerebral arteries.

MICROSCOPIC DESCRIPTION

Heart: The anterior left ventricular wall and left main coronary artery show myocardial hypertrophy, focal myocardial scarring, and moderate atherosclerosis. The anterior left ventricular wall and left anterior descending artery show myocardial hypertrophy, increased interstitial and perivascular fibrosis, and marked atherosclerosis with 80% luminal occlusion. The anterolateral left ventricular wall and left circumflex arteries show myocardial hypertrophy, perivascular fibrosis, and moderate atherosclerosis with 60% luminal occlusion. The lateral left ventricular wall, posterolateral left ventricular wall, posterior left ventricular wall, and posterior interventricular wall show myocardial hypertrophy and perivascular fibrosis. The mid-interventricular septum shows myocardial hypertrophy. The anterior interventricular septum shows myocardial hypertrophy and perivascular fibrosis. The anterior right ventricular wall and right coronary artery demonstrate mild atherosclerosis. The posterior right ventricular wall shows no significant histopathology.

Lungs: The right lung periphery shows marked congestion and edema, as do the right lung hilum, left lung periphery, and left lung hilum.

Esophagus, stomach, small and large intestines: There is autolysis present.

Liver: The liver shows centrilobular congestion.

Spleen and pancreas: The spleen shows congestion. The pancreas demonstrates autolysis.

Kidneys and adrenals: There is autolysis and occasional totally sclerosed glomeruli of the right and left kidneys and adrenals.

Bladder, prostate, right and left testes: Benign prostatic hypertrophy is present.

Aorta and bone marrow: Mild to moderate atherosclerosis is demonstrated.

Brain: Serial coronal sections of the cerebral hemispheres show symmetrical lateral ventricles which are covered by a smooth ependymal lining. The cerebral cortex and white matter are unremarkable. The corpora striata, thalami, and hippocampi reveal no gross pathology. Serial horizontal sections of the brain stem demonstrate no gross lesions. Upon serial sagittal sections, the cerebellum is unremarkable.

(continued)

CAMPBELL, ALEXANDER
#111313
Expired: 10/14/XXXX
Page 3

MAJOR PATHOLOGIC DIAGNOSES
1. Moderate to marked atherosclerosis, coronary arteries and distal abdominal aorta.
2. Cardiomegaly (560 g).
3. Marked bilateral pulmonary congestion and edema.
4. Passive congestion of liver and spleen with splenomegaly (380 g).
5. Diabetes mellitus.

CAUSE OF DEATH
Atherosclerotic heart disease.

JAMES WATT, MD

JW:hpi

d&t: 10/15/XXXX

NEEL, SUSAN ELLEN
#291863
Surgery: 9/10/XXXX

GROSS DESCRIPTION

Specimen #1 is received in the fresh state and consists of a nodular-shaped fragment of dark brown, firm, friable tissue. The received specimen measures 1.9 x 1.5 x 0.8 cm in greatest dimension. On sectioning there is noted an area that has a tannish-brown color and a firm, friable consistency. This area measures 1.2 cm in diameter. A frozen section is performed on the specimen and is submitted in entirety for histologic study and labeled "1A." Additional sections are submitted for histologic study and are labeled "1B."

Specimen #2 is received in the fresh state and consists of a segment of right colon with cecum and attached segment of terminal ileum. The segment of right colon measures 46 cm in length. The segment of terminal ileum measures 8.9 cm in length. The serosal adipose tissue is marked by irregular focal areas of surgical trauma. There is noted an obstructing napkin-ring-shaped lesion within the right colon. This lesion measures 3.9 cm in greatest dimension. It shows edges which are rolled. There is central ulceration in this lesion. This lesion is located 17.5 cm from the distal margin of resection and 30 cm from the ileocecal valve. The proximal and distal margins of resection are seen to be free of tumor. The segment of right colon, which is proximal to this obstructing lesion, is dilated. There is marked hyperemia to the mucosal surface. No polyps are seen. An irregular globular-shaped fragment of omental tissue is seen attached to the surface of the colon. The omental tissue shows focal areas of hemorrhage. There is not seen any gross area of metastatic tumor. Representative sections are submitted from the following areas for histologic study:
A) primary lesion; B) proximal margin of resection; C) distal margin of resection; D) serosal surface over the lesion; E) mesenteric lymph nodes; F) omental tissue.

FROZEN TISSUE DIAGNOSIS

Biopsy of right hepatic nodule: Metastatic adenocarcinoma.

MICROSCOPIC EXAMINATION

Specimen #1 consists of multiple sections of biopsy of a right hepatic nodule. The sections demonstrate, within the parenchyma, a metastatic focus of hyperchromic nuclei with prominent nucleoli. Atypical mitoses are seen. The majority of the tumor shows distinct gland formation. Within the malignant glandular structures, the cells show loss of orientation and polarity. There is evidence of mucin production within the malignant glandular structures. The adjacent liver parenchyma shows no evidence of any hepatitis or granulomatous disease.

Specimen #2: Multiple sections from the primary lesion within the right colon show a moderately well differentiated adenocarcinoma arising from the mucosal surface. This is moderately well differentiated adenocarcinoma which extends into the lamina propria. There is extension into the muscularis. There is minimal extension into the adenocarcinoma. Proximal and distal margins of resection are free of adenocarcinoma. Several sections from the right colon show several distinct diverticula. Sections from 17 mesenteric lymph nodes are examined histologically. One of the 17 lymph nodes is positive for metastatic adenocarcinoma. A section from omental tissue shows edema and congestion to the omental tissues. The omental tissue shows no evidence of any metastatic adenocarcinoma.

(continued)

NEEL, SUSAN ELLEN
#291863
Surgery: 9/10/XXXX
Page 2

PATHOLOGIC DIAGNOSES
1. Biopsy right hepatic dome nodule: Metastatic mucin-secreting adenocarcinoma. (56-8146, I)
2. Right colon (extended): Moderately well differentiated adenocarcinoma arising from the mucosal surface of the right colon. This is an obstructing napkin-ring-shaped, moderately well differentiated adenocarcinoma. The proximal and distal margins of resection are free of adenocarcinoma. Several diverticula are seen both proximal and distal to the adenocarcinoma. One of 17 mesenteric lymph nodes is positive for metastatic adenocarcinoma. The received omental tissue shows edema and congestion with no areas of metastatic adenocarcinoma. (67-8143, I)

HENRY GODDARD, MD

HG:hpi
d&t: 9/10/XXXX

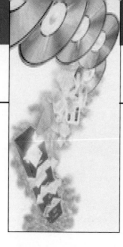

Transcription Practice

Key Words

The following terms appear in the pathology dictations. Before beginning the medical transcription practice for Chapter 16, look up each term below in a medical or English dictionary and write out a short definition.

appendix
autopsy
bladder washings
cytology
ear lesion
endocervix
epidermal inclusion cyst
frozen section
Gleason score
gangrenous ulceration
gross examination
liver biopsy

lymph nodes
microscopic examination
nevus
Nuclepore preparation
pinna lesion
prostate
punch biopsy
rosette formation
ruptured cyst
transitional cell carcinoma
TURP

After completing all the readings and exercises in Chapter 16, transcribe the pathology dictation. Proofread your transcribed documents carefully, listening to the dictation while you read your transcripts.

Transcribe (*not* retype) the same reports again without referring to your previous transcription attempt. Initially, you may need to transcribe some reports more than twice before you can produce an error-free document. Your ultimate goal is to produce an error-free document the first time.

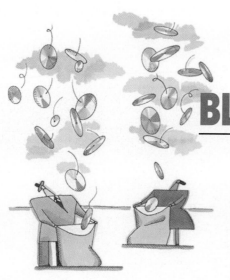

BLOOPERS

Incorrect	Correct
The tumor is attached to the mucosal surface by a broad pedestal and a tapering stock.	The tumor is attached to the mucosal surface by a broad pedicle and a tapering stalk.
Cause of death: Subarachnoid hemorrhoid due to trauma.	Cause of death: Subarachnoid hemorrhage due to trauma.
Vocal hemorrhages are grossly visible throughout both cerebral hemispheres.	Focal hemorrhages are grossly visible throughout both cerebral hemispheres.
Anasarca and widespread visceral edema indicate longstanding watery tension.	Anasarca and widespread visceral edema indicate longstanding water retention.
There is a zone of ecchymosis and crepitus overlying the left-off septal boss.	There is a zone of ecchymosis and crepitus overlying the left occipital boss.
Received informally is a mess of partially decomposed tissue with prominent vascular elephants.	Received in formalin is a mass of partially decomposed tissue with prominent vascular elements.

Radiology

Chapter Outline

Learning Objectives

- Spell and define common radiology terms.
- Define various diagnostic radiologic procedures.
- Identify and describe imaging techniques that do not involve x-rays.

- Demonstrate knowledge of anatomical and medical terms by accurately completing the exercises in this chapter.

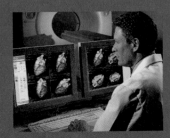
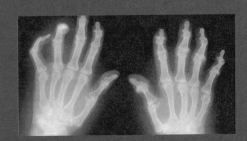
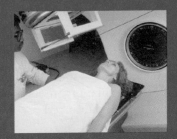

Transcribing Radiology Dictation

Radiology, known as Diagnostic Imaging, is the branch of health sciences that deals with radioactive substances and radiant energy, and with the diagnosis and treatment of disease by means of both ionizing (e.g., x-rays) and non-ionizing (e.g., ultrasound) radiations.

Anatomy in Brief

Imaging studies are used to view virtually all anatomic structures of the body. From simple x-rays to MRI to SPECT scans, nearly every bone and organ can be imaged for diagnostic purposes. Following are some commonly dictated anatomic structures.

ankle mortise The normal articulation between the talus and the distal tibia and fibula.

collateral vessels Vascular channels newly formed from existing ones to maintain the circulation of a tissue or organ whose normal blood supply has been impaired by disease or injury.

collecting system The nonexcretory portions of the kidney, which collect newly formed urine and conduct it to the ureter; the minor and major calices and the renal pelvis.

deglutition mechanism The coordinated sequence of muscular contractions in the mouth, pharynx, and esophagus involved in normal swallowing, as demonstrated in a barium swallow or upper gastrointestinal series (UGI).

duodenal bulb Onion-shaped dilatation of the duodenum immediately below its origin at the pylorus.

duodenal C-loop C-shaped loop formed by the duodenum as it courses around the head of the pancreas.

duodenal sweep The normal course of the duodenum, from the pylorus and around the head of the pancreas to the ligament of Treitz, as visualized with contrast medium in an upper GI series.

great vessels The major vascular trunks entering and leaving the heart: the superior and inferior venae cavae, the pulmonary arteries and veins, and the aorta.

origin of a vessel The commencement of a vessel as it branches off from a larger vessel.

peristaltic wave A wave of muscular contractions passing along a tubular organ, such as the intestine, by which its contents are advanced.

pole of kidney The upper or lower extremity of a kidney.

posterior sulcus The groove formed by the intersection of the diaphragm and the posterior thoracic wall, as seen in a lateral chest x-ray.

pulmonary vascular markings As seen on chest x-ray, the normal radiographic appearance of the branches of the pulmonary arteries and veins about the hila of the lungs.

subcutaneous fat line The radiographic appearance of the subcutaneous fat layer.

tail of breast A wedge-shaped mass of normal breast tissue extending toward the axilla.

takeoff of a vessel The origin of a branch from a larger vessel, as demonstrated radiographically with injected contrast medium.

tibial plateau The flattened surface at the upper end of the anterior aspect of the tibia.

Terminology Review

acoustical shadowing The inability of ultrasound to reach and delineate structures located in the "shadow" of an organ or tissue that reflects a large amount of ultrasound.

air-fluid level A line representing the level of a collection of fluid seen in profile, with air or gas above it.

air-space disease As seen on chest x-ray, disease or abnormality of lung tissue that encroaches on space normally filled by air.

blood pool The circulating blood, into which radionuclides are injected for various types of circulatory scans.

blunted costophrenic angle On chest x-ray, a costophrenic angle that is flattened or distorted by scarring or pleural fluid.

bony island Benign developmental abnormality consisting of a localized zone of increased density in a long bone.

bowel gas pattern On abdominal film, the normal radiographic appearance of gas in the intestine.

bridging osteophytes Osteophytes on adjacent vertebrae that meet and fuse, forming a "bridge" across the joint space.

consolidative process An abnormal process that increases the density of a tissue or region.

contiguous images A series of scans without intervals of unexamined tissue between them.

correlate radiographic findings clinically Interpret x-ray appearance in light of the patient's medical history and objective findings on physical examination and laboratory testing.

cut A CT section or image; a scan.

demineralization Reduction in the amount of calcium present in bone, due to disease or immobilization.

echo characteristics The frequency, intensity, and distribution of echoes produced by a structure or region on ultrasound examination.

echo pattern The ultrasonographic appearance of a structure as seen on a visual display.

effacement Abnormal flattening of the contour of a structure.

esophageal dysmotility Seen on upper GI series; abnormality in the strength or coordination of peristaltic movements in the esophagus.

extravasation of contrast Leakage of contrast medium from the structure into which it is injected through a perforation or other abnormal orifice.

filling defect A zone within a tubular structure that is not filled by injected contrast medium (usually a tumor or abnormal mass).

free air Air or gas in a body cavity where it does not belong, usually after escape from the GI tract.

gadolinium A nonradioactive metallic element that acts as a contrast agent in MRI studies by enhancing the signal of areas or tissues in which it is present. After intravenous injection it can show up narrowed areas or malformations in blood vessels, vascular tumors, and areas of hemorrhage. It can also be used to delineate joint spaces in arthrography.

gas density line A linear band of maximal radiolucency, representing or appearing to represent a narrow zone of air or gas.

gastroesophageal reflux Abnormal backflow of material from the stomach into the lower esophagus.

gated view An image obtained by a technique synchronized with motions of the heart to eliminate blurring.

high field strength scanner An MRI device using a static magnetic field of maximal intensity.

hypoaeration Abnormal reduction in the amount of air in lung tissue.

hypokinesis Abnormal reduction of mobility or motility; reduced contractile movement in one or both cardiac ventricles.

ileus Small bowel obstruction due to failure of peristalsis.

impingement Contact or pressure, generally abnormal, between two structures.

internal fixation device Any appliance placed surgically in or on a bone to stabilize a fracture during healing.

interstitial markings The radiographic appearance of lung tissue, as opposed to the appearance of air contained in the lung.

interval change Change in the radiographic appearance of a structure or lesion in the interval between two examinations.

label To render a substance radioactive by incorporating a radionuclide in it; also, to cause a tissue or organ to take up radioactive material.

loculated effusion A collection of fluid in a body cavity whose distribution is limited by adjacent normal or abnormal structures.

lucent defect An abnormal zone of decreased resistance to x-rays.

lytic (osteolytic) lesion A disease or abnormality resulting from or consisting of focal breakdown of bone, with reduction in density.

mass effect The radiographic appearance created by an abnormal mass in or adjacent to the area of study.

mass lesion Anything that occupies space within the body and is not normal tissue.

midline shift Displacement of a structure that is normally seen at or near the midline of the body, such as the pineal gland or the trachea.

opacification An increase in the density of a tissue or region, with increased resistance to x-rays.

origin of a vessel The commencement of a vessel as it branches off from a larger vessel.

orthopedic hardware Wires, pins, screws, plates, and other devices of metal or other material that are implanted in or attached to bone in the course of a surgical procedure.

partial saturation technique A magnetic resonance technique in which single excitation pulses are delivered to tissue at intervals equal to or shorter than T1.

peribronchial cuffing Thickening of bronchial walls by edema or fibrosis, as seen in asthma, emphysema, cardiac failure, and other acute and chronic respiratory and circulatory disorders.

peristaltic wave A wave of muscular contractions passing along a tubular organ (such as the intestine), by which its contents are advanced.

pleural effusion An abnormal accumulation of fluid in the pleural cavity.

probe Ultrasound transducer.

pulmonary vascular redistribution Increased prominence of upper pulmonary vessels and reduced prominence of lower pulmonary vessels at the lung hila in left ventricular failure and other disturbances of circulatory dynamics.

radiolucent Offering relatively little resistance to x-rays (by analogy with *translucent*).

radionuclide Radioactive isotope; a species of atom that spontaneously emits radioactivity.

radiopaque Resisting penetration by x-rays.

reconstitution Maintenance of flow in an artery beyond an area of narrowing or obstruction by establishment of collateral circulation.

runoff The flow of blood and contrast medium through the branches of an artery into which the medium has been injected.

sacralization Abnormal bony fusion between the fifth lumbar vertebra and the sacrum.

sensitize To introduce radioactive material into a fluid, tissue, or space for purposes of performing a radioactive scan; essentially the same as *label*. See *label*.

serial scans A series of scans made at regular intervals along one dimension of a body region.

signal intensity The strength of the signal or stream of radiofrequency energy emitted by tissue after an excitation pulse.

small bowel transit time The time required for swallowed contrast medium to pass through the small bowel and appear in the colon.

sonolucent Offering relatively little resistance to ultrasound waves (as air or fluid) and hence generating few or no echoes.

spurring Formation of one or more jagged osteophytes, as in osteoarthritis.

stacked scans Same as *contiguous images*.

strandy infiltrate A pulmonic infiltrate that appears as strands or streaks of increased density.

subcutaneous emphysema Air or gas in subcutaneous tissue.

suboptimal Not as good as might have been expected; usually referring to technical factors in an x-ray study, such as positioning, film quality, and patient cooperation.

surface coil In MRI, a simple flat coil placed on the surface of the body and used as a receiver.

tag Same as *label*.

TE (echo time) The interval between the first pulse in a spin echo examination and the appearance of the resulting echo.

technetium (Tc 99m) A synthetic radioisotope with wide applications in nuclear imaging. In a HIDA (hepatobiliary iminodiacetic acid) scan, an intravenously administered technetium compound outlines the biliary tract more precisely than is possible with conventional radiology or ultrasound. Other technetium compounds are used in scanning the scrotum to diagnose testicular torsion and in performing bone and other scans to identify local areas of inflammation such as abscesses or zones of osteomyelitis.

tenting of hemidiaphragm On chest x-ray, a distortion of the diaphragm by scarring, in which an up-pointing angular configuration (like a tent) replaces all or part of the normal curved contour of a hemidiaphragm.

tertiary contractions Aberrant contractions of the esophagus, occurring after the primary and secondary waves of normal swallowing.

T1 On MRI, the time it takes for protons to return to their orientation to a static magnetic field after an excitation pulse.

TR (repetition time) On MRI, the interval between one spin echo pulse sequence and the next.

T2 On MRI, the time it takes for protons to go out of phase after having been shifted in their orientation by an excitation pulse.

uptake Absorption or concentration of a radionuclide by an organ or tissue.

ventricular ejection fraction That portion of the total volume of a ventricle that is ejected during ventricular contraction (systole); usually expressed as a percent rather than a fraction.

volvulus Intestinal obstruction due to twisting or obstruction of the bowel.

washout phase Scintiscanning of the lungs at the conclusion of the inhalation phase of a lung scan, after an interval during which all inhaled radionuclide would be expected to have been exhaled.

Lay and Medical Terms

| x-ray | radiograph, roentgenogram, roentgenograph |

Medical Readings

A Doctor's View

Diagnostic Radiology

by John H. Dirckx, M.D.

X-rays are a form of electromagnetic radiation having a wavelength between that of gamma rays and that of ultraviolet rays. The importance of x-rays in medicine arises from their ability to penetrate most of the tissues of the human body and to expose photographic film in a manner similar to light. Like gamma rays, x-rays have potentially harmful effects on living tissue, particularly actively growing or reproducing tissue. The power of x-rays to shrink or destroy certain kinds of tumor has been put to use in therapeutic radiology. Because x-rays are also capable of inducing tumors in certain tissues, and of damaging any tissue after excessive exposure, they must be used with the greatest caution and restraint.

In diagnostic radiology, x-rays are produced in a high-voltage electron tube (Coolidge tube) with equipment that controls the intensity of the beam, its direction and shape, and the duration of emission. X-rays pass through the part of the body under study and create an image on a sheet of film that is protected from light

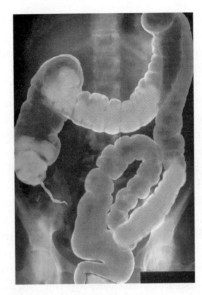

Figure 17-2
Barium Enema Exam with Enhanced Color X-ray of Colon

in a filmholder or cassette. Since no lenses are used to focus x-rays, the image is of about the same size as the subject, and correspondingly large sheets of film must be used (Figure 17-1).

X-rays can also be used with cinematographic equipment to make moving pictures of internal organs such as the heart, lungs, and digestive system. In **fluoroscopy**, a continuous stream of x-rays passing through a part of the body is made to create an image on a sensitive screen. Modern fluoroscopic equipment electronically enhances this image and projects it on a television screen so that the dose of radiation can be kept to a minimum (Figure 17-2).

The fact that x-ray images are made by rays that have passed through the subject accounts for several important differences between x-ray and conventional photography. Different tissues offer different amounts of resistance to the passage of x-rays and produce correspondingly light or dark images on film. When x-rays encounter little resistance, as in passing through a zone of gas in the bowel, they expose the film to a maximal extent. After developing, this area of the film will be dark gray or black. When x-rays are stopped, as by a bone or a metallic foreign body, the corresponding area on the film is left unexposed, and after developing appears white (translucent).

The radiologist can distinguish only four degrees of density in tissue: *metal density* (bone, gallstones, urinary calculi, metallic foreign bodies, orthopedic pins, screws, and wires); *water density* (body fluids and most soft tissues other than fat); *fat density*; and *air* or *gas density* (air in respiratory passages, gas in digestive passages, or either of these in inappropriate places). Shapes or outlines

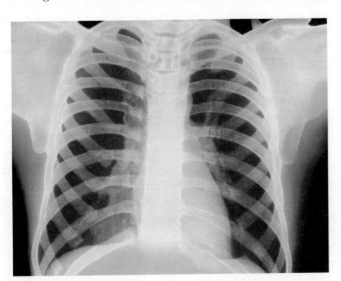

Figure 17-1
Normal Chest X-ray (with Enhanced Color) in an 11-Year-Old Boy

appear in an x-ray image only where two zones of contrasting density touch or overlap.

Radiologists can see the outline of a bone (which is of metal density) because it is silhouetted against surrounding soft tissues of water density. They can usually see a bubble of air in the stomach because it, too, is surrounded by water density tissue. But where two structures of like density (e.g., two muscles, or the spleen and pancreas) are contiguous, no silhouette is produced, and the border or interface between them is not represented in the image.

This limitation of radiography has been overcome to some extent by the use of **contrast media**, solutions of metallic salts or iodides that are opaque to x-rays. Introduced into the body, they can outline a hollow structure such as the stomach or the colon, or a tubular system such as the circulation, the bile ducts, or the urinary tract. Contrast media can be swallowed, injected, or introduced through a tube, catheter, or enema apparatus.

In light photography, a positive print is made from the film negative. In radiology, the film itself is used. For examination or "reading," the film is placed on a backlighted view box that provides bright, even illumination. Unlike a photograph, an x-ray picture gives no information about the depth or contours of the subject. An x-ray picture is literally a shadow or group of shadows. Everything is represented in an absolutely flat, two-dimensional image (Figure 17-3).

An x-ray film of a right hand, when turned over, cannot be distinguished from an x-ray of a left hand. For this reason, an x-ray picture of any part of an extremity is normally labeled *L* or *R* at the time of exposure. A metal letter

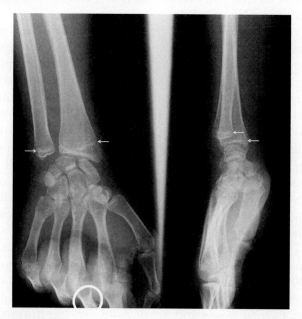

Figure 17-3
Epiphyseal Plate (arrows)

clipped to a corner of the filmholder becomes a part of the image.

When x-rays leave their source, they tend to radiate in all directions. Their direction and lateral spread can be controlled with metal housings, deflectors, and cones, but any x-ray beam (like any beam of light), no matter how narrow, will tend to spread out the further it gets from its source. This has an effect on the fidelity with which an x-ray picture reproduces the internal structures through which the rays have passed. The closer an object is to the source of x-rays (and the further from the film), the larger and less distinct it will appear. Hence for maximum clarity the zone of interest is placed as close to the x-ray film as possible. A standard chest x-ray is taken with the front of the patient's chest against the filmholder and the x-ray source behind the patient. (This is called a **postero-anterior** or **PA view**.) This technique gives maximum definition to the heart shadow while blurring and dulling the shadow of the spinal column. When the thoracic spine is the center of interest, the same part of the body is x-rayed with the patient's back nearest the filmholder (**antero-posterior** or **AP view**).

As x-rays pass through tissue, they tend to be deflected to some extent from their straight course, much as light waves are when passing through murky fluid. This phenomenon (**soft tissue scatter**) causes a certain blurring of images, which may limit the value of a study performed on an obese subject or in certain body regions. In order to reduce soft tissue scatter and the effects of lateral spreading (radiation), a **Bucky grid** may be placed between the subject and the film. This grid consists of very thin metal strips arranged in parallel with very narrow spaces between them. Rays that are still traveling comparatively straight after passing through the subject get through the grid and expose the film. Deflected (oblique) rays cannot get through to add their blurring effect to the image. During the fraction of a second that the film is being exposed, the grid is set in motion by an automatic mechanism so that the grid itself will not appear in the image.

Tomography is a technique for focusing on a particular site or level within the subject. While the subject remains stationary, the x-ray source and the filmholder rotate in an arc around the subject, in opposite directions, during exposure of the film. The point within the subject about which this rotation occurs will produce an image of maximum clarity on the film, while tissues closer to and further away from the film will be blurred or invisible. In effect, a tomogram is an x-ray of a narrow slice of the subject. Typically a series of tomograms or "cuts" are made, each focused at a different plane. Tomography is used primarily in defining and localizing abnormal masses and foreign bodies. This technique should not be confused with **computerized tomography** (CT).

Diagnostic Procedures

angiography (arteriography) The radiographic study of arteries into which radiopaque medium has been injected. Still pictures may be taken immediately after injection, or motion pictures may be made showing the flow of blood and contrast medium through vessels.

barium enema (BE) The standard radiographic examination of the large intestine by introduction of barium solution into the rectum. Indications for barium enema are unexplained lower abdominal pain, change in bowel habits, hematochezia, detection of occult blood in stool, unexplained anemia or weight loss, and history of colonic polyps or cancer.

chest x-ray (CXR) The standard PA chest film is the most frequently performed of all plain radiographic examinations. It provides diagnostic information on solid tumors and abnormal accumulations of fluid when they encroach on lung tissue, and shows the heart and great vessels sharply silhouetted against lung tissue.

cine (for cinematograph) view A moving picture of the cardiac cycle, constructed from individual frames, each of which is a composite image of one point in the cardiac cycle obtained by cardiac gating.

computed tomography (CT) scan Also **computerized axial tomography (CAT) scan.** An application of computer technology to diagnostic radiology (Figures 17-4 and 17-5). Instead of exposing a film after passing

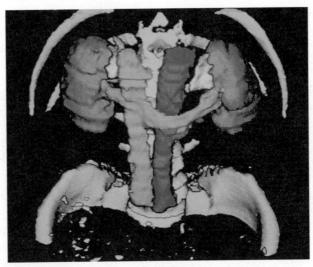

Figure 17-5
Enhanced-Color CAT Scan of Kidneys (in red)

through the subject, x-rays are detected and recorded by a scintillation counter. The x-ray tube moves around the subject on a frame called a gantry, rotating through an arc and "cutting" across one plane of the subject. A series of scintillation counters are so placed that each detects the rays passing through the subject at a different angle. (Alternatively a single counter may rotate in perfect alignment with the x-ray source.) Data on the amount of x-ray that penetrates the subject at each angle are collected from the counters, digitized, stored, and analyzed by a minicomputer programmed to generate a cross-sectional image of the subject corresponding to the plane cut by the moving x-ray beam. Contrast medium may be injected into the circulation immediately before CT scanning. IV contrast enhances the sensitivity of CT scanning of certain structures and body regions and improves the visibility of some tumors.

coned-down view A study limited to a small area by the use of a cone that narrows and "focuses" the x-ray beam.

double-contrast technique A modification of the barium enema (BE) procedure. After the standard barium enema examination has been completed, the patient expels most of the barium, and the colon is then inflated with air. The coating of barium remaining on the surface may outline masses or defects not seen during the standard examination.

first-pass view An image or set of images obtained immediately after injection of radionuclide into the circulation, when its concentration in the blood pool is at its highest.

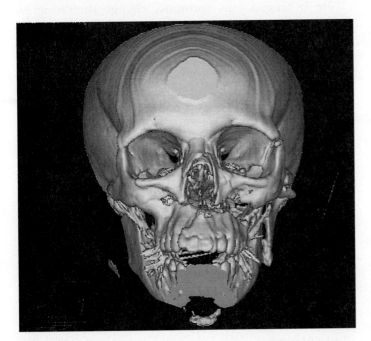

Figure 17-4
Facial Fracture, Three-dimensional Computed Tomography

frogleg view An x-ray of one or both hip joints for which the patient lies supine with thighs maximally abducted and externally rotated and knees flexed so as to bring the soles of the feet together.

full-bladder technique An ultrasonographic examination of the pelvic region performed while the subject's bladder is distended with urine. This is done to improve the recognition of the bladder outline, which cannot be distinguished adequately when the bladder is empty.

full-column barium enema Barium enema examination in which the contrast medium is injected into the colon under full pressure, by elevation of the barium reservoir to the maximum safe height.

intravenous pyelogram (IVP) The delineation of the urinary tract (renal pelves, ureters, bladder, and urethra) by means of a contrast agent injected intravenously and then excreted by the kidneys can reveal urinary obstruction, bleeding from the urinary tract, or abdominal trauma, and can identify and localize renal calculi as well as tumors or cysts both within the urinary tract and close adjacent to it. Also called *intravenous urogram (IVU)* and *excretory urogram (XU)*.

kidneys, ureters, bladder (KUB) film. A plain film often done to screen for a stone in the urinary tract.

low-dose screen film technique A radiographic technique used in mammography to provide adequate imaging with less radiation than is used in conventional techniques.

magnetic resonance imaging (MRI) A method of obtaining cross-sectional "pictures" of the human body electronically (Figure 17-6). It is based on physical principles altogether different from those used in x-ray and ultrasonography. Although the theoreti-

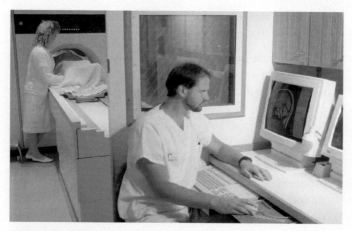

Figure 17-6
MRI Laboratory

cal basis of magnetic resonance imaging is abstruse and complex, the practical applications and terminology can be grasped without difficulty.

As in an x-ray or ultrasound examination, this diagnostic technique depends on variations in the physical properties of tissues; for example, bone vs. muscle, and normal liver vs. neoplasm. However, instead of detecting varying resistances to penetration by x-rays or sound waves, the MRI technique detects varying concentrations or densities of hydrogen atoms (ions) from one tissue to another. The attraction of a magnet for iron and iron-containing alloys is familiar to everyone. A magnet will attract, to some degree, any atoms which, like those of iron, have an unequal number of protons and neutrons in their nuclei.

The degree to which such an atom will respond to magnetic attraction depends on its nuclear structure and is expressed as a physical constant called **spin**. The simplest of all atoms is that of hydrogen, which, with but a single proton in its nucleus, possesses spin and responds to magnetic attraction. If the human body is placed in a static magnetic field of sufficient strength, its hydrogen atoms align themselves with this field like so many infinitesimal compass needles.

In a magnetic resonance examination, the patient is placed inside a static magnetic field generated by a large and powerful magnet. A pulse of radio waves (**excitation pulse**) is then used to create for a brief period of time a second magnetic field at a right angle to the static field. While this second field is present, the hydrogen ions (protons) change their orientation, and when the second field is removed, they go back to their previous orientation to the static magnetic field. In doing so they give off a stream of radiofrequency energy or "**signal**," which can be detected by a suitably placed receiving **coil**. The intensity of the signal given off by any tissue is proportional to its hydrogen concentration or proton density. Muscle emits a very high signal, bone a very low one, air almost none.

The time it takes for the protons to return to their former orientation after an **excitation pulse** is called **T1**. This **time interval**, a fraction of a second, is in direct proportion to the hydrogen ion density of the sample. Purely by way of analogy, one might think of the time it takes a roomful of people to come back to order after a sudden disturbance as a measure of the number of people in the room. When the **excitation pulse** is applied, all of the protons in the sample respond together, or in **phase**, in taking up their new orientation.

After the excitation pulse ceases, but before the protons have all come back to their former orientation with the static magnetic field, they tend to get out of phase with each other because of the interaction of many adjacent molecules. Once the protons go out of phase, a signal can no longer be detected by the **receiving coil**. The time it takes for the protons to go out of phase is called **T2**. Because both T1 and T2 vary in proportion to the proton density of the sample, they can be used by a computer to generate an image of it. However, direct measurement of T1 is not possible, since the signal is lost as soon as the protons go out of phase.

There are also technical obstacles to precise measurement of T2. Some of these obstacles have been eliminated by the **spin echo technique**, in which the excitation pulse is followed, after a brief interval, by a second and stronger pulse. This results in the production of an **echo signal** from which T2 can be determined. The time that elapses between the first pulse and the appearance of the echo is called the **echo time (TE)**.

In order to obtain **cross-sectional images**, it is necessary to modify the magnetic resonance system by adding yet a third magnetic field. This gradient magnetic field, created by a separate coil, introduces a positional element into the signals detected by the receiver. A computer decodes and analyzes the signals, generating two-dimensional cross-sectional images of the subject in much the same way that cross-sectional x-ray images are generated in computed tomography. In practice, a number of different pulses and time intervals are used in predetermined series called pulse sequences, and the resulting spin-echo signals are averaged. **Repetition time (TR)** is the interval between one pulse sequence and the next. An image generated with a pulse sequence using a relatively short TR is called a **T1-weighted image** because it reflects the T1 to a greater extent than the T2 of the specimen. An image generated with a longer TR is called a **T2-weighted image.**

mammography Radiologic evaluation of the female breast, primarily to search for or evaluate abnormal masses that may be malignant. Special equipment and techniques have been devised to limit radiation exposure and enhance the diagnostic value of the procedure.

multi-echo images On MRI, a series of spin-echo images obtained with various pulse sequences.

multiple gated acquisition (MUGA) scan A study of cardiac shape and dynamics in which a radionuclide is introduced into the circulation. Radioactive emissions from the heart are electronically monitored, stored, and analyzed, resulting in a composite scan consisting of a series of successive images all taken at the same point in the cardiac cycle.

open-mouth odontoid view A view of the odontoid process of the second cervical vertebra, for which the x-ray beam is aimed through the patient's open mouth.

plain film A radiographic study performed without contrast medium.

portable film An x-ray picture taken with movable equipment at the bedside or in the emergency department or operating room when it is not feasible to move the patient to the radiology department.

positron emission tomography (PET) A diagnostic imaging procedure that uses positron-emitting radioisotopes to assess the metabolic activity and physiologic function of organs and tissues rather than their anatomic structure; particularly useful in diagnosis of subtle cerebral and cardiac lesions (Figure 17-7).

radionuclide scans The essence of any radioactive scan procedure is the introduction into the body of a radioactive substance whose distribution in tissues, vessels, or cavities can be detected and recorded by a device that senses radiation. A variety of radioactive substances (radionuclides, isotopes) are used in scanning procedures. In some cases the choice of material is governed by the tendency of certain organs or tissues to take up (absorb, concentrate) certain elements or compounds. Radionuclides may be swallowed, inhaled, or injected into a body cavity or into the circulation. Scanning may be performed immediately after the material is administered (as in studies of blood flow) or after an interval (as when absorption or concentration

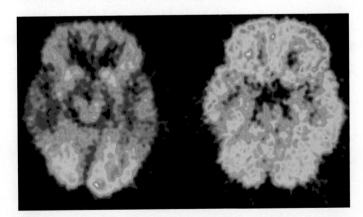

Figure 17-7
PET Scan Comparing the Metabolic Activity Levels of a Normal Brain (right) **and the Brain of an Alzheimer Patient** (left). Red and yellow colors indicate high activity levels, while blue colors represent low activity levels.

of a substance in an organ must occur first). The standard lung scan procedure includes two separate scans of the lungs, one after inhalation of a radionuclide and the other after injection of a second radionuclide into the circulation. The scanning is done with a scintillation camera (scintiscanner, gamma camera) which creates a picture on film representing the distribution and intensity of gamma radiation emitted by the subject.

real-time examination Ultrasonographic examination performed by sweeping the ultrasound beam through the scan plane at a rapid rate, generating up to 30 images per second. The display of images at this frequency is in effect a motion picture, providing visualization of movement of internal structures as it actually occurs.

reconstruction study Generation of an image by computer processing of scan data.

resolution The ability of an optical, radiographic, or other image-forming device to distinguish or separate two closely adjacent points in the subject. In CT, resolution is measured in lines per millimeter. The higher the resolution, the sharper and more faithful the image.

single-photon emission computed tomography (SPECT) A form of nuclear imaging using computer software to generate two- and three-dimensional images. Used to evaluate regional blood flow, assess disorders of the heart and lungs, and evaluate head injuries, seizure disorders, stroke, brain tumors, and dementia.

spin-echo image An MRI obtained by the spin-echo technique. With this technique, T2 is determined indirectly, as a function of TE, the echo time.

stress cystogram A radiographic study of the bladder intended to demonstrate stress incontinence. Contrast medium is instilled into the bladder and films are taken while the subject coughs and bears down.

sunrise view of the patella X-ray study of the knee region in which the patella is visualized above the distal femur and appears like a rising or setting sun.

swimmer's view An oblique view of the thoracic spine in which the arm nearer to the x-ray source hangs at the patient's side and the opposite arm is upraised.

T1-weighted image On MRI, a spin-echo image generated by a pulse sequence using a short TR (0.6 seconds or less).

T2-weighted image On MRI, a spin-echo image generated by a pulse sequence using a long TR (2.0 seconds or more).

ultrasonography (US) A means of visualizing internal structures by observing the effects they have on a beam of sound waves. The sound used for this procedure is at a higher frequency (pitch) than the human ear can detect. Ultrasound waves pass through air, gas, and fluid without being reflected. However, they bounce back from rigid structures such as bone and gallstones, creating an "echo" that can be detected by a receiver. Solid organs such as the liver and kidney partially reflect ultrasound waves in predictable patterns. Waves are also reflected from the interface between two structures.

Ultrasonography might be compared to taking a flash photograph. Light from the flashbulb bounces off the subject and comes back to create an image on film of the surface contours of the subject. In ultrasonography, however, the echo must be converted electronically to a visible image before it can be interpreted. Sophisticated electronic equipment permits ultrasound scanning of a body region with generation of a two-dimensional picture of internal structures. In practice, the same device (a transducer) that generates the sound waves also acts as the receiver. Although it emits signals at a rate of 1000 per second, the transducer is actually functioning as a receiver 99.9% of the time.

upper gastrointestinal (GI) series Barium sulfate is given orally to outline the esophagus, stomach, and duodenum on x-ray film.

upper GI (UGI) series and small-bowel follow through An upper GI series is done, and x-ray films are taken over a period of time to visualize the barium as it moves through the small bowel.

working orthopedic surgery film A radiographic study done during the course of an operation; for example, to monitor the reduction of a fracture or the placement of a fixation device.

Pharmacology

contrast medium A substance that is introduced into or around a structure and, because of the difference in absorption of x-rays by the contrast medium and surrounding tissues, allows radiographic visualization of the structure.

iodinated contrast medium A contrast medium containing iodine rather than a metallic salt; used in angiography, intravenous pyelography, oral cholecystography, and other studies.

Spotlight on

The Radiology Transcriptionist

by Kathryn Stewart

I was transcribing in the hospital radiology department, my earphones hooked up to the transcribing unit, when a transcriptionist from the medical records department spoke to me. "Kathy, how can you stand to transcribe x-rays all day? How boring it must be!" She was on her way home after spending her day transcribing histories and physicals, consultation and operation reports, and discharge summaries. She thrived on the diversity and had told me more than once that she would probably die of boredom if she had to transcribe the same thing over and over.

That was about 15 years ago, and I still specialize in radiology. And I still don't find it boring. To the contrary, because of the many advances in computer and medical technology, radiology transcription has become one of the most exciting areas in which to work. The chorus of "It's boring" is no longer sung. Many transcriptionists are humming a new tune.

Over 25 years ago, I moved to California from Ohio with three years of a college English major and four years as a newspaper ombudsman under my belt and no plans for the future. I landed my first job in the medical field as an orderly and darkroom technician for a community hospital's x-ray department. The hospital was small, with only 67 patient beds. The radiology department had one room where the x-rays were taken, a darkroom for developing them, and an office where they were read by a radiologist. The office also did duty as the reception area, the chief tech's office, and the transcription area.

Because of the size of the department, from the beginning I was exposed to more than the specialized x-ray terminology. I was present when the radiologists explained their findings to a patient's attending physician and when the reports were dictated. I heard the technologists discuss positions and views among themselves and with the radiologists. I listened in when the interning students from the community college radiology technology program were taught about both the technical and medical aspects of the various x-ray exams. I learned a great deal about the importance of positioning and the reasons for an adequate preparation for certain tests.

I had been on the job for about six months when I was asked if I would be interested in learning transcription. I received on-the-job training, learning new terminology as I went on to other radiology departments and as the field of radiology itself advanced and expanded. Many radiologists are eager to help the transcriptionist with further explanation of the terms or exams, and many techs will take the time to review what positions a patient was placed in or what views

were taken. The availability of previous reports has many times helped me to decipher something in the dictation.

It is true there are days when a radiology transcriptionist hears no more exciting dictation than normal chest x-rays and a few decidedly uninteresting broken bones (just as there are days when the generalist transcribes nothing but normal H&Ps and a few decidedly uninteresting metatarsal resections). But the ever-advancing field of radiology, with all of its new technologies, has become one of the most exciting specialties a medical transcriptionist can choose.

References. My personal reference library consists of three sections: the basics, which I think any medical transcriptionist should have; a second classification of materials which each medical transcriptionist chooses to add to the basics; and those materials which deal exclusively with radiology.

The third segment of my reference library consists of those materials which relate to radiology. In addition to these books, my radiology reference material includes copies of all the "normal" reports used by all the radiologists for whom I've ever transcribed (A "normal" is a report for any exam which failed to show any abnormalities on the radiologist's reading. Each radiologist usually has an individual normal for each exam done in the department.); lists of isotopes which I obtained from a radiopharmaceutical company; and lists of patient positions, film views, and body planes gleaned from the offices of several chief x-ray techs for whom I've worked.

Over the years, each medical transcriptionist builds up a personal medical reference library from newly published texts and by adding to the terminology notebook begun by each of us in our first days on our first transcription job. We network with our peers to ensure that our knowledge of our specialty is kept up-to-date. We do all of this because we find our work exciting and we see ourselves as professionals.

Transcription practices. There is another aspect of the radiology specialty which is unlike most other areas of medical transcription, and which can separate the truly professional medical transcriptionist from one who looks on the radiology specialty as merely a boring job.

The professional radiology transcriptionist uses an extensive reference library, other medical professionals, sales representatives, catalogs, magazines, newsletters, seminars, conventions, and a good dose of initiative to track down the elusive term, the garbled dictation, the new procedure. Doing so guarantees work far removed from the complaints of boredom I used to hear. Doing so also gives the radiology transcriptionist a real sense of the importance of a professional job professionally done.

Source: *The SUM Program Radiology Transcription Unit*

TRANSCRIPTION**TIPS**

1. Directions can be expressed as adverbs by adding the suffix *ly*.

anterior	anteriorly
distal	distally
inferior	inferiorly
lateral	laterally
medial	medially
posterior	posteriorly
proximal	proximally
superior	superiorly

2. A combining vowel can be used to join directional and positional adjectives into a single word; the adjectives can also be combined using a hyphen. Notice the spelling changes in the combined forms. *Note:* The choice is the dictator's, not the transcriptionist's. The term should be transcribed as dictated.

anterior-posterior	anteroposterior
anterior-lateral	anterolateral
posterior-anterior	posteroanterior
posterior-lateral	posterolateral
superior-lateral	superolateral

3. The direction *transverse* is an adjective. Do not confuse it with the verb *traverse*, which means "to go across."

   A transverse view of the joint was obtained.
   The ultrasound probe traversed the entire abdomen.

4. The term *sagittal* is often misspelled. Remember that it has one *g* and two *t*'s.

5. Like many other adjectives in medical terminology, the word *navicular*, meaning boat-shaped (from the Latin *navicula*, "little boat"), is often used without a noun, becoming in effect a noun itself. There are naviculars (navicular bones) in both the wrist and the ankle.

   Prominent spurs were seen off the anterior surface of the talus and the navicular.

6. The term *x-ray* is transcribed using a lowercase *x* and a hyphen. It is occasionally spelled with a capital *X* in nonmedical publications; however, *x-ray* is the accepted medical style.

7. The term *x-ray* can be used as a noun (the photographic image) or a verb (the radiologic procedure).

   An x-ray was taken of the abdomen.
   The patient was x-rayed after admission.
   The patient was re-x-rayed on the second hospital day.

8. Translate the following slang terms when encountered in dictation.

C spine	cervical spine
L spine	lumbar spine
LS spine	lumbosacral spine
sono	sonogram
T spine	thoracic spine
tib	tibia, tibial
fib	fibula, fibular
tib-fib	tibia and fibula, tibiofibular

9. The following terms have more than one acceptable spelling.

Preferred	*Acceptable*
anulus	annulus
distention	distension
disk	disc
transected	transsected

10. Some radiologists dictate "colon mark" to indicate the colon as a mark of punctuation, so as to avoid confusion with the colon (the large intestine).

11. Radiologists often dictate in the present tense because they are interpreting their findings as they actually view the films. It is not unusual for them to switch from present tense to past tense within the same report, particularly when they are dictating their findings on a procedure in which they actively participated, such as a barium enema or an ultrasound examination.

    PA and lateral views were obtained, and they show a transverse fracture.
    The barium was seen to flow smoothly through the colon, and there is no sign of diverticula.

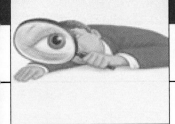

Proofreading Skills

Instructions: In the paragraphs below, circle the errors. Identify misspelled and missing medical and English words and punctuation errors, and write the correct words and punctuation in the numbered spaces opposite the text.

1 AIR CONTRAST BARIUM ENEMA

2

3 Under fluoroscopic control the Barium was allowed to

4 flow in a retrograde manner to fill the cecum. Using a

5 double-contrast technique, multiple films was obtained.

6 Several small diverticula are noted. There is some

7 lateral displacement of the sigmoid towards the left.

8 There is also some elevation of the small bowel. A

9 defuse soft tissue density is seen within the lower

10 adbomen. No mucosal ulcerations or polypoid lesions

11 are identified.

12

13 IMPRESSION

14 Air contrast study shows displacement of bowel

15 suggestive of a pelvic mass. Posibility of an enlarged

16 bladder should be considered. No evidence of

17 polypoid lesions or masses are seen within the colon.

1 _____

2 _____

3 _barium_____

4 _____

5 _____

6 _____

7 _____

8 _____

9 _____

10 _____

11 _____

12 _____

13 _____

14 _____

15 _____

16 _____

17 _____

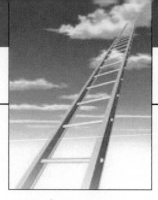

Skills Challenge

Medical Terminology Matching Exercise

Instructions: Match the definitions in Column A with their terms in Column B.

Column A

1. ___ x-ray of breast
2. ___ general term for any radioactive substance used in x-ray imaging
3. ___ contrast medium used in studies of GI tract
4. ___ uses sound waves to show differences in tissue density
5. ___ x-rays appear on fluorescent screen rather than x-ray film
6. ___ image produced by gamma camera after injection of radio-nuclide
7. ___ the image produced by ultrasound
8. ___ image produced after injection of radionuclide that shows rates of tissue metabolism
9. ___ roentgenogram
10. ___ x-ray of spinal cord using contrast medium
11. ___ chemical symbol for technetium
12. ___ x-ray of urinary system using contrast medium

Column B

A. x-ray
B. barium
C. fluoroscopy
D. intravenous pyelogram
E. myelogram
F. mammogram
G. ultrasound
H. sonogram
I. radionuclide
J. Tc 99m
K. scan
L. PET

Abbreviations Exercise

Instructions: Define the following radiology abbreviations and memorize the definitions in order to increase your speed and accuracy in transcribing radiology reports.

AP view _____
CAT _____
CT _____
CXR _____
IVP _____
KUB _____
MRI _____
PA view _____
PET _____
SPECT _____
UGI _____

Directions Matching Exercise

Instructions: Match the directions in Column A with their definitions in Column B.

Column A

1. ___ further away from the midline of the body
2. ___ further away from the center of the body or some other point of reference
3. ___ higher, upward
4. ___ lower, downward
5. ___ higher in the body
6. ___ nearer to the center of of the body or some other point of reference
7. ___ lower in the body
8. ___ pertaining to or in the direction of the front surface of the body
9. ___ rear, toward the back
10. ___ front, toward the front of the body
11. ___ pertaining to or in the direction of the back
12. ___ nearer to the midline of the body

Column B

A. anterior
B. caudal
C. cranial
D. distal
E. dorsal
F. inferior
G. lateral
H. medial
I. posterior
J. proximal
K. superior
L. ventral

Dictation Exercises

Prior to transcribing the dictations, complete these activities.

1. **Using Chapter 3, Style Guide**
   a. Many radiology studies are abbreviated (CT, MRI, PET); do these abbreviations ever need to be expanded? If so, when?
   b. When, according to the Style Guide, do you expand brief forms and abbreviations?
   c. What is the correct way to transcribe the letter-number combinations indicating interspaces of the vertebral spine? Give examples.
   d. What does the Style Guide recommend when a term contains a subscript or superscript?
   e. Review the section in the Style Guide on subject-verb agreement and prepositions. What does it say about prepositions and the subject of a sentence? What determines the number of the verb when certain specific words like *part, all,* or *none* are used with prepositions?
   f. What symbol is substituted for the word *per* in units of measure?

2. **Problem Solving**
   a. There are numerous good radiology sites on the Internet. Many include actual images and point out the anatomical structures and abnormalities that can be seen on the images. Perform a Google search for "best Radiology sites Web" without the quotation marks. Take the time to check out the first 5 to 10 "hits." Pay particular attention to those sites that are anatomy and vocabulary "rich." Bookmark your favorites for future reference.
   b. You hear the dictator say something that sounds like "curly lines" on a chest x-ray. On listening closer, you hear a *z* sound at the end of the word that sounds like "curly." What does hearing the *z* sound at the end make you think? What letter besides *c* could make the sound at the beginning of the word that sounds like "curly"? How can you research this term in order to find the correct spelling?
   c. Like pathology, radiology terminology is very heavy with anatomical terms. Find some good resources for anatomy.
   d. The Style Guide gives guidelines for the transcription of combined anatomical and directional terms, but does that mean you can combine any two anatomical or directional terms, just because they're dictated adjacent to each other? When you can't really tell by listening whether a dictator is saying two separate words or joining them (usually with an *o* in the middle, but sometimes the *o* is indistinct), how can you be reasonably sure you're transcribing the term(s) correctly?

   e. How can you improve your understanding of foreign accents?
   f. *Vertebra* and *vertebrae* can be difficult to distinguish in dictation. What kinds of context clues can you look for to help you determine whether to use the singular or plural form?

3. **Preparatory Research**
   a. The field of radiology has expanded in recent years and might be more aptly referred to now as imaging. How many different types of imaging procedures can you document that are not, strictly speaking, radiologic procedures?
   b. How many synonyms can you find for the word *x-ray*?
   c. What is meant by *tenting of the hemidiaphragm*?
   d. What types of lung conditions are most likely to be associated with fibrosis?
   e. What structures in the chest form the *costophrenic angles*?
   f. Where is the *olecranon* located?
   g. What does *bony resorption* mean?
   h. What is the difference in meaning between *callus* and *callous*?
   i. What is the difference between open reduction and internal fixation and open reduction and external fixation (of a fracture)?
   j. What is the plural of *foramen*? Define *atlantoaxial articulation*.
   k. Define *radiopaque*.
   l. What is a *spur* or *spurring* on a vertebra?
   m. What is a *scout film*?
   n. Define the following: *pedicle* (of the vertebra), *diverticulum, extravasation*.
   o. Define the following: *Spalding sign, sonolucent, menstrual age, abruption*. (*Hint:* On the phrases, look in the dictionary under the noun.)
   p. Define the following: *bifurcation, mesentery, obturator*.
   q. Where is the *sella turcica*? What gland is located there?
   r. What is the difference in meaning between *discreet* and *discrete*? Which is more likely to be used in a radiology report?
   s. Research the *imaging techniques* and planes associated with *magnetic resonance imaging*.
   t. Define the following: *microadenoma, prolactinoma*.
   u. Describe how a *myelogram* is performed.
   v. What is a *duplex scan*?
   w. Define *plaque* (as in an artery).
   x. Define the following: *attenuation, tracer, gating* (in tomography), *dyskinesis, ischemia*.
   y. What is the difference in meaning between *profusion* and *perfusion*? Between *injection* and *ejection*? (*Hint:* Think about the context of an imaging study of the heart.)
   z. List the arteries of the lower extremities.

Sample Reports

Sample radiology reports appear on the following pages, illustrating a variety of reports. Fictional names are provided for illustration of proper format, and no resemblance to actual persons is intended. Sample transcripts were prepared according to the *AAMT Book of Style*, where possible.

Radiology Report

GETZ, STANLEY
#122541
9/13/XXXX
Attending: Michael Kalm, MD

CHEST, PA AND LATERAL

The heart is normal in size. Trachea is at midline. Normal pulmonary vascular markings. Opaque sutures are seen in the projection of the right upper chest, and there are minimal fibrotic changes in the right lung. Lungs are expanded, and no active infiltrate is otherwise seen.

IMPRESSION
Presence of opaque sutures in the projection of the right upper chest and minimal fibrotic changes in the right lung. No active cardiopulmonary disease is otherwise demonstrated at this time.

SCOTT JAFFE, MD

SJ:hpi
d&t: 9/13/XXXX

MUGGELBERG, MARY
#111332
9/13/XXXX
Attending: Hiyas Fonte, MD

LOW-DOSE MAMMOGRAPHY

CLINICAL HISTORY
There is no family history of breast cancer. Patient had onset of menses at age 12 years, and her last menstrual period (LMP) was at age 50 years. Patient is a gravida 4, para 3, ab 1. Currently she is asymptomatic. There is no history of previous breast surgery. She is on intermittent estrogen therapy.

Bilateral mammographic examination reveals atrophic breasts with minimal fibrocystic residuals, predominantly fibrotic. There are no dominant mass lesions. No abnormal calcifications are detected. Small intramammary lymph nodes are noted in the tail of each breast. The skin and subcutaneous fat lines appear smooth. Vascularity is normal and symmetrical.

IMPRESSION
1. Atrophic breasts with minor fibrocystic residuals.
2. No evident malignant mass lesion.
3. Annual mammography is recommended in this age group.

MAX GREMILLION, MD

MG:hpi
D&T: 9/13/XXXX

TERASHIMA, DANIEL
#111332
9/13/XXXX
ATTENDING: Nora Roberts, MD

LIMITED SINUSES

Upright Waters and Caldwell views demonstrate apparent air-fluid level in the left maxillary sinus, consistent with sinusitis. However, I certainly cannot exclude this representing a polyp or cyst. The remainder of the visualized paranasal sinuses, soft tissue, and bony structures are unremarkable.

IMPRESSION
Demonstration of an apparent air-fluid level in the left maxillary sinus, consistent with sinusitis. Please correlate clinically.

CT SCAN OF THE SINUSES

Multiple 4-mm sections at 4-mm intervals were taken in coronal projection without iodinated intravenous contrast. Air-fluid level is seen in the right maxillary sinus, suggesting a right maxillary sinusitis. No bony abnormality is seen about the paranasal sinuses. No soft tissue or bony abnormality is seen near the ostia of the maxillary sinuses. The soft tissues and bones of the face, which are also visualized, are grossly normal.

IMPRESSION
Right maxillary sinusitis with no variation or abnormality seen.

TOAN LAM, MD

TL:hpi:

D&T 9/13/XXXX

Radiology Report

FERREIRA, LARRY
#36592
9/13/XXXX
Attending: Thomas Boettger, MD

KIDNEYS, URETERS, BLADDER (KUB)
The spinous processes, transverse processes, and pedicles of the lumbar vertebrae are fairly well maintained. A minimal amount of degenerative disease is seen within the hips. A large amount of gas and feces is noted throughout the colon. Some gas is noted within the small bowel. Calcified phleboliths are seen within the pelvis. There is also a large 2 x 4-cm mass of increased density in the midportion of the true pelvis.

IMPRESSION
Density within the midpelvis of undetermined etiology. In this first film on this patient, the possibilities include (1) a suppository, (2) residual barium from a previous study, (3) a foreign body.

INTRAVENOUS PYELOGRAM
The KUB study shows the 4-mm calcification in the lower midpole of the right kidney and is unchanged in the interval since our comparison study. The right kidney also appeared normal at that time. The left kidney showed exactly the same configuration on the outside study presented for review, with an irregular right upper pole and two small cystic changes lateral to the upper pole caliceal system, measuring 2 cm and 2.5 cm in diameter. The curvilinear displacement of the caliceal systems also suggests a larger cystic change in the parapelvic region, measuring approximately 5 cm in diameter. The compression of the renal pelvis and deviation of the left upper ureter are essentially the same as seen on the intravenous pyelogram. The bladder again appears normal with a minimal residual.

IMPRESSION
Right renal lithiasis and slight right nephroptosis on the upright study; otherwise normal-appearing right upper urinary tract and ureter. Deformity of the upper pole of the left kidney with some blunting of the caliceal system and the formation of cystic calices lateral to the main upper pole caliceal system suggests a pyelonephritis. Tuberculosis should be considered as an etiology. A larger parapelvic cyst is also noted, displacing the renal pelvis inferiorly and causing some deformity but no evident amputation of the middle or lower pole caliceal systems. The study is consistent with the same findings as on our recent intravenous pyelogram.

ALLISON BARKER, MD

AB:hpi

d&t: 9/13/XXXX

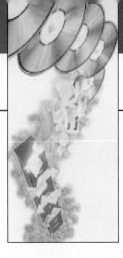

Transcription Practice

Key Words

The following terms appear in the radiology dictations. Before beginning the medical transcription practice for Chapter 17, look up each term below in a medical or English dictionary and write out a short definition.

adenopathy
anterolateral infarct
arterial system
attenuation
axial CT views
barium enema
cardiomegaly
cervical spine
CT scan of chest, abdomen, and pelvis
diverticula
diverticulitis
duplex scan

fetal demise
fibrosis
hematoma
KUB film
lumbar myelogram
MRI scan
myocardial imaging
obstetrical ultrasound
olecranon fracture
pituitary microadenoma
retroperitoneal mass
sella turcica

After completing all the readings and exercises in Chapter 17, transcribe the radiology dictation. Proofread your transcribed documents carefully, listening to the dictation while you read your transcripts.

Transcribe (*not* retype) the same reports again without referring to your previous transcription attempt. Initially, you may need to transcribe some reports more than twice before you can produce an error-free document. Your ultimate goal is to produce an error-free document the first time.

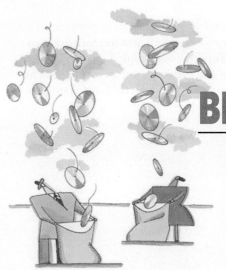

BLOOPERS

Incorrect	Correct
The x-ray was frantically normal.	The x-ray was practically normal.
There were many radio loosened stones.	There were many radiolucent stones.
Excess study of the GI tract.	X-ray study of the GI tract.
The patient had an intrapenis pyelogram.	The patient had an intravenous pyelogram.
Mugger study.	MUGA study (for nuclear medicine).
X-rays of the vertebral column showed bunny fur formation.	X-rays of the vertebral column showed bony spur formation.

Resources

Abba, Elaine Aamodt, "Promoting Wellness, Preventing Injury," *Perspectives on the Medical Transcription Profession*, Winter 1992-93, pp. 10-11.

Cadigan, Carolyn, "Tips on Transcribing Orthopedic Dictation," *The SUM Program Orthopedic Transcription Unit* (Modesto, Ca.: Health Professions Institute, 1988).

Campbell, Linda C., "Confidentially Speaking . . . ," *Perspectives on the Medical Transcription Profession*, Spring 1995, pp. 11-13.

Diehl, Marcy, ""Criticism," *Beginning Medical Transcription* (Modesto, Ca.: Health Professions Institute, 1989).

Dirckx, John H., M.D., "Acid Backwards: Perspectives on Gastroesophageal Reflux," *Perspectives on the Medical Transcription Profession*, Spring 2001, pp. 31–36.

Dirckx, John H., M.D., "Brainstorms: Perspectives on Epilepsy," *Perspectives on the Medical Transcription Profession*, Winter 2001-2002, pp. 32-37.

Dirckx, John H., M.D., "Dealing with Hazardous Waists: Trends in the Management of Obesity," *Perspectives on the Medical Transcription Profession*, Winter 1999-2000, pp. 36-42.

Dirckx, John H., M.D., "Dictation and Transcription: Adventures in Thought Transference," *Perspectives on the Medical Transcription Profession*, Summer 1990, pp. 34-37.

Dirckx, John H., M.D., "Downside: Adverse Effects of Drug Therapy," *Perspectives on the Medical Transcription Profession*, Summer 2000, pp. 30-39.

Dirckx, John H., M.D., *H&P: A Nonphysician's Guide to the Medical History and Physical Examination*, 3rd ed. (Modesto, Ca.: Health Professions Institute, 2001).

Dirckx, John H., M.D., "The Honeyed Siphon: Diabetes Mellitus Past, Present, and Future," *Perspectives on the Medical Transcription Profession*, Fall 1998, pp. 35-41.

Dirckx, John H., M.D., *Human Diseases*, 2nd ed. (Modesto, Ca.: Health Professions Institute, 2003).

Dirckx, John H., M.D., "It's Breathtaking! Perspectives on Asthma," *Perspectives on the Medical Transcription Profession*, Fall 2001, pp. 30-36.

Dirckx, John H., M.D., *Laboratory Tests and Diagnostic Procedures in Medicine* (Modesto, Ca.: Health Professions Institute, 2004).

Dirckx, John H., M.D., "Mental Illness: It's All in Your Body," *Perspectives on the Medical Transcription Profession*, Winter 1995-1996, pp. 32-39.

Dirckx, John H., M.D., "Much More Than Just a Filter: Perspectives on Renal Function," *Perspectives on the Medical Transcription Profession*, September 2003, pp. 18-22.

Dirckx, John H., M.D., "Sexually Transmitted Diseases: Update 1993," *Perspectives on the Medical Transcription Profession*, Winter 1992-1993, pp. 41-47.

Dirckx, John H., "Wake Me When It's Over: Sleep and Its Disorders," *Perspectives on the Medical Transcription Profession*, Spring 2000, pp. 28-35.

Donneson, Kathy, "Professionalism and the Medical Transcriptionist," *Beginning Medical Transcription* (Modesto, Ca.: Health Professions Institute, 1989).

D'Onofrio, Mary Ann, "The Ophthalmology Medical Transcriptionist," *Perspectives on the Medical Transcription Profession*, Fall 1990, pp. 22-24.

D'Onofrio, Mary Ann, and Elizabeth D'Onofrio, "Curve Balls," *Perspectives on the Medical Transcription Profession*, Summer 1990, pp. 4-6.

Dooley, Susan, and Ellen Drake, "Foreign Accents Revisited," *Perspectives on the Medical Transcription Profession*, Winter 1995-1996, pp. 30-31.

Drake, Ellen, "Job Searching," *Medical Transcription Fundamentals & Practice*, 2nd ed. (Upper Saddle River, N.J.: Prentice Hall Health, 2000).

Drake, Ellen, and Randy Drake, *Saunders Pharmaceutical Word Book* (Philadelphia: W.B. Saunders Co., 2006).

Ellis, Michael A., M.D., "Orthopedic Practice and Surgery," *The SUM Program Orthopedic Transcription Unit* (Modesto, Ca.: Health Professions Institute, 1988).

Green, Georgia, "Feeling the Need for Speed," *Perspectives on the Medical Transcription Profession*, Fall 2001, pp. 6-8.

Hinickle, Judy, "Employment Enigmas," *Perspectives on the Medical Transcription Profession*, Spring/Summer 1991, pp. 22-23.

Klass, Perri, M.D., "Medical Short-Tongue," *Journal of AAMT*, Summer 1985.

Largen, Thomas L., M.D., FACS, "A Surgeon's View of Gastroenterology and Practice," *The SUM Program Gastrointestinal Transcription Unit* (Modesto, Ca.: Health Professions Institute, 1989).

Lederer, Richard, Ph.D., "Jest for the Health of It," *Perspectives on the Medical Transcription Profession*, Spring 1999, p. 21.

Lederer, Richard, Ph.D., "A Little Bit of Comma Sense," *e-Perspectives on the Medical Transcription Profession*, Summer 2006. Excerpted from Richard Lederer's and John Shore's *Comma Sense: A Fun-damental Guide to Punctuation* (New York City: St. Martin's Press, 2005).

Marshall, Judith, "What Is a Medical Transcriptionist?", pp. 1-3; "Tape Dancing," pp. 4-9; "Fat Chance," pp. 27-32; "Confessions of an Addict," pp. 33-41; "Kits and Caboodle," pp. 42-50, *Medicate Me* (Modesto, Ca.: Health Professions Institute, 1987).

Marshall, Judith, "Whining and Dining," pp. 35-38; "Call Me Madam," pp. 58-60; "It's All Right to Laugh," pp. 99-102, *Medicate Me Again* (Modesto, Ca.: Health Professions Institute, 1994).

Martin, April, "Evolution of the Healthcare Documentation Specialist," *Plexus*, November 2005, pp. 8-9).

The Medical Transcription Workbook (Modesto, Ca.: Health Professions Institute, 1999).

Moormeister, Sidney K., Ph.D., "Careers in Death Investigation—Is One Right for You?," *Perspectives on the Medical Transcription Profession*, Spring/Summer 1993, pp. 30-35.

O'Donnell, Michael J., M.D., "Cardiology and Cardiovascular Surgery," *The SUM Program Cardiology Transcription Unit* (Modesto, Ca.: Health Professions Institute, 1989).

Pitman, Sally C., "Humor in Medicine: Bloopers," first published as an introduction to *The eMpTy Laugh Book* (Modesto, Ca.: American Association for Medical Transcription, 1991).

Pitman, Sally C., "The Fire Within," *Perspectives on the Medical Transcription Profession*, Winter 2001-2002, p. 2.

Pitman, Sally C., "The Racetrack," *Perspectives on the Medical Transcription Profession*, Fall 1996, p. 2.

Pitman, Sally C., "Seeing Is Believing," *Perspectives on the Medical Transcription Profession*, Summer 1996, pp. 4-5.

Priest, Renee, "The Gourmet Medical Transcriptionist," *Perspectives on the Medical Transcription Profession*, Spring 1999, p. 40.

Priest, Renee, "It's All in the Tushie," *Perspectives on the Medical Transcription Profession*, Winter 1999-2000, pp. 47-48.

Priest, Renee, "Seasoned Medical Transcriptionist's Syndrome," *Perspectives on the Medical Transcription Profession*, Winter 2000-2001, p. 40.

Priest, Renee, "Slaplingopathy," *Perspectives on the Medical Transcription Profession*, Spring 2001, p. 40.

Pyle, Vera, *Vera Pyle's Current Medical Terminology*, 10th ed. (Modesto, Ca.: Health Professions Institute, 2005).

Sims, Lea, "The Competitive Edge," *JAAMT*, August 2005, p. 203.

Stevens, Cindy, illustrations in *Medicate Me* (Modesto, Ca.: Health Professions Institute, 1987).

Stewart, Kathryn, "The Radiology Transcriptionist," *The SUM Program Radiology Transcription Unit* (Modesto, Ca.: Health Professions Institute, 1987; rev. 1990).

Stewart, Kathryn, "Transcriptionists Are People, Too," *Perspectives on the Medical Transcription Profession*, Fall 1991, p. 25.

Taylor, Bron, "How I Became a Medical Transcriptionist," *Perspectives on the Medical Transcription Profession*, Winter 1996-1997, pp. 10-12.

Taylor, Bron, "Transcribing Gastroenterology Dictation," *The SUM Program Gastrointestinal Transcription Unit* (Modesto, Ca.: Health Professions Institute, 1989).

Turley, Susan M., *Medical Language* (Upper Saddle River, N.J.: Pearson Prentice Hall, 2007). **http://www.prenhall. com/turley** A text-specific, interactive on-line workbook.

Turley, Susan M., *Understanding Pharmacology for Health Professionals*, 3rd ed. (Upper Saddle River, N.J.: Prentice Hall Health, 2003).

Turley, Susan M., "Who Nose?", *Perspectives on the Medical Transcription Profession*, Fall 1991, p.27.

Woods, Kathleen Mors, "Transcribing Cardiology Dictation," *The SUM Program Cardiology Transcription Unit* (Modesto, Ca.: Health Professions Institute, 1989).

Web Sites

http://www.hpisum.com/ Free downloads for students and teachers available from Health Professions Institute.

http://www.prenhall.com/medtrans/ Medical Transcription Central, Prentice Hall Health's free Web site featuring software downloads, dictation bloopers, up-to-date word lists, and more.

http://www.aamt.org/ American Association for Medical Transcription, information on the RMT and CMT credentials.

http://www. geocities.com/gene_moutoux/diagrams. htm/ Sentence diagramming.

http://webster.commnet.edu/grammar/index.htm/ Comprehensive grammar site and quizzes hosted by Capital Community College.

http://www.ismp.org/ List of error-prone abbreviations.

http://www.jcaho.org/accredited+organizations/patient+ safety/04+npsg/04_faqs.htm/ List of error-prone abbreviations.

http://www.emedicine.com/specialties Register free. Much free information for students on diagnosis, disease, and treatment. Often has accompanying illustrations.

http://www.fpnotebook.com/index.htm/ Discusses physical findings and treatment.

http://www.labcorp.com/datasets/labcorp/html/chapter/ On-line lab data.

http://www.onelook.com/ Good on-line dictionary, wild card searches, and reverse lookup (using the definition instead of the word). **Onelook** will find medical and nonmedical words.

http://www.ritecode.com/free_opreports/opreport_free_index.htm/ Sample operative reports.

http://www.mtdesk.com/ops.shtml Sample operative reports.

http://spwb.com/ Web site for *Saunders Pharmaceutical Word Book*. Once you've purchased the CD, you can get free monthly updates.

http://www.bartleby.com/ A great all-round Web site for a number of different on-line references. Usage, grammar, dictionary, thesaurus, etc.

Glossary

abdominoperineal resection Removal of the entire lower bowel, including the anus.

ablation Total removal of a part, normal or abnormal, by surgical or chemical means.

abscess A localized zone of inflammation, generally due to infection, in which pus forms in a tissue space walled off from surrounding tissues by fibrin, coagulated tissue fluids, and eventually fibrous tissue.

absence ("ab sáhnce") **seizure (petit mal)** Brief loss of attention and perception.

absorption tests Based on determination of blood or stool levels of substances that have been ingested in measured amounts.

abulia Diminished ability to make decisions.

accessory muscles of respiration Neck and upper chest muscles not needed for normal breathing.

acetone, urinary Acetone in the urine can be measured with a dipstick. Small amounts are found in starvation and other abnormal metabolic states, larger amounts in uncontrolled diabetes mellitus.

acid-fast stain A staining procedure in which sputum, tissue, or other material is exposed to fluorochrome dye and then washed with acid-alcohol. Organisms of the genus *Mycobacterium* and some others retain the dye and are said to be acid-fast.

acoustical shadowing The inability of ultrasound to reach and delineate structures located in the "shadow" of an organ or tissue that reflects a large amount of ultrasound.

acromegaly Abnormal growth of the body, especially facial features and extremities.

acute pharyngitis Sore throat.

adenoma A benign tumor arising from glandular epithelium.

adipocere A waxy substance that forms in a dead body after prolonged immersion.

adnexa Organs adjacent to the uterus—ovaries and tubes.

affect One's prevailing mood or emotional state, pleasant or unpleasant, particularly as perceived by the examiner: basic emotional state, and emotional content of responses to examiner (apathetic, blunted, depressed, elated, euphoric, flat, inappropriate, labile).

agglutinins, cold Antibodies formed by persons with mycoplasmal pneumonia, which cause red blood cells to clump when chilled but not at room or body temperature.

agglutinins, febrile A group of antibody tests, each for a specific febrile (fever-causing) infectious disease, used as a screening procedure in patients with fever of unknown origin (FUO).

air-fluid level A line representing the level of a collection of fluid as seen in a radiographic image, with air or gas above it.

air-space disease As seen on chest x-ray, disease or abnormality of lung tissue that encroaches on space normally filled by air.

AK amputation Above-the-knee amputation.

akathisia Extreme restlessness, inability to remain seated.

alkaline phosphatase An enzyme whose level in the serum is often increased in bone disease and obstructive liver disease. When "alk phos" is dictated, it must be expanded in transcription.

alopecia Local or widespread loss of scalp hair.

ALT (alanine aminotransferase) Formerly called *SGPT*. An enzyme whose level in the serum is elevated in hepatitis, cirrhosis, and other liver diseases.

altered level of consciousness Varying from slight drowsiness or inattentiveness to confusion and disorientation to deep coma from which the subject cannot be aroused by any stimulus.

amblyopia Dulling of vision that cannot be corrected with a lens.

amenorrhea Absence of menstruation.

amino acid A relatively simple nitrogen-containing organic compound. Of the 20 amino acids that are essential to human metabolism, half can be manufactured in the body and the others must be obtained in the diet.

ammonia, serum A breakdown product of protein metabolism, increased in hepatic failure.

amnesia Loss of memory, recent, remote, or total.

amniocentesis A procedure to withdraw amniotic fluid through a needle from the uterus of a pregnant woman. The fetal cells and chemicals in the fluid are studied to identify fetal abnormalities.

amylase, serum An enzyme whose level is increased in pancreatitis and mumps.

ANA (antinuclear antibody) An antibody detected by immunofluorescence in patients with rheumatoid arthritis, lupus erythematosus, and other autoimmune diseases.

anaplastic Referring to tumor tissue containing primitive, undifferentiated cells, unlike the structurally differentiated cells of normal tissue.

anastomosis Surgical joining of two organs or vessels.

anatomic pathology Concerned with the gross and microscopic changes brought about in living human tissues by disease.

anemia Deficiency of red blood cells.

anencephaly Absence of cerebral hemispheres.

anesthesia Total loss of sensation on one or more parts of the body surface.

aneurysm Abnormal dilatation of a blood vessel.

aneurysm resection Surgical removal of a segment of vessel that has an abnormal ballooning and threatens to rupture.

angiography May be used to show cranial vasculature with injected contrast medium. In digital subtraction angiography, x-ray images of the head with and without contrast medium are processed by a computer, which deletes all shadows common to both films (skull bones, soft tissue profiles and interfaces), leaving only the vascular system visible.

anhedonia Inability to experience pleasure from normally pleasurable activities.

anion gap Referring to electrolytes.

ankle mortise The normal articulation between the talus and the distal tibia and fibula.

ankylosis Immobility and consolidation of a joint due to disease, injury, or surgical procedure.

anorexia nervosa A compulsive reduction of body weight to an unhealthful level by rigorous dieting, often supplemented by strenuous exercise, self-induced vomiting, or the use of diuretics or laxatives.

anovulation Failure of ovulation to occur at the expected times.

anterior drawer test With the patient supine, the injured knee is bent to 90 degrees. The physician then grasps the upper end of the tibia and pulls it anteriorly. Excessive movement means the anterior cruciate ligament within the knee joint is damaged or torn.

anxiety disorders Social phobia, agoraphobia, panic disorder, obsessive-compulsive disorder.

aphasia Impairment of the ability to communicate through spoken or written language, or to understand spoken or written language, or both.

apophysis Bony outgrowth.

appendectomy Surgical excision of the vermiform appendix.

Argyll Robertson pupil A pupil that constricts when the subject focuses on a near object, but not when the eye is stimulated with light; due to central nervous system disease, most often syphilis.

arrhythmia Irregular rhythm of the heartbeat, with or without an abnormally slow or fast rate.

arterial blood gases (ABGs) So-called because they are usually measured in a specimen of blood drawn from an artery. See *blood gases.*

arteriography The radiographic study of arteries into which radiopaque medium has been injected. Still pictures may be taken immediately after injection, or motion pictures may be made showing the flow of blood and contrast medium through vessels.

arthroscopy A surgical procedure which involves an incision into a joint and the insertion of an arthroscope to view the structures inside the joint.

ascites Swelling of the abdomen due to effusion of fluid into the peritoneal cavity.

ASO titer A test to detect and measure antistreptolysin O in serum. This antibody is present during and shortly after streptococcal infections. The value is measured in Todd units.

AST (aspartate aminotransferase) Formerly called *SGOT.* An enzyme whose level in the serum is elevated in myocardial infarction, liver disease, and other conditions.

ataxia Impairment of complex movements due to loss of proprioceptive impulses from the muscles of the trunk or limbs.

atelectasis Collapse of lung tissue.

athetosis Slow, writhing, involuntary movements of the face or limbs.

astigmatism Distortion of images by warping of the cornea out of the normal spherical shape.

audiography A precise measurement of the faintest loudness (in decibels) that the subject can hear, each ear tested separately at each of several pitches (for example, 250, 500, 1000, 2000, 3000, 4000, 6000, and 8000 Hz); this can be performed by a trained technician with carefully calibrated testing equipment, or by automated machinery activated by the subject.

auscultation Listening to the chest, particularly breath sounds, with the use of a stethoscope.

auscultation of the heart The physician notes the quality and loudness of heart sounds heard through a stethoscope at the four valve areas.

autoinoculation Implantation of infective viral material at new sites, with spread of lesions.

autopsy The examination of a body after death, consisting of detailed visual observations of external body tissues and internal organs, and microscopic analyses of the internal organs and structures following tissue dissection. Also called *postmortem examination, necropsy, "post."*

AV (arteriovenous) nicking Tapering of a venule where an arteriole crosses it as seen on funduscopy.

avascular necrosis Death of tissue due to loss of blood supply.

aversion therapy A form of behavior therapy that associates an objectionable or undesirable pattern of behavior with an unpleasant experience or consequence, so as to reduce or extinguish the behavior.

avian flu A term used to describe the influenza viruses that infect birds, including wild birds such as ducks, and domestic birds such as chickens. Many forms of avian flu virus cause only mild symptoms in the birds or no symptoms at all. However, some of the viruses produce a highly contagious and rapidly fatal disease, leading to severe epidemics. These virulent viruses are known as "highly pathogenic avian influenza," and it is these viruses that cause particular concern. Until 1997 avian flu was believed to infect only birds; however, in 1997 it was discovered that the virus can occasionally infect people who have been in close contact with live birds in markets or farms. It is possible that a highly pathogenic avian flu virus could merge with a human flu virus and create a new virus that could be easily passed between humans.

avulsion The ripping or tearing away of a part.

axes See *multiaxial assessment.*

Babinski reflex Consists of dorsiflexion of the great toe and flaring of the other toes in response to stroking the sole of the foot toward the toes; an indication of disease or injury affecting a corticospinal tract. A normal reflex is downgoing, except in newborns and infants, in which the normal Babinski reflex is upgoing.

backward failure Inability of the heart to distend adequately during diastole, with resulting increase of pressure in the venous system.

bacterial vaginosis A mixed vaginal infection that causes a thin grayish discharge with a foul fishy odor but little vulvar irritation or itching.

bagged Manually ventilated with an Ambu bag.

Baker cyst Fluctuant swelling of the bursa behind the knee joint.

balloon angioplasty Stretching or breaking up atherosclerotic plaques in coronary arteries.

band forms, bands Immature neutrophils whose nuclei appear as bands, in contrast to mature neutrophils whose nuclei are segmented or lobed.

barium enema (BE) Standard radiographic examination of the large intestine by introduction of barium solution into the rectum.

barrel chest In pulmonary emphysema the anteroposterior diameter of the chest is often increased so that the rib cage approaches a cylindrical shape.

Barrett esophagus A metaplasia (transformation) of normal squamous esophageal epithelium into columnar epithelium; some cases of Barrett esophagus progress to adenocarcinoma.

Bartholin glands Secretory glands lateral to the vaginal vestibule.

basal body temperature Daily determination of oral temperature on arising is useful in confirming and dating ovulation. Daily graphing of basal body temperature will show a rise of 0.75-1.0°F (0.2-0.5°C) approximately one day after ovulation.

basos An acceptable brief form for *basophils.*

basilar Pertaining to the bases (lowermost parts) of the lungs.

behavior (behavioral) therapy Any type of psychotherapy that focuses on the alteration or correction of undesirable behavior, including such responses to external stimuli as anxiety, depression, and physical symptoms of emotion (tachycardia, muscle tension, sweating). Behavior therapy uses conditioning, muscle relaxation techniques, meditation, breathing retraining, biofeedback, guided learning, and other methods.

belching Burping.

benign Not malignant.

beta HCG See *HCG.*

Bethesda system A uniform system for reporting findings on Pap (Papanicolaou) smear of the uterine cervix.

bilirubin, conjugated (direct) Bilirubin that has been conjugated (combined with glucuronic acid) by the liver. Because it is water-soluble, it can be excreted in the urine, and reacts directly with testing chemicals. Its level is increased in biliary obstruction.

bilirubin, unconjugated (indirect) Bilirubin in the serum that has not been conjugated (combined with glucuronic acid) by the liver. Because unconjugated bilirubin is lipid-soluble but not water-soluble, it is not excreted in the urine and does not react directly with testing chemicals. Its level is increased in disorders that impair the function of liver cells.

bilirubin, urinary Bilirubin in the urine; it can be measured with a dipstick. Any amount is considered abnormal; usually it indicates obstructive liver disease or hepatitis.

bilirubinuria, choluria Bilirubin in the urine.

biopsy Surgical removal of tissue from a living patient for histologic examination to identify neoplasm, infection, or other abnormality.

biopsy, excisional Complete removal of a lesion or neoplasm for histologic study. Some adjacent, normal-appearing tissue is also removed for comparison.

biopsy, incisional Partial removal of a lesion by making an incision into the lesion and removing a section of it as well as some adjacent, normal-appearing tissue for comparison.

biopsy punch A cylindrical instrument used to obtain a plug of tissue for examination.

biopsy, punch Removal of one section of a lesion using a sharp surgical instrument known as a punch.

biopsy, skin Removal of all or part of a skin lesion. The tissue is sent to the pathology laboratory for histologic diagnosis and to determine whether it is malignant.

BK amputation Below-knee amputation.

blast forms, blasts Very immature cells, particularly leukocytes, not normally found in peripheral blood but present in acute leukemia.

bleeding time The number of minutes it takes for a small incision in the skin, made with a lancet, to stop bleeding. Either the Duke method (puncture of the earlobe) or the Ivy method (puncture of the forearm) may be used.

blepharitis Inflammation of one or both eyelids.

blepharospasm Spasm of the eyelids, usually due to local irritation, photophobia, or both.

bloating An overly full, distended feeling, usually from excessive intestinal gas.

blood gases Oxygen and carbon dioxide, the principal gases dissolved in the blood. Sometimes called arterial blood gases because they are usually measured in a specimen of blood drawn from an artery. Blood gas measurements include partial pressures of oxygen (pO_2) and of carbon dioxide (pCO_2) and oxygen saturation. From these data and the serum pH, it is possible to calculate the bicarbonate level. Alternatively, the base excess may be reported as the variation from a neutral blood pH.

blood pool The circulating blood, into which radionuclides are injected for various types of circulatory scans.

blood sugar Determination of the concentration of glucose in circulating blood.

blood type A genetically determined and permanent characteristic of a person's red blood cells based on the presence of certain antigens. Two blood type systems of clinical importance are the ABO (comprising types A, B, AB, and O) and the Rh (comprising Rh-positive and Rh-negative). Blood for transfusion must be typed and then cross-matched (experimentally combined) with the prospective recipient's blood to avoid reactions due to incompatibility of bloods. Other red cell antigens not used for type and cross-matching include Duffy, Kell, Kidd, and Lewis. These are often used when blood typing is used as evidence of nonpaternity.

blunted costophrenic angle On chest x-ray, a costophrenic angle that is flattened or distorted by scarring or pleural fluid.

body mass index (BMI) A measure of the proportion of fat to lean body mass.

bone marrow Site of production of red blood cells, white blood cells, and platelets.

bone scan A nuclear imaging test which, following the intravenous administration of radioisotope, uses a scanning device to detect areas of abnormal uptake in the bones to identify fracture, infection, or malignancy.

bone wax Gel-like material that is exactly like wax that you would use in the kitchen. It has the ability to seal little pores in the bone that are exuding blood.

bony island Benign developmental abnormality consisting of a localized zone of increased density in a long bone.

borborygmus (pl. **borborygmi**) Audible rumbling and gurgling sounds in the digestive tract due to intestinal activity.

bowel gas pattern On abdominal film, the normal radiographic appearance of gas in the intestine.

bradyarrhythmia A pulse that is both irregular and abnormally slow.

bradycardia Abnormal slowness of the heartbeat (pulse less than 60/min).

brain scan An examination based on the distribution of a radioactive isotope injected systemically.

bridging Formation of a bridge from one bone to another by abnormal calcium deposition, as in osteoarthritis.

bridging osteophytes Osteophytes on adjacent vertebrae that meet and fuse, forming a "bridge" across the joint space.

bronchiectasis Abnormal, irreversible dilatation of bronchi, related to chronic infection.

bronchoalveolar lavage (BAL) Obtaining of material from lung tissue by washing.

bronchoscopy Inspection of the interior of the trachea and main bronchi with a fiberoptic instrument. Specimens and biopsies can be taken through the instrument.

Brudzinski sign Passive flexion of the neck causes active flexion of the hip and knee.

bruit A rough vascular sound, synchronous with the heartbeat, heard with a stethoscope over a narrowing in an artery.

buffalo hump Soft tissue prominence over upper back.

bulimia nervosa A common behavioral disorder of young women characterized by recurrent episodes of binge eating. The typical patient engages in uncontrollable gorging with high-carbohydrate food several times a week.

bulla (pl. **bullae**) A blister; a fluid-filled epidermal sac larger than a vesicle.

burr cell An abnormal red blood cell with a jagged contour.

bursas Purselike cushions containing a little fluid to protect underlying surfaces and reduce friction.

BUS Bartholin glands, urethra, and Skene glands.

bx (biopsy).

bypass See *coronary artery bypass graft.*

calcitonin, serum A hormone produced by the thyroid gland and affecting the metabolism of calcium. It is markedly elevated in certain malignancies of the thyroid and lung.

callus formation An unorganized meshwork of woven bone, which is formed following fracture of a bone and is normally replaced by hard adult bone.

calorie A measurement of the energy released by food.

Campylobacter pylori Older name for the organism now called *Helicobacter pylori*.

Candida albicans A yeastlike fungus capable of causing superficial infection in the mouth (thrush) or vagina and on the skin.

candidiasis Infection of skin and mucous membranes with the yeastlike fungus *Candida albicans*. Also, *candidosis*.

carbohydrate One of three basic food types, it is the source of energy in the diet which is consumed in the form of starches and sugars.

carbuncle A spreading lesion made up of furuncles communicating by subcutaneous passages.

carcinoembryonic antigen (CEA) Not a reliable diagnostic indicator of colon cancer, but useful in watching for recurrence or metastatic disease after surgery.

carcinoma A malignant tumor arising from epithelial cells.

cardiac catheterization A procedure that involves passing a flexible catheter through the femoral artery and into the heart to measure pressures within the heart's chambers. Dye is then injected to show patency or obstruction of the coronary arteries.

cardiomegaly Enlargement of the heart.

cardiopulmonary resuscitation (CPR) The use of external compression of the heart coupled with breathing techniques to revive a victim whose heart and respirations have stopped.

carotid endarterectomy Removal of hardened plaque from an obstructed carotid artery.

carpopedal spasm Painful cramps of wrists and ankles.

catatonic schizophrenia Statue-like posturing, rigidity, or stupor.

catheterized specimen Obtained by urethral catheter.

causalgia Burning or stinging due to irritation or inflammation of nerves.

CBC (complete blood count) A group of blood tests, including counts of red blood cells, white blood cells, and platelets; a differential count of the various types of white blood cells; and a determination of hemoglobin and hematocrit.

cellulitis A type of infection occurring in soft tissues, including the skin, whose cardinal features are diffuse and spreading tissue swelling, redness, pain, and fever; often caused by streptococci.

cervical Pertaining to the neck or to the uterine cervix.

cesarean section Removal of the fetus (usually term or near-term) surgically though an incision in the abdomen and uterus.

Chaddock reflex Extension of the great toe elicited by tapping the ankle behind the lateral malleolus, a sign of disease or injury of a corticospinal tract.

chandelier sign The term fancifully implies that the pain on the physician's palpation of the uterine adnexa causes the patient to leap into the air and cling to the chandelier.

cheilosis Chapping and fissuring of lips.

chemosis Marked watery edema and bulging of the conjunctiva.

chem-7 Seven different blood chemistry tests.

chest x-ray (CXR) X-rays of the chest are taken to assess the clarity of the lung fields. Milky or opaque shadows in the lung fields can denote edema or mucus secretions. An anterior-posterior (anteroposterior) (AP) film shows the lungs as the x-rays pass from the front of the body (anterior) to the back (posterior). A posterior-anterior (posteroanterior) (PA) film shows the lungs as the x-rays pass from the back of the body to the front.

Chlamydia trachomatis A gram-negative intracellular bacterium that causes sexually transmitted infections of the genital tract and other types of infection.

chocolate agar A culture medium containing blood which, when autoclaved, turns chocolate brown. It is used to culture *Neisseria gonorrhoeae* and *Haemophilus influenzae*.

choked disk Edema of the optic disk due to increased intracranial pressure caused by intracranial hemorrhage, neoplasm, or disturbance of cerebrospinal fluid circulation.

cholecystectomy Surgical removal of the gallbladder. It can be done either through an open incision or through minimally invasive laparoscopy.

cholecystitis Inflammation of the gallbladder.

cholesterol, serum A lipid (fatty) material formed in the liver and transported in the blood, which serves as a building block for various hormones and other substances. Elevation of serum cholesterol, which is usually due to an inherited disturbance of lipid metabolism, is associated with increased risk of atherosclerosis. See *HDL, LDL, VLD.*

cholesteatoma A benign but locally invasive growth of the tympanic membrane caused by prolonged negative pressure (partial vacuum) in the middle ear.

chorea Rapid, jerky, purposeless involuntary movements of one or several muscle groups.

Chvostek test, sign Twitching of the face after percussion over the facial nerve in front of the ear, a sign of latent tetany due to hypocalcemia.

cicatrix (scar) A zone of fibrous tissue occurring at the site of a healed injury or inflammatory or destructive lesion extending into the dermis.

cine (for cinematograph) view A moving picture of the cardiac cycle, constructed from individual frames, each of which is a composite image of one point in the cardiac cycle obtained by cardiac gating.

client The recipient of psychotherapy; a term preferred to "patient" when the therapist is not a physician.

client-centered therapy A form of psychotherapy in which the client is encouraged, with a minimum of direction by the therapist, to discover the sources of distressing mental symptoms and means of resolving them.

clinical pathology Refers to the laboratory examination of bodily fluids and waste products such as blood, spinal fluid, urine, and feces.

CLO (*Campylobacter*-like organism) test To detect *H. pylori* in acid peptic disease.

clotting factors See *factors, blood clotting.*

clotting time The time needed for a clot to form in a tube of freshly drawn blood under standard conditions. The Lee-White method is the one most often used.

clubbing Club-shaped deformity of fingertips, seen in chronic pulmonary disease.

coags Slang term for *coagulation studies.*

cobblestoning Coarsely granular appearance of the conjunctiva.

Coca-Cola urine Urine of smoky brown color often indicates the presence of hemolyzed blood.

cognitive therapy A form of psychotherapy based on promoting the client's rational understanding of the source of distressing emotions, thought patterns, and undesirable behaviors, and correction of these by adoption of more mature, balanced, and realistic attitudes.

colectomy Surgical excision of part or all of the colon.

colic Sharp, crampy pains.

collateral vessels Vascular channels newly formed from existing ones to maintain the circulation of a tissue or organ whose normal blood supply has been impaired by disease or injury.

collecting system The nonexcretory portions of the kidney, which collect newly formed urine and conduct it to the ureter; the minor and major calices and the renal pelvis.

coloboma (iridis) A congenital defect in the iris, in which a wedge-shaped segment is absent, giving a keyhole appearance to the pupil; similar defects are created by certain types of ocular surgery.

colon Term that can mean part or all of the large intestine.

colonoscopy Endoscopic procedure to view the colon using a flexible (fiberoptic) endoscope.

colostomy A surgically created opening from the colon to the abdominal wall, through which feces are passed rather than by the rectum; may be temporary or permanent.

colposcopy Examination of the cervix with an illuminated low-power microscope, which facilitates identification of suspicious cervical lesions requiring biopsy.

commissurotomy Surgical enlargement of the aperture of a stenotic heart valve, particularly the mitral, by stretching or cutting.

compensation (overcompensation) A mechanism by which one covers up a defect or weakness by exaggerating or overdeveloping some other property or faculty.

complete blood count See *CBC*.

complex seizure Impaired alertness or unconsciousness; sometimes with psychic symptoms or automatisms.

computed tomography (CT) scan Also *computerized axial tomography (CAT) scan*. An application of computer technology to diagnostic radiology. Instead of exposing a film after passing through the subject, x-rays are detected and recorded by a scintillation counter. The x-ray tube moves around the subject on a frame called a gantry, rotating through an arc and "cutting" across one plane of the subject. A series of scintillation counters are so placed that each detects the rays passing through the subject at a different angle. (Alternatively a single counter may rotate in perfect alignment with the x-ray source.) Data on the amount of x-ray that penetrates the subject at each angle are collected from the counters, digitized, stored, and analyzed by a minicomputer programmed to generate a cross-sectional image of the subject corresponding to the plane cut by the moving x-ray beam. Contrast medium may be injected into the circulation immediately before CT scanning. IV contrast enhances the sensitivity of CT scanning of certain structures and body regions and improves the visibility of some tumors.

coned-down view A study limited to a small area by the use of a cone that narrows and "focuses" the x-ray beam.

confabulation Invention of stories about one's past, often bizarre and complex, to fill in gaps left by amnesia; a typical feature of Korsakoff syndrome in chronic alcoholics.

conization of the cervix Removal of a cone of tissue from the cervix for microscopic examination.

consolidative process An abnormal process that increases the density of a tissue or region.

constipation Firm, difficult stools.

contiguous images A series of scans without intervals of unexamined tissue between them.

Coombs test, direct A test to determine whether the patient's red blood cells have become coated with an antiglobulin. The test is positive in newborns with hemolytic disease due to Rh incompatibility and in others with acquired hemolytic disease.

Coombs test, indirect A test to determine whether the patient's serum contains antiglobulin to red blood cells. This test is positive in the mother of an infant with hemolytic disease due to Rh incompatibility and in others with acquired hemolytic disease.

copper-wire or **silver-wire**. Appearance of narrowed arteries in the retina. Seen in some patients with arteriosclerosis in the funduscopic examination.

cor pulmonale Dilatation, hypertrophy, or failure of the right ventricle due to acute or chronic pulmonary disease.

coronary artery bypass graft (CABG) Surgical procedure done to bypass one or more occluded coronary arteries by using a vein graft (often from the leg).

correlate radiographic findings clinically Interpret x-ray appearance in light of the patient's medical history and objective findings on physical examination and laboratory testing.

corticosteroid Cortisol or aldosterone (hormones of the adrenal cortex), or any synthetic drug having similar effects.

coryza Common cold, including acute rhinitis.

cough May be variously described as brassy, bubbling, croupy, hacking, harsh, hollow, loose, metallic, nonproductive, productive, rasping, rattling, or wracking.

CPK (creatine phosphokinase).

CPR (cardiopulmonary resuscitation) The use of external compression of the heart coupled with breathing techniques to revive a victim whose heart and respirations have stopped.

craniectomy Surgical removal of part of the bone of the skull.

craniotomy Surgical incision into the cranium, which necessitates drilling a hole through the bone of the skull.

creatine phosphokinase (CPK) A serum enzyme that can be chemically distinguished into three isoenzymes or fractions: the BB isoenzyme is elevated in cerebral infarction, the MM in muscular dystrophy and muscle crush injury, and MB in myocardial infarction. When separated in the laboratory by electrophoresis, these isoenzymes appear as distinct bands in a visual display. Hence, the expression *MB band* is roughly synonymous with *MB isoenzyme*. Do not confuse *creatine* with *creatinine*.

Creutzfeldt-Jakob disease A degenerative disease of the cerebral cortex caused by a prion.

crepitant rale A fine crackling rale.

crepitus Rubbing, grating, grinding, or crunching sounds.

crossed (or contralateral) straight leg raising With the patient supine, the unaffected leg is held straight and flexed at the hip. If sciatica is present, the patient will experience pain in the opposite, affected side.

crust A hard, friable, irregular layer of dried blood, serum, pus, tissue debris, or any combination of these adherent to the surface of injured or inflamed skin; a scab.

cryoprobe A cryosurgical instrument containing a circulating refrigerant, which can be rapidly chilled so as to deliver subfreezing temperature to tissues.

cryosurgery The application of liquid nitrogen (at a temperature of -196 degrees Celsius) to destroy superficial skin lesions.

cryotherapy Local treatment of neoplasms or other lesions by freezing with liquid nitrogen or a cryoprobe.

CSF (cerebrospinal fluid) The fluid medium of the central nervous system (brain and spinal cord), which can be sampled by lumbar puncture (spinal tap) for chemical testing, cell counts, and culture.

cuffing, peribronchial Thickening of bronchial walls as seen on chest x-ray.

cul-de-sac Lowermost part of pelvic cavity, between uterus and rectum.

culdoscopy Endoscopic inspection of the cul-de-sac (pouch of Douglas), the lowermost part of the peritoneal cavity, which lies between the uterus and the rectum. The instrument is introduced vaginally under anesthesia.

culture Exudate, pus, crusts, or scrapings for bacteria, fungi, or viruses.

cupping of the disk The normal optic nerve head has a slight central depression (physiologic cupping). Increase in the depth of the cup occurs with increased intraocular pressure (glaucoma) or atrophy of the optic nerve.

curettage A surgical scraping.

cut A CT section or image; a scan.

cyanosis Bluish color of skin, particularly lips and nail beds, due to presence of excess unoxygenated blood in the circulation.

cyclothymia Abnormal lability of mood, which varies between excitement and depression without becoming severe enough to be called bipolar disorder.

cystocele Bulging of the urinary bladder through the anterior vaginal wall.

cytology Study of cells that have been detached from a surface for microscopic study, such as a Pap smear.

cytomegalovirus (CMV) A herpesvirus that is often not symptomatic but can cause infections, particularly virulent in persons with AIDS, resulting in CMV retinitis.

dark-field microscopy A microscopic technique using special lighting that makes it easier to identify *Treponema pallidum*, the organism that causes syphilis.

debridement Successive scraping away of dead skin down to viable tissue that bleeds, especially for burns.

decibel A measure of the loudness of sound; one tenth of a bel (named for Alexander Graham Bell).

decreased skin turgor Loss of normal consistency and fullness.

deep tendon reflexes Also called *muscle stretch reflexes*; occur in response to sudden stretching of a muscle, usually induced by tapping a tendon with a rubber-headed reflex hammer. Tendon reflexes are tested in several muscles of the upper and lower extremities, with comparison of the two sides.

deglutition mechanism The coordinated sequence of muscular contractions in the mouth, pharynx, and esophagus involved in normal swallowing, as demonstrated in a barium swallow or upper gastrointestinal series (UGI).

delusion A distorted belief or perception, such as thinking that one is a famous historical figure (Jesus, Napoleon) or that one is the object of persecution.

dementia Deterioration of mental function.

demineralization Reduction in the amount of calcium present in bone, due to disease or immobilization.

denial A mechanism by which one refuses to believe, remember, or accept an unpleasant fact or circumstance, such as a past painful experience or the fact of being ill.

densitometry Determination of variations in density (for example, bone density) by comparison with that of

another material or with a certain standard. See *dual photon densitometry*.

dependent edema Edema of the lower extremities, aggravated by the dependent (downward hanging) position.

dermatitis Inflammation of the skin.

dermatographism The property of abnormally sensitive skin by which strokes or writing with a pointed object are reproduced on the skin surface as raised red lines.

dermatosis A general term for any abnormal condition of the skin, but usually excluding inflammatory conditions, which are called dermatitis.

Diagnostic and Statistical Manual of Mental Disorders (DSM) A description and classification of mental disorders based on objective categories. Recognized as a diagnostic standard and widely used for reporting, coding, and statistical purposes, *DSM* is published by the American Psychiatric Association. The current (fourth) edition (*DSM-IV*) appeared in 1994.

diaphoresis Sweating.

diarrhea Abnormal frequency, urgency, and looseness of stools.

diascopy Inspection of red or purplish lesions through a transparent plastic or glass plate, which compresses the skin. If the color is due to dilated blood vessels, it blanches (fades) with compression; color due to deposition of pigment, including blood pigment, in tissues is not altered by surface pressure.

diener The morgue attendant.

differential white blood cell count A determination of the relative numbers of the six types of white blood cells normally found in peripheral blood. When the count is performed visually, a technician observes 100 white blood cells in a stained smear of whole blood and reports the number of each cell type found as a percent. The differential count can also be done electronically. The six types of white blood cells are segmented neutrophils (PMNs or segs), band neutrophils (bands, representing the immature form), eosinophils (eos), basophils (basos), lymphocytes (lymphs), and monocytes (monos).

digital clubbing Enlargement of fingertips with elevation of proximal parts of nails, due to chronic pulmonary disease.

dilatation and curettage (D&C) Scraping of the endometrium, after stretching of the cervix with graded dilators, to obtain specimen material for the diagnosis of endometrial disease. This procedure, performed under anesthesia (general, spinal, or intravenous), is also used therapeutically for various endometrial disorders.

diplopia Double vision; seeing two overlapping two-dimensional images instead of one three-dimensional image; may result from injury or disease of one or both eyes or from failure of fusion of images in the cerebral cortex, due to alcohol, drugs, fever, infection, neoplasm, or trauma.

discoid Consisting of small, flat plaques.

disorganized (hebephrenic) schizophrenia Severe breakdown of mental function and incongruous or silly behavior.

diverticulum An abnormal outpouching of a hollow organ such as the colon.

double-contrast technique A modification of the barium enema (BE) procedure. After the standard barium enema examination has been completed, the patient expels most of the barium, and the colon is then inflated with air. The coating of barium remaining on the surface may outline masses or defects not seen during the standard examination.

dual photon densitometry A quantitative assessment of a patient's bone density, and comparison with normal ranges for persons of the same age and sex.

Duke bleeding time See *bleeding time.*

dullness to percussion Muffling on percussion due to consolidation of lung tissue by infection or neoplasm, or to fluid in the pleural space.

duodenal bulb Onion-shaped dilatation of the duodenum immediately below its origin at the pylorus.

duodenal C-loop C-shaped loop formed by the duodenum as it courses around the head of the pancreas.

duodenal sweep The normal course of the duodenum, from the pylorus and around the head of the pancreas to the ligament of Treitz, as visualized with contrast medium in an upper GI series.

dysequilibrium Loss of balance sense; tendency to fall without support.

dysfunctional uterine bleeding Irregular, unpredictable menstrual flow (too frequent or too infrequent, too heavy or too light), or amenorrhea, occurring in the absence of pregnancy, infection, or neoplasm.

dysmenorrhea Pain occurring with menstruation, typically felt low in the pelvis and in the low back, and often severe. The lay term for dysmenorrhea is "menstrual cramps."

dyspareunia Pain in the vulva, vagina, or pelvis with sexual intercourse.

dysphagia Difficulty swallowing.

dysphoria A general feeling of mental or emotional discomfort.

dysplasia Cell abnormalities heralding eventual development of malignancy.

dyspnea Shortness of breath.

dyspareunia Pain with intercourse.

dysthymia A depressed mood, usually chronic or recurrent, that is not severe enough to be called major depression.

dysuria Pain in the urethra or vulva with urination.

early satiety Feeling that the stomach is full after only one or two mouthfuls of food.

eburnation Increased density of articular ends of bone.

ECG, EKG (electrocardiogram) A tracing of the electrical activity of the heart. An EKG traces the conduction of the electrical impulse generated by the SA node as it travels through the atria (P wave on the EKG) and through the ventricles (QRS complex on the EKG). Then, during the recovery period as the heart prepares to contract again, the T wave is evident on the EKG.

echo characteristics The frequency, intensity, and distribution of echoes produced by a structure or region ion ultrasound examination.

echo pattern The ultrasonographic appearance of a structure as seen on a visual display.

echocardiography A noninvasive diagnostic procedure in which an ultrasonic beam is directed at the heart and the returning echoes are recorded and analyzed; valuable for the measurement of cardiac chambers (wall thickness and cavity volume), assessment of ventricular function, and identification of valvular malfunction.

ectropion Eversion (turning outward) and drooping of the lower eyelid, exposing the conjunctival surface and allowing overflow of tears.

eczema An acute or chronic inflammation of the skin with itching, redness, blistering, weeping, crusting, and scaling.

edema Swelling due to the presence of fluid in tissue spaces.

effacement Abnormal flattening of the contour of a structure.

effusion An abnormal accumulation of fluid in a body cavity, such as the pericardium.

ejection fraction (EF) The percentage of the blood contained in a ventricle at the end of diastole that is ejected from the heart during the succeeding systole, normally 65% or higher.

electroconvulsive (electroshock) therapy Delivery of controlled electric shocks to the brain to alter electrochemical function, primarily in depression. The treatment, administered only by a physician, causes convulsions and loss of consciousness; the patient awakens in a state of disorientation. Several treatment sessions may be necessary before improvement is noted.

electrodesiccation See *fulguration.*

electroencephalography (EEG) Measurement and recording of electrical activity of the brain. Electrodes are attached with fine needles to standard sites on the scalp and the record is made on a strip of moving paper. Tracings are usually made after administration of a short-acting sedative (with the subject asleep, if possible). The effects of hyperventilation and of photic stimulation (exposure to a flashing light) are recorded also. The EEG is particularly useful in identifying and classifying seizure disorders.

electrolytes, sweat Sodium and chloride ions in the sweat, increased in persons with cystic fibrosis.

electromyogram (EMG) Test to determine the response pattern of muscles when stimulated by an electrical impulse from a needle electrode inserted into the muscle.

electron microscopy The study of specimens with an electron microscope.

electrophysiologic studies Measurement of electrical activity in nerves and muscles. Electromyography (EMG) involves insertion of fine needle electrodes into voluntary muscles. Nerve conduction velocity (NCV) is measured by timing the passage of nerve impulses between a stimulating and a recording electrode, which are a precisely measured distance apart.

embolism Obstruction of a blood vessel by a detached blood clot, air, fat, or injected material.

encephalopathy Any organic disease or damage of the brain, particularly the cerebral cortex, that causes impairment of mental or physical functioning; often due to degenerative diseases (Alzheimer disease, Creutzfeldt-Jakob disease) or chemical intoxications (alcohol, lead).

endocrine gland A gland that secretes internally (directly into the circulation): pituitary, thyroid, adrenal, pancreas, gonads.

endolymph The fluid medium contained in the inner ear.

endometriosis The presence of abnormal implants of endometrial tissue outside the uterus, chiefly involving the pelvic peritoneum, ovaries, and lower bowel.

endorectal Inside the rectum; said of diagnostic or therapeutic instruments or procedures.

endoscopy Insertion of a tube with a light source into a body cavity to view and often to biopsy internal structures. Common types of endoscopies are esophagoscopy, gastroscopy, gastroduodenoscopy, anoscopy, sigmoidoscopy, and colonoscopy.

enterocolitis Inflammatory disease of both the small and large intestines.

entropion Inward turning of the margin of the lower eyelid, often so that the lower lashes touch the eyeball.

eos Brief form for *eosinophils*.

epiglottis A flexible valve that closes the respiratory passage during swallowing of food or drink.

epiphora Chronic overflow of tears from the lower eyelid onto the cheek; may be due to blockage of the nasolacrimal duct or to deformity of the lower lid (ectropion).

epiphysis The expanded articular end of a long bone.

erectile dysfunction (impotence) Failure of the penis to become erect after sexual stimulation, or to maintain sufficient rigidity for intercourse.

erosion A surface defect in the epidermis produced by rubbing or scratching.

eructation Belching; burping.

erythrocyte A mature red blood cell. Compare *reticulocyte*.

erythrocyte sedimentation rate (ESR, sed rate) The rate at which red blood cells settle to the bottom of a specimen of whole blood that has been treated with anticoagulant. The rate is expressed in millimeters per hour (mm/h), as measured in a standard glass column. Elevation of the sedimentation rate occurs in various inflammatory and malignant diseases but is diagnostic of none. An acceptable brief form is *sed rate*.

eschar The crust that forms on a burn.

esophageal dysmotility Seen on upper GI series; abnormality in the strength or coordination of peristaltic movements in the esophagus.

esophageal hiatus hernia Weakness or dilatation of the opening in the diaphragm where the esophagus passes through, with herniation of part or all of the stomach into the thorax; often asymptomatic.

esophagogastroduodenoscopy (EGD) Endoscopic procedure to view the esophagus, stomach, and duodenum.

esophoria Inward deviation of one eye.

essential amino acids Amino acids that cannot be made in the body and must be obtained from diet.

estradiol The principal estrogen (female hormone) secreted by the ovary. Measurement of its level in serum gives an estimate of ovarian function.

euthyroid Normal thyroid.

exacerbation An increase in the severity of a disease, particularly when occurring after a period of improvement (remission).

examination of stool For occult blood, fat, pathogens (bacteria, fungi, parasites), abnormal constituents.

excisional biopsy The surgical removal of an entire tumor, lesion, or diseased organ from a living patient.

excoriation Abrasion of the epidermal surface by scratching.

exercise stress test Test during which the patient exercises on a treadmill to stress the heart and reproduce symptoms of angina and EKG changes.

exophoria Outward deviation of one eye.

exophthalmos Abnormal bulging of the eye between the lids; may be due to local disease (orbital cellulitis or neoplasm) or (when bilateral) to systemic disease (Graves disease).

exploratory laparotomy Inspection of the abdominal and pelvic cavities through an incision in the abdominal wall.

external auditory meatus A tube that conducts sound waves from the pinna to the middle ear.

extra-articular Affecting or pertaining to structures other than joints.

extracorporeal shock wave lithotripsy (ESWL) Can be used to break renal calculi into fragments, which then pass with the urine.

extravasation of contrast Leakage of contrast medium from the structure into which it is injected through a perforation or other abnormal orifice.

exudate A material deposited in or on tissues as a result of inflammation or degeneration and consisting of protein-rich fluid, inflammatory cells, and tissue debris.

factors, blood clotting Substances present in the blood that participate in the clotting process.
Factor I fibrinogen
Factor II prothrombin
Factor III tissue thromboplastin
Factor IV calcium
Factor V labile factor (proaccelerin)
Factor VI (term not in current use)
Factor VII stable factor (proconvertin)
Factor VIII antihemophilic globulin (AHG)
Factor IX Christmas factor
Factor X Stuart-Prower factor
Factor XI plasma thromboplastin antecedent
Factor XII Hageman factor
Factor XIII fibrin-stabilizing factor

family therapy Psychotherapy that treats the family as a unit and seeks to promote understanding and correction of pathologic attitudes and relationships among members of the unit.

fasciculations Repeated twitching of small groups of voluntary muscle fibers.

fasting blood sugar (FBS) Determination of serum glucose in a specimen drawn from a patient who has been fasting for several hours, usually overnight.

fat One of three basic food types, also called lipid. It is an oily or greasy substance built up of fatty acids (long, straight-chain organic acids).

fecalith Stonelike mass of hardened feces.

femoral-popliteal bypass Implantation of a vessel graft (real or artificial) into the femoral and popliteal arteries to bypass one or more blockages.

FEV$_1$ (forced expiratory volume in one second) The amount of air that can be forcefully exhaled in one second following maximum inspiration.

fibrillation Rapid, random, ineffectual twitching of cardiac muscle, instead of normal regular systolic contractions, due usually to metabolic or coronary vascular disease; whereas atrial fibrillation can continue for years without serious impairment of health, ventricular fibrillation is rapidly fatal.

filling defect A zone within a tubular structure that is not filled by injected contrast medium (usually a tumor or abnormal mass).

fine-needle aspiration A technique used to remove cells by suction from certain structures such as the prostate, subcutaneous lymph nodes and other neck masses, and breast masses.

finger-to-nose test The patient extends the arms outward laterally, closes the eyes, and tries to touch the finger to the nose. Tests coordination.

FiO$_2$ (fractional inspired oxygen or inspired flow of oxygen). Note the lowercase *i*.

first-pass view An image or set of images obtained immediately after injection of radionuclide into the circulation, when its concentration in the blood pool is at its highest.

fissure A linear defect or crack in the continuity of the epidermis.

fistula Abnormal passage or communication between organs, or from an organ through to the outside surface of the body.

Fitz-Hugh–Curtis syndrome Localized peritonitis in the region of the liver, due to chlamydia or gonococcus.

5'-nucleotidase (pronounced "five prime nucleotidase") A serum enzyme whose level increases in biliary obstruction. Testing for this enzyme helps to distinguish liver disease from bone disease as possible causes of elevated serum alkaline phosphatase.

fixation device See *internal fixation device*.

fixative A fluid used to arrest the process of decomposition that begins almost at once in devitalized tissue, to kill bacteria and fungi in or on the specimen, and to begin hardening the tissue to facilitate preparation for microscopic study.

flaccidity Absence of muscle tone and absence of reflexes.

flare and cell Diminished clarity of the aqueous humor due to protein leakage from the iris; swirls of inflammatory cells in the anterior chamber due to inflammation.

flatulence Excessive intestinal gas.

fluctuancy The sensation of contained fluid on palpation.

forensic pathology Involves the application of clinical and anatomical pathology to certain issues in civil and criminal law.

forward failure Inability of the heart to pump blood at a volume that is adequate for the needs of tissues.

free air Air or gas in a body cavity where it does not belong, usually after escape from the GI tract.

friable Crumbly; fragmenting or bleeding easily on touch or manipulation; said usually of diseased tissue.

frogleg view An x-ray of one or both hip joints for which the patient lies supine with thighs maximally abducted and externally rotated and knees flexed so as to bring the soles of the feet together.

frozen section Specimen that is quick-frozen so that it can be examined under the microscope.

FSH (follicle-stimulating hormone) A hormone secreted by the anterior pituitary gland that stimulates ovulation in women and spermatogenesis in men. Measurement of serum FSH is part of the evaluation of a patient for infertility or gonadal dysfunction.

FTA (fluorescent treponemal antibody) test An indirect immunofluorescence test, highly specific for syphilis.

fulguration The application of an electrical current to destroy superficial skin or mucosal lesions.

full-bladder technique An ultrasonographic examination of the pelvic region performed while the subject's bladder is distended with urine. This is done to improve the recognition of the bladder outline, which cannot be distinguished adequately when the bladder is empty.

full-column barium enema Barium enema examination in which the contrast medium is injected into the colon under full pressure, by elevation of the barium reservoir to the maximum safe height.

fundus The rear of the interior of the eye, consisting of the retina, its blood vessels, and the optic nerve head.

furuncle A deep, solitary abscess.

FVC (forced vital capacity) The total amount of air that can be exhaled forcefully following maximum inspiration.

gadolinium A nonradioactive metallic element that acts as a contrast agent in MRI studies by enhancing the signal of areas or tissues in which it is present.

gallop rhythm A cardiac rhythm that simulates the sound of a galloping horse on auscultation, usually due to the presence of a third or fourth heart sound, or both.

gangrene Tissue death due to compromise of blood supply.

Gardnerella vaginalis A gram-negative organism, formerly called *Haemophilus vaginalis*, which causes bacterial vaginosis.

gas density line A linear band of maximal radiolucency, representing or appearing to represent a narrow zone of air or gas.

gastrectomy Excision of a portion or all of the stomach.

gastroesophageal reflux Abnormal backflow of material from the stomach into the lower esophagus.

gastroscopy Endoscopic procedure to view the stomach.

gated view An image obtained by a technique synchronized with motions of the heart to eliminate blurring.

generalized seizure A seizure in which the entire cerebral cortex is involved.

glaucoma Any of several related disorders in which sustained elevation of increased intraocular pressure can lead to irreversible impairment of vision.

Gleason score A grading for prognosis in carcinoma of the prostate, on a scale of 1 through 5, from well differentiated to poorly differentiated. The test is done twice, in different areas, and the results added together (for example, 2+3 = 5 Gleason grade cancer). A combined score of 10, for example, would give a grave prognosis.

Glucometer A small, portable device from Bayer used to measure blood sugar.

glucose A 6-carbon sugar that is the most plentiful in the blood and the principal fuel of cellular energy metabolism.

glucose tolerance test (GTT) Measurements of blood sugar made at various intervals after ingestion of a standard carbohydrate meal.

glucose, urinary Should be negative. Glucose (sugar) in the urine usually indicates diabetes mellitus or other endocrine dysfunction.

glycosuria Glucose in the urine.

glycosylated hemoglobin (hemoglobin A1c) Measurement of the amount of glucose bound to the hemoglobin of red blood cells. Useful in monitoring long-term control of diabetes mellitus.

goiter Enlarged thyroid gland.

GPT (glutamic-pyruvic transaminase) An older name for *ALT (alanine transferase)*.

graft An organ or tissue transplanted from one part of the body to another, or from one person to another.

grand mal seizure See *tonic-clonic seizure.*

granulocytes White blood cells with conspicuous cytoplasmic granules. According to the staining properties of these granules, the cells are classified as neutrophils, eosinophils, and basophils.

gravida (G) Pregnant.

great vessels The major vascular trunks entering and leaving the heart: the superior and inferior venae cavae, the pulmonary arteries and veins, and the aorta.

gross description The report of the pathologist's findings after examining a specimen with the naked eye.

group therapy Psychotherapy administered to several persons at once, making use of sharing of perceptions, experiences, and feelings, group dynamics, and mutual understanding and support.

GTT (glucose tolerance test).

guilt A sense of having done wrong, of having failed to meet one's own or others' expectations or standards, or of being inferior or inadequate; as used in psychiatry and psychoanalysis, guilt is a distinct concept from moral guilt, which arises from deliberate violation of ethical principles or civil law.

Haemophilus vaginalis Older name for *Gardnerella vaginalis.*

hallucination A sensory experience, usually auditory or visual, without any physical basis—for example, seeing snakes floating in the air, or hearing voices urging one to do something.

H&E Hematoxylin and eosin, the most commonly used combination of stains in histology.

H&H Slang abbreviation for *hemoglobin and hematocrit.* The hemoglobin level is usually dictated first.

Hashimoto thyroiditis Intrinsic thyroid disease.

HCG (human chorionic gonadotropin) A hormone produced by the placenta and detected in various blood and urine tests for pregnancy. A more specific test detects only the beta subunit of this hormone, hence the term *beta HCG.*

Hct, HCT (hematocrit).

HDL (high-density lipoproteins).

headache Local or generalized, intermittent or constant; can result from infection, neoplasm, or hemorrhage within the cranium, obstruction to the flow of cerebrospinal fluid, trauma, or migraine.

heartburn Burning pain in the epigastrium or chest due to digestive disorders.

Heberden nodes Small firm nodules at the distal interphalangeal joints of the fingers in osteoarthritis.

heel-to-shin test With the patient standing straight, the heel of one foot is placed against the shin of the opposing leg. Tests coordination.

Helicobacter pylori A gram-negative organism formerly known as *Campylobacter pylori,* which is the cause of many peptic ulcers.

hematemesis Vomiting blood.

hematochezia Passage of blood from the rectum.

hematocrit (Hct, HCT) The percentage of a blood sample that consists of cells. The sample is spun in a centrifuge, which quickly drives all of the cells to the bottom of the tube. The length of the column of cells is expressed as a percent of the total length of the specimen. Red and white blood cells and platelets are all included, but red blood cells far outnumber the other formed elements.

hematocrit, central A hematocrit value determined by using a blood sample drawn from a central line catheter.

hemicolectomy Surgical excision of approximately half the colon.

Hemoccult Test for occult blood in the stool.

hemoglobin (Hgb, HGB) The oxygen-carrying complex of iron and protein in red blood cells. The hemoglobin level is reduced in anemia.

hemoglobin A1 Normal adult hemoglobin.

hemoglobin F Normal fetal hemoglobin, found also in adults with certain forms of anemia and leukemia.

hemoglobin S The abnormal hemoglobin found in the red blood cells of persons with sickle cell anemia.

hemoptysis Coughing up blood from respiratory passages.

hemorrhoidectomy Surgical excision of hemorrhoids (anal varicose veins).

hemorrhoids Anal varicose veins.

hepatic Referring to the liver.

hepatojugular reflux Increase in jugular venous distention when the liver is compressed.

hepatomegaly Enlargement of the liver.

hernia Protrusion of organ or tissue through an abnormal opening.

herniorrhaphy Surgical repair of a hernia.

herpes simplex virus (HSV), type 1 The herpesvirus that causes cold sores, pharyngitis, conjunctivitis, and some skin infections.

herpes simplex virus (HSV), type 2 The herpesvirus that causes genital herpes.

heterotropia A persistent deviation of one or both eyes, due to congenital ocular muscle weakness or imbalance.

high field strength scanner A magnetic resonance imaging device using a static magnetic field of maximal intensity.

high-density lipoproteins (HDL) Lipid-carrying serum proteins associated with a relatively low risk of cholesterol deposition in arteries.

histology The division of anatomy concerned with the microscopic study of tissues.

Holter monitoring A continuously recorded EKG as monitored by a portable EKG machine worn by the patient. This procedure is done on an outpatient basis for 24 hours to detect arrhythmias.

Homans sign Calf pain or tightness on passive dorsiflexion of the foot.

hormone A chemical messenger or mediator produced by a cell, tissue, or gland.

hot and cold testing Assessing the subject's ability to recognize hot and cold (via test tubes of hot and cold water) on various parts of the body surface (a sensory examination).

hydranencephaly A more severe form of microcephaly, with very little cerebral cortex remaining.

hyperactivity Restlessness, fidgeting, or squirming instead of sitting or standing still; excessive talking.

hypercalcemia Abnormally high level of calcium in the blood.

hyperglycemia Elevated blood glucose.

hyperkalemia Elevation of serum potassium.

hyperlucency Reduced resistance to passage of x-rays in lung tissue.

hypermenorrhea Abnormally high volume of menstrual discharge.

hyperplasia An increase in the number of cells in a tissue or organ.

hyperprolactinemia Abnormal elevation of prolactin.

hyperresonance Accentuation or increased hollowness of the percussion note due to a cavity within lung tissue or air in the pleural space.

hypertension Elevation of blood pressure.

hypertriglyceridemia Abnormally high level of triglycerides in the blood.

hypertrophic Overgrown, usually as a result of increase in the size of cells.

hypertrophy, cardiac Enlargement of a heart chamber due to increase in the thickness of its muscular wall.

hypesthesia Partial loss of sensation on one or more parts of the body surface.

hyphema Presence of blood in the anterior chamber of the eye.

hypnosis A technique in which the therapist places the client into a sleeplike trance in which outside stimuli are reduced to a minimum, the subconscious is more directly accessible, and the client is more susceptible to the influence of the therapist's suggestions and advice.

hypoaeration Abnormal reduction in the amount of air in lung tissue.

hypocalcemia Drop in serum calcium.

hypoglycemia Low level of blood glucose.

hypokinesis Abnormal reduction of mobility or motility; reduced contractile movement in one or both cardiac ventricles.

hypomenorrhea Abnormally low volume of menstrual discharge.

hypopyon Presence of pus in the anterior chamber.

hypotension Abnormally low blood pressure.

hypovolemia Reduced blood volume due to hemorrhage, dehydration, severe burns, ascites.

hypoxia Deficiency of oxygen in circulating blood.

hysterectomy Surgical removal of the uterus.

hysterosalpingogram A test to assess infertility in which radiopaque dye is injected into the uterus and uterine tubes, and x-rays are taken to show if the tubes are patent (clear) or obstructed.

Hz (hertz) A measure of the frequency of a vibration, particularly one producing sound; equivalent to one cycle (or double vibration) per second. The normal human ear can detect sounds ranging in pitch from 20 to 20,000 Hz.

identification A mental process whereby one takes on the properties or actions of another with whom an emotional tie exists (a boy walking and talking like his father; a woman dressing and behaving like a movie idol).

ileus Small bowel obstruction due to failure of peristalsis.

imaging studies Methods and techniques that render the internal structure of the body visible for diagnostic purposes, including x-ray and its varieties (fluoroscopy, CT, contrast studies), ultrasound, MRI, and nuclear imaging.

impaction Plugging of an orifice with a dense mass of some material, as cerumen in the external auditory meatus.

impingement Contact or pressure, generally abnormal, between two structures.

Implanon A single matchstick-like implant inserted into the upper arm as a contraceptive device; it releases a low dose of progestin into the body to block ovulation and thicken cervical mucus so that sperm cannot enter for up to three years.

impulsiveness Blurting out one's thoughts without adequate reflection, butting in front of others in waiting lines.

IMV (intermittent mandatory ventilation) Usually followed by a number, e.g., IMV of 5.

inattentiveness Short attention span, distractibility, inability to complete tasks undertaken, difficulty in following directions, tendency to lose personal articles, disregard for personal safety.

incisional biopsy Refers to the surgical removal of part of a tumor, lesion, or diseased organ for pathologic study.

incoordination Jerkiness and awkwardness in activities requiring smooth coordination of several muscles.

infarction Death of tissue due to interruption of its blood supply.

infiltrate Diffusion of inflammatory fluid or exudate into air cavities of the lung, or their walls, producing cloudiness of lung tissue on chest x-ray.

influenza An acute respiratory infection caused by any of several related viruses. Onset is abrupt, with fever, chills, myalgia, and cough. Inflammation of lower respiratory mucosa often progresses to pneumonitis, and bacterial superinfection is common.

insertion of collar button (ventilation) tubes Surgical placement of a tiny tube in the tympanic membrane to prevent chronic ear infections.

inspection of the throat With a focused light, often with the aid of a tongue depressor (tongue blade) to press the tongue out of the field of vision.

insulin pump A portable or implantable electronic device that delivers insulin from a reservoir through an indwelling subcutaneous catheter.

intention tremor Tremor occurring only during voluntary movement.

intercostal retractions Sucking in of muscles between ribs on inspiration.

internal fixation device A plate, pin, nail, or screw used to hold fracture fragments in place.

interrogation of pacemaker Downloading monitoring information stored on a chip in the pacemaker.

interstitial markings The radiographic appearance of lung tissue, as opposed to the appearance of air contained in the lung.

interval change Change in the radiographic appearance of a structure or lesion in the interval between two examinations.

intradermal test The injection between layers of the skin of a chemical or other type of substance known to produce an allergic reaction in sensitive individuals. This creates a wheal which is outlined with a pen and/or measured. The area is examined again in 30 minutes. A reddened, enlarged area at the site of the injection indicates a positive allergic reaction of that chemical or allergen.

intravenous pyelogram (IVP) The delineation of the urinary tract (renal pelves, ureters, bladder, and urethra) by means of a contrast agent injected intravenously and then excreted by the kidneys can reveal urinary obstruction, bleeding from the urinary tract, or abdominal trauma, and can identify and localize renal calculi as well as tumors or cysts both within the urinary tract and closely adjacent to it. Also called *intravenous urogram (IVU)* and *excretory urogram (XU)*.

introitus Entrance to the vaginal vault.

intussusception Prolapse of one part of the intestine into another.

involuntary guarding Spasm of abdominal muscles on palpation.

ischemia Inadequate blood supply.

isoenzyme Any of a group of enzymes having similar chemical effects but differing in structure and often arising from different sources in the body. See *CPK, LDH*.

IUD Intrauterine device. Examples: Mirena, a T-shaped device the size of a quarter, contains a type of progestin called levonorgestrel, which blocks sperm and alters the lining of the uterus; it provides protection for 5 years. ParaGard T 380A contains copper which kills sperm; it provides protection for 10 years. See also *Implanon implant*.

Janeway spots Painless red spots of palms and soles.

jaundice Discoloration of skin and sclerae by excessive bile pigment.

"jelling" Stiffness of the joints after prolonged inactivity (overnight).

Keith-Wagener-Barker classification Often used to grade (using Roman numerals I through IV) hypertensive retinopathy on funduscopic observations.

keloid A firm, nodular, irregular, often pigmented mass of fibrous tissue representing a hypertrophic scar.

keratic precipitates (KPs) Whitish deposits of inflammatory cells on the posterior surface of the cornea.

Kernig sign Inability to extend the knee when the thigh is flexed, a sign of meningitis.

ketoacidosis, diabetic Accumulation of ketone bodies in the body tissues and fluids from abnormal metabolization of fat.

ketones, serum A group of waste products resulting from abnormal metabolism of fat in uncontrolled diabetes mellitus. Ketones may be called ketone bodies or simply "acetone."

kidneys, ureters, bladder (KUB) film A plain film often done to screen for a stone in the urinary tract.

Koebner phenomenon Formation of lesions at sites of trauma.

KUB x-ray Plain x-ray to image the kidneys, bladder, and ureters (hence *KUB*).

kyphosis Forward hunching of the upper spine.

label To render a substance radioactive by incorporating a radionuclide in it; also, to cause a tissue or organ to take up radioactive material.

Lachman test Similar to the anterior drawer test, but performed with the patient's knee flexed only to 15 or 20 degrees. Also used to evaluate anterior cruciate ligament stability.

lacrimation (tearing) Increased flow of tears.

lactation Producing milk from the breasts.

lactic dehydrogenase See *LDH.*

laminectomy Surgical cutting through the posterior arch of one or more vertebrae and removal of herniated disk material.

laparoscopy Inspection of pelvic viscera through a laparoscope, a tubular instrument with illumination and magnification, inserted through a small incision in the abdominal wall. Surgical procedures can be performed through the instrument.

laryngopharynx The lowermost part of the throat.

larynx The voice box, containing the vocal cords and situated between the laryngopharynx (the lowermost part of the throat) and the trachea (windpipe).

Lasègue sign or test See *straight leg raising.*

laser ablation Eradication or destruction of a lesion with a laser.

LDH (lactic dehydrogenase). An isoenzyme. LDH1 is found in heart muscle; levels are increased after myocardial infarction. LDH2 is normally found in higher amounts in the serum than is LDH1. When the level of LDH1 surpasses that of LDH2, this is called a "flipped LDH."

LDL (low-density lipoproteins).

LE cell prep Lupus erythematosus cell test.

left shift See *shift to the left.*

Leopold maneuvers Palpation of the gravid uterus to determine the position in which the fetus lies within the uterus.

leukocytes White blood cells (WBCs).

LFTs (liver function tests).

libido Sexual desire or drive; often, more generally, the totality of pleasure-directed energy or activity.

lichenification Thickening, coarsening, and pigment change of skin due to chronic irritation, usually scratching.

lid lag Slowness of upper eyelids to move with eye movements.

lientery Passage of undigested food in stools.

light touch test Assessing the subject's ability to recognize a wisp of cotton drawn across the skin on various parts of the body surface (a sensory examination).

lipid Fat.

lipoproteins, serum Serum proteins that bind and transport lipid materials including cholesterol.

liver span The width of liver dullness between lung and bowel resonances.

livor mortis A purplish discoloration of the skin due to engorgement of capillaries that occurs shortly after death.

lobectomy Surgical removal of one lobe of a multilobed organ such as the liver, the thyroid gland, or a lung.

loculated effusion A collection of fluid in a body cavity whose distribution is limited by adjacent normal or abnormal structures.

long bones Hollow, with bone marrow in their cavities.

low-density lipoproteins (LDL) Lipid-carrying serum proteins associated with a relatively high risk of cholesterol deposition in arteries.

low-dose screen film technique A radiographic technique used in mammography to provide adequate imaging with less radiation than is used in conventional techniques.

lucent defect An abnormal zone of decreased resistance to x-rays.

lumbar Pertaining to the midback.

lumbar puncture (LP) Withdrawal of a specimen of cerebrospinal fluid from the subarachnoid space by inserting a needle between two vertebrae (usually L4 and L5) at the lower end of the spinal cord. A manometer (graduated glass tube) is used to measure the pressure of the fluid at the beginning of the procedure (opening pressure) and the end (closing pressure).

lumen The hollow interior of a vessel or other tubular structure.

luteinizing hormone (LH) A hormone produced by the anterior pituitary gland. In women it stimulates ovulation and formation of the corpus luteum, and in men it stimulates production of androgens in the testicle. Measurement of LH is part of the evaluation of a patient for infertility or gonadal dysfunction.

lymphocytosis Increase in the percentage of lymphocytes among white blood cells, and in their total number.

lymphoma Development of a malignant solid neoplasm of lymphoid tissue.

lytic (osteolytic) lesion A disease or abnormality resulting from or consisting of focal breakdown of bone, with reduction in density.

macule A flat patch or mark differing in color from surrounding skin.

magnetic resonance imaging (MRI) A method of obtaining cross-sectional "pictures" of the human body electronically. It is based on physical principles altogether different from those used in x-ray and ultrasonography.

malaise A vague sense of being unwell.

malar Pertaining to or situated on the cheeks.

malignant Tending to become worse; having the properties of anaplasia, invasion, and metastasis. Carcinoma is an example of malignancy.

mammogram, mammography Radiologic evaluation of the female breast, primarily to search for or evaluate abnormal masses that may be malignant. Special equipment and techniques have been devised to limit radiation exposure and enhance the diagnostic value of the procedure. Used as a screening test in large numbers of women, particularly those over age 40, to detect breast carcinomas.

Mantoux test Skin test for tuberculosis (**TB**). A needle is inserted intradermally, and a small amount of purified protein derivative (**PPD**) from the bacterium *Mycobacterium tuberculosis* is inserted under the skin. A Mantoux test is a definitive test and is usually done to confirm a previously positive tine test. A positive reaction means the patient has or has had tuberculosis.

Marshall-Marchetti-Krantz (MMK) procedure An operation for urinary stress incontinence, performed retropubically.

mass effect The radiographic appearance created by an abnormal mass in or adjacent to the area of study.

mass lesion Anything that occupies space within the body and is not normal tissue.

MB bands See *creatine phosphokinase.*

McBurney point About one third of the distance from the right anterior superior iliac spine to the umbilicus. It corresponds with the normal position of the appendix and is tender in acute appendicitis.

MCH (mean corpuscular hemoglobin) The average weight of hemoglobin per red blood cell, calculated from the hemoglobin level and the red blood cell count.

MCHC (mean corpuscular hemoglobin concentration) The average concentration of hemoglobin in red blood cells, calculated from the hemoglobin level and the hematocrit.

mcL (microliters) Used in cell counts to avoid using such abbreviations as μL or mm^3 or 10^3 because special characters and symbols used in medical transcripts do not transmit well electronically.

MCV (mean corpuscular volume) The average volume of a red blood cell, calculated from the hematocrit and the red blood cell count.

McMurray test or sign Extension of the knee from full flexion with the leg and foot externally rotated causes an audible or palpable snap in medial meniscus tear; extension with the leg and foot internally rotated causes a snap in lateral meniscus tear.

mechanism (also defense mechanism, ego-defensive mechanism, mental mechanism, unconscious mechanism) An automatic, unconscious mental process whereby repressed emotions (painful feelings, sexual urges) generate new beliefs or attitudes to protect the ego from a sense of guilt, inadequacy, or other negative feelings; see compensation, identification, projection, rationalization, repression, sublimation.

meconium Stool formed in the fetal intestine before birth.

melena Black stools (often due to the presence of blood).

menarche The onset of the first menstrual period.

Ménière disease Hearing loss, tinnitus, and vertigo resulting from nonsuppurative disease of the labyrinth with edema.

menometrorrhagia Excessive menstrual bleeding occurring both during menses and at irregular intervals.

menopause The cessation of regular menstrual periods.

menorrhagia Regularly occurring menstrual flow that is excessive in volume and lasts longer than a normal menstrual period.

metastasis Having the properties of recurrence and spreading to other sites in the body.

metrorrhagia Menstrual bleeding occurring at irregular but frequent intervals.

microcephaly Abnormally small, maldeveloped cerebral hemispheres, typically associated with mental and motor retardation.

microhematocrit A hematocrit measurement performed on a small specimen of blood obtained by finger stick and centrifuged in a capillary tube.

microscopic description The pathologist's findings upon examination of a specimen under the microscope.

microscopic examination of scrapings from the skin To identify fungal material, the mites of scabies, and distinctive kinds of scales; skin scrapings are usually treated with potassium hydroxide (KOH) and heat, which partially or completely dissolve human tissue but leave fungal elements unchanged.

midline shift Displacement of a structure that is normally seen at or near the midline of the body, such as the pineal gland or the trachea.

millimeters of mercury (mmHg).

miosis Sustained constriction of the pupil, which may be due to ocular or nervous system disease or to the effect of drugs (pilocarpine, morphine).

mittelschmerz Intermenstrual pain due to peritoneal irritation by a small volume of blood escaping from the ovary at the time of ovulation.

mmHg (millimeters of mercury).

monos Brief form for *monocytes.*

MUGA (multiple gated acquisition) scan A study of cardiac shape and dynamics in which a radionuclide is introduced into the circulation. Radioactive emissions from the heart are electronically monitored, stored, and analyzed, resulting in a composite scan consisting of a series of successive images all taken at the same point in the cardiac cycle.

multiaxial assessment As outlined in *DSM-IV*, provides for a comprehensive diagnostic formulation of mental illness that includes consideration of five distinct domains or axes.

multi-echo images On MRI, a series of spin-echo images obtained with various pulse sequences.

mural thrombus A localized clot adjacent to the infarcted area of ventricular wall.

murmur An abnormal sound, synchronous with the heartbeat, due to flow of blood through a valve or other passage in the heart. Murmurs are distinguished as to sound quality (harsh, blowing, high-pitched); timing (systolic, mid-systolic, late diastolic); loudness (grade 1 to 6 in one system, 1 to 4 in another; 1/6 = grade 1 on a scale of 1 to 6, a barely audible murmur); radiation (to apex, carotids, left axilla); where best heard (left sternal border, aortic valve area); effect of position (squatting, standing, recumbency); and effect of respiratory movements (inspiration, expiration, breath-holding).

"musical chest" In asthma, rhonchi of many different pitches may be heard together.

mydriasis Sustained dilatation of the pupil, which may be due to ocular or nervous system disease or to the effect of drugs (atropine, cyclopentolate).

myelocytes White blood cells formed in bone marrow: neutrophils, basophils, eosinophils, and monocytes.

myelography Visualization of the spinal canal (the tubular enclosure of the spinal cord formed collectively by the vertebrae) by x-ray with contrast medium introduced into the subarachnoid space by lumbar puncture.

myoclonic seizures Repeated shocklike, often violent contractions in one or more muscle groups.

myoclonus Involuntary jerking or twitching of certain muscles or muscle groups.

myomectomy Surgical removal of small or solitary myomas.

myringotomy Surgical puncture of the tympanic membrane to drain fluid from the middle ear.

myxedema Abnormal swelling of the skin due to deficiency of thyroid hormone.

narcissism Extreme self-love; excessive preoccupation with oneself and one's own concerns and needs, to the exclusion of normal emotional ties with others.

nasal smear Examination of a stained smear of scrapings from the nasal mucosa for evidence of infection (neutrophilic leukocytes) or allergy (eosinophilic leukocytes).

needle biopsy A needle is passed through the skin directly into the organ to be studied, and an inner cutting needle slices and removes a core of tissue.

Neisseria gonorrhoeae The gram-negative diplococcus that causes gonorrhea.

nephrolithiasis Kidney stones. See also *urolithiasis.*

nephrostomy Draining urine from the renal pelvis.

nerve conduction velocity (NCV) Measured by timing the passage of nerve impulses between a stimulating and a recording electrode, which are a precisely measured distance apart.

neurosis A mental disorder in which the patient experiences, and gives evidence of, emotional distress, but remains in touch with reality at all times.

neurotransmitter A normal chemical substance produced in minute quantities by nerve tissue and involved in the transmission of electrical impulses from one nerve cell to another; the effect of a neurotransmitter may be to stimulate or inhibit the nerve cell on which it acts; well-known neurotransmitters include acetylcholine, dopamine, epinephrine, gamma-aminobutyric acid (GABA), norepinephrine, and serotonin.

neutrophil, segmented A mature neutrophil with a segmented or lobulated nucleus. Also called *polymorphonuclear leukocytes* or *polys* or *segs.*

nevus (1) A pigmented lesion of the skin. (2) A skin lesion present since birth (birthmark).

nocturia The need to rise from bed to urinate during the night.

NSAID Nonsteroidal anti-inflammatory drug.

nulliparity Never having borne a viable child.

nutrition The intake and use of foods by the body.

nyctalopia Marked reduction of visual acuity at night (that is, under conditions of near-darkness). Also called *night blindness.*

nystagmus A rhythmic back-and-forth movement of the eyes usually due to congenital abnormality or central nervous system disease.

obstipation Total inability to pass stool.

obstructive urinary symptoms Decreased force and caliber of urinary stream, hesitancy, intermittency.

occult Hidden; not obvious, but sometimes able to be inferred from indirect evidence.

occult blood Blood present in quantities too small to be detected by naked-eye observation but detected by microscopic or chemical examination.

ocular discharge A serous, mucous, or purulent material formed on conjunctival surfaces, often gluing the eyelids together and producing crusting of the eyelashes; usually due to infection or allergy.

odynophagia Pain on swallowing.

oligomenorrhea Infrequent or scanty menstrual bleeding.

oophorectomy Surgical removal of an ovary.

opacification An increase in the density of a tissue or region, with increased resistance to x-rays.

open reduction, internal fixation (ORIF) A surgical procedure to correct a fracture that requires alignment and fixation with a plate, pin, or screw. Also, **open reduction, external fixation (OREF).**

open-mouth odontoid view A view of the odontoid process of the second cervical vertebra, for which the x-ray beam is aimed through the patient's open mouth.

ophthalmoscope An instrument with a light source and a set of changeable lenses to enable the examiner to focus on the fundus regardless of refractive errors in the subject's lens.

optic neuritis Intrinsic eye disease.

origin of a vessel The commencement of a vessel as it branches off from a larger vessel.

orthopedic hardware Wires, pins, screws, plates, and other devices of metal or other material that are implanted in or attached to bone in the course of a surgical procedure.

O$_2$ saturation The amount of oxygen being carried by the hemoglobin, compared to the amount that could be carried, and expressed as a percent (100% being total saturation). When the slang form "O$_2$ sat" is dictated, it should be expanded.

Osler nodes Tender purplish lumps in fingers, toes.

osseous Bony.

osteophytes, osteophyte formation Outgrowths of bone from the surface.

otosclerosis Bony changes in inner ear structures (bony labyrinth, cochlea), sometimes also involving the stapes.

otoscope An instrument that directs a light into the ear through a conical speculum, and is equipped with a magnifying lens.

otoscopy Inspection of the external auditory meatus and tympanic membrane with an otoscope; mobility of the tympanic membrane can be assessed when the subject swallows or performs the Valsalva maneuver (or when, in children, the examiner blows a puff of air into the ear).

ovalocytosis Abnormal oval shape of red blood cells, seen in various congenital disorders of red blood cell formation, including elliptocytosis.

pacemaker implantation Placement of pacemaker electrodes to the heart to correct heart block or control persistent irregular rhythms.

pain in the eye May be a superficial irritation or scratchy feeling on the cornea or sclera (as from an abrasion or ulcer) or a deep, throbbing pain within the eyeball (as in acute glaucoma).

pain test Assessing the subject's ability to recognize a prick from a sterile needle on various parts of the body surface (a sensory examination).

palliative Directed to the relief of symptoms rather than the elimination of their cause.

palpitation(s) Various abnormal sensations accompanying heartbeat; unduly rapid heartbeat; noticeably irregular beat; a feeling that some or all heartbeats are unusually strong; a sense of missed beats; or intermittent flip-flop sensations in the heart.

Pap (Papanicolaou) smear Removal of superficial cells from the vagina and cervix for cytologic examination, to judge hormonal effect and to identify abnormal cell changes due to inflammation, infection, dysplasia, or actual malignancy. Specimens are taken from three areas: 1) the vaginal vault, with a flat wooden spatula; 2) the squamocolumnar junction (transition line between the squamous epithelium of the vagina and the columnar epithelium of the endocervical canal), with a specially shaped wooden spatula (Ayre spatula); 3) the endocervical canal, with a bristle brush to ensure sampling of columnar epithelial cells.

papilledema Swelling of the optic disk, as observed with an ophthalmoscope; usually due to increased intracranial pressure ("choked disk") (caused by intracranial hemorrhage, neoplasm, or disturbance of cerebrospinal fluid circulation) or intrinsic eye disease (optic neuritis). The disk appears edematous and perhaps injected, and the retinal vessels as they emerge from the swollen disk appear to be kinked ("stepping" of vessels).

papule A small elevated zone of skin.

para (P) Live birth.

paracentesis Removal of peritoneal fluid with a needle passed through the abdominal wall.

paralysis Complete loss of muscular function.

paranasal sinuses Cavities within the bones of the skull, somewhat variable in size and shape, and lined with mucosa like that of the nose.

paranoid schizophrenia Prominent delusions of persecution or grandeur, often reinforced by hallucinations.

parathyroidectomy Surgical removal of one or more of the parathyroid glands.

paresis Muscle weakness.

paresthesia A sense of tingling or prickling ("pins and needles") on a part of the body surface. The lay term "numbness" is applied indiscriminately to hypesthesia, anesthesia, and paresthesia.

paroxysmal Occurring in sudden attacks or seizures (paroxysms).

paroxysmal nocturnal dyspnea Sudden attacks of labored breathing awakening the patient from sleep.

partial saturation technique A magnetic resonance technique in which single excitation pulses are delivered to tissue at intervals equal to or shorter than T1.

partial seizure Seizure in which only part of one cerebral cortex is involved.

patch test The application to the skin of a piece of filter paper containing a chemical or other type of substance known to produce an allergic reaction in sensitive individuals. Many patches are taped to the skin and labeled. After 24-48 hours the skin underneath is examined. Reddened, raised areas of skin indicate a positive allergic reaction to that chemical or allergen.

pathologic reflexes Present only in neurological disorders, such as Babinski reflex or Chaddock reflex.

PCP (*Pneumocystis* pneumonia). Due to *Pneumocystis jiroveci* (formerly *P. carinii*).

PE (polyethylene) tubes Placed in the tympanic membrane(s) to aerate the middle ear(s) and allow for escape of purulent secretion.

percutaneous transluminal angioplasty Procedure used to dilate an occluded artery, usually a coronary artery, by passing a catheter (with a deflated balloon section) to the site of the occlusion and inflating the balloon to compress the obstruction and enlarge the lumen of the vessel.

perfusion Delivery of oxygen and nutrients to tissues by the circulatory system, with removal of carbon dioxide and other wastes.

peribronchial cuffing Thickening of bronchial walls by edema or fibrosis, as seen in asthma, emphysema, cardiac failure, and other acute and chronic respiratory and circulatory disorders.

pericarditis Inflammation of the pericardium, the membranous sac surrounding the heart.

peripheral edema Edema of the extremities.

peristaltic rushes Urgent-sounding series of squeaking or gurgling sounds occurring with overactive peristaltic movements.

peristaltic wave A wave of muscular contractions passing along a tubular organ, such as the intestine, by which its contents are advanced.

peritoneal lavage Injection of fluid through a needle passed through the abdominal wall, followed by its withdrawal and laboratory examination.

permanent section Prepared, stained, and fixed specimen that is ready for microscopic examination.

petechia (pl. **petechiae**) A very small spot of hemorrhage under the surface of skin or mucous membrane, usually multiple, due to a local or systemic disorder.

petit mal seizure (absence seizure) Characterized by brief loss of attention and perception.

pH A measure of the acidity or alkalinity of a substance. A pH of 7.0 indicates neutrality. Numbers above 7.0 indicate alkalinity, numbers below indicate acidity. The p is always a lowercase letter. When the term *pH* begins a sentence, insert the article *The* before it.

Phalen sign Reproduction of pain or paresthesia in carpal tunnel syndrome when both wrists are flexed with the hands firmly pressing one another back-to-back for 60 seconds.

pharmacotherapy Treatment with drugs, generally prescription drugs.

photophobia Aversion to bright light, which causes a sense of pain in the eye, usually because of irritability or spasm of the iris.

physiologic cupping The slight central depression normally seen in the optic nerve head.

pica Eating nonfood materials such as clay.

pinkeye Acute epidemic conjunctivitis.

pinna The cartilaginous appendage on either side of the head, which collects sound waves like a funnel.

"pins and needles" (paresthesia) A sense of tingling or prickling on a part of the body surface.

pit A small depression in the skin resulting from local atrophy or scarring after trauma or inflammation.

pitting edema Edema that retains the mark of the examiner's fingers after release of pressure.

pivot-shift test With the patient supine, the foot is held in the physician's hand. The physician then turns the foot inward while pushing on the outside of the knee with the opposite hand, at the same time flexing and extending the patient's leg. This test is also used to evaluate anterior cruciate ligament stability.

plain film A radiographic study performed without contrast medium.

plantar (not planter's) Pertaining to the sole of the foot.

plastic surgery Surgery concerned with the restoration, reconstruction, correction, or improvement in the shape and appearance of body structures that are defective, damaged, or misshapen by injury, disease, or growth and development.

platelets Noncellular formed elements in circulating blood, produced in bone marrow and active in blood coagulation. Also called *thrombocytes*.

play therapy A form of psychotherapy used with children, in which structured or unstructured play settings with dolls and other toys enable the therapist to identify and correct false or unhealthy attitudes and behavior patterns.

pleura A delicate serous membrane lining the thoracic cavity and covering the lungs.

pleural effusion An abnormal accumulation of inflammatory fluid in the pleural cavity.

pleural exudates Fluid higher in protein than transudates and also containing LDH.

pleural friction rub A creaking, grating, or rubbing sound caused by friction between inflamed pleural surfaces during breathing.

pleural or lung biopsy Either by percutaneous (needle) or open procedure.

pleural transudates Fluid relatively low in protein.

pleuritic chest pain Sharply localized, stabbing pain in the chest that is aggravated by taking a deep breath, and virtually abolished by breathholding. It typically results from irritation of the pleura due to pleurisy, pneumonia, pulmonary infarction, or chest wall injury.

PMNs (polymorphonuclear leukocytes).

pneumothorax Air in the pleural space.

pneumotympanometry Assessment of the mobility of the tympanic membrane by applying pressure to its outer surface with a device fitting tightly in the external meatus.

poikilocytosis An abnormally wide variation in the shapes of red blood cells as seen in a stained smear.

point of maximal intensity (PMI) The point on the chest wall where the impulse of the beating heart is most distinctly felt by the examiner's fingers.

pole of kidney The upper or lower extremity of a kidney.

polycythemia Increase in number of circulating red blood cells.

polydipsia Excessive thirst.

polymenorrhea Menstrual bleeding that occurs with abnormal frequency.

polymorphonuclear leukocytes (PMNs, polys) White blood cells with segmented or lobulated nuclei. An acceptable brief form is *polys*. The term is often used synonymously with *neutrophils*, although eosinophils and basophils are also polymorphonuclear leukocytes.

polyps Massive overgrowths of chronically inflamed mucosa.

polypectomy The surgical removal of outgrowths (polyps).

polyphagia Excessive hunger.

polys Brief form for *polymorphonuclear leukocytes.*

polyuria Excessive urination.

porencephaly One or more cysts or cavities in a cerebral hemisphere communicating with the ventricular system. There may be little or no neurologic impairment.

portable film An x-ray picture taken with movable equipment at the bedside or in the emergency department or operating room when it is not feasible to move the patient to the radiology department.

portacaval shunt Surgical procedure allowing portal vein blood to bypass the liver and empty directly into the inferior vena cava.

positron emission tomography (PET) A diagnostic imaging procedure that uses positron-emitting radioisotopes to assess the metabolic activity and physiologic function of organs and tissues rather than their anatomic structure; particularly useful in diagnosis of subtle cerebral and cardiac lesions.

post Short for *postmortem.*

posterior rhinoscopy Inspection of posterior nares with angled mirror placed in the oropharynx.

posterior sulcus The groove formed by the intersection of the diaphragm and the posterior thoracic wall, as seen in a lateral chest x-ray.

postictal state After awakening from seizure, subject is drowsy and amnesic for a variable period.

postprandial After meals.

postrenal azotemia Increase of nitrogenous wastes in the circulation due to obstruction of the outflow of urine from the kidney.

"powder burn" lesions on peritoneal surfaces Endometrial implants appearing as hemorrhagic cysts.

PPD test See *Mantoux test, tine test.*

precordial In front of the heart.

pregnancy test See *HCG.*

prerenal azotemia Increase of nitrogenous wastes in the circulation due to reduction of renal blood flow.

pressured speech Rapid, strained speech as if the subject's mouth can't keep up with the flow of thoughts.

presyncope Feeling dizzy, light-headed, and about to faint.

primary amenorrhea Failure of menses to start at puberty (by age 14-16).

probe Ultrasound transducer.

production of sputum Phlegm from the respiratory passages. Can be watery, viscous, or purulent.

projection A mechanism whereby one unconsciously attributes one's own thoughts and attitudes (usually negative or unpleasant) to others as a means of dealing with a sense of guilt or inadequacy.

proprioception test Tested by having the subject report whether a toe or finger is moved up or down by the examiner.

prostate specific antigen (PSA) Blood test to screen for prostatic carcinoma.

protein One of three basic food types, made up of long strands of amino acids. Proteins are responsible for maintenance and repair of tissues and organs, and for production of intracellular enzymes, hormones, and other substances.

proteinuria Protein in the urine.

pruritus, pruritic Itching.

pseudocysts Pockets of inflammatory fluid and debris between the pancreas and surrounding tissues.

pseudomembranous enterocolitis Due to toxin-producing *Clostridium difficile*, often following treatment with antibiotics that kill normal intestinal flora.

psyche A vague term roughly equivalent to "mind."

psychiatry The branch of medicine concerned with the diagnosis and treatment of mental disorders; all psychiatrists are physicians.

psychoanalysis A school of clinical psychology founded by Sigmund Freud and based on lengthy, searching analysis of the patient's mental life, including particularly the content of the subconscious, which can be made manifest by hypnosis, dream interpretation, free association (nondirected reflections voiced by the patient), and other methods; many psychiatrists are psychoanalysts, but not all psychoanalysts are psychiatrists (physicians).

psychodrama A type of group therapy in which clients resolve conflicts and distressing emotional states by acting out their fantasies and fears in the setting of a dramatic performance before an audience of fellow clients.

psychology Broadly, the study of all mental processes and functions (perception, memory, judgment, learning ability, mood, social interaction, communication, and others). Clinical psychology is a professional discipline concerned with the nonmedical treatment of mental disorders; a clinical psychologist ordinarily does not hold a medical degree.

psychomotor retardation Delayed development in muscle strength and coordination and impairment in the ability to understand and learn.

psychosis A mental disorder in which, in addition to emotional distress, the patient experiences a break with reality, manifested by delusions, hallucinations, and grossly bizarre or socially inappropriate behavior.

psychotherapy Any method or technique, except the administration of medicines, used in the treatment of mental disorders.

PTCA (percutaneous transluminal coronary angioplasty).

PT, pro time (prothrombin time) The time required for a clot to form in blood treated with certain reagents. The result may be reported as both a time (in seconds) and a percent of normal prothrombin activity as detected by the same test in a control. The prothrombin time is prolonged in deficiency of certain coagulation factors and after treatment with heparin or coumarin anticoagulants.

ptosis Drooping of an upper eyelid that cannot be fully corrected by voluntary effort. Adjective: ptotic.

PT/PTT Prothrombin time and partial thromboplastin time.

PTT (partial thromboplastin time) The time required for a clot to form in blood treated with certain reagents. Abnormal prolongation of this time occurs in deficiency of various coagulation factors and after treatment with heparin.

pulmonary function tests (PFTs) To measure the rate and volume of gas exchange in the respiratory system by means of finely calibrated instruments.

pulmonary vascular markings As seen on chest x-ray, the normal radiographic appearance of the branches of the pulmonary arteries and veins about the hila of the lungs.

pulmonary vascular redistribution Increased prominence of upper pulmonary vessels and reduced prominence of lower pulmonary vessels at the lung hila in left ventricular failure and other disturbances of circulatory dynamics.

pulse The heartbeat, and by extension the rate of heartbeat, as measured at the wrist (radial pulse), the cardiac apex (apical pulse), or elsewhere.

purulent Containing or consisting of pus.

pyloroplasty Incision of the pylorus and reconstruction of the pyloric channel to relieve pyloric obstruction.

pyoderma General term for any purulent (pus-forming) infection of the skin.

quadriceps exercises Repeatedly bringing the knee into full extension, with tensing of the muscles of the front of the thigh.

quadriceps femoris muscle The large four-headed muscle on the front of the thigh that extends the knee joint.

radical mastectomy Removal of the entire breast as well as surrounding and underlying tissues and axillary lymph nodes.

RA test Rheumatoid arthritis test. See *rheumatoid factor*.

radiolucent Offering relatively little resistance to x-rays (by analogy with *translucent*).

radionuclide Radioactive isotope; a species of atom that spontaneously emits radioactivity.

radionuclide scans The essence of any radioactive scan procedure is the introduction into the body of a radioactive substance whose distribution in tissues, vessels, or cavities can be detected and recorded by a device that senses radiation.

radiopaque Resisting penetration by x-rays.

rale An irregular discontinuous sound, like bubbling fluid, crackling paper, or popping corn. Rales are heard on auscultation of the lungs and are due to passage of air through fluid—mucus, pus, edema fluid, or blood—or to the sudden expansion of small air passages that have been plugged or sealed by mucus.

rapidly alternating movements test A test for coordination, this test has the patient perform rapid alternating movements of the hands or feet.

rasp, raspatory A surgical file.

rational therapy A form of treatment in which mental disorders, which are thought to result from misinformation, wrong belief systems, and distorted logic, are improved by the therapist's use of direct, positive teaching and advice.

rationalization A mental process of justifying some act or omission through logical reasoning or argumentation, usually as a means of reducing feelings of guilt or inadequacy.

RBCs (red blood cells) The most numerous cells of the blood, which carry oxygen from the lungs to the tissues, and carbon dioxide from the tissues to the lungs.

reality testing An individual's ability to perceive reality as it is, not as distorted by abnormal thought processes, disorders of perception, delusions, or hallucinations.

real-time examination Ultrasonographic examination performed by sweeping the ultrasound beam through the scan plane at a rapid rate, generating up to 30 images per second. The display of images at this frequency is in effect a motion picture, providing visualization of movement of internal structures as it actually occurs.

rebound tenderness Additional stab of pain when pressure on abdomen is released, often indicating peritoneal irritation.

reconstitution Maintenance of flow in an artery beyond an area of narrowing or obstruction by establishment of collateral circulation.

reconstruction study Generation of an image by computer processing of scan data.

rectocele Bulging of the rectum through the posterior vaginal wall.

rectovaginal exam With the patient in the lithotomy position, the examiner inserts one finger in the vagina and another in the rectum at the same time.

red blood cell count The number of red blood cells per cubic millimeter of blood, as counted by a technician using a microscope or by an electronic cell counter. The count may be reported either as a simple numeral (e.g., 5,300,000/mcL [microliter]) or as the product of a number less than ten and 10^6 (e.g., 5.3×10^6). The count may be dictated simply as 5.3 and may be so transcribed or may be expanded to 5,300,000.

red blood cells, nucleated Immature red blood cells, released from the bone marrow before disappearance of their nuclei. Mature RBCs have no nuclei.

red blood cell indices Measures of the volume and hemoglobin content of red blood cells, derived by calculating from the hemoglobin, hematocrit, and red blood cell count. The red cell indices are the MCV, MCH, and MCHC.

redness of the eye Due either to local inflammation and hyperemia of the conjunctiva or to hemorrhage in the anterior chamber.

reflex A muscular contraction occurring in response to a sensory stimulus.

Reiter syndrome Arthritis, conjunctivitis, mucocutaneous lesions.

releasing hormone Promotes release of a specific hormone into the circulation.

renal azotemia Parenchymal or intrinsic; disease of the kidney proper.

repression The mental process of thrusting out of consciousness impulses or desires that are perceived as incompatible with one's own standards or sense of fitness, and that therefore generate unpleasant emotions; repressed material occupies a large part of the subconscious.

resection Surgical removal.

residual schizophrenia History of schizophrenia but only mild, nonpsychotic residual impairment of mental function.

resolution The ability of an optical, radiographic, or other image-forming device to distinguish or separate two closely adjacent points in the subject. In CT, resolution is measured in lines per millimeter. The higher the resolution, the sharper and more faithful the image.

respiratory distress Indicated by increased effort to breathe, pursing of lips, and use of accessory muscles of respiration.

resting tremor Tremor occurring only when the affected muscles are not being used for purposeful activity.

reticulocyte An immature red blood cell whose cytoplasm contains an irregular network of degenerating nuclear material. An increase in the number of reticulocytes indicates increased red blood cell production in response to blood loss or hemolysis.

retinitis Inflammation of the retina, the light-sensitive membrane at the back of the eyeball.

rheumatoid factor (RF) An antibody present in the serum of patients with rheumatoid arthritis and other autoimmune disorders.

rhinitis Inflammation of the nasal mucous membrane.

rhinophyma Enlargement and deformity of the external nose, usually as a result of rosacea.

rhinoplasty Surgical correction of nasal deformities for functional or cosmetic purposes ("nose job").

rhinoscope An instrument for examining the interior of the nose.

rhonchus (pl. rhonchi) Whistling or honking sounds resulting from passage of air through a respiratory passage narrowed by bronchospasm (in asthma), swelling, thickened secretions, or tumor. Rhonchi vary widely in pitch and intensity; in asthma, rhonchi of many different pitches may be heard together ("musical chest").

rigor mortis Stiffening of the muscles that comes on within a few hours after death and passes off after another few hours.

Rinne test The sound of a vibrating tuning fork positioned so that the tines are near the pinna (air conduction) should be heard by the subject even after the sound sensed when the shank of the tuning fork is placed on the mastoid process behind the ear (bone conduction) can no longer be heard; when bone conduction is heard longer than air conduction in an ear with reduced hearing, the hearing loss is due to obstruction of the meatus or disease of the middle ear.

Romberg test Has the subject stand with feet together and eyes open, then eyes closed, to assess position sense in the trunk and legs.

Roth spots Retinal exudates.

RPR (rapid plasma reagin) Test for antibody to *Treponema pallidum*. Used in the diagnosis of syphilis.

runoff The flow of blood and contrast medium through the branches of an artery into which the medium has been injected.

sacral Pertaining to the sacrum, a wedge-shaped mass of bone at the lower end of the spine that represents the fusion of five vertebrae and articulates with the pelvic bones.

sacralization Abnormal bony fusion between the fifth lumbar vertebra and the sacrum.

salpingectomy Surgical removal of a uterine tube.

saucerization Radical surgical excision of infected bone.

scab See *crust*.

scale A flake of epidermis shed from the skin surface.

scar See *cicatrix*.

scintillating scotomas Transitory visual field defects.

scoliosis Lateral curvature of the spine.

scotoma A blind spot; a gap in the visual field of one or both eyes in which objects cannot be seen. A scotoma that appears identical in each eye is always due to a disease or condition of the central nervous system (for example, migraine headache). A scotoma may appear as a black hole or may show flashes or swirls of white or colored light.

scratch test The application, to a superficial scratch made in the skin, of a chemical or other type of substance known to produce an allergic reaction in sensitive individuals. Many scratches are made in the skin, and the area is examined again in 30 minutes. Reddened, raised areas of skin indicate a positive allergic reaction.

secondary amenorrhea Cessation of menses that have been normal in the past.

sections Small samples of representative tissue used by the pathologist for gross examination.

sed rate See *erythrocyte sedimentation rate*.

segs An acceptable brief form for *segmented neutrophils*.

seizures Sudden, transitory impairment of central nervous system function, with or without loss of consciousness, and with or without local or generalized tonic and clonic contractions of voluntary muscles.

sella turcica The saddle-shaped bony depression in which the pituitary gland rests.

semen analysis Examination of semen to determine the number, shape, and motility of spermatozoa as a part of an infertility evaluation.

sensitize To introduce radioactive material into a fluid, tissue, or space for purposes of performing a radioactive scan; essentially the same as label.

serial scans A series of scans made at regular intervals along one dimension of a body region.

serial sections Multiple slices of a specimen to provide a three-dimensional concept of a tissue or lesion.

serous gland One producing a thin, watery secretion, not containing mucus.

17-ketosteroids Urinary breakdown products of adrenal cortical hormones, increased in certain disorders of the adrenal gland.

SGOT (serum glutamic-oxaloacetic transaminase) An older name for *AST*.

SGPT (serum glutamic-pyruvic transaminase) An older name for *ALT*.

shave biopsy A thin layer of skin consisting mostly or entirely of epidermis is removed with a blade held approximately parallel to the surface.

shift to the left An increase in the relative number of immature neutrophils, as detected in a differential white blood count. The various types of cells were formerly recorded on forms arranged in columns, the more immature neutrophils being recorded at the extreme left of the form.

shock (precordial) An abnormally strong thrust applied to the chest wall by the beating heart, as detected by the examiner's fingers.

shortness of breath Feeling out of breath; breathlessness; difficulty catching one's breath.

sickle cell An abnormal red blood cell found in persons with sickle cell anemia; the cell assumes a sickle or crescent shape at reduced oxygen levels.

sickling An abnormal sickle or crescent shape observed in red blood cells on a blood smear.

signal intensity The strength of the signal or stream of radiofrequency energy emitted by tissue after an excitation pulse.

simple seizure No unconsciousness; local twitching or jerking; perception of flashing lights or other abnormal sensory phenomena.

Sjögren syndrome Symptom complex marked by keratoconjunctivitis sicca.

skip areas Intervening zones of normal mucosa on sigmoidoscopy and colonoscopy.

small bowel transit time The time required for swallowed contrast medium to pass through the small bowel and appear in the colon.

smear Material spread thinly over a microscopic slide.

smear and culture Microbiologic study of secretions or other materials from the cervix, vagina, urethra, rectum, or from superficial lesions, to identify causes of infection.

somatostatin A hormone that inhibits production and release of growth hormone.

sonogram See *ultrasound*.

sonolucent Offering relatively little resistance to ultrasound waves (as air or fluid) and hence generating few or no echoes.

sounds Clicking, popping, rubbing, grating.

spasm Sustained contraction, usually painful, of a muscle.

spasticity Tight muscles with resistance to manipulation and hyperactive reflexes.

SPECT (single photon emission computed tomography) A form of nuclear imaging using computer software to generate two- and three-dimensional images. Used to evaluate regional blood flow, assess disorders of the heart and lungs, and evaluate head injuries, seizure disorders, stroke, brain tumors, and dementia.

speculum An instrument for inspecting a body cavity or orifice, often equipped with a light source, a magnifying lens, or both.

spherocytosis Abnormal spherical shape of red blood cells as noted in a stained smear of whole blood on microscopic examination.

sphincterotomy through the scope Cutting the sphincter of Oddi, which is located in the second portion of the duodenum through which the pancreatic duct and the common bile duct enter the small intestine.

spina bifida A failure of closure of one or more vertebrae in the posterior midline, which may be associated with bulging of meninges (meningocele) or of spinal cord and meninges (meningomyelocele).

spinal tap See *lumbar puncture*.

spin-echo image An MRI obtained by the spin-echo technique. With this technique, T2 is determined indirectly, as a function of TE, the echo time.

spinnbarkeit When the estrogen level is high but the progesterone level is low (the conditions existing just before and just after ovulation), a specimen of cervical mucus can be drawn out into strings or strands several centimeters in length. This property is called *spinnbarkeit* (German, "ability to be drawn out into a string"). When both estrogen and progesterone are present in large amounts, cervical mucus loses this property, and attempts to draw it out into a string fail.

spirochete A spiral-shaped bacterium. The organisms that cause syphilis and Lyme disease are spirochetes.

splenectomy Surgical removal of the spleen, usually precipitated by splenic injury.

splenomegaly Enlargement of the spleen.

spline Flat nail that is placed across a fracture or osteotomy to hold it in place.

splitting Separation of the first or second heart sound, or both, into two distinctly audible components.

spondylolisthesis Forward displacement of one vertebra over another.

spondylolysis A congenital defect in the pars interarticularis of a lumbar vertebra (usually L5) that predisposes to spondylolisthesis.

spontaneous pneumothorax Sudden leakage of air from a lung into the pleural space.

spurring Formation of one or more jagged osteophytes, as in osteoarthritis.

sputum May be variously described as blood-streaked, bloody, clear, foul-tasting, frothy, gelatinous, green, purulent, putrid, ropy, rusty, viscid, viscous, watery, or yellow.

sputum examination For pathogenic organisms (by smear and culture), neoplastic cells, or other abnormal findings.

stabs Another name for *bands* (immature neutrophils). The German word *Stab* means *staff* or *rod*, referring to the unsegmented nucleus of an immature neutrophil.

stacked scans Same as contiguous images.

status asthmaticus Severe refractory asthma.

status epilepticus Series of grand mal seizures without waking intervals.

status post A Latin phrase meaning *state or condition after or following*. Sometimes *status* is omitted from the expression *status post* but is understood.

STD Sexually transmitted disease.

STD screen Sexually transmitted diseases screen.

steatorrhea Excessive amounts of fat in the feces.

stenosis Abnormal narrowing of a passage or vessel.

stereognosis test Test of the patient's ability to recognize an object by handling it.

stigma (pl. **stigmata**) A structural or functional peculiarity or abnormality that is characteristic of an inherited or acquired condition, and may be useful in its diagnosis.

stool for ova and parasites (O&P) Examination of stool for parasites or their ova (eggs).

strabismus A general term for any condition in which the direction of gaze is different in the two eyes, as noted by an observer.

straight leg raising With the patient supine, the leg is elevated with the knee straight to the point where pain is experienced in the back or leg itself, or dorsiflexion of the foot causes an increase in pain. This test is done to determine if nerve root irritation is present. Also known as *Lasègue sign* or *test*.

strandy infiltrate A pulmonic infiltrate that appears as strands or streaks of increased density.

strangulation Ischemia of the involved portion of bowel.

"strawberry cervix" Erythema of the cervix.

strep screen Faster than culture, but detecting only beta-hemolytic streptococci. *Strep* is an acceptable brief form for streptococcus.

stress cystogram A radiographic study of the bladder intended to demonstrate stress incontinence. Contrast medium is instilled into the bladder and films are taken while the subject coughs and bears down.

string sign Regional narrowing of the lumen of the bowel as shown on barium enema.

STS (serologic test for syphilis) A general term referring to any test used to identify syphilis by a serologic method.

subconscious (mind) Elements of one's personality (feelings, attitudes, prejudices, desires, behavior patterns) of which one is unaware; a general and somewhat vague term including but not always identical to what Freud called the unconscious (*Unbewusstsein*).

subcutaneous emphysema Air or gas in subcutaneous tissue.

subcutaneous fat line The radiographic appearance of the subcutaneous fat layer.

sublimation Diversion of sexual energy or impulses into higher or more socially acceptable activities.

suboptimal Not as good as might have been expected; usually referring to technical factors in an x-ray study, such as positioning, film quality, and patient cooperation.

suicidal ideation Thoughts of committing suicide as a relief from mental distress, without actual attempts at suicide.

sunrise view of the patella X-ray study of the knee region in which the patella is visualized above the distal femur and appears like a rising or setting sun.

superficial reflexes Muscle contractions in response to stroking the skin; those of the abdominal wall are tested as part of a complete neurologic examination.

surface coil In MRI, a simple flat coil placed on the surface of the body and used as a receiver.

swimmer's view An oblique view of the thoracic spine in which the arm nearer to the x-ray source hangs at the patient's side and the opposite arm is upraised.

syncope (fainting) Sudden loss of consciousness, usually transitory, due to circulatory or neurologic abnormality, including central nervous system intoxication or injury, but frequently the result of strong emotion in the absence of organic disease.

syncope Sudden loss of consciousness; fainting.

synovial membrane A delicate, highly vascular connective tissue that secretes a lubricating fluid in small amounts; surrounding a joint.

tachyarrhythmia A pulse that is both irregular and abnormally rapid.

tachycardia Rapid heart rate (over 100/min).

tachypnea Increased respiratory rate.

tactile fremitus Transmission of vocal vibrations to the examiner's hand on the chest wall.

tag Same as *label.*

tail of breast A wedge-shaped mass of normal breast tissue extending toward the axilla.

takeoff of a vessel The origin of a branch from a larger vessel, as demonstrated radiographically with injected contrast medium.

tandem walking test Tests the subject's ability to walk with one foot in front of the other in a straight line. A coordination test, often used by police officers to assess drivers for substance abuse.

tardive dyskinesia Irreversible neurologic disorder causing twitching and writhing movements, particularly in the lips and tongue.

target cell An abnormal red blood cell with a bull's-eye appearance due to flattening of the cell with a prominent spot of hemoglobin in the center.

TE (echo time) The interval between the first pulse in a spin echo examination and the appearance of the resulting echo.

technetium (Tc 99m) A synthetic radioisotope with wide applications in nuclear imaging. In a HIDA (hepatobiliary iminodiacetic acid) scan, an intravenously administered technetium compound outlines the biliary tract more precisely than is possible with conventional radiology or ultrasound. Other technetium compounds are used in scanning the scrotum to diagnose testicular torsion and in performing bone and other scans to identify local areas of inflammation such as abscesses or zones of osteomyelitis.

telangiectases Visible patches of dilated skin vessels.

telangiectatic Pertaining to telangiectasia; a permanent dilatation of small blood vessels (capillaries, arterioles, venules), visible through a skin or mucous surface.

tenesmus Straining at stool, usually without result and often painful.

TENS unit Transcutaneous electrical nerve stimulator, a device used in the treatment of chronic pain.

tenting of hemidiaphragm On chest x-ray, a distortion of the diaphragm by scarring, in which an up-pointing angular configuration (like a tent) replaces all or part of the normal curved contour of a hemidiaphragm.

tertiary contractions Aberrant contractions of the esophagus, occurring after the primary and secondary waves of normal swallowing.

test To locate specific tests in a medical dictionary, look under *test, sign, maneuver,* or under the name of the test itself listed alphabetically.

tetralogy of Fallot Pulmonary stenosis, ventricular septal defect, dextroposition of the aorta, and right ventricular hypertrophy.

T4, T$_4$ (thyroxine) Thyroid hormone.

Thayer-Martin agar A culture medium containing denatured blood and antibiotics, intended to facilitate the growth of *Neisseria gonorrhoeae.*

thenar The fleshy part of the palm proximal to the thumb and index finger.

therapeutic blood level Tests the amount of measurable drug in the serum. Many drugs have optimum levels where they are most effective (therapeutic range).

therapist One who treats; in mental health, anyone administering psychotherapy.

thoracic Pertaining to the chest.

thoracentesis Needle puncture of chest wall with aspiration of fluid by syringe.

thrill An abnormal sensation felt by the examiner over the heart when blood jets through an anomalous or narrowed orifice.

throat culture To identify bacterial pathogens.

thrombocytes See *platelets*.

thyroid panel A group of laboratory tests used to detect or identify disease of the thyroid gland.

thyroidectomy Surgical removal of the thyroid gland.

thyroid-stimulating hormone (TSH) Hormone secreted by the anterior pituitary gland that stimulates the thyroid gland and promotes its normal function.

thyroxine Principal hormone of the thyroid gland. Also called T4.

tibial plateau The flattened surface at the upper end of the anterior aspect of the tibia.

tic A rapid involuntary muscle twitch, typically recurrent and stereotyped, affecting one or several body areas.

tilt test Moving the patient from recumbent to erect position to measure a rise in pulse and drop in blood pressure.

time interval Fraction of a second.

tinea capitis Ringworm of the scalp.

tinea cruris Jock itch.

tinea pedis Athlete's foot.

tinea unguium Onychomycosis.

tinea versicolor Caused by *Malassezia furfur*, consists of variable numbers of white to tan macules with very fine scales.

tine test Skin test for tuberculosis. A multiple-puncture device is used to pierce the skin and insert a small amount of purified protein derivative (PPD) from the bacterium *Mycobacterium tuberculosis*. A positive reaction is confirmed by doing a Mantoux test. The four small blades used to puncture the skin are called tines because they resemble the tips or tines of a fork.

Tinel sign Shocklike pain when the volar aspect of the wrist is tapped; indicative of carpal tunnel syndrome.

TMJ Temporomandibular joint.

TNTC (too numerous to count). This usually refers to a very large number of red blood cells or white blood cells seen on microscopic examination of urine. Because any number higher than 15-20 cells per high-power field indicates significant hematuria or pyuria, an exact count of 50 or more cells would provide no additional useful information. Doctors frequently dictate simply *TNTC*.

T1 On MRI, the time it takes for protons to return to their orientation to a static magnetic field after an excitation pulse.

T1-weighted image On MRI, a spin-echo image generated by a pulse sequence using a short TR (0.6 seconds or less).

tonic-clonic seizure In the tonic phase, the victim becomes rigid, often cries out, loses consciousness, falls, stops breathing. In the clonic phase there is generalized muscular jerking; may bite tongue or lips, may be incontinent of urine or stool. Also, *grand mal seizure*.

tonsillectomy and adenoidectomy (T&A) Surgical removal of the palatine tonsils and adenoids in the throat due to chronic episodes of infection and hypertrophy.

tophi Nodular deposits of urate crystals with local inflammation, typical in gout.

topical Referring to a medicine applied directly to skin or mucous membrane.

torr A unit of pressure equal to 1.0 mmHg.

toxic dilatation Extreme dilatation of the colon, compounded by effect of bacterial toxins; a complication of ulcerative colitis.

TPI (*Treponema pallidum* immobilization) A diagnostic test for syphilis.

TR (repetition time) On MRI, the interval between one spin echo pulse sequence and the next.

transference The development, on the part of the client, of an emotional bond (positive or negative) with the therapist.

transrectal Said of a diagnostic or surgical procedure that is performed through the rectum.

treadmill stress test See *exercise stress test*.

tremor(s) Shaking of parts of the body supplied by voluntary muscles, principally the arms, forearms, and hands.

Treponema pallidum The spirochete that causes syphilis.

trichiasis A growing inward of some eyelash hairs, with resultant irritation of the eye.

Trichomonas vaginalis A protozoan parasite that causes vaginitis.

triglycerides, serum The level of fat in the serum, usually measured in the fasting state.

tropic hormone Stimulates the cells of a remote gland to produce its secretion.

Trousseau test, sign Spastic contraction of the hand after application of a constricting cuff to the arm, a sign of latent tetany.

T3, T₃ (triiodothyronine) Thyroid hormone.

T2 On MRI, the time it takes for protons to go out of phase after having been shifted in their orientation by an excitation pulse.

T2-weighted image On MRI, a spin-echo image generated by a pulse sequence using a long TR (2.0 seconds or more).

tubal ligation Surgical division of the uterine tubes to obtain sterility.

(tunica) intima The innermost layer or lining of an artery.

24-hour urine specimen Consists of all the urine passed by the patient during a 24-hour period.

two-point discrimination test Test of the patient's ability to distinguish two points close together on the skin.

tympanites Hollow percussion note due to distention of bowel with gas.

tympanocentesis Puncture of the tympanic membrane and withdrawal of fluid from the middle ear for examination, including culture.

tympanoplasty Surgical repair for chronic perforation of the tympanic membrane.

typed and cross-matched Blood for transfusion must be typed and then cross-matched (experimentally combined) with the prospective recipient's blood to avoid reactions due to incompatibility of bloods.

Tzanck smear A stained smear of material from a cutaneous or mucosal lesion, intended to identify changes due to viral infection from herpes simplex or varicella.

ulcer A cutaneous defect extending into the dermis.

ultrasonography (US) A means of visualizing internal structures by observing the effects they have on a beam of sound waves. The sound used for this procedure is at a higher frequency (pitch) than the human ear can detect. Ultrasound waves pass through air, gas, and fluid without being reflected. However, they bounce back from rigid structures such as bone and gallstones, creating an "echo" that can be detected by a receiver. Solid organs such as the liver and kidney partially reflect ultrasound waves in predictable patterns. Waves are also reflected from the interface between two structures. Ultrasonography might be compared to taking a flash photograph. Light from the flashbulb bounces off the subject and comes back to create an image on film of the surface contours of the subject. In ultrasonography, however, the echo must be converted electronically to a visible image before it can be interpreted. Sophisticated electronic equipment permits ultrasound scanning of a body region with generation of a two-dimensional picture of internal structures. In practice, the same device (a transducer) that generates the sound waves also acts as the receiver. Although it emits signals at a rate of 1000 per second, the transducer is actually functioning as a receiver 99.9% of the time.

undifferentiated schizophrenia Without defining features.

upper GI (UGI) series and small-bowel follow-through Barium sulfate is given orally to outline the esophagus, stomach, and duodenum on x-ray film. Films are taken over a period of time to visualize the barium as it moves through the small bowel.

uptake Absorption or concentration of a radionuclide by an organ or tissue.

uric acid, serum A breakdown product of purine metabolism, increased in gout and other disorders.

urolithiasis A general term for the formation or presence of calculi (stones, gravel) anywhere in the urinary tract. Most stones are formed in the kidneys (**nephrolithiasis**) but don't give trouble until they obstruct a ureter (**ureterolithiasis**) or reach the bladder and cause dysuria, bleeding, or obstruction.

Valsalva maneuver Attempt at forced expiration, with the lips and nostrils closed; this drives air into the auditory tubes unless they are obstructed.

valve replacement Excision and replacement of a valve of the heart because of stenosis or insufficiency.

vascular Pertaining to one or more blood vessels.

vasculitis Inflammation of blood vessels.

vasoconstrictor A medicine that constricts blood vessels, either when applied topically or through systemic action.

VDRL (Venereal Disease Research Laboratory) A serologic test for syphilis.

vector An animal (for example, a rat) that transmits a pathogenic organism from one host to another.

vein stripping Surgical removal of (usually) the saphenous leg vein and its branches to treat varicose veins.

venipuncture Insertion of a needle into a vein for the purpose of removing blood for testing, or to inject fluids, medicines, or diagnostic materials.

ventilation-perfusion (V-P) scan A nuclear scan so named because it studies both airflow (ventilation) and blood flow (perfusion) in the lungs. The purpose of this test is to look for evidence of a blood clot in the lungs, called a pulmonary embolus, that lowers oxygen levels, causes shortness of breath, and sometimes is fatal. *V-Q* is an incorrect abbreviation for *ventilation-perfusion*. The initials *V-Q* (Q = quotient) are used in mathematical equations that calculate airflow and blood flow.

ventricular aneurysm Extreme dilatation and thinning of the ventricle, with loss of contractile power.

ventricular ejection fraction That portion of the total volume of a ventricle that is ejected during ventricular contraction (systole); usually expressed as a percent rather than a fraction.

vertigo A subjective sense of spinning. Dysequilibrium and vertigo sometimes occur together, and both are indiscriminately referred to as dizziness by lay persons.

vesicle A small thin-walled sac containing clear fluid.

vibratory sense test Test of the patient's ability to sense the vibration of a tuning fork when the stem is placed on a bone near the surface, such as the elbow or the shin.

visual field defect See *scotoma*.

vitamin An organic compound normally present in many foods that the human body needs in trace amounts, usually to serve as boosters or catalysts in essential metabolic processes.

VLDL (very low-density lipoproteins).

volvulus Intestinal obstruction due to twisting or obstruction of the bowel.

washout phase Scintiscanning of the lungs at the conclusion of the inhalation phase of a lung scan, after an interval during which all inhaled radionuclide would be expected to have been exhaled.

WBC (white blood [cell] count) See *leukocytes* and *white blood cell count*.

WBCs (white blood cells) See *leukocytes* and *white blood cell count*.

Weber test A vibrating tuning fork placed against a bony surface of the head at the midline sends vibrations through the bones of the skull. These should be heard equally in the two ears; if there is hearing loss due to blockage of the external auditory meatus or to injury or disease of the middle ear, the tone of the fork will be heard louder in the affected ear; in hearing loss due to damage to the inner ear or acoustic nerve, however, the tone will be heard louder in the more normal ear.

Wechsler Adult Intelligence Scale (WAIS) A group of tests for assessment of intellectual functioning in adults.

Wechsler Intelligence Scale for Children (WISC) A group of tests for assessment of intellectual functioning in children ages 5 to 15.

Wechsler Memory Scale, Form 1 (WMS-1).

West Nile virus disease An infection of wild crows and jays transmitted by several species of mosquito. Human infection, first recognized in the U.S. as recently as 1999, has now spread throughout most of the contiguous states. The highest incidence of human infections occurs during the mosquito season (late spring, summer, and early fall).

wheal (weal, welt) The characteristic lesion of hives. A small zone of edema in skin, which may be red or white; wheals are typically multiple and appear and disappear abruptly.

wheezing Whistling sound made in breathing.

white blood cell count (WBC) (white count, white cell count) The number of white blood cells per cubic millimeter of blood, as counted by a technician using a microscope or by an electronic cell counter. The count may be reported as either a simple numeral (e.g., $7,200/mm^3$ or mcL [microliter]) or as the product of a small number and 10^3 (e.g., 7.2×10^3). In the latter case, the report may be dictated simply as 7.2 and may be so transcribed or may be expanded to 7,200.

Wood light An ultraviolet lamp with a filter that selects wavelengths under which certain funguses infecting skin or hair fluoresce brightly.

working orthopedic surgery film A radiographic study done during the course of an operation; for example, to monitor the reduction of a fracture or the placement of a fixation device.

xerophthalmia Abnormal dryness of the eye, usually due to decreased flow of tears.

x-ray To identify foreign bodies, masses, or abnormalities of the airway due to injury or disease.

yeast A one-celled fungus; often interchangeably used with *Candida albicans*.

Quick-Reference Word List

AAA (abdominal aortic aneurysm)

AAA (diagnostic arthroscopy, operative arthroscopy, and operative arthrotomy)

AAMT (American Association for Medical Transcription)

A&P (anterior and posterior) vaginal repair

ab, Ab (abortion)

abate

abdominoplasty

ABGs (arterial blood gases)

ablation

ablation of neuromata

ablative measures for VIN (vulvar intraepithelial neoplasia)

ABO (comprising types A, B, AB, and O) blood type system

abrasion

abscess

absorbable suture

abutting

a.c. (before meals)

Accu-Chek

Accupril

Accutane

Accuzyme

Ace bandage

Aceon

Achilles tendon

AcipHex

ACLS (advanced cardiac life support)

acne vulgaris

AcrySof intraocular lens

ACTH (adrenocorticotropic hormone)

Actos

acuity (pl. acuities)

acute depressed mood

ADA (American Diabetes Association) diet

ADD (attention deficit disorder)

adenocarcinoma

adenomatous colon polyp

adenopathy

adenosine stress test

adenosine study

adequate hemostasis

ADH (antidiuretic hormone)

ADHD (attention-deficit hyperactivity disorder)

adherent gallbladder

adhesive tape

adipose tissue

ADLs (activities of daily living)

adnexal cyst

adnexal mass

Advair

adventitious breath sounds

adverse effects

Advil

"aerosol pentam" (slang for *aerosolized pentamidine*)

AFI (amniotic fluid index)

"a fib" (slang for *atrial fibrillation*)

AFP (alpha fetoprotein)

Afrin

aftercare

agitation

AHIMA (American Health Information Management Association)

Ahmed valve

AIDS (acquired immunodeficiency syndrome)

air bag

air leak

AK (above-knee) amputation

akinesia

akinesis

albuterol inhaler

Alcon AcrySof intraocular lens

Aldactone

alertness for details within environment

alkaline phosphatase

"alk phos" (slang for *alkaline phosphatase*)

ALL (acute lymphocytic leukemia)

allopurinol

alpha$_1$-antitrypsin

alpha-blocker

alpha fetoprotein (AFP)

alpha-fetoprotein (AFP) level

ALT (alanine aminotransferase)

Altace

altered awareness

altered functioning

alternating

alveolar spaces

alveolar walls

Ambien

amikacin

amoxicillin

"amp" (slang for *ampule, ampicillin*)

amplitude

ANA (antinuclear antibody)

anal canal

ANCA (anti-neutrophil cytoplasmic antibody) lab test

anemic

anesthetized

aneurysmal dilatation

angiography

AngioJet

anicteric

anion gap

ankle fracture

ankle jerks

anorexia nervosa

anterior chamber

anterior lip of the cervix

anteroapical infarction

anterolateral infarct

anterolateral region

anterolateral segment

anterolateral wall

anteroseptal infarction

anteverted uterus

anticoagulation

antihelix

antihemophilic globulin (AHG)

antipsychotic drugs

antitachycardia pacing

antral gastritis

antral mucosa

antrum

anulus (*not* annulus)

anxiety

anxiolytic (tranquilizer) drugs

aortic bruit

AP (anteroposterior)

apex of heart

Apgar score (Apgars)

A positive blood type

appendectomy

appendiceal lumen

appendiceal orifice

appendicitis

"appy" (slang for *appendectomy*)

arch hypoplasia

Aricept

arm board

arm twitching

Armstrong tube

arterial blood flow

arterial system

arteriovenous (see *AV*)

arthroscopy

Arthrotec
articulation
ascites
ascitic fluid
ASC-US (abnormal squamous cells
    of undetermined significance)
ASCVD (arteriosclerotic cardio-
    vascular disease)
aseptic debridement
ASHD (arteriosclerotic heart
    disease)
aspiration
assistive device
associate learning
AST (aspartate aminotransferase)
asthma
ASTM (American Society
    for Testing of Materials)
asymptomatic
Atacand
ataxia
ataxic gait
atelectasis
atenolol
Ativan
atlantoaxial articulation
atraumatic
atrial fibrillation
atrial tachycardia
atrioventricular (see *AV*)
attenuation-correction software
attic cholesteatoma
attic perforation
attic pocket
atypical
atypical ductal hyperplasia
auditory hallucinations
Augmentin
auscultation
Avandia
Avapro
aVL (augmented voltage, left arm)
AV (arteriole-venule) ratio
AV (arteriovenous)
    AV access
    AV aneurysm
    AV fistula
    AV malformation
    AV nicking
AV (atrioventricular)
    AV block
    AV nodal ablation
    AV node
AVNRT (atrioventricular nodal
    reentrant tachycardia)
Avonex

aVR (augmented voltage, right arm)
axial CT views
axilla
axonal degeneration

Bactroban
BAL (bronchoalveolar lavage)
balanced salt solution
bands (brief form for *banded
    neutrophils*)
bare metal stent
Barrett esophagus
BAs (business associates)
basal cell carcinoma
basal cell nevus syndrome
base of the hemorrhoid
baseline
Basic Four (history and physical
    examination, consultation report,
    operative report, discharge
    summary)
basilar rales
basos (brief form for *basophils*)
Battle sign
BCC (basal cell carcinoma)
BCG (bacille Calmette-Guérin)
    immunotherapy
BE (barium enema)
Beaver blade
beta-blocker
Betadine
Betadine prep
Betadine solution
beta-hemolytic strep
beta-hydroxybutyrate
beta-lactamase-producing strains
Betaseron
"bicarb" (slang for *bicarbonate*)
b.i.d. (twice a day)
bifurcation
bigeminy
"bili" (slang for *bilirubin*)
biopsy-proven carcinoma
BiPAP (bilevel positive airway
    pressure)
Bishop forceps
bite block
BK (below-knee) amputation
bladder function
bladder repair with mesh
bladder washings
bleeding internal hemorrhoids
block construction skills
block design
blood in the vagina
blood pressure cuff

blue collar button tube
blurred vision
BM (bowel movement)
BMI (body mass index)
BMP (basic metabolic panel)
BNP (brain natriuretic peptide) level
boarded and collared
bolster
bone bank bone
bone flap
bone grafting of the scaphoid
bone plug
bony callus formation
bony integrity
bony resorption
bony structures
borderline cardiomegaly
borderline hypertension
Botox injection
bovied
Bovie electrocautery
bowel function
bowel gas pattern
bowel loop
bowel obstruction
bowel resection
bowel sounds
BP (blood pressure)
BPD (biparietal diameter)
BPH (benign prostatic hyperplasia)
brain metastases
breast biopsy
breast cyst biopsy
Breslow classification of thickness
    of tumor
bridle suture
brisk carotids
bronchial breath sounds
bronchial resection
bronchitis
bronchodilators
bronchoscopy
bruising
bruit
BSS (balanced salt solution)
BSS Plus solution
Bucky grid
Buddha position
bulbar conjunctiva
bulging soft palate
bulging tympanic membrane
bulimia nervosa
BUN (blood urea nitrogen)
bundle branch block
buried knots
buried sutures

BUS (Bartholin glands, urethra, and Skene glands)
buttock area
by (*x* as in 2 x 3 x 4 cm)

"ca" (slang for *carcinoma*)
"cabbage" (CABG, coronary artery bypass graft)
CABG ("cabbage") (coronary artery bypass graft)
C&S (culture and sensitivity)
CA 125 level in ovarian cancer
CA-1919
cachexia (wasting)
calcaneus (pl. calcanei)
calcification
calculus
calf tenderness
callus
Candida albicans
candidiasis
cannula
capsular bag
capsulorhexis *or* capsulorrhexis
Carbastat
carbidopa-levodopa
cardia
cardiac "cath" (catheterization)
cardiac serum markers
Cardiolite stress test
cardiomyopathy
Cardizem
carotid bruit
carotid bulge
carotid duplex ultrasound
carotids
carpal tunnel decompression
carpal tunnel release
carpal tunnel syndrome (CTS)
cartilage
"cath," "cath'd" (slang for *catheterization, catheterized*)
CAT scan (also, CT scan)
cataract
catty-corner
cavity dilatation
CBC (complete blood count)
CBC with differential
CBD (common bile duct)
CC (chief complaint)
cc (cubic centimeter) (used in laboratory values but not in drug doses) (equivalent to mL, milliliter)
CDC (Centers for Disease Control)
C. difficile (*Clostridium difficile*)
CE (covered entity)

CEA (carcinoembryonic antigen) test; titer
Ceclor
cecum
cefotetan
cellulitis
Celsius
central conduction
central retinal artery
central zones
cephalexin oral suspension
cerebellar stroke
cerebral atrophy
cerebral concussion
cerebral contusion
cerebral hemisphere
cerebral laceration
cerebral MRI
cerumen (earwax)
cervical adenopathy
cervical motion tenderness
cervical spine
cervix
cesarean section (C-section)
channel ulceration
Charcot-Marie-Tooth disease
cheek biting
chemo (brief form for *chemotherapy*)
chem-7 (7 different chemical tests)
chemotherapy
chest tube
CHF (congestive heart failure)
chiropractic manipulation
"chole" (slang for *cholecystectomy*)
cholecystectomy
cholecystitis
cholesteatoma
cholesterol emboli
cholesterol profile
chondromalacia patellae
chorda tympani nerve
chronic depression
"circ" (slang for *circumflex* artery)
circumferential manner
circumferentially
circumstantiality
cirrhosis
Clark classification of the depth of invasion of the tumor
claudication
clavus (pl. clavi)
cleansed
clear watery fluid
clicking in ears
clicking teeth
clipped wire
CLL (chronic lymphocytic leukemia)

CLO (*Campylobacter*-like organism) test
clonidine
closed cervix
closed reduction of fracture
closing pressure
closure
closure of foramen ovale
Cloward fusion
clubbing, cyanosis, or edema
cm (centimeter)
CML (chronic myelogenous leukemia)
CMT (Certified Medical Transcriptionist)
CMV (cytomegalovirus) retinitis
CNS (central nervous system)
CO_2, CO2 (carbon dioxide)
CO_2/gadolinium angiography
"coags" (slang for *coagulation tests* or *studies*)
coagulate
coarctation of aorta
coarse rales
cobalt treatment
cocaine pledgets
cognitive decline
cogwheel rigidity
cohesive qualities
colectomy
colitis
collar button tube
collateral laxity
collateral stability
colon polyp
colonoscopy
colonoscopy with polypectomy
colposcopic examination
columnar epithelium
Combivent
comedone
comfort care
commonalities between objects
Compazine
completion amputation
complex partial seizure
compression plate and screws
conchal bowl
conduction block
condyloma acuminatum (pl. condylomata acuminata)
configuration
congested vessels
congestion of lungs
congestive heart failure (CHF)
conjunctiva (pl. conjunctivae)

conjunctival flap
conjunctival pallor
conjunctivitis
connective tissue
conscious sedation
continuity
continuous suture
contusion
convexity
Copaxone
COPD (chronic obstructive pulmonary disease)
copious irrigation
copiously irrigated
Coreg
cornea
coronary stenting
coronary syndrome
cortex (pl. cortices)
cortical cancellous bone grafting
cortical cataract
cortical remnants
cortices
Coumadin
counterstain
couplets
Cozaar
CPAP ("see-pap") (continuous positive airway pressure)
CPK (creatine phosphokinase)
CPM (continuous passive motion) machine
CPR (cardiopulmonary resuscitation)
cranial nerves
craniotomy
crimping
"crit" (slang for *hematocrit*)
Crohn disease
cross section (noun)
cross-section (verb)
cross-sectional images
crusted lashes
crusting
cryotherapy
C-section (cesarean section) delivery
C7-T1 disk space
CSF (cerebrospinal fluid)
C-spine (cervical spine)
CTS (carpal tunnel syndrome)
CT (computed tomography) scan
cup-to-disk ratio (also, cup:disk)
curet
curvilinear incision
CUSA (Cavitron ultrasonic aspirator)

cutaneous lacerations
CV (cardiovascular)
CVA (cerebrovascular accident)
CVA (costovertebral angle) tenderness
CVP (central venous pressure) catheter
CXR (chest x-ray)
cyanosis
cyanosis, clubbing, or edema
cyst
"cysto" (slang for *cystoscopy*)
cystotome
cytology
cytoplasm
Cytospin preparation

daily (alternative for *q. day*)
D&C (dilatation and curettage)
D&E (dilatation and evacuation)
D/C, DC (transcribe *discharge* or *discontinue*)
D/C'd, DC'd (transcribe *discharged* or *discontinued*)
debrided
debridement of nails
debris
debulking of tumor
decolorizer
decomposed
decompression
decongest
decongested
decubitus position
deep tendon reflexes
defatted
defervesced
deflated tourniquet
deformity
degenerative joint disease
degree (°)
dehydrated
dehydration
Dejerine-Sottas disease
delayed scaphoid union
delirium
delusions of grandiosity
delusions of persecution
delusions of reference
demeanor
dementia
Demerol
demyelinating
Depakote
dependent edema
Depo-Provera

depression
dermatitis
descending duodenum
descent
Desenex
desensitization
deteriorated
Detrol LA
Dewecker scissors
DEXA (dual-energy x-ray absorptiometry)
diabetes mellitus type 1
diabetes mellitus type 2
diabetic ketoacidosis
diabetic toe ulcer
diagonal branch
diaphoresis
diastolic dysfunction
diazepam
DIC (disseminated intravascular coagulation)
"didge," "dig," "didg" (slang for *digoxin*)
"diff" (slang for *differential count*)
differential diagnosis
diffuse pulmonary edema
diffuse swelling
digit span
digit symbol
DigiTrace
digoxin
Dilantin
dilated cervix
Dilaudid
diltiazem
DIP (distal interphalangeal) joint
diplopia
direction of arterial flow
disarray
discoid lupus
discrete area
discrete rounded mass
dissected
dissected out
distal
distally
distention
diuretics
diverticular disease
diverticular ostia
diverticulitis
diverticulum (pl. diverticula)
divide-and-conquer technique
dizzy spells
DJD (degenerative joint disease)
DKA (diabetic ketoacidosis)

DOE (dyspnea on exertion)
dominant nodule
donor site
dopa agonists
dopamine
Doppler ultrasound
dorsal lithotomy position (incorrect but commonly dictated term for *lithotomy position*)
dorsalis pedis pulse
dorsiflexion
dorsum
dose-response curve
downward gaze
doxycycline
draining cyst
drawer sign
dry gauze
dry sterile dressing
DS (discharge summary)
DSM-IV (*Diagnostic and Statistical Manual of Mental Disorders*, 4th edition)
DTs (delirium tremens)
ductal hyperplasia of breast
dull tympanic membrane
duodenal bulb
duodenal mucosa
duodenal turn
duplex scan
duplex ultrasound
dura
dura mater
DVT (deep vein thrombosis)
Dx (diagnosis)
Dyazide
dysarthria
dysarthric speech
dysfunctional uterine bleeding
dyskinesis
dysmenorrhea
dysphagia
dysplasia
dyspnea
dyspnea on exertion (DOE)
dysthymia
dysuria

ear block
ear drum
earwax (cerumen)
easy fatigability
EBL (estimated blood loss)
eburnation
EBV (Epstein-Barr virus)
ECC (endocervical curettage)
ecchymoses around the umbilicus

ECG, EKG (electrocardiogram)
echo (echocardiogram)
echocardiogram
echo signal
E. coli (*Escherichia coli*)
Ecotrin
ectopic beats
edema of extremities
edema of lungs
edematous
ED, ER (emergency department, emergency room)
EEG (electroencephalogram)
EF (ejection fraction)
EGD (esophagogastroduo-denoscopy)
egress of aqueous
EHL (extensor hallucis longus) muscle
EHR (electronic health record)
ejection fraction
ejection systolic murmur
EKG, ECG (electrocardiogram)
electrocautery dissection
electrodiagnostic findings
electroshock (electroconvulsive) therapy
elevated
ELISA (enzyme-linked immuno-sorbent assay)
elliptical incision
elongated nails
emanating
embedded
embryonal cell carcinoma
emergent biliary drainage
EMG (electromyogram, electro-myography)
emotionally labile
EMR (electronic medical record)
EMT (emergency medical techni-cian)
enalapril
en bloc
encased
endocervical curettage
endocervical polyp
endocervix
end-of-the-day sock line edema
endometrial ablation
endometrial adenocarcinoma
endometrial biopsy
endometrial cavity
endometrial or "chocolate" cysts in ovaries
endometriosis
energy disturbance

enlarged heart
ENT (ears, nose, and throat)
entirety
EOM (extraocular movements)
EOMI (extraocular muscles intact)
eos (brief form for *eosinophils*)
epidermal inclusion cyst
epidermal tissue
epidermis
epidural
epigastric abdominal pain
epilepsy
epinephrine 1:100,000
epistaxis (nosebleed)
epithelialization
epithelialized
ER, ED (emergency room, emergency department)
eradication
ERCP (endoscopic retrograde cholangiopancreatogram)
erectile dysfunction (impotence)
eroding
erosion
erratic sleep
erythema
erythematous conjunctivae
erythematous tympanic membrane
erythromycin ointment
erythromycin ophthalmic ointment
ESL (English as a second language)
Esmarch bandage
esophageal diaphragmatic hiatus
esophageal mucosa
esophagectomy
esophagogastroduodenoscopy (EGD)
esophagogastroduodenoscopy with biopsy
ESR (erythrocyte sedimentation rate; sed rate)
estimated blood loss
estimated fetal weight
ESWL (extracorporeal shock wave lithotripsy)
ET (enterostomal therapy) nursing
etiology
eustachian tube dysfunction
evacuated
event monitor
exacerbation
exam (examination)
exam under anesthesia
excision
excision of cervical disk and spur
excision of hematoma
excision of neuromata

excitation pulse
exertional chest pain
exploratory laparotomy
external fixator
extradural hemorrhage
extraocular motility
extraocular movements
extravasation of barium
extravasation of contrast
extubated
exudate
eye patch
eye shield

FA (fluorescent antibody)
failure of descent
fascia
fast beats
fatty vacuoles
FBS (fasting blood sugar)
febrile episode
fecal incontinence
femoral bruit
femoropopliteal graft
"fem-pop" (slang for *femoral-popliteal*)
fentanyl epidural
festinating gait
festination in propulsion
fetal anomaly
fetal demise
fetal heart rate
fetal heart tones
FEV-1, FEV$_1$ (forced expiratory
    volume in 1 second)
FH (family history)
"fib flutter" (slang for *atrial fibrilla-
    tion/flutter*)
fibrinous exudate
fibrofatty tissue
fibrosis
fibrous capsule
fibrous pleuritis
fibrovascular adhesion
fibular head
fibular shaft fracture
field deficits
15 blade
15-blade scalpel
filmy adhesions
fingersticks
FiO$_2$ (fractional inspired oxygen or
    inspired flow of oxygen)
first-degree AV block
first trimester
fissure
fixation
Flagyl

flattened
fleeting suicidal thinking
Flexeril
flexible Olympus video gastroscope
flight of ideas
Flonase
Florinef
flow pattern
fluconazole
"fluctuance" (use *fluctuancy*)
fluctuancy (*not* fluctuance)
fluffs
fluid analysis cytology
fluid in pleural space
fluid intelligence
flu-like symptoms
fluttering
FNA (fine-needle aspiration)
foam doughnut
FOBT (fecal occult blood test)
focal areas
focal infiltrates
focally
focally hemorrhagic adipose tissue
foci (plural of *focus*)
focus of organized pneumonia
Foley catheter
Foley gallbladder
Foley to gravity
follicular carcinoma
follicular hyperplasia
follicular neoplasm
fontanelle
foot mole excision
foreign body in the anterior
    chamber of the eye
foreign body reaction
formalin
formed tissue
fornix-based conjunctival flap
fornix-based peritomy
Fosamax
4/5 strength ("four over five")
4-0 silk stitches
4-pillow orthopnea
fourchette
fracture fragments
frail-appearing
free bone flap
free fascia
free reflux
freestanding surgery center
free T4, T$_4$
free tie
Friedreich ataxia
frontal sinus
frontoparietal region

frozen pathology
frozen section
FSH (follicle-stimulating hormone)
FTA (fluorescent treponemal
    antibody) test
FTP (file transfer protocol)
full-bladder technique
full-column barium enema
full-scale IQ
full-thickness skin graft
fundal
fundus (pl. fundi)
funduscopic examination
FUO (fever of undetermined origin)
furosemide
fusion
fusion and plating
FVC (forced vital capacity)
F wave
F-wave latency
Fx (fracture)

g (gram)
G (gravida) (as in G1, P1)
GABA (gamma-aminobutyric acid)
gadolinium
gait and station
gait disturbance
gait impairment
gait stable
gallbladder wall thickness
gallstones
ganglion cyst
gangrene
gangrenous gallbladder
gangrenous ulceration
gastric antrum
gastric body
gastric cardia
gastric contents
gastric fundus
gastric mucosa
gastritis
gastroesophageal reflux disease
    (GERD)
gated tomographic study
GC (gonorrhea)
GE (gastroesophageal) junction
generalized tonic-clonic seizures
gentamicin
GERD (gastroesophageal reflux
    disease)
GI (gastrointestinal)
giant cells
girth
glandular structures
glaucoma

Gleason grade (score) for prostate cancer
glipizide
global systolic ventricular function
glomerulus (pl. glomeruli)
glucose out of control
glucose tolerance test (GTT)
gluteus
glyburide
goiter
grade 1-2/6 murmur
grade 2/6 murmur
grade 2/6 systolic ejection murmur
grandiosity
granular cell layer
granulation tissue
grasped
gravida (G) (G1, P1)
gravida 2, para 1-0-0-1 (G2, P1-0-0-1)
gravid uterus
Greenfield filter
grenz zone
grimaces with movement
gross description
group A beta-hemolytic strep
GTT (glucose tolerance test)
GU (genitourinary)
guarding
guidewire
Guillain-Barré syndrome
Gyn (gynecology)

hallucinations
hammer digits
hallucinations
handheld
H&E (hematoxylin and eosin)
"H&H" (slang for *hemoglobin and hematocrit*)
H&P (history and physical examination)
HAV (hepatitis A virus)
hay fever (allergic rhinitis)
H$_2$ blocker
HBV (hepatitis B virus)
HCG, hCG (human chorionic gonadotropin)
Hct, HCT (hematocrit)
HCTZ (hydrochlorothiazide)
HCV (hepatitis C)
HDL (high-density lipoprotein)
HDL cholesterol
HDN (hemolytic disease of the newborn)
Healon
heel and toe walk

heel pain
HEENT (head, eyes, ears, nose, and throat)
Helicobacter pylori (*H. pylori*) test
helix
hematocrit
hematological disorder
hematoxylin and eosin (H&E)
hemifacial spasm
hemisphere
hemodynamically
hemoglobin (Hgb)
hemoglobin A$_{1c}$ (glycosylated hemoglobin)
hemoptysis
hemorrhage into alveoli
hemorrhage occurring post partum (noun, two words) (cf., postpartum hemorrhage [adj.])
hemorrhagic adipose tissue
hemorrhagic ulcer
hemorrhoid
hemorrhoidectomy
hemostasis
hemostatic wound
hepatic vein thrombosis
hepatitis B vaccination
hepatitis titer
hepatojugular reflux
hepatosplenomegaly
herald
herniated disk
herniated disk and spur, C7-T1
herniated disk extrusion
herpesvirus type 1 (oral, labial, facial herpes)
herpesvirus type 2 (genital herpes)
Hgb, HGB (hemoglobin)
HGSIL (high-grade squamous intraepithelial lesion)
hiatal hernia
HIDA (hepatobiliary iminodiacetic acid) scan
high-dose radiation
high-grade dysplasia
high-resolution CT scan
high-volume spinal tap
hilar soft tissue
HIM (health information management)
HIPAA (Health Insurance Portability and Accountability Act)
HIV (human immunodeficiency virus) disease
HIV test

hives
HMO (health maintenance organization)
HNP (herniated nucleus pulposus)
Hodgkin disease
Holter monitor
Holter scan
home oxygen (home O$_2$)
homicidal ideation
horizontal gaze
Hospice home care
hpf (high power field)
HPI (history of present illness)
HPV (human papillomavirus)
H. pylori (*Helicobacter pylori*)
H reflex
HRT (hormone replacement therapy)
HS (half-strength)
h.s. (at bedtime) (do not use *q.h.s.*)
HSP (human papillomavirus)
HSV-1 (type 1 herpes simplex virus)
HSV-2 (type 2 herpes simplex virus)
human bite
humeral fracture
Humulin N insulin
Humulin R insulin
hydrocele
hydrocephalus
hydrochlorothiazide
hydrodelineation
hydrodissection
hydrogel dressings
hydrosalpinx
hydrothermal endometrial ablation
hydroxybutyrate (see *beta-hydroxybutyrate*)
hypercholesterolemic
hyperchromatic nuclei
hyperlipidemia
hypermenorrhea
hypermetabolic uptake
hyperparathyroidism
hyperprolactinemia
hypertension
hypertrophic cardiomyopathy
hypertrophic tonsils
hypocontractile
hypodensities
hypoglycemic reaction
hypostatic bronchopneumonia
hypothyroidism
hysterectomy
Hyzaar
Hz (hertz)

I&D (incision and drainage)
IBD (inflammatory bowel disease) (includes Crohn disease as well as ulcerative colitis)
IBS (irritable bowel syndrome)
ibuprofen
IC (independent contractor)
ICD (implantable cardioverter-defibrillator)
ICU (intensive care unit)
idiopathic epilepsy
Ig (immunoglobulins)
ileoanal pouch anastomosis
ileocecal valve
iliac nodal chain
iliac node
iliofemoral venous thrombosis
IM (intramuscular)
image quality
impetigo
Implanon implant for contraception
impotence (erectile dysfunction)
IMV (intermittent mandatory ventilation)
incarceration (inability to reduce hernia),
incision packed open
incision site
incudostapedial joint
incus
Indocin
induration
infarction
inferior
inferior flap
inferior wall myocardial ischemia
inferomedially
infiltrate
infiltrating
infiltration of anesthetic
infiltration of the mesentery
inflammation
inflammatory cells
inflated
influenza
infrapatellar area
infusion
inguinal nodes
INR (international normalized ratio) on blood test
insertion site
inspection
insufflated
intact hymen
intellectual functioning
interlobular fibrofatty tissue
intermittent claudication

intermittent stitches
internal iliac node
internal sclerostomy
interrogation
interrupted sutures
interstitial edema
interstitial lung disease
interstitial opacities
interstitial tissues
intra-abdominal bleeding
intra-abdominal hemorrhage
intra-abdominal mass
intracutaneous fistula
intradermal nevus
intraocular lens (IOL)
intraocular lens implantation
intraocular pressure (IOP)
intraoperative complications
intraperitoneal free fluid
intrapleural catheter
intrauterine fetal demise
intrauterine fetus
intrauterine pregnancy
introitus
intubated
intussusception
investing fascia
iodinated contrast
iodinated contrast infusion
IOL (intraocular lens)
IOP (intraocular pressure)
iridectomy
iron deficiency anemia
iron stores
irrigant
irrigation-aspiration instrument
irritative urinary symptoms (frequency, urgency, nocturia)
ischemia
ischemic disease of the brain
ISMP (Institute for Safe Medication Practices)
IT (information technology)
ITP (idiopathic thrombocytopenic purpura)
ITT (internal tibial torsion)
IU (international unit)
IUD (intrauterine device)
IV (intravenous)
IVC (inferior vena cava) filter
IVC (intravenous cholangiography)
IVIG (intravenous immunoglobulin)
IVP (intravenous pyelogram)
IVU (intravenous urogram)

JAAMT (Journal of the American Association for Medical Transcription)

JCAHO (Joint Commission on Accreditation of Healthcare Organizations)
jejunal limb
joint space narrowing
JP (Jackson-Pratt) drain
J tube
JVD (jugular venous distention)
JVP (jugular venous pressure)

K (potassium)
KCl
K-Dur
Keflex
Kerley lines
Kerlix
Kerlix and Ace bandage wrap
ketones
kg (kilogram)
"kilo" (slang for kg, kilogram)
kissing tonsils
Kling
Kling wrap
knee jerks
knife handle
KOH (potassium hydroxide)
KPs (keratic precipitates)
KUB (kidneys, ureters, and urinary bladder)

L (liter)
LA (long acting)
lab (laboratory)
labile
laceration
Lactulose
LAD (left anterior descending) coronary artery
LADD (left anterior descending diagonal) artery
Lamictal
laminaria placement
laminated keratotic debris
Lantus insulin
"lap" (slang for laparoscopy)
laparoscopic cholecystectomy
laparoscopic ileostomy
laparotomy
"lap chole" (slang for laparoscopic cholecystectomy)
laryngeal nerve
LASIK (laser-assisted in situ keratomileusis)
Lasix
lateral aspect
lateral decubitus position
lateral-medial helix

lateralmost portion
lateralward
LDH (lactic dehydrogenase)
LDL (low-density lipoprotein)
LE (lupus erythematosus) cell prep
lead impedance
leaking
left axis deviation
left shift
leg bypass surgery
leiomyoma uteri
lens nucleus
LES (lower esophageal sphincter)
lesion
Lexapro
L5 nerve root
L5-S1 (fifth lumbar vertebra and first sacral vertebra)
L4 nerve root
L4-5 disk
LFTs (liver function tests)
LGSIL (low-grade squamous intra-epithelial lesion)
LH (luteinizing hormone)
lid block
lid fissures
lidocaine 1%
lid speculum
ligature
light-headed
light-headedness
light perception only
light touch
limb coordination
limbal area
linear incision
lipid arcus
lipid panel
lipid profile
Lipitor
liquid green stool
lisinopril
liters
lithotomy position
liver biopsy
liver function studies
liver panel
livor mortis
LLQ (left lower quadrant)
LMP (last menstrual period)
lobectomy
lobular pattern of pancreas
local field block
localized needle biopsy
localized pain
longitudinally incised
long-standing history

long-term care
long TR
loop recorder
loose body
loose associations
Lortab
Lovenox
low columnar epithelium
lower back strain
lower esophageal sphincter (LES)
low-grade dysplasia
LP (lumbar puncture)
LUL (left upper lobe)
lumbar spine fusion
lumbar stenosis
lumbar strain
lumbosacral area
lung primary
lung resection
Lupron
lupus
LVAD (left ventricular assist device)
LVEF (left ventricular ejection fraction)
LVF (left ventricular function)
LVH (left ventricular hypertrophy)
Lyme disease
Lyme titer
lymph node dissection
lymphadenopathy
lymphohistiocytic infiltrate
lymphs (brief form for *lymphocytes*)
"lytes" (slang for *electrolytes*)

MAC (Marcaine, adrenaline, and cocaine) anesthesia
MAC (monitored anesthesia care)
MAC anesthesia
macular dystrophy
MAI, MAC (*M. avium intracellulare* complex)
Maisonneuve-type ankle injury
major tranquilizer drugs
malignant cells
malleus
malpighian bodies
malunion
mammography suite
manic-depressive disorder (bipolar disorder)
manipulation
manometer
Marcaine 0.5% ("half percent")
Marcaine with epinephrine
Marcaine without epinephrine
margin
marked hypertrophy

mask facies
MAST (military antishock trousers)
mastoidectomy
mastoiditis (invasion of mastoid air cells)
mattress suture
McBurney point
mcg (micrograms)
MCH (mean corpuscular hemo-globin)
MCHC (mean corpuscular hemo-globin concentration)
mcL (microliter)
McMurray test
MCP (metacarpophalangeal) joint
mcU/mL (microunits per milliliter)
MCV (mean corpuscular volume)
MD, M.D. (doctor of medicine)
MDI (metered-dose inhaler)
Mebron
"med," "meds" (slang for *medications*)
medial border of patella
medial joint line
medial-lateral direction
medial nerve
median nerve decompression
median nerve distribution
mediastinal adenopathy
mediastinal lymph nodes
mediastinoscopy
mediastinum
Mefoxin
melanoma
memory impairment
memory passage
menorrhagia
menses
mental status
mentation
mEq (milliequivalent)
mesenteric adenopathy
mesenteric caking
metachromatic stain
metastasis (pl. metastases)
metastatic adenocarcinoma
metastatic carcinoma
metastatic ovarian cancer
metformin
metolazone
metoprolol
"mets" (slang for *metastases*) to the brain
"Metz" (slang for *Metzenbaum scissors*)
Metzenbaum scissors
mg (milligram)
mg/dL (milligrams per deciliter)

mg/kg (milligrams per kilogram)
mg/mL (milligrams per milliliter)
MI (myocardial infarction)
microdiskectomy fusion and plating
microgram (mcg)
micro pituitary rongeur
midline
midline trachea
midthoracic area
migraine with aura
migraine without aura
migratory headache
milligram (mg)
millimeters of mercury (mmHg)
mini mental status examination
minimal rigidity
minocycline
minor tranquilizer drugs
Miradon
Mirapex
Mirena IUD (intrauterine device)
MIS (manager of information
    systems) director
mitomycin
mitral regurgitation
mitral valve repair
mL (milliliter)
mL/h (milliliters per hour)
mm (millimeter)
mmHg (millimeters of mercury)
MMK (Marshall-Marchetti-Krantz)
    procedure
mobilized
Mohs technique
monitored anesthesia care (MAC)
"mono" (slang for *mononucleosis*) test
monocular
monos (brief form for *monocytes*)
monotherapy
morbid obesity
mordant
Morison pouch
morphine
mortise
motion tenderness
motor amplitude
motor conduction velocity
motor polyneuropathy
MQ (memory quotient)
MRA (magnetic resonance
    angiography)
MRCP (magnetic resonance
    cholangiopancreatography)
MRI (magnetic resonance imaging)
MS (multiple sclerosis)
msec (millisecond)
MT (medical transcriptionist)

MTA (metatarsus adductus)
MTF&P (*Medical Transcription Funda-
    mentals & Practice*), 3rd edition
µg (microgram) (transcribe *mcg*)
Mucinex
mucosal surface
mucosal ulceration
mucous membranes
MUGA (multiple gated acquisition)
    scan
multiaxial assessment
multinodular thyroid gland
"multip" (slang for *multipara*)
multiple sclerosis (MS)
multisystem review
murmur
murmur, gallop, rub, or cardiac
    enlargement
murmur, grade 1-2/6 ("one to two
    over six")
Murphy ball
mV (millivolt)
myalgia
myasthenia gravis
myelitis
myelogram
myocardial fibers
myocardial imaging
myocardial infarction
myocardial perfusion scan
myocardial tracer uptake
myomectomy
myringotomy

naris (pl. nares)
nasal balloon
nasal bones
nasal fracture
nasal pack
nasogastric (NG) tube
nasolabial fold
NCV (nerve conduction velocity)
near-occlusion
near total thyroidectomy
necrotic debris
necrotic gallbladder
needle EMG
needlepoint electrocautery
negative for tumor
neonatal jaundice
neoplasm
nerve compression
nerve conduction studies
nerve conduction study
nerve root cutoff
nerve roots
neural foramina

neuroleptic drugs
neuromata
Neurontin
neuropathy
neurovascular status
neutralizing antibodies
nevus cells
Nexium
NG (nasogastric) tube
Niaspan
NICU ("nick-yoo") (neonatal
    intensive care unit)
nightly (use for *q.h.s.*)
NIH (National Institutes of Health)
"nitro" (slang for *nitroglycerin*)
NKDA (no known drug allergies)
nodularity
nodule
nondistended abdomen
nonjaundiced
nonproductive cough
nonpurulent
nonreactive NST (nonstress test)
nonreassuring
non-small cell carcinoma
nonspecific abnormality
nonspecific T2 hyperintensities
nonspecific T-wave abnormality
nontender uterus
nontoxic
nonunion
nonweightbearing
    acceptable alternatives:
        non-weightbearing
        non-weight-bearing
Norflex
normal pressure hydrocephalus
normoactive bowel sounds
normocephalic
Norvasc
Norwood repair for hypoplastic
    left-sided heart syndrome
nosebleed (epistaxis)
nostril
novel stimuli
NPH insulin
n.p.o. (nothing by mouth)
NSAIDs (nonsteroidal anti-
    inflammatory drugs)
NST (nonstress test)
NSVD (normal spontaneous vaginal
    delivery)
nuclear sclerotic
nuclear study
Nuclepore (*not* Nucleopore) prepa-
    ration
nucleus (pl. nuclei)

numbness and tingling
nylon suture

O₂ (oxygen)
O&P (ova and parasites)
O'Brien lid block
object assembly
obstruction
obturator and pelvic lymph node
    dissection
obturator nodal chain
occluded
occluded tympanic membrane
occlusion of artery
OCD (obsessive-compulsive
    disorder)
OCG (oral cholecystogram)
ocular migraine
OD (overdose)
OD (translate: right eye)
off-loaded
OGTT (oral glucose tolerance test)
ohms
olecranon fracture
olfactory hallucinations
oligohydramnios
Olympus video gastroscope
1 to 2+ pulses
onychomycosis
oozing
open angle glaucoma
open cholecystectomy
opening pressure
open wound of lower extremity
ophthalmoplegia
optic enhancement
optic nerve
Optison
orbital inflammatory pseudotumor
OREF (open reduction and external
    fixation)
organomegaly
orientation
oriented x3
ORIF (open reduction and internal
    fixation)
orifice
oropharynx
"ortho" (orthopedics)
orthopnea
orthostatic drop of blood pressure
OS (translate: left eye)
OSHA (Occupational Safety and
    Health Administration)
ossicular chain
"osteo" (slang for *osteomyelitis*)
osteomyelitis

osteopenia
osteopenia of spine and hip
osteoporotic
ostomy
otitis media
"O₂ sat" (slang for *oxygen saturation*)
OTC (over-the-counter)
    medications
OT (occipitotransverse) position of
    the fetus
OU (each eye)
outpatient
ova and parasites (O&P)
ovarian cancer
ovarian cyst
overlying bowel gas
oversewing of atrial appendage
oversuturing
oxybutynin
oxygen saturation

PA (posteroanterior)
PACs (premature atrial contractions)
PACU ("pack-yoo" or "p-a-c-u")
    (postanesthesia care unit)
pallor
palmar fascia
palmar mass
palpation
palpebral conjunctiva
palpitation
pancolonic diverticulosis
pancreas
pancreatic mass
P&A (percussion and auscultation)
Pap smear
papilledema
papule
paracentesis (pl. paracenteses)
paracentesis tracts
ParaGard T 380A copper IUD
paragenital lesion
paramediastinal region
parapatellar region
paraspinous muscular spasm
parathyroid glands
paratubal cyst
paresthesias
Parkinson disease
passing blood from rectum
PAT (paroxysmal atrial tachycardia)
patchy infiltrates
patellar margin
patellar tracking
patellofemoral joint
patency of artery
patent artery

Paxil
p.c. (after meals)
PCA (patient-controlled analgesia)
pCO₂, PCO₂, PCO2 (partial pressure
    of carbon dioxide)
PCP (*Pneumocystis [jiroveci]* pneu-
    monia)
PDA (posterior descending [coro-
    nary] artery)
PDA (posterior ductus arteriosus)
PD (posterior descending) ligation
PDS sutures
PE (physical examination)
PE (pulmonary embolism,
    embolus)
PE (polyethylene) tubes
peak level
peak stress images
pear capsulorhexis
pedal pulses
pedicles
"peds" (slang for *pediatrics*)
PEG (percutaneous endoscopic
    gastrostomy)
pelvic ultrasound
pelvis (pl. pelves) of kidney
penicillin V potassium (*not* "pen
    VK")
"pentam" (slang for *pentamidine*)
"pen VK" (use *penicillin V potassium*)
Pepcid
perceptional organizational skills
Percocet
perforated appendix
perforation
performance IQ
performance subtest
perfusion abnormality
perfusion defect
perianal area
perianal condylomata
perianal lesion
periaortic lymph node
periaortic node dissection
periapical abscess with caries
pericardial effusion
perichondrium
peri-infarct ischemia
periorbital area
periosteal flap
peripheral edema
peripheral iridectomy
peripheral nerve disorders
peripheral neuropathy
peripheral polyneuropathy
peripheral pulses
peripheral vascular disease

perirectal area
peristalsis
peritoneal carcinomatosis
peritoneal dialysis catheter
peritonitis
peritonsillar abscess
periumbilical ecchymoses
permanent section
peroneal nerve
per os (use *p.o.*, *by mouth*, or *orally*)
PERRL (pupils equal, round, and reactive to light)
PERRLA (pupils equal, round, reactive to light and accommodation)
persecution
Perspectives on the Medical Transcription Profession (published by Health Professions Institute)
perusal
PET (positron emission tomography) scan
PFT, PFTs (pulmonary function test)(s)
pH (hydrogen ion concentration)
phacoemulsification
pharmacologic intervention
pharynx (throat) (oropharynx, nasopharynx, laryngopharynx)
Phenergan
PHI (protected health information)
PHR (personal health record)
phthisis (wasting)
physical therapy (PT)
physiotherapy
picture arrangement
picture completion
PID (pelvic inflammatory disease)
pinhole
pinkeye (acute epidemic conjunctivitis)
pinna lesion
pin prick
pituitary adenoma
pituitary fossa
pituitary microadenoma
pituitary stalk
PKU (phenylketonuria)
placenta
plantar fasciitis
plantar flexion
plaque in carotid system
platelet count
platysma
Plavix
pledgets
pleural adhesion

pleural aspect
pleural effusion
pleural space
Plexus (published by the American Association for Medical Transcription)
PMH (past medical history)
PMI (point of maximal intensity, or impulse)
PMNs (polymorphonuclear neutrophils) (also, polys)
PMS (premenstrual syndrome)
PND (paroxysmal nocturnal dyspnea)
PND (postnasal drip)
pneumococcal pneumonia
Pneumocystis jiroveci pneumonia
pneumonia
pneumothorax
p.o. (may also use *by mouth* or *orally*)
pO$_2$, PO$_2$, PO2 (partial pressure of oxygen)
podiatry consult
polychrome stain
polys (brief form for *polymorphonuclear leukocytes*) (also, PMNs)
polycystic ovary syndrome
polypoid filling defect
Polysorb suture
Polysorb Vicryl suture
popliteal flexion crease
portal spaces
Portex tracheostomy tube
postabortal pain
postauricular incision
"postchemo" (slang for *postchemotherapy*)
postcoital bleeding
postdate induction
posterior chamber intraocular lens implantation
posterior descending (coronary) artery (PDA)
posterior fourchette
posterior placenta
posterior pressure
posterolateral
posteromedial
postmenopausal bleeding
postop (postoperative)
postpartum hemorrhage (adj.)
post partum (noun)
postprandial (PP)
potassium chloride
potentiated
PP (postprandial)

PPD (purified protein derivative)
Pratt dilator
Pravachol
prednisone
prenatal complications
preop (preoperative)
prepped and draped
presumptive diagnosis
presyncopal
presyncope
prevertebral adenopathy
primary C-section
primary low transverse cesarean section
"primip" (slang for *primipara*)
p.r.n. (as needed)
Procardia XL
Procrit
"procto" (slang for *proctoscopy*)
proctocolectomy
Profile 1
Profile 2
Profore wrap
prolactinoma
prolapsed bladder
Prolene stitch
proliferative retinopathy
prolonged latency
ProMod
pronator drift
prone
Propionibacterium acnes
proptosis
protein-rich fluid
proteinuria
pro time (prothrombin time)
Protonix
Proventil inhaler
Provera
proximal
proximal-distal direction
proximally
Prozac
pruritic
PSA (prostate-specific antigen)
pseudotumor
"psych" (slang for *psychiatric*, *psychiatry*)
PT (prothrombin time)
PTA (percutaneous transluminal angioplasty)
PTC (percutaneous transhepatic cholangiography)
PTCA (percutaneous transluminal coronary angioplasty)
PTH (parathyroid hormone)

PT/INR or PT-INR (pro time/international normalized ratio)
PTT (partial thromboplastin time)
PUD (peptic ulcer disease)
puff
pull test
pulmonary adenocarcinoma
pulmonary edema
pulmonary fibrosis
pulmonary homograft
pulmonary infiltrates
pulmonary insufficiency
pulmonary nodule
pulmonary vascular redistribution
pulse oximetry
pulse sequence
pulses +2/4 ("plus two over four")
pulses 2+/4 ("two plus over four")
punch biopsy
purulent drainage
purulent fluid
purulent material
pustule
PUVA (psoralen + ultraviolet wavelength A)
PVCs (premature ventricular contractions)
pylorus
pyramidal lobe

q. (each; every)
    Acceptable
        q.a.m. (every morning)
        q. day (daily; every day)
        q.4 h. (every 4 hours)
        q.i.d. (4 times a day)
    Unacceptable
        "q.d." (use "daily" or "every day")
        "q.h.s." (use "nightly")
        "q.o.d." (use "every other day")
Q (= blood flow [in mL/min] in ventilation-perfusion scan)
quadriceps
"quarter percent" (0.25%)
questionable
Questran
quinapril
quinolone
quinsy (peritonsillar abscess)
Q waves

RA (rheumatoid arthritis)
RAD (reactive airways disease)
radial aspect of digit
radial pulse
radial styloid

radiation
radicular symptoms
radiculopathy
radiocarpal arthritis
radiofrequency signal
radiolucent areas
radiopaque calculus
radius
ranitidine
Rapid Strep
RAST (radioallergosorbent test)
Rastelli procedure
rate-controlled
rbc/hpf (red blood cells per high power field)
RBCs (red blood cells)
RCA (right coronary artery)
RDA (recommended daily allowance)
reactive pupils
reapproximated
rebound
receiving coil
recreational drugs
rectal mass
rectal mucosal surface
rectovaginal fistula
rectovaginal septum
recurrent bleeding
redness
reduced air entry
reflected anteriorly
reflux
reflux disease
regional anesthesia
regional wall motion
regression
rehab (rehabilitation)
reimplantation
remote memory
renal artery stenosis
renal artery stenting
renal artery ultrasound
renal disease
renal failure
renal function
renal insufficiency
repeat C-section
Requip
resection
residual
residual clot
respiratory distress
resting study
restless legs syndrome
retained products of conception
retinopathy

retraction of the scalp
retrobulbar lid block
retroflexed view
retromembranous hematoma
retroperitoneal mass
return of bowel function
return of bowel sounds
revascularization
revascularization of finger
RF (rheumatoid factor)
Rh (Rh-positive blood and Rh-negative blood)
RHIA (Registered Health Information Administrator)
rhinorrhea
RHIT (Registered Health Information Technician)
RhoGAM
rhythm
rhythmic tremor
RIA (radioimmunoassay)
right bundle/left anterior axis
right-hand dominant
right-hand-dominant patient
right hemisphere perceptional organizational skills
rigor mortis
RLL (right lower lobe)
RLQ (right lower quadrant)
RMT (Registered Medical Transcriptionist)
Rocaltrol
ROM (range of motion)
Romberg test
"romied" (verb form of ROMI [rule out MI])
room air
ROS (review of systems)
rosacea
rosette formation
rotund abdomen
round pupils
Roux-en-Y gastric bypass
Rovsing sign
RPR (rapid plasma reagin) test for syphilis
RSI (repetitive stress injury)
RSV (respiratory syncytial virus)
RUL (right upper lobe)
running stitch
running suture
ruptured cyst
RUQ (right upper quadrant)
RV (right ventricular) to PA (pulmonary artery) conduit
R waves

sacroiliac
sacrum
SAD (seasonal affective disorder)
saline bolus
saline containing bacitracin
saline-soaked lap pad
salvos
SARS (severe acute respiratory syndrome)
"satting" (slang for *oxygen saturation*)
saucerization
SBE (subacute bacterial endo-carditis) prophylaxis
SBFT (small bowel follow-through)
"SC," "sq," "subQ" (slang for *subcuta-neous*) (use "subcu" if dictated)
scaphoid bone
scaphoid healing
scaphoid nonunion
scaphoid tenderness
Schiotz tonometry
schizophrenic thought processes
sciatica
scintiscanner
sclera
scleral flap
scleral icterus
scleral patch graft
scleritis
sclerosis
sclerostomy
scout film
screening examination
"script" (prescription)
scutum
seat belt
sed rate (ESR, erythrocyte sedimen-tation rate)
segs (brief form for *segmented neutrophils*; *segmented mature RBCs*)
segmented neutrophils (segs)
seizures
sella turcica
sensation
sense of reality testing
sensorimotor response
sensorium
sensory polyneuropathy
sensory potential
sensory response
sepsis
septal deviation
septal hematoma
septal wall myocardial infarction
sequencing of skills
sequential compression devices
serial

Seroquel
serous fluid
sessile polyp
S_4 gallop
S4, S_4 heart sound
SH (social history)
sharp costophrenic angles
sharp dissection
sharply dissected
shin
Shirley wound drain
shish kebab effect of the fibrous flexor sheath in digital avulsion injuries
shish kebab operation
short gut syndrome
short-term memory
short TR
shortness of breath
shotty lymphadenopathy
shotty nodes (*not* shoddy)
shunt disconnection/malfunction
sibilant (whistling) rhonchi
side effects
SIDS (sudden infant death syndrome)
signal intensity
silk suture
Simcoe irrigation-aspiration instrument
simvastatin
single-chamber St. Jude ICD (implantable cardioverter-defibrillator)
single-toothed tenaculum
sinus bradycardia
sinus histiocytosis
sinusoids
sinus rhythm
sinus tachycardia
sinus washes
skin crease lines
skin graft
skipped beats
sleep apnea
SMAC ("smack") panel (Sequential Multiple Analyzer plus Computer)
small cell carcinoma
small vessel ischemic disease
snare cautery
SOAP (subjective, objective, assess-ment, plan)
SOB (shortness of breath)
sock-line edema
soft apical murmur
soft S_4
soft tissue

soft tissue scatter
soft tissue swelling
Solu-Medrol
somatosensory evoked potential
S1, S2, S3, S4 (S_1, S_2, S_3, S_4) heart sounds
S1 nerve root
sonolucent rim
sonorous (humming) rhonchi
soundalike
SPA (single-photon absorptiometry)
Spalding sign
spastic gait
spasticity
specimen
SPECT (single photon emission computed tomography) scan
spectrum
spectrum beta-lactamase-producing strain
spell-checker
spell-checking
spike fevers
spinal cerebral atrophy
spinal fluid leak
spinal stenosis surgery
spinal tap
spin echo signal
spin echo technique
spinous processes
Spiriva inhaler
splenectomy
splint
sponge and needle counts
spur at C7-T1
spurring
SR (slow release)
SS (soap suds) enema
ST and T-wave abnormalities
stab incision
stage 1 ulcer of lower extremity
staging of tumor
Stalevo
stapes
staples
Stargardt disease
start hesitation
STD (sexually transmitted disease)
stenosis in artery
stenting
sterile drapes
sterile gauze
Steri-Strips
sternal apex
sternal border
steroid injection
steroids

St. Jude ICD (implantable cardioverter-defibrillator)
S3 heart sound
stitch
stomach inflated with air
stomach maximally insufflated
straight leg raise
straight leg raising
straight suction curet
straps
strength 5/5
strength and coordination
strep pharyngitis
"stress and cath" (slang for *stress test and catheterization*)
stress echo (echogram)
stress fracture
stress steroids
stretching of the foot
stricture
stride
stroke
stroke prevention
STS (serologic test for syphilis)
ST-segment configuration
S2 heart sound
stye (hordeolum)
subacute bacterial endocarditis (SBE)
subarachnoid hemorrhage
subcarinal adenopathy
subconjunctival hemorrhage
subconjunctivally
subcu (transcribe *subcutaneous*)
subcutaneous tissue
subcuticular stitch
subdural fluid
subdural hematoma
subdural hemorrhage
submucosally
suboccipital incision
suboccipital wound
subperiosteally
"subQ," "sq," or "SC" (transcribe *subcu or subcutaneous(ly)*)
suction curet
suction curettage
suction D&C (dilatation and curettage)
suctioned
suicidal ideation
sulfa
superficial
superior flap
superior pole vessels
superior rectus bridle suture
supine position

supraclavicular region
supranuclear palsy
suprapatellar area
supraventricular ectopic beats
supraventricular ectopy
supraventricular rhythm
supraventricular tachycardia
sural latency
sural nerve
sural sensory potential
sural sensory response
swimmer's view
symptomatology
syncope
syndesmosis injury
syndesmotic screws
Synthroid
systemic

"tab" (tablet)
TAB (therapeutic abortion)
tachycardic
tactile hallucinations
TAH-BSO (total abdominal hysterectomy and bilateral salpingo-oophorectomy)
Tambocor
T&A (tonsillectomy and adenoidectomy)
tandem walk
tangentiality in thought processes
taper
TB (tuberculosis)
TBG (thyroid binding globulin)
TCC (transitional cell carcinoma)
TE (echo time)
technetium (Tc 99m)
Techni-Care
TED hose
Temodar
temp (brief form for *temperature*)
temporal lobe
tendon sheath ganglion
tenesmus
TENS (transcutaneous electrical nerve stimulator)
tenting of hemidiaphragm
term intrauterine pregnancy
terminal ileum fat stranding
tetanus shot
T4, T_4 (thyroxine)
theophylline
thickened alveolar walls
thickened appendix
thickened nails
thoracotomy
thought processes

threadlike
throat culture
throat swab
thrombotic thrombocytopenic purpura (TTP)
thrombus
thyroid nodule
thyroid vein
TIA (transient ischemic attack)
TIBC (total iron-binding capacity) test
"tib-fib" (slang for *tibia-fibula*)
tibial nerve
"tic" (slang for *diverticulum*)
t.i.d. (3 times a day)
tilt table test
tingling
titrate
titrated
titrating
TKO (to keep [the vein] open)
"T max" (slang for *maximum temperature*)
TMJ (temporomandibular joint) disease
TMs (tympanic membranes)
TNM (tumor, nodes, metastases)
TNTC (too numerous to count) white cells
toe cellulitis
toes downgoing
T1-weighted coronal images
T1-weighted image
T1-weighted sagittal images
tongue biting
tonic-clonic seizures
tonsillectomy
Toprol
tortuosity of aorta
tortuous (coiled, twisted)
total cholesterol
total knee replacement
tourniquet
TPI (*Treponema pallidum* immobilization)
tPA (tissue plasminogen activator)
TPN (total parenteral nutrition)
T-PRK (tracker-assisted photorefractive keratectomy)
TR (repetition time)
trabeculectomy
trace ankle edema
trace dorsalis pedis pulses
trace edema
tracer uptake
"trach" (slang for *tracheostomy*)
trachea

tracheobronchial angle
tracheobronchitis
tracheostomy
tracking
transhiatal
transient episode of altered
    awareness
transient stress-induced cavity
    dilatation
transitional cell carcinoma of
    bladder
transmural myocardial infarction
transverse carpal ligament
transverse incision
transverse myelitis
transverse processes
traumatic amputation
traumatic tap
traversed
trazodone
Trental
"trep" (slang for *Treponema*) titer
treponema titer
trial of labor
triangular density
"trich" (slang for *Trichomonas*)
Tricor
tricuspid regurgitation
tricuspid valve repair
triglyceride, triglycerides
trimalleolar ankle fracture
troponin
trough level
truncal ataxia
TSH (thyroid stimulating hormone)
TTP (thrombotic thrombocytopenic
    purpura)
T3, T$_3$ (triiodothyronine)
T2 hyperintensities in the white
    matter
T2-weighted image
T tube
tube feeds
tubules
tumor invasion
tunneled
TUR (transurethral resection)
TURP (transurethral resection
    of the prostate)
12 cranial nerves (I through XII)
12-lead EKG
12 o'clock position
2+ pitting edema
tympanic attic

tympanomeatal flap
tympanoplasty
type 1 diabetes mellitus
type 2 diabetes mellitus

U (unit)
UA (urinalysis)
UGI (upper GI) series
ulcerating
ulceration
ulcerative colitis
ulcerative colitis with dysplasia
ulna
ulnar aspect of digit
ulnar nerve
ulnar styloid
ultrasound
ultrasound guidance
uncertain etiology
UPJ (ureteropelvic junction)
upper quadrant pain
uptake
upward gaze
URI (upper respiratory infection)
US (ultrasound)
urine culture
uterine artery embolization
uterine sound
UTI (urinary tract infection)
Utrata forceps
UVJ (ureterovesical junction)

vacuolated cytoplasm
vaginal bleeding
vaginal candidiasis
vaginitis
Vagisil
valproate monotherapy
valvular surgery
Vannas scissors
variable
vascular compression techniques
vascularized bone graft
vasoconstriction
VBAC (vaginal birth after cesarean
    [section])
VD (venereal disease)
VDRL (Venereal Disease Research
    Laboratory)
vein ligation and stripping
vein thrombosis
velocity (pl. velocities)
venous insufficiency of lower
    extremity
venous stent

"vent-dependent" (ventilator-
    dependent)
ventral hernia repair with mesh
ventricular cavity dilatation
ventricular cavity size
ventricular ectopic beats
ventricular ectopy
ventricular ejection fraction
ventricular hypertrophy
ventricular pacing threshold
ventricular systolic function
ventriculopleural shunt
verapamil
verbal IQ
verbal subtest
Versed
vertebral artery
vertebrobasilar insufficiency
vertebrobasilar stroke
vertical mattress sutures
vertigo
"V fib" (slang for *ventricular fibrilla-
    tion*)
Vicodin
Vicryl mattress suture
Vicryl running suture
Vicryl suture
video gastroscope, Olympus
VIN (vulvar intraepithelial
    neoplasia)
VIR (vascular and interventional
    radiology)
viral illness
viral syndrome
visceropleural adhesion
Viscoat
visual acuity
visual analytical skills
visual field
visual hallucinations
visual memory
visual reproduction
visualization
vital signs
VLDL (very low-density lipoproteins)
volar aspect
volar plaster splint strips
V-P (ventilation-perfusion) scan
    V-Q (Q = blood flow) scan
VR (voice recognition)
VSD (ventricular septal defect)
    repair
"V tach" (slang for *ventricular
    tachycardia*)
vulva
vulvar lesion

WAIS (Wechsler Adult Intelligence Scale)
WAIS-R (Revised Wechsler Adult Intelligence Scale)
wasting (cachexia; phthisis)
Watco brace
Waterhouse-Friderichsen syndrome
water seal
WBC (white blood count)
wbc/hpf (white blood cells per high power field)
weaned
Webril
Weck-cel sponge
weightbearing, weight bearing, weight-bearing
weight lifting
Wellbutrin
well-differentiated adenocarcinoma
well-healed incision

well-healed scar
West Nile virus disease
wet-field cautery
wet fluff
wheeze, rale, or rhonchi
widened sinusoids
wire sutures
WISC (Wechsler Intelligence Scale for Children)
WMS (Wechsler Memory Scale)
WMS-1 (Wechsler Memory Scale, Form 1)
wobbling
word-finding difficulties
worsening
wrist fusion

x (*by*, as in 1 x 2 x 3 cm)
x (*times*, as in oriented x3)
Xalatan

xanthochromia
Xeroform
XR (extended release)
XRT (status post radiation therapy)
Xylocaine 0.5%
Xylocaine 1% without epinephrine

YAG (yttrium-aluminum-garnet) laser
Y-shaped incision

Zarontin
Zaroxolyn
Zetia
Z-line of the esophagus
Zocor
Zoloft
Zonegran

Normal Lab Values

Tests Performed on Whole Blood, Plasma, or Serum

Note. Test results depend on methods used. Normal ranges and other interpretive data given in this book are intended solely for purposes of orientation and should not be applied to actual test results.

Analyte or Procedure	Normal Range (Metric)	Normal Range (SI)
acid phosphatase	< 0.6 U/L	< 0.6 U/L
ACTH (adrenocorticotropic hormone)	10-50 pg/mL	2.2-11.1 pmol/L
A/G (albumin-globulin) ratio	1.5-3.0	1.5-3.0
albumin	3.5-5.0 g/dL	35-50 g/L
aldolase	2.5 U/L	2.5 U/L
aldosterone, recumbent	3-16 ng/dL	0.08-0.44 nmol/L
upright	7-30 ng/dL	0.19-0.83 nmol/L
alkaline phosphatase (slang "alk phos")	20-120 U/L	20-120 U/L
alpha$_1$-antitrypsin (AAT)	100-300 mg/mL	20-60 mmol/L
alpha fetoprotein (AFP)	< 15 ng/mL	< 15 mcg/L
ALT (alanine aminotransferase) (formerly SGPT)	8-45 U/L	8-45 U/L
ammonia, serum	15-45 mcg/dL	11-32 mcmol/L
amylase	< 125 U/L	< 125 U/L
anion gap	12-20 mEq/L	12-20 mmol/L
AST (aspartate aminotransferase) (formerly SGOT)	< 35 U/L	< 35 U/L
B cells	5-15%	5-15%
bands (banded neutrophils)	4-8%	4-8%
basophils (basos)	0-1%	0-1%
bicarbonate	24-30 mEq/L	24-30 mmol/L
bilirubin, direct	0.1-0.4 mg/dL	0.1-0.5 mg/dL
bilirubin, indirect	0.1-0.9 mg/dL	1.7-6.8 mcmol/L
bilirubin, total	1.7-8.5 mcmol/L	1.7-15.3 mcmol/L
bleeding time	< 4 minutes	< 4 minutes
BNP (brain natriuretic peptide)	< 50 pg/mL	< 50 ng/L
BUN (blood urea nitrogen)	5-20 mg/dL	1.8-7.1 mcmol/L
calcitonin, male	0-15 pg/mL	0-4.20 pmol/L
calcium	8.2-10.2 mg/dL	2-2.5 mmol/L
CD4 cell count	500-1500 cells/mm^3	0.5-1.5 x 10^9 cells/L
CEA (carcinoembryonic antigen)	< 2.5 ng/mL	< 2.5 mcg/L
chloride	100-106 mEq/L	100-106 mmol/L

Analyte or Procedure	Normal Range (Metric)	Normal Range (SI)
cholesterol	< 200 mg/dL	< 520 mmol/L
cholinesterase (pseudocholinesterase)	8-18 U/L	8-18 U/L
clotting time, Lee-White	6-17 minutes	6-17 minutes
copper	0.7-1.5 mcg/mL	11-24 mmol/L
cortisol, 8 a.m.	5-23 mcg/dL	138-635 nmol/L
4 p.m.	3-16 mcg/dL	83-441 nmol/L
creatinine	0.6-1.2 mg/dL	50-100 mcmol/L
electrolytes: see individual values for sodium, potassium, chloride, and bicarbonate		
eosinophils (eos)	2-4%	2-4%
EPO (erythropoietin)	5-30 mcU/mL	5-30 U/L
erythrocyte sedimentation rate, Westergren	0-20 mm/hr	0-20 mm/hr
Wintrobe	0-15 mm/hr	0-15 mm/hr
erythropoietin (EPO)	5-30 mcU/mL	5-30 mcU/mL
estradiol	24-149 pg/m	90-550 pmol/L
ferritin	20-200 ng/mL	20-200 mcg/L
fibrin degradation products (fibrin split products)	< 3 mcg/mL	< 3 mg/L
5´-nucleotidase	< 12.5 U/L	< 12.5 U/L
follicle-stimulating hormone (FSH), female	1.1-24 ng/mL	5.0-108 U/L
male	0.5-4.5 ng/mL	2.2-20.0 U/L
free fatty acids (FFA)	8-20 mg/dL	0.2-0.7 mmol/L
free T_4 index	0.9-2.1 ng/dL	12-27 pmol/L
FSH (follicle-stimulating hormone), female	1.1-24 ng/mL	5.0-108 U/L
male	0.5-4.5 ng/mL	2.2-20.0 U/L
FSP (fibrin split products)	< 3 mcg/mL	< 3 mg/L
gamma-glutamyl trans-peptidase (GGT)	< 65 U/L	< 65 U/L
gastrin	21-125 pg/mL	10-59.3 pmol/L
GFR (glomerular filtration rate)	90-135 mL/min per 1.73 m^2	0.86-1.3 mL/sec per m^2
GGT (gamma-glutamyl transpeptidase)	< 65 U/L	< 65 U/L
globulin, total	1.5-3.0 g/dL	15-30 g/L
glomerular filtration rate (GFR)	90-135 mL/min/1.73 m^2	0.86-1.3 mL/sec/m^2
glucagon	50-200 pg/mL	14-57 pmol/L
glucose	60-115 mg/dL	3.3-64 mmol/L
glycosylated hemoglobin (hemoglobin A$_{1C}$), normal	4-7%	4-7%
acceptable diabetic control	< 8%	< 8%

Analyte or Procedure	Normal Range (Metric)	Normal Range (SI)
haptoglobin	40-180 mg/dL	0.4-1.8 g/L
HDL (high density lipoprotein) cholesterol	35-80 mg/dL	1-2 mmol/L
hematocrit	40-48%	40-48%
hemoglobin	12-16 g/dL	7.5-10 mmol/L
hemoglobin A_{1C} (glycosylated hemoglobin), normal	4-7%	4-7%
acceptable diabetic control	< 8%	< 8%
hexosaminidase A	2.5-9 U/L	2.5-9 U/L
high density lipoprotein (HDL) cholesterol	35-80 mg/dL	1-2 mmol/L
homocysteine	< 1.6 mg/L	< 12 mcmol/L
insulin	5-25 mcU/mL	34-172 pmol/L
iron, males	50-160 mcg/dL	9.0-28.8 mcmol/L
females	45-144 mcg/dL	8.1-26 mcmol/L
iron-binding capacity	250-350 mcg/dL	45-63 mcmol/L
lactate dehydrogenase (LDH)	< 110 U/L	< 110 U/L
lactic acid	4.5-19.8 mg/dL	0.5-2.2 mmol/L
LDH (lactate dehydrogenase)	< 110 U/L	< 110 U/L
LDL (low density lipoprotein) cholesterol	40-130 mg/dL	1-3 mmol/L
leucine aminopeptidase, serum (SLAP)	< 40 U/L	< 40 U/L
LH (luteinizing hormone), females	0.5-2.7 mcg/mL	4.5-24.3 U/L
males	0.4-1.9 mcg/mL	3.6-17.1 U/L
lipase	< 1.5 U/L	< 1.5 U/L
low density lipoprotein (LDL) cholesterol	40-130 mg/dL	1-3 mmol/L
luteinizing hormone (LH), females	0.5-2.7 mcg/mL	0.4-1.9 mcg/mL
males	4.5-24.3 U/L	3.6-17.1 U/L
lymphocytes	25-40%	25-40%
magnesium	1.5-2.3 mg/dL	0.6-1.0 mmol/L
MCH (mean corpuscular hemoglobin)	27-31 pg/cell	27-31 pg/cell
MCHC (mean corpuscular hemoglobin concentration)	32-36 g/dL	320-360 g/L
MCV (mean corpuscular volume)	82-92 mcm^3	82-92 fL
mean corpuscular hemoglobin (MCH)	27-31 pg/cell	27-31 pg/cell
mean corpuscular hemoglobin concentration (MCHC)	32-36 g/dL	320-360 g/L
mean corpuscular volume (MCV)	82-92 mcm^3	82-92 fL

Analyte or Procedure	Normal Range (Metric)	Normal Range (SI)
melatonin, 8 a.m.	0.8-7.7 pg/mL	3.7-23.3 pg/mL
midnight	3.5-33 pmol/L	16-100 pmol/L
methemoglobin	< 3%	< 3%
monocytes	4-6%	4-6%
myeloid/erythroid ratio	2.0-4.0	2.0-4.0
myoglobin	14-51 mcg/L	0.8-2.9 mol/L
osmolality, serum	280-295 mOsm/kg	280-295 mOsm/kg
oxygen saturation	95-100%	95-100%
parathyroid hormone	11-54 pg/mL	1.2-56 pmol/L
partial pressure of carbon dioxide (pCO_2)	35-45 torr	35-45 torr
partial pressure of oxygen (pO_2)	75-100 torr	75-100 torr
partial thromboplastin time (PTT)	22-37 seconds	22-37 seconds
pCO_2 (partial pressure of carbon dioxide)	35-45 torr	35-45 torr
pepsinogen	124-142 ng/mL	124-142 mcg/L
pH	7.35-7.45	7.35-7.45
phenylalanine	2-4 mg/dL	121-242 mcmol/L
phosphorus	2.5-4.5 mg/dL	0.8-1.5 mmol/L
platelets	150,000-400,000/mm^3	150-400 x 10^9/L
pO_2 (partial pressure of oxygen)	75-100 torr	75-100 torr
potassium	3.5-5.0 mEq/L	3.5-5.0 mmol/L
progesterone	0.1-28 ng/mL	0.3-89 nmol/L
prolactin (nonpregnant)	2.5-19 ng/mL	1.1-8.6 nmol/L
PSA (prostate specific antigen)	< 4 ng/mL	< 4 mcg/L
pseudocholinesterase (cholinesterase)	8-18 U/L	8-18 U/L
PT (prothrombin time)	12-14 seconds	12-14 seconds
PTT (partial thromboplastin time)	22-37 seconds	22-37 seconds
RDW (red cell distribution width)	< 15%	< 15%
red blood cells	4,800,000-5,600,000/mm^3	4.8-5.6 x 10^{12}/L
red cell distribution width (RDW)	< 15%	< 15%
renin, reclining	0.2-2.3 ng/mL	1.6-4.3 ng/mL
upright	4.7-54.5 pmol/L	38-102 pmol/L
reticulocytes	0.5-1.5%	0.5-1.5%
sedimentation rate (see *erythrocyte sedimentation rate*)		
segmented neutrophils	40-70%	40-70%

Analyte or Procedure	Normal Range (Metric)	Normal Range (SI)
serum glutamic pyruvic transaminase (SGPT) (now ALT)	8-45 U/L	8-45 U/L
SGGT (see *GGT*)		
SGOT (serum glutamic oxaloacetic transaminase) (now AST)	< 35 U/L	< 35 U/L
SLAP (serum leucine aminopeptidase)	< 40 U/L	< 40 U/L
sodium	136-145 mEq/L	136-145 mmol/L
somatotropin, child	5-10 ng/mL	< 2.5 ng/mL
adult	232-465 pmol/L	< 116 pmol/L
T cells	55-65%	55-65%
T_3	70-190 ng/dL	1.1-2.9 nmol/L
T_3 uptake	25-38%	0.25-0.38
T_4 (thyroxine)	4.5-12.0 mcg/dL	58-154 nmol/L
testosterone, male	300-1200 ng/d	10.5-42 nmol/L
thyroxine (T_4)	4.5-12.0 mcg/dL	58-154 nmol/L
transferrin	250-430 mg/dL	2.5-4.3 g/L
triglycerides	< 160 mg/dL	< 1.80 mmol/L
troponin I	< 1.5 ng/mL	< 1.5 mcg/L
troponin T	< 0.029 ng/mL	< 0.029 mcg/L
TSH (thyroid stimulating hormone)	0.4-4.2 mcU/mL	0.4-4.2 mU/L
two-hour (2-hour) postprandial glucose	< 140 mg/dL	< 7.7 mmol/L
uric acid	3.4-7 mg/dL	202-416 mcmol/L
vasopressin	2-12 pg/mL	1.85-11.1 pmol/L
white blood cells	5000–10,000/mm^3	5-10 x 10^9/L
zinc	0.75-1.4 mcg/mL	11.5-21.6 mcmol/L

Index

gastritis, 255
gastroenteritis, 257
gastroesophageal reflux disease (GERD), 254-255
gastrostomy or jejunostomy, 25
genital herpes, 122, 341, 344-345
genital warts, 341, 345-346
genus and species, 99-100
GERD drugs, 267
GI dictation, 270-271
GI spasm drugs, 267
GI stimulants, 267
Giardia lamblia, 257
gigantism, 293
Glasgow Coma Scale, 420
glaucoma, 166-167; drugs, 171
Gleason grade or sco re, 88
glossary, 495-520
glomerulonephritis, 315-316
gold salts, 383-384
gonorrhea, 319-320, 344
gout, 380; drugs, 385
grade, stage, type, 100
Green, Georgia, "Feeling the Need for Speed," 60-63
Grey Turner sign, 264
gross exam of tissue, 454-458
Guillain-Barré syndrome, 410

Haemophilus influenzae, 143
H&E stain, 457
hay fever, 144
H$_2$ blockers, 267
head injuries, 415-416
headings, 87, 98, 98-99
healthcare record, 5
hearing loss, 144
heart, 208f
heart attack, 216
heart transplant, 214
heart valves, 212
Helicobacter pylori, 255; drugs, 267
helper T cells, 225
hematology, 225-226
hemolytic disease of the newborn, 227
hemophilia, 375
hemorrhoids, 260
hepatitis A, 261
hepatitis B, 261-262
hepatitis C, 262
hepatojugular reflux, 217
hernia, 260-261
herniated nucleus pulposus, 377
herniated disk, 377
herpes simplex, 122, 122f, 345f
herpesvirus type 1, 122
herpesvirus type 2, 122
heterophoria, 168
heterotropia, 168
Hinickle, Judy, "Employment Enigmas," 66-67
hip replacement, 375

HIPAA, 6
histopathology lab, 456
history and physical examination, 8, 19-21, 37-38, 119-120, 135, 142-143, 163, 186-187, 211-212, 242-243, 252-253, 280-281, 291, 306, 312-315, 331, 340, 365, 372-373, 432-436
history of present illness (HPI), 8
hives, 124
HMG CoA reductase inhibitors, 224
Hodgkin disease, 229, 229f
Homans sign, 219
hordeolum, 165
hospitals and medical centers, 17
human papillomavirus (HPV), 122, 345, 346
hydrocephalus, 409-410, 410f
hyperadrenocorticism, 295
hyperopia, 168
hypertension, 218
hyperthyroidism, 293-294
hyphens, 100-105, 113
    adverb-adjective combinations, 100
    ages, 100
    clarity, 100-101
    compound modifiers in a series, 101
    compounds, 101
    double letters, 102
    numbers, 101
    prefixes and suffixes, 102
    ranges, 102
    single letters, 102
hypoparathyroidism, 294
hypothyroidism, 293

id reaction, 121
ileitis, 258
ileus, 260
immunosuppressants, 268
impetigo, 120, 121f
impotence, 320
inconsistencies, 96
independent contractors (ICs), 17
infective endocarditis, 215
influenza, 189
inguinal hernia, 261
inhalation, 26
initial office evaluation, 8
insertions, 92
insomnia drugs, 419-420
insulin, 298-299
insulin pump, 299
interjections, 92
internship, 19
intestinal obstruction, 259
intra-arterial, 27
intra-articular, 27
intracardiac, 27
intradermal, 27
intramuscular (IM), 27
intrathecal, 27
intravenous (IV), 27

intussusception, 254, 259
iridectomy, 167
iron deficiency anemia, 226
irritable bowel syndrome, 257; drugs, 268
itching, 128
IUD (intrauterine device), 342, 344
IV drip, 27
IV piggyback, 27
IV push, 27

JCAHO, 5
job searching, 63
jock itch, 121
joints, 380f

Keith-Wagener-Barker changes, 167, 218
keratitis, 166
kerion, 121
keyboards, 13
kidneys, 312- 314, 315, 316-317, 455f, 479f
Klass, Perri, M.D., "Medical Short-Tongue," 81-82

laboratory, 6
laboratory procedures, 127, 148, 170, 193, 222, 230, 266, 297-298, 321, 350, 381, 458
laboratory tests, 21-23
laboratory values, normal, 538-542
laparoscopy, 254
Largen, Thomas L., M.D., "A Surgeon's View of Gastroenterology and Practice," 253-254
lasers, 214
laser trabeculectomy, 166
LASIK, 169
late luteal phase dysphoria, 342
laxatives, 267
lay and medical terms, 119, 142, 162, 211, 252, 291, 312, 339, 372, 406, 432, 453, 477
Lederer, Richard, Ph.D.
    "A Little Bit of Comma Sense," 90
    "Jest for the Health of It," 71-72
Legg-Calvé-Perthes disease, 376
letter, 7, 64, 134, 155, 179, 278
leukemia, 227, 228f
leukotriene receptor antagonists, 194
lists, 104
lithotripsy, 263
Lou Gehrig disease, 410-411
lumbar puncture, 418, 418f
lupus erythematosus (LE), 381
lymphocytes, 225

M. avium intracellulare complex (MAI), 190, 195
Malassezia furfur, 121
male reproductive organs, 311f
mammary dysplasia, 347
manic-depressive disorder, 437